Clinical Consult to Psychiatric Nursing for Advanced Practice

Jacqueline Rhoads, PhD, APRN-BC, CNL-BC, PMHNP-BE, FAANP, is a professor of nursing at University of Texas Medical Branch at Galveston School of Nursing, and has held many faculty positions during her career. She has taught in nurse practitioner (NP) programs since 1994. She has been awarded major research funding for a variety of research projects and continues to foster an evidence-based practice implementing outcomes-focused care. Dr. Rhoads earned her PhD from the University of Texas, Austin, and has earned post-master's degrees in acute care NP, community health primary care adult NP, gerontology NP, and psychiatric/mental health NP, and recently earned her clinical nurse leader certification. She is a fellow in the American Academy of Nurse Practitioners, and was awarded numerous commendations and medals for meritorious service in the U.S. Army Nurse Corps. Dr. Rhoads has authored three books for major nursing publishers as well as numerous articles. Her recent publication, *Nurses' Clinical Consult to Psychopharmacology*, won first place as AJN Book of the Year Award, 2012. Her textbook, *Clinical Consult to Psychiatric Mental Health Care*, won second place as AJN Book of the Year Award in 2011.

Patrick J. M. Murphy, PhD, is an assistant professor at the Seattle University College of Nursing, where he teaches introduction to pharmacology (Bachelor of Science in Nursing students), and advanced pharmacological application in primary care and psychopharmacology in advanced practice nursing (Master's of Science in Nursing/nurse practitioner students), among other courses. He holds an MS and PhD in pharmacology from the University of Michigan. He has served as the scholar-in-residence, Hope Heart Institute (Seattle, Washington), and as a visiting scientist at Fred Hutchinson Cancer Research Center, also in Seattle. Previously, he served as a research fellow, University of Michigan Medical School, and guest lecturer, University of Michigan School of Nursing. He has published 22 peer-reviewed journal articles and multiple book chapters, as well as having presented 15 podium presentations and numerous invitational lectures. He is the co- or the primary investigator on six funded research projects. Dr. Murphy is the recipient of multiple honors and awards, notably the Outstanding Teacher of the Year Award (2009, Seattle University), Outstanding Graduate Student Teaching Award (2001, University of Michigan Medical School), and a Horace H. Rackham Fellowship from the University of Michigan Graduate School. He is a member of the Phi Sigma Tau Academic Honorary Society and the Phi Eta Sigma Academic Honorary Society.

Clinical Consult to Psychiatric Nursing for Advanced Practice

Jacqueline Rhoads, PhD, APRN-BC, CNL-BC, PMHNP-BE, FAANP

Patrick J. M. Murphy, PhD

Consultants

Tammie Lee Demler, BS, PharmD, MBA, BCPP
Sandra J. Wiggins Petersen, DNP, FNP, GNP-BC

SPRINGER PUBLISHING COMPANY

NEW YORK

Springer Publishing Company, LLC
11 West 42nd Street
New York, NY 10036
www.springerpub.com

Acquisitions Editor: Margaret Zuccarini
Composition: Newgen Knowledge Work

ISBN: 978-0-8261-9595-1
Ebook ISBN: 978-0-8261-9596-8

14 15 16 17 18/ 5 4 3 2 1

The author and the publisher of this Work have made every effort to use sources believed to be reliable to provide information that is accurate and compatible with the standards generally accepted at the time of publication. Because medical science is continually advancing, our knowledge base continues to expand. Therefore, as new information becomes available, changes in procedures become necessary. We recommend that the reader always consult current research, specific institutional policies, and current formularies or drug guides before performing any clinical procedure or prescribing or administering any drug(s). The author and publisher shall not be liable for any special, consequential, or exemplary damages resulting, in whole or in part, from the readers' use of, or reliance on, the information contained in this book. The publisher has no responsibility for the persistence or accuracy of URLs for external or third-party Internet Web sites referred to in this publication and does not guarantee that any content on such Web sites is, or will remain, accurate or appropriate.

Library of Congress Cataloging-in-Publication Data
Rhoads, Jacqueline, author.
   Clinical consult to psychiatric nursing for advanced practice / Jacqueline Rhoads, Patrick J.M. Murphy.
      p. ; cm.
   Includes bibliographical references and index.
   ISBN 978-0-8261-9595-1 — ISBN 978-0-8261-9596-8 (e-book)
   I. Murphy, Patrick J. M., author. II. Title.
   [DNLM: 1. Mental Disorders—nursing. 2. Mental Disorders—therapy. 3. Psychiatric Nursing—methods. 4. Psychopharmacology—methods. WY 160]
   RC440
   616.89′0231—dc23
                                                                            2014015684

Printed in the United States of America by McNaughton & Gunn.

This book is dedicated to all those suffering from a mental health disorder and to those who care for them.

Contents

---

*All psychopharmacology treatment guidelines and drug selection tables are incorporated into each applicable disorder.

---

*All psychopharmacology treatment guidelines and drug selection tables are incorporated into each applicable disorder.

Contributors

Contributors to Clinical Consult to Psychiatric Mental Health Care

Athena J. Arthur, MS, LCDC
Doctoral Student
Fielding Graduate University
Santa Barbara, California

Renee R. Azzouz, ARNP
Overland Park, Kansas

Sandra S. Bauman, PhD, ARNP, LMHC
Lecturer
School of Nursing and Health Studies
University of Miami School
Coral Gables, Florida

Virginia Brooke, RN, PhD
University of Texas Medical Branch
    Medical School
Galveston, Texas

**Deonne J. Brown-Benedict, DNP, ARNP,
    FNP-BC**
Assistant Professor and Family
    Nurse Practitioner Track Clinical
    Coordinator
College of Nursing
Seattle University
Seattle, Washington

Angela Chia-Chen Chen, PhD, RN
Assistant Professor
College of Nursing and Health
    Innovation
Arizona State University
Phoenix, Arizona

Lawrence S. Dilks, PhD
Clinical Neuropsychologist
Lake Charles, Louisiana

Susan O. Edionwe, MD
University of Texas Medical Branch
    Medical School
Galveston, Texas

Elizabeth Hite Erwin, PhD, APRN-BC
Assistant Professor
School of Nursing
University of Virginia
Charlottesville, Virginia

Deborah Gilbert-Palmer, EdD, FNP-BC
Associate Professor of Nursing and FNP
    Program Coordinator
Department of Nursing
Arkansas State University
State University, Arizona

Nnenna I. Igbo, MD
University of Texas Medical Branch
    Medical School
Galveston, Texas

Jose Levy, MA, BCBA, CBIST
Fielding Graduate University
Austin, Texas

Jo-Ann Summitt Marrs, EdD, FNP-BC
East Tennessee State University
Johnson City, Tennessee

Patrick J. M. Murphy, PhD
College of Nursing
Seattle University
Seattle, Washington

Meena Patel, ARNP, DNP (Candidate)
Overland Park, Kansas

Nancy Pierce, ARNP
Psychiatric and Counseling Associates
Leawood, Kansas

Theresa Raphael-Grimm, PhD, RN, CS
University of North Carolina
Chapel Hill, North Carolina

**Jacqueline Rhoads, PhD, ACNP-BC,
ANP-C, CNL-BC, PMHNP-BE, FAANP**
Professor of Nursing
University of Texas at Galveston Health
Science Center School of Nursing
Galveston, Texas

Judy Rice, BSN, MSN FNPCS
Johnson City, Tennessee

**Victoria Soltis-Jarrett, PhD, PMHCNS/
NP-BC**
Clinical Associate Professor and Coordinator
University of North Carolina
Chapel Hill, North Carolina

Kimberly Swanson, PhD
Research Interventionalist
University of Washington School of
Social Work
Seattle, Washington

Hisn-Yi (Jean) Tang, PhD, APRN
Assistant Professor
College of Nursing
Seattle University
Seattle, Washington

Kristen Vandenberg, MSN, ARNP, FNP-BC
University of North Florida
Jacksonville, Florida

Alma Vega, EdD, MSN, ARNP-BC
Assistant Professor
School of Nursing and Health Studies
University of Miami
Coral Gables, Florida

Lucinda Whitney, MSN, ARNP-BC
Overland Park, Kansas

Elizabeth Willford
University of Texas Medical Branch
Medical School
Galveston, Texas

Contributors to Nurses' Clinical Consult to Psychopharmacology

Sandra S. Bauman, PhD, ARNP, LMHC
Lecturer
School of Nursing and Health Studies
University of Miami School
Coral Gables, Florida

**Deonne J. Brown-Benedict, DNP, ARNP,
FNP-BC**
Assistant Professor
Family Nurse Practitioner Track Clinical
Coordinator
Seattle University College of Nursing
Seattle, Washington

**Angela Chia-Chen Chen, PhD, RN,
PMHNP-BC**
Assistant Professor
Arizona State University
College of Nursing and Healthcare
Innovation
Phoenix, Arizona

Karen Crowley, DNP, APRN-BC, WHNP, ANP
Assistant Professor
Regis College
School of Nursing, Sciences and Health
Professionals
Weston, Massachusetts

Deborah Gilbert-Palmer, EdD, FNP-BC
Associate Professor
Arkansas State University
State University, Arkansas

Lori S. Irelan, FNP, APRN, MSN
Wilmington University
New Castle, Delaware

Mitsi H. Lizer, PharmD, BCPP, CGP
Associate Professor Pharmacy Practice,
Shenandoah University School of
Pharmacy
Winchester, Virginia

JoAnn Marrs, EdD, FNP-BC
East Tennessee State University
Johnson City, Tennessee

Patrick J. M. Murphy, PhD
Assistant Professor
Seattle College of Nursing
Seattle, Washington

Sandra J. Peterson, PhD, RN
Professor Emeritus
Bethel University
St. Paul, Minnesota

Stephanie Ann Plummer, DNP, APRN,
PMHNP-BC
Assistant Clinical Professor
UCLA School of Nursing
Fayetteville, Arkansas
Department of Psychiatry
VAMC—Jay CBOC
Jay, Oklahoma

Jacqueline Rhoads, PhD, ACNP-BC, ANP-C,
CNL-BC, PMHNP-BE, FAANP
Professor of Nursing
University of Texas at Galveston Health Science
Center School of Nursing
Galveston, Texas

Ester Ruiz, PhD, RN
Professor Emeritus
Arizona State University
Tempe, Arizona

Barbara Sartell, EdD, RN, CANP
Wilmington University
New Castle, Delaware

Antiqua Smart, BSN, MN, APRN, FNP-BC, CPE
Southern University and A&M College
Baton Rouge, Louisiana

Sandra J. Wiggins Petersen, DNP, FNP, GNP-BC
Program Track Administrator
UTMB Masters in Nursing Leadership Program,
UTMB
School of Nursing
Galveston, Texas

Hsin-Yi (Jean) Tang, PhD, APRN-BC, PMHNP
Assistant Professor
College of Nursing
Seattle University
Seattle, Washington

Kristen M. Vandenberg, DNP, ARNP
Advanced Nurse Practitioner
Colorado West, Inc.
Grand Junction, Colorado

Lisa Waggoner, DNP, FNP-BC
Arkansas State University
State University, Arkansas

Veronica Wilbur, PhD, FNP-BC, CNE
Associate Professor
Wilmington University
New Castle, Delaware

Contributors *to* Clinical Consult to Psychiatric Nursing for Advanced Practice

Susan Basset, MS
Instructor
Mental Health, Nursing Education, Gerontology
South Dakota State University
Rapid City, South Dakota

Sandra S. Bauman, PhD, ARNP, LMHC
Lecturer
School of Nursing and Health Studies
University of Miami School of Nursing
Coral Gables, Florida

Julie Bertram, MSN, RN, PMHCNS-BC
Instructor
Saint Louis University School of Nursing
St. Louis, Missouri

Leslie Binford, RN, MSN, PMHNP-BC
Instructor
Vanderbilt University
School of Nursing
Nashville, Tennessee

Angela Chia-Chen Chen, PhD, RN
Associate Professor
Arizona State University
Phoenix, Arizona

Neva L. Crogan, PhD, GNP-BC,
FNGNA, FAAN
Professor of Nursing
Gonzaga University
Spokane, Washington

Kay Foland, PhD, RN, PMHNP-BC, PMHCNS-BC, CNP
Professor
South Dakota State University
    College of Nursing
West River Department
Rapid City, South Dakota

Deborah Gilbert-Palmer, EdD, FNP-BC
Associate Professor of Nursing and FNP
    Program Coordinator
Department of Nursing
Arkansas State University
Batesville, Arkansas

Patricia Hentz, EdD, PMHNP-BC, CRNP
Associate Clinical Professor
Rutgers, The State University of
    New Jersey
School of Nursing
Newark, New Jersey

LaKeetra Josey, MSN, CRNP, PMHNP, BC
Associate Program Director
University of Pennsylvania
    School of Nursing
Philadelphia, Pennsylvania

JoAnn Marrs, PhD, RN, FNP, BC
Professor and Clinical Coordinator RODP
East Tennessee State University
School of Nursing
Johnson City, Tennessee

Michele A. Martens, APN, PMHCNS-BC
Instructor
Vanderbilt University School of Nursing
Nashville, Tennessee

Elizabeth Pasquariello, MSN/ED, BSN
Instructor
ANCC-Certified Psychiatric/Mental
    Health Nurse
South Dakota State University
Rapid City, South Dakota

Judy Rice, BSN, MSN, FNPCS
Assistant Professor
East Tennessee State University,
    School of Nursing
Johnson City, Tennessee

Lynn Shell, PhD, MSN
Clinical Assistant Professor
Rutgers, The State University of New Jersey
Newark, New Jersey

Janet A Sobczak, PhD, PMHNP-BC, PMHCNS-BC, NPP
Associate Professor
State University of New York
College of Nursing
Syracuse, New York

Preface

The devastation of the Gulf Coast after Hurricane Katrina has been imprinted in our memories not only by the sensational news coverage but also by the personal experiences of many health care providers who volunteered countless hours in helping the people affected by this disaster. I was one of the providers who responded. From that experience came a realization of how many people were and are affected by mental illness, and how little I knew of the protocols that could be used to provide mental health care to those I served. I went back to school for my post-master's degree in psychiatric mental health and saw the lack of published information that would lend assistance to those caring for people with mental disorders.

As a result of this realization, the *Clinical Consult to Psychiatric Mental Health Care* was published in October 2010, and provides "what to do next" guidelines when working with and beginning the treatment of a patient with a mental health disorder. But this was only the first step: the next step was to publish the *Nurses' Clinical Consult to Psychopharmacology* in January 2012. This important psychopharmacology reference is customized to reflect particular prescribing and management considerations for a wide range of psychiatric disorders. These two resources together provide evidence-based guidelines to consider when assessing and caring for persons with a mental health disorder.

Now, these two essential clinical references are combined into one "complete" clinical resource for use by nurse practitioners and others caring for patients in clinical practice. Compiled by expert practitioners in psychiatric care, this work provides an overview of the management of the major *Diagnostic and Statistical Manual of Mental Disorders, fifth edition* (American Psychiatric Association, 2013) disorders *across the life span* and delivers complete clinical guidelines for their diagnosis, treatment options, and psychopharmacologic management.

We have constructed each chapter using a bullet format for quick reference within a structured approach. This reference is organized into two major sections: The first is the overview of the principles of clinical psychiatry (interview, clinical decision making, diagnostic evaluation, and treatment planning), psychotherapeutic management, behavioral therapy and cognitive behavioral therapy, and the principles of psychopharmacology (neurotransmitters, receptors, neuroanatomy, pharmacokinetics, and pharmacodynamics), and syndromes and treatment in adult psychiatry and syndromes and treatment in child and adolescent psychiatry. The second section presents nearly 90 monographs representing current major drug therapies for the major disorders that benefit from drug intervention.

A clinically useful drug selection table appears with each disorder for which psychopharmacology is an appropriate intervention and *identifies the first and second line of drug therapy along with adjunctive therapies.* It is important to note that the order in which drugs are listed within the drug classification on the drug table is significant in helping to guide drug choice. Additionally, it is important to note that not every drug within a classification is included for all disorders; rather, drugs that have been shown to have clinical efficacy are listed in a priority fashion to help guide the drug choice by the prescriber.

Essential drug information that is needed to safely prescribe and monitor the patient's response to those drugs includes the following: drug name, brand name, and generic name; drug class, usual and customary dosage, and administration of the drug; availability (e.g., as tablet, injection, intravenous, capsule); side effect, drug interaction, pharmacokinetics, precautions; patient education; and special populations. The special populations section includes management of those who are pregnant, breastfeeding, older adults, children, adolescents, and patients with impaired renal, hepatic, or cardiac function.

The book provides a concise, complete, easy-to-access clinical resource so the primary care provider can quickly access the following:

▦ Diagnostic criteria and differential diagnoses for each disorder
▦ The range of therapeutic interventions useful for managing disorders, including psychotherapeutic management, psychotherapy, and cognitive behavioral therapy
▦ The overarching principles of pharmacodynamics and pharmacokinetics to consider when prescribing a drug
▦ The main psychotropic medications, when to prescribe, and how to select the most efficacious drug for each patient
▦ Special considerations for patient populations, including older adults, those who are pregnant, breastfeeding, children, and adolescents
▦ Clinical considerations for prescribing in patients with impairment of renal, hepatic, and/or cardiac function
▦ Easy-to-read drug-selection tables for reliable clinical consultation
▦ Extensive references for further reading

Pharmacology knowledge and applied clinical practices are constantly evolving due to new research and applied science, which expand our diagnostic capabilities and treatments. Therefore, it must be emphasized that practitioners carry an important responsibility to ensure that the treatment they select reflects current research and is appropriate according to manufacturer drug information for drugs selected; that dosages, route of administration, effects/precautions have been taken into consideration; and also that interactions and use in special populations are all accurate and appropriate for each patient. The practitioner is ultimately responsible to know each patient's history, to have conducted a thorough physical examination, and to consult appropriate diagnostic test results so as to ascertain best possible pharmacotherapeutic actions for optimal patient outcomes and appropriate safety procedures.

The contributors to this text have worked hard to present current and applicable content that is of therapeutic value in the understanding of specific mental health disorders. We are very grateful to the contributors of this text for their hard work and focused support.

Jacqueline Rhoads
Patrick J. M. Murphy

Acknowledgments

I wish to acknowledge several individuals for the help and support they provided in the creation of this book. First to Joanne Jay, vice president of production, at Springer. Her dedication and work on this book and its publication made the book possible.

Second, I would like to acknowledge all the expert input by the reviewers, which has produced a high level of excellence.

Third, to the contributors who provided their time and competent knowledge in the development of the chapter content.

Lastly, to my mother, who was instrumental in providing me with the love and support that gave me direction and courage to persevere when times were so difficult.

Jacqueline Rhoads

Clinical Consult to Psychiatric Nursing for Advanced Practice

Part I
General Psychiatry

Chapter 1

The Psychiatric Interview and Diagnosis

The Psychiatric Interview

INTRODUCTION

- The psychiatric interview is the core of proper psychiatric evaluation. It plays an important role not only in clinical assessment but also in therapy. The interviewer should come to understand the patient's behaviors, emotions, experiences, and psychological, social, religious influences, and motivations through verbal and nonverbal communication with the patient.
- The psychiatric interview can be divided into the following stages: building an alliance with the patient, psychiatric history, diagnostic evaluation, and treatment plan formulation.
- As with all interviews, the patient–provider relationship is very important. An intact relationship between the interviewer and the patient increases the patient's confidence and willingness to disclose the personal or sensitive information necessary for diagnosis and facilitates patient compliance.
- The psychiatric interview depends on more than verbal communication; it requires that the physician be observant and listen. Nonverbal communication can provide insight necessary for the patient's clinical assessment and diagnosis, especially in patients significantly impaired by psychiatric disease.
- The extent of psychiatric impairment may necessitate that the interviews occur in multiple sessions or depend on information from additional persons such as family members or friends.
- The interview should begin with an open-ended approach.
- A structured interview approach combines the psychiatric interview with diagnostic criteria in attempts to derive a thorough psychiatric history.

THE PATIENT–PROVIDER RELATIONSHIP: BUILDING AN ALLIANCE

- The patient–provider relationship is fundamental to providing excellent care, improving patient outcomes, and the healing process. It has special significance in psychiatry, where the "stigma" of psychiatric treatment can make even seeking treatment difficult.
- A solid patient–clinician relationship requires optimization of the following seven components:
  - Communication
  - Office experience
  - Hospital experience
  - Patient education
  - Integration (information sharing among all members of the treatment team)
  - Shared decision making
  - Outcomes
- The patient–provider relationship involves a working or therapeutic alliance, which is an agreement between provider and patient, based on mutual rapport and trust, to undertake treatment together.
- The interviewer must be sensitive to the importance of empathy, respect, and trust to develop a good working alliance.
- Distrust is a common reason for noncompliance. In fact, most instances of noncompliance come from interruption of the provider–patient relationship.
- The interviewer should develop a rapport with the patient:
  - Remain attentive:
    - Maintain eye contact
    - Minimize distractions such as excessive note taking or interrupting the patient while speaking
  - Be empathic:
    - Show the patient an understanding and appreciation for his or her situation.
    - Reinforce what the patient is feeling. One way to do this is by making statements such as, "I can see that was a very difficult time for you."
  - Listen! Listen! Listen!

THE INTERVIEW: NONVERBAL COMMUNICATION

- Active observation of the patient should occur within the first few minutes of the interview, before names have been exchanged and the "formal" interview has begun.
- Actively process the patient's nonverbal communication, such as the following:
  - How does the patient first greet the interviewer?
  - Does the patient make eye contact?
  - What items (books or pictures, etc.) are present?
  - What is the patient wearing and is his or her appearance disheveled or neat?
  - What (if any) unusual sounds or smells are in the room?
- Observation of the patient should continue throughout the interview. The interviewer should take note of the patient's body language and emotional expressions during responses to the questions.
- For example, a patient who becomes emotional when asked about a spouse may be depressed about a recent divorce or loss of a loved one.

- Certain kinds of nonverbal communication are included in diagnostic criteria and the interviewer should be cognizant of their presence.
- Active observation becomes increasingly important with increases in psychiatric impairments.

THE INTERVIEW: VERBAL COMMUNICATION

- Open-ended questions
    - After formally introducing yourself and your role in the patient's care, start by asking open-ended questions.
    - Examples of open-ended questions include the following:
        - Tell me what brings you here.
        - Tell me what kinds of problems you have had, lately.
    - Three reasons why an open-ended manner of interviewing is important are as follows:
        - It strengthens the patient–provider relationship by showing that the interviewer is interested in the concerns of the patient.
        - It provides insight into the patient's condition.
        - It allows the interviewer to understand what is most important to the patient rather than making assumptions.
    - The interviewer should engage in active listening as the patient responds to questions.
- Diagnosis-specific questions
    - As the history develops, specific questions such as, "Do you see things that others cannot see?" (hallucinations) or "Have you ever tried to harm yourself?" (suicidal ideations) become necessary. Follow up on the responses.
    - These specific questions aim at gathering information necessary for diagnosis based on *Diagnostic and Statistical Manual of Mental Disorders,* fifth edition (*DSM-5*; American Psychiatric Association, 2013) criteria.
    - The interviewer should be able to transition from open-ended questions to more specific ones.
        - For example, "Now I would like to ask you about several psychological symptoms that patients might experience."

STRUCTURED INTERVIEWS

- A structured interview uses a series of questions that couple the interview method with the *DSM-5* diagnostic criteria in attempts to explore the signs and symptoms necessary for diagnosis.
- Examples include the following:
    - The MINI-International Neuropsychiatric Interview (MINI[-Plus])
    - Structured Clinical Interview for *DSM-5* disorders (SCID)
    - Composite International Diagnostic Interview (CIDI)
    - Schedules for Clinical Assessment in Neuropsychiatry (SCAN)

PSYCHIATRIC INTERVIEW ICD-10

- ICD-10 Code: **Z046 (Z04.6)** Code Type: **Diagnosis**

The Diagnostic Encounter

PHASES OF THE DIAGNOSTIC ENCOUNTER

The diagnostic encounter is divided into three phases:
- Opening phase
- Body of the interview
- Closing phase

Opening Phase
- Initial 5 to 10 minutes
- Goals
  - Introductions
  - Preinterview preparation
    - For example, ease patient's fears or concerns about the necessity for the interview
  - Building a therapeutic alliance
  - Keeping questions open ended and allowing the patient to speak uninterrupted for an appropriate amount of time

Body of the Interview
- 30 to 45 minutes
- Goals
  - Psychiatric history
  - Diagnosis-specific questions such as, "Does this patient meet *DSM-5* criteria for diagnosis?"
  - Mental status examination (MSE)
  - Physical examination
  - Additional investigations

Closing Phase
- 5 to 10 minutes
- Goals
  - Review your assessment with the patient
  - Collaborate with the patient on a treatment and follow-up plan

PSYCHIATRIC HISTORY

- *Identifying data*: collecting basic details about the patient, such as name, gender, age, religion, educational status, occupation, relationship status, and contact details.
- *Chief complaint* (CC): the reason for the patient's presentation.
- *History of present illness* (HPI): the interviewer attempts to gain a clear understanding of the full history of the patient's problems, such as when they started, what they entail, worsening symptoms, or associated symptoms. The HPI allows the interviewer to formulate preliminary hypotheses as to a diagnosis.
- *Past medical history* (PMH): the interviewer should explore the PMH to look for surgical or medical diseases or medications that cause, contribute to, or mimic psychiatric disease.

■ *Past psychiatric history*: explore previous diagnoses, treatments, and outcomes.

■ *Family history* (FH): explore familial psychiatric disorders or medical conditions as a cause of or contributing factors to psychiatric disorders.

■ *Social history* (SH): document the social circumstances of the patient, such as finances, housing, relationships, drug and alcohol use, and problems with the law, as these can contribute to the cause of psychiatric disease.

■ *Development history*: past, present, family, social, and cultural.

■ *Review of systems* (ROS): explore pertinent systems associated with the onset of psychiatric disease.

MENTAL STATUS EXAMINATION

■ *Appearance*: physique, grooming, dress, habits, nutritional status, posture, nervousness, and eye contact.

■ *Attitude/rapport*: attitude toward the examiner. For example, is the patient friendly, cooperative, bored, or defensive?

■ *Mood*: the patient's emotions. Elicit by asking the patient questions such as, "How have you been feeling on most days?" List the mood in the patient's own words. Moods include being depressed, angry, anxious, stressed, or elevated.

■ *Affect*: defined by the interviewer. Observable emotion: euthymic (normal), neutral, euphoric, dysphoric, or flat (no variation in emotion); the range: full, constricted, or blunted; appropriateness: appropriate or labile.

■ *Speech*: quality, quantity, rate, and volume.

■ *Thought process*: the organization of the patient's thoughts
  ○ *Logical*: normal thought process
  ○ *Loose associations*: the patient slips off the track from one idea to an unrelated one.
  ○ *Flight of ideas*: verbally skipping from one idea to another before the previous one has been concluded
  ○ *Tangentiality*: the responses never approach the point of the questions.
  ○ *Thought blocking*: patient stops abruptly in the middle of a thought.
  ○ *Circumstantiality*: delay in getting to the point because of unnecessary details and irrelevant remarks
  ○ *Neologism*: patient creates new words.

■ Thought content
  ○ *Suicidal ideation*: assess plan and previous attempts
  ○ *Homicidal ideation*: assess plan and previous attempts
  ○ Obsessions and compulsions
  ○ Phobias
  ○ Paranoia

■ Perceptual disturbances

■ *Hallucinations*: perception of a stimulus in the absence of a stimulus; auditory (hearing things), visual (seeing things), olfactory (smelling things), tactile (feeling things), and gustatory (tasting things)

■ *Delusions*: grandiosity, religious delusion, persecution, jealousy, thought insertion (belief that someone is putting ideas or thoughts into his or her mind), ideas of reference (belief that irrelevant, unrelated phenomena in the world refer to him or her directly or have special personal significance)

■ *Illusions*: erroneous interpretation of a present stimulus

■ *Insight*: the patient's understanding of his or her illness

▦ *Judgment*: estimate the patient's judgment on the basis of the history or on an imaginary scenario. Ask the following question: "What would you do if you smelled smoke in a crowded theater?" (adequate response is, "Call 911" or "Get help"; poor response is, "Do nothing" or "Watch the smoke rise").
▦ *Impulsivity*: the degree of the patient's impulse control
▦ *Reliability*: determine whether the patient seems reliable, unreliable, or if it is difficult to determine.

PHYSICAL EXAMINATION

▦ Medical conditions (central nervous system [CNS] malignancy, hypothyroidism, or pancreatic cancer) can mimic a psychiatric illness. A thorough physical examination (usually except genitourinary examination), including full neurological examination, should be documented.

ADDITIONAL INVESTIGATIONS

▦ Lab investigations
▦ Additional information from accompanying friend or family members
▦ Other forms of pertinent information

Clinical Decision Making

▦ The decision-making process has been broken down into a systematic and individualized process involving the following:
  ▦ State-mandated criteria: clinical practice guidelines, *DSM-5*, and so on.
  ▦ Investigation of alternatives: for example, ruling out medical conditions that mimic psychiatric disease through lab investigations
  ▦ Shared decision making: requires an adequate patient–clinician relationship
  ▦ Intuitive reasoning and experiences such as years of experience or exposure to previous psychiatric disorders
  ▦ Connection with the client, caution, and inability to control all contingencies
▦ Strategies of clinical reasoning and decision making include the following:
  ▦ Tolerate uncertainty, avoid premature closure, and consider alternatives.
  ▦ Separate cue from inference; be able to refer inferences to the salient cues from which they were derived.
  ▦ Be aware of personal reactions to the patient.
  ▦ Be alert for fresh evidence, particularly evidence that demands a revision or deletion of a hypothesis or diagnosis.
  ▦ Value negative evidence above positive evidence.
  ▦ Be prepared to commit to a diagnosis when enough evidence has been gathered.
▦ Historically, decision making has shown variability among practitioners. As a result, efforts have been made to create practice guidelines, processes, and recommendations that will result in consistency in the diagnostic evaluation and, subsequently, in the treatment of psychiatric disease.
▦ Trend toward evidence-based clinical decision making:
  ▦ Use of *DSM-5* guidelines
  ▦ Goals

- More clinical research independent of pharmaceutical companies
- An efficient means of making evidence-based data easily accessible to clinicians

Diagnostic Formulation, Treatment Planning, and Modes of Treatment

PUTTING IT ALL TOGETHER: DIAGNOSTIC FORMULATION

- Diagnostic formulation has been traditionally described as a summary of the relevant genetic, constitutional, and personality factors and their interaction with the etiological factors, taking into account the patient's life situation, together with a provisional diagnosis.
- Essentially, the full encounter, including psychiatric history, MSE, labs, referral information, additional information from family members/friends, and physical examination, is assessed to yield a diagnosis.
- Currently, a diagnostic formulation is best accomplished using the *DSM-5* multiaxial system of assessment.

DSM-5 DISORDERS AND ICD-10 CODES

- These disorders will be listed as Axis I or Axis II on the multiaxial system assessment.
- Adjustment disorders
  - Adjustment Disorder Unspecified (F43.20)
  - Adjustment Disorder with Anxiety (F43.22)
  - Adjustment Disorder with Depressed Mood (F43.21)
  - Adjustment Disorder with Disturbance of Conduct (F43.24)
  - Adjustment Disorder with Mixed Anxiety and Depressed Mood (F43.23)
  - Adjustment Disorder with Mixed Disturbance of Emotions and Conduct (F43.25)
- Anxiety disorders
  - Acute Stress Disorder (F43.0)
  - Agoraphobia (without a history of Panic Disorder) (F40.02)
  - Generalized Anxiety Disorder (GAD; [F41.1])
  - Obsessive-Compulsive Disorder (OCD; [F42])
  - Panic Disorder—with Agoraphobia (F40.01) or without Agoraphobia (F41.0)
  - Social Phobia (F40.10)
  - Posttraumatic Stress Disorder (PTSD; [F43.1])
- Dissociative disorders
  - Dissociative Amnesia (F44.0)
  - Dissociative Fugue (F44.1)
  - Dissociative Identity (Multiple Personality) Disorder (F44.81)
  - Depersonalization-Derealization Syndrome (F48.1)
- Eating disorders
  - Anorexia Nervosa (F50.0)
  - Bulimia Nervosa (F50.2)

- Impulse control disorders
  - Intermittent Explosive Disorder (F63.81)
  - Kleptomania (F63.2)
  - Pathological Gambling (F63.0)
- Mood disorders
  - Bipolar Disorder (F31.0)
  - Cyclothymic Disorder (F34.0)
  - Dysthymic Disorder (F34.1)
  - Major Depressive Disorder (F32.0)
- Sexual disorders
  - Exhibitionism (F65.2)
  - Fetishism (F65.0)
  - Frotteurism (52.8)
  - Pedophilia (F65.4)
  - Sexual Masochism (F65.51)
  - Sexual Sadism (F65.52)
  - Transvestic Fetishism (F65.1)
  - Voyeurism (F65.3)
- Sleep disorders
  - Primary Insomnia (F51.01)
  - Primary Hypersomnia (F51.11)
  - Narcolepsy (G47.4)
  - Nightmare Disorder (F51.5)
  - Sleep Terror Disorder (F51.4)
  - Sleepwalking Disorder (F51.3)
- Psychotic disorders
  - Brief Psychotic Disorder (F23)
  - Delusional Disorder (F22)
  - Schizoaffective Disorder (F29.5)
  - Schizophrenia
    - Schizophrenia, Catatonic Type (F20.2)
    - Schizophrenia, Disorganized Type (F20.1)
    - Schizophrenia, Paranoid Type (F20)
    - Schizophrenia, Residual Type (F20.5)
    - Schizophrenia, Undifferentiated Type (F20.5)
  - Schizophreniform (F20.81)
  - Shared Psychotic Disorder (F24)
- Sexual dysfunctions
  - Dyspareunia (F52.6)
  - Female Orgasmic Disorder (F52.31)
  - Female Sexual Arousal Disorder (F52.31)
  - Gender Identity Disorder (F52.22)
  - Hypoactive Sexual Desire Disorder (F64.2)
  - Male Erectile Disorder (F52.21)
  - Male Orgasmic Disorder (F52.8)
  - Premature Ejaculation (F52.4)
  - Sexual Aversion Disorder (F52.1)
  - Vaginismus (F52)
- Somatoform disorders
  - Body Dysmorphic Disorder (F45.22)

  - Conversion Disorder (F44.9)
  - Hypochondriasis Disorder (F45.21)
  - Pain Disorder (F45.19)
  - Somatization Disorder (F45.20)
- Substance disorders
  - Substance Abuse (F19.18)
  - Substance Dependence (F19.28)
- Personality disorders
  - Antisocial Personality Disorder (F60.2)
  - Borderline Personality Disorder (F60.3)
  - Narcissistic Personality Disorder (F60.81)
  - Dependent Personality Disorder (F60.7)
  - Histrionic Personality Disorder (F60.4)
  - Paranoid Personality Disorder (F60)

TREATMENT PLANNING

- Treatment planning is the next step after a diagnosis is evident.
- Selection of a therapeutic method depends on the mode, time, and setting of treatment.
- Patient involvement is necessary in formulating a treatment plan.
- Treatment plan goals
  - To clarify treatment focus
    - What the treatment is meant to accomplish and through what means
  - To set realistic treatment expectations and goals
    - Treatment goals should have criteria for achievement, be achievable, and collaboratively developed and prioritized.
    - Expectations should adequately clarify to patients what they can realistically expect from a treatment course.
    - Clarify patient and provider roles, setting ground rules for therapy and establishing realistic goals agreed on by the patient.
  - To establish a standard for measuring treatment progress
    - Include a plan for reevaluation or follow-up.
  - To facilitate communication among professionals
  - For the purposes of managed health care, treatment plans also serve to support treatment authorization, to document quality assurance efforts, and to facilitate communication with external reviewers.

MODES OF TREATMENT

- Pharmacotherapy
  - *Antidepressants*: used to treat depression, panic attacks, OCD, PTSD, social anxiety disorder, anxiety, premenstrual dysphoric disorder, nicotine withdrawal symptoms
  - *Mood stabilizers*: used to treat bipolar disorder, dementia (anticonvulsants), severe agitation, aggression, severe impulsive behavior, mania, and disinhibition
  - *Neuroleptics*: used to treat schizophrenia, mania, delusional disorder, symptoms of psychosis, Tourette's disease, Asperger's syndrome

- *Anticholinergics*: used for anxiety and stress reactions. Also used to offset extrapyramidal symptoms (EPS) for patients experiencing these symptoms while on antipsychotics.
- *Anxiolytics*: used to treat anxiety disorders
- *Sedative hypnotics*: used to treat insomnia and sleep disorders
- Electroconvulsive therapy
  - Major depression with or without psychotic features
  - Bipolar illness (used to treat both depressed and manic phases)
  - Catatonic schizophrenia
  - Schizophrenia with strong affective components or schizophrenia highly resistant to treatment
- Behavior therapy and cognitive therapy
  - Used to help patients eliminate target behaviors; refer to additional texts for more information
- Group psychotherapy
  - Used to treat the following disorders in a group setting:
    - Most personality disorders
    - Most anxiety disorders
    - Somatoform disorders
    - Substance-related disorders
    - Schizophrenia and related psychotic disorders
    - Stable bipolar disorders
    - PTSD
    - Eating disorders
    - Medical illness
    - Depressive disorders
    - Adjustment disorders
- Family/marital therapy

The Diagnostic Evaluation

THE PROCESS OF DIAGNOSTIC EVALUATION

- A complete diagnostic evaluation involves obtaining a complete psychiatric history, including the presence of specific symptoms, course, and duration, in addition to the mental status exam (MSE), physical examination, pertinent labs, and other additional information. Diagnosis-specific questions for *DSM* criteria during the diagnostic encounter are the key.

Diagnosis-Specific Questions
- As the interviewer develops hypotheses for a diagnosis, diagnosis-specific questions are asked to elicit *DSM-5* criteria for diagnosis as follows:
  - *How long have you felt depressed?*—the *DSM-5* diagnosis for a major depressive disorder (MDD) requires at least 2 weeks of symptoms.
  - *Do you still derive pleasure from doing your favorite activities?*—the *DSM-5* diagnosis for MDD must include the presence of lack of pleasure (anhedonia) or a depressed mood.
  - *Are you able to function during the day on little to no sleep?*—a decreased need for sleep is one of the possible criteria for a diagnosis of bipolar disorder.

- *Do you have flashbacks or nightmares of the traumatic event?*—reexperiencing a trauma (via nightmares, flashbacks, obsessive thoughts) is part of the *DSM-5* criteria of diagnosis for PTSD.
- The interview may refer to additional diagnosis-specific screening questionnaires such as the following:
  - Mini-Cog—instrument to assess dementia
  - Mini-Mental State Examination—screening tool for cognitive function and impairment
  - Clock drawing test—screening tool to assess executive function
  - Beck Depression Inventory
  - Hamilton Depression Scale
  - Prime clinician instruments based on *DSM* criteria (intended for and sufficiently diagnostic in primary care settings)

THE DIAGNOSTIC AND STATISTICAL MANUAL OF MENTAL DISORDERS

Diagnostic Criteria

- Standard classification of mental health disorders used by mental health professionals in the United States.
- Designed for use across settings, such as inpatient, outpatient, partial hospital, clinic, private practice, and primary care; with community populations; and by psychiatrists, psychologists, nurses, occupational and rehabilitation therapists, counselors, social workers, medical students, and other health and mental health professionals.
- Necessary tool for collecting and communicating accurate public health data.
- Three major components: the diagnostic classification, the diagnostic criteria sets, and the descriptive text.
- For each disorder in the *DSM*, a set of diagnostic criteria indicates inclusion criteria (symptoms and length of presence) and exclusion criteria to qualify for a particular diagnosis.

Psychological Testing in Psychiatry

WHAT IS PSYCHOLOGICAL TESTING?

Psychological testing offers objective data about mental functioning. It involves administration, scoring, and interpretation of specific tasks in a controlled fashion. Tests must be

- Normed on a representative population
- Administered in a controlled environment
- Administered in a standard fashion
- Reliable and valid
- Culturally fair
- Scored according to standardized procedures
- Interpreted according to acceptable professional practices by a trained professional

WHAT INFORMATION DOES PSYCHOLOGICAL TESTING PROVIDE, AND FOR WHOM IS IT APPROPRIATE?

Psychological testing has the ability to provide useful diagnostic information regarding level of intellectual functioning, identify and describe the nature of a mental health disorder, and indicate underlying motivation, personality attributes, and other variables.

- The patient must be able to participate in the assessment. Grossly confused or psychotic patients are not good candidates for psychological testing.
- Psychological testing is useful in treatment planning and outcome evaluation.
- Psychological testing is useful when objective data are required to establish a suspected diagnosis (sanity boards, interdiction).

TYPES OF PSYCHOLOGICAL TESTS

Many types of psychological tests are available to qualified users, which include the following:

- Measures of intellectual functioning
- Personality questionnaires
- Projective techniques
- Neuropsychological tests
- Measures of cognitive impairment

Associated tests include the following:

- Psychodiagnostic screening tests
- Educational diagnostic tests
- Aptitude tests
- Interest inventories

HOW TO DETERMINE THE APPROPRIATE TYPES OF PATIENTS FOR PSYCHOLOGICAL TESTING

- Almost anyone who possesses a reasonable reality orientation and is nonpsychotic is an appropriate candidate for psychological testing.
- Individuals with better mental statuses are capable of participating in more complex psychological testing procedures.
- Not all patients are capable of participating in all psychological tests. Physical handicaps, language barriers, and illiteracy may limit the available testing procedures.
- The willingness of the patient has an influence on the procedure. Angry or deceptive individuals may distort the outcome data. There are specific psychological tests to detect malingering and deception.
- Very specific referral questions allow for the selection of instruments (measures) to specifically address the reason for referral for testing.

HOW LONG SHOULD PSYCHOLOGICAL TESTING TAKE?

- The time to complete psychological testing depends on the referral questions and the number of testing procedures performed. The time may be as short as 2 hours or as long as 8 hours.

- Testing can be expedited by prearranging appointments, providing relevant records and history, clear referral questions, and, when necessary, preapproval by third-party payers.
- Testing may be delayed when a third-party payer has questions as to the necessity of testing procedures, schedules are full, referral questions are vague, funding is unavailable, or the client is inappropriate for assessment.

WHO PERFORMS PSYCHOLOGICAL TESTS?

- A licensed psychologist or a technician under the supervision of a licensed clinical psychologist conducts psychological testing.
- Not all psychologists provide psychological testing and referrals are frequently made to specialists, especially in the case of neuropsychological assessment.
- Some states allow psychological testing to be conducted by nonpsychologists for specific purposes or in limited environments.

IMPORTANT ISSUES IN PSYCHOLOGICAL TESTING

- Reliability
- Validity
- Cultural bias
- Confidentiality
- Qualified examiners and assistants
- Explaining test results to referral sources

PSYCHOLOGICAL TESTS AND PROCEDURES OF IMPORTANCE IN PSYCHIATRY

The WAIS-IV
- The gold standard in the assessment of intellectual functioning
- Cross-culturally normed and can be used with any U.S. population above the age of 16 years
- Requires 60 to 90 minutes to administer
- Provides several IQ and index scores for different realms of intellectual ability

The MMPI-2
- The most widely investigated and empirically validated personality questionnaire available
- The self-report format consists of 556 true-and-false questions requiring 1 to 2 hours for completion.
- Has built-in validity scales to detect malingering and deception
- Consists of 10 basic clinical scales and supplemental scales to assess personality
- Has a number of presentation formats: paper, short form, and computer administration
- Optic scan options are available, which can then generate a written report for rapid review

The Rorschach
- The classic inkblot projective technique
- The patients are instructed to provide a description of what they see in an ambiguous picture
- The responses have been correlated with personality variables and psychopathology
- Requires specialized training and supervised practice to administer and interpret
- Computer programs are available to assist with scoring and interpretation

Self-Report Instruments
- Typically, self-report inventories are pencil-and-paper tests, wherein the patient endorses items either with a true/false or Likert-scale format.
- These reports can also be done in an interview format.
- They come in "short" and "long" versions, which take time to complete.
- These have been empirically validated with various clinical populations and demographic groups.

Common Measures
- The Beck Depression Inventory
- The Beck Anxiety Inventory
- The Hamilton Depression Scales
- The Hamilton Anxiety Scale

NEUROPSYCHOLOGICAL TEST BATTERIES
- A group of tests that describe brain–behavior relationships.
- Some tests are preselected and referred to as structured batteries while others are selected by the neuropsychologist as per the referral question and are known as flexible batteries.
- Individual tests assess psychological functions in different regions of the brain.
- The test results can be assembled to draw conclusions about damaged and persevered cognitive realms and abilities.
- Tests are useful in assessing the loss secondary to neurological insult and making predictions about recovery.
- Neuropsychological testing requires up to 8 hours of testing time.
- Specialized training is required to administer, score, and interpret measures used in neuropsychological assessment.

QUESTIONS FOR REFERRAL SOURCES TO ASK IN MAKING A REFERRAL
- Will psychological testing answer the questions I have about my patient?
- How soon will the psychologist see my patient?
- How long will the testing take?
- Is the procedure covered by my patient's insurance?
- Does your office have a payment plan?
- How long will it take to get the results?

▪ Will the psychologist go over the results with my patient and me?

▪ If my patient has difficulty in understanding the results, can he or she come and see the psychologist for further review?

▪ Will the results include recommendations that I can implement?

▪ How will my patient's confidentiality and privacy be protected.

REFERENCE

American Psychiatric Association. (2013). *Diagnostic and statistical manual of mental disorders* (5th ed.). Washington, DC: American Psychiatric Press.

BIBLIOGRAPHY

American Medical Association. (2013). *AMA physician ICD-10-CM2010* (Vols. 1 and 2). Chicago, IL: American Medical Association Press.

American Psychiatric Association. (2000). *Diagnostic and statistical manual of mental disorders*, fourth edition, text revision. Washington, DC: American Psychiatric Press.

Andronikof, A. (2008). Exneriana-II—The scientific legacy of John E. Exner, Jr. *Rorschachiana, 29*, 81–107.

Carlat, D. J. (2004). *The psychiatric interview: A practical guide to psychiatry* (2nd ed.). Chicago: Lippincott Williams & Wilkins.

Ebert, M. H., Loosen, P. T., Nurcombe, B., & Leckman, J. F. (Eds.). (2008). *Current diagnosis and treatment psychiatry* (2nd ed.). New York: McGraw-Hill.

Gillis, M. M., Haaga, D. A. F., & Ford, G. T. (1995). Normative values for the Beck Anxiety Inventory, Fear Questionnaire, Penn State Worry Questionnaire, and Social Phobia and Anxiety Inventory. *Psychological Assessment, 7*, 450–455.

LeBlond, R. F., DeGowin, R. L., & Brown, D.D. (Eds.). (2009). *DeGowin's diagnostic examination* (9th ed.). New York, NY: McGraw-Hill.

Meyer, G. J., Riethmiller, R. J., Brooks, R. D., Benoit, W. A., & Handler, L. (2000). A replication of Rorschach and MMPI-2 convergent validity. *Psychological Assessment, 74*, 175–215.

Moras, K., di Nardo, P. A., & Barlow, D. H. (1992). Distinguishing anxiety and depression: Reexamination of the reconstructed Hamilton scales. *Psychological Assessment, 42*, 224–227.

Pearson Education, Inc. (2008). *Introducing the WAIS-IV*. Upper Saddle River, NJ: Author.

Scheiber, S. C. (2004). The psychiatric interview, psychiatric history, and mental status examination. In R. A. Hales, S. C. Yukovsky, & J. A. Talbott (Eds.), *Essentials of clinical psychiatry* (2nd ed.). Washington, DC: American Psychiatric Press.

Valenstin, M., Dalack, G., Blow, F., Figueroa, S., Standiford, C., & Douglass A. (1997). Screening for psychiatric illness with a combined screening and diagnostic instrument. *Journal of General and Internal Medicine, 12*(11), 679–685.

Psychotherapeutic Management

Establish a Philosophy of Management

Management of the psychotherapeutic process is a multidimensional endeavor that requires the following:

- Staff management
- Patient well-being
- Coordination with other professionals
- Time management

Establish a fundamental philosophy guiding both outpatient and inpatient treatment as follows:

- What are the variables that influence service delivery?
- How can you ensure services meet a level of excellence?
- How will staff teamwork be accomplished?
- Selection of the appropriate psychotherapy
- Risk management

The interactions of the above factors with other relevant factors, such as those given below specific to the patient's environment, will determine the ultimate process of intervention.

- How can patient outcome be optimal?
- How can the service program become accountable?
- How can the treatment program become flexible and adaptable?
- How can the program achieve total fairness and mutual respect?

Standards of Care in Psychotherapy Management

In the realm of psychotherapy, surrounding issues are not as well established as in other realms of medicine. This is changing as more becomes known about the process and utility of different forms of intervention. Current influences on the standard of care include the following:

- Laws and current statutes
- Regulations passed by state licensing boards
- Precedent and case law

■ Professional codes of ethics
■ Opinions of consumers and other professionals

The three standards of care established in mental health are as follows:

■ Duty to report abuse
■ The case of *Tarasoff v. the Board of Regents of the University of California*
■ Health Insurance Portability and Accountability Act (HIPAA) guidelines

Psychotherapy: Initial Interview

Presentation by the patient includes the following:

■ Attire
■ Overall attitude
■ Gross motor skills
■ Speech
■ Language
■ Hygiene

Initial assessment includes the following:

■ Presentation of the problem
■ Secondary problems
■ Medical history
■ Work with patient to determine whether there were any past "manic or hypo-manic" episodes—Drug and alcohol history
■ Legal history
■ Developmental history
■ Educational history
■ Employment history
■ Marital status and history
■ Abuse issues

Mental status examination includes the following:

■ Alertness
■ Coherence
■ Mental organization
■ Thought processing
■ Delusions
■ Obsessions
■ Suicidal/homicidal ideation
■ Affect and mood
■ Illusions
■ Hallucinations
■ Orientation
■ Memory
■ Fund of information
■ Abstraction

Psychotherapy Record Management and the Standard of Care

At a minimum, a psychotherapy chart or file should include history of severe adverse drug reactions and allergies.

- Diagnosis
- Presentation of problem
- Mental status examination
- History of past mental illness
- Background information
- Treatment goals
- Progress notes

If appropriate, the chart or notes should display the following:

- Psychological test results
- Psychiatric consultation
- Relevant medical tests or history
- Consultations
- Unscheduled communications with the patient

Special population notes should include the following:

- Nature of the condition
- Concurrent problems
- Potential for violence
- Crisis intervention procedures
- Detailed notes concerning abuse or neglect

Psychotherapeutic Management of Disorders

PERSONALITY DISORDERS

The management of personality disorders presents an unusual challenge because many of the maladaptive features that have caused the patient pain and suffering are fundamental components of the personality structure. Key features in management include the following:

- Maintaining strict boundaries between the patient and the psychotherapist
- Establishing a clear reimbursement plan
- In writing, establishing the responsibility of the patient and the responsibility of the psychotherapist
- Setting rules and consequences for tardiness in the outpatient setting
- Enacting a no-suicide contract
- Agreeing on a plan of action if the patient becomes suicidal
- Always promptly addressing patient's threat to discontinue treatment
- Always assessing secondary issues such as drug and alcohol use
- Becoming alert to issues of secondary gain and disruptive behavior

- Addressing self-destructive behaviors
- Working on enhancing adaptive behaviors and social skills
- Focusing on educating the patient to cause-and-effect relationships
- Helping establish personal, spiritual, and vocational goals of a long-term nature
- Minimizing self-disclosure
- Not accepting excuses

SUBSTANCE ABUSE

Substance abuse disorders require the clinicians to wear many hats and address many different aspects of the patient's experiences.

- Treatment goals should be simple and clear.
- Patients should be actively involved in treatment.
- Therapists should structure a supportive environment.
- Patients must take responsibility for their behavior.
- Therapists should emphasize self-direction.
- Confrontation must be appropriate to the client's tolerance level.
- Empathy should be conditional and measured.
- Avoid arguing with patients.
- Involve the significant other whenever possible.
- Always emphasize the patient's motivation.
- Enhance awareness of problem behaviors.
- Focus on self-destructive cyclic behaviors.
- Educate about the physical destructiveness of substances.
- Engage the family in treatment.
- Help the patient identify feelings and express them appropriately.

DEMENTIA

Management of dementia is achieved in both inpatient and outpatient settings. A multidisciplinary team approach is necessary to manage most cases effectively.

- Address physical safety issues.
- Gauge psychotherapy to the level of impairment.
- Address issues of incontinence in counseling.
- Enhance mobility.
- Educate as to the dangers of falling.
- Address depression in both individual and group sessions.
- Offer orientation counseling to low-functioning patients.
- Offer family consultation and counseling to all family members.
- Address end-of-life issues in group therapy.
- Carefully investigate drug and alcohol issues.
- Consult with family about driving privileges.
- Assess memory repeatedly.
- Stress a wellness model.
- Prepare to address sundowning problems.
- Establish smoking and obesity groups.
- Offer counseling for depression and loss.

DEPRESSION

Depression is the most common illness in the general population. There are numerous diagnostic categories for the depressive disorders but some basic management principles apply to all forms of depression.

- Assess the depth of the depression.
- Establish the etiology, duration, and frequency of the depression.
- Assess vegetative signs.
- Assess suicide risk.
- Stabilize the affect and mood with medication management.
- Educate the patient as to the nature of the illness.
- Reduce guilt.
- Initiate a supportive therapy to stabilize.
- Look for cultural influences that maintain depression.
- Reduce stressors.
- Enhance self-esteem.
- Build problem-solving skills.
- Manage self-defeating thoughts.
- Help explore self-defeating behaviors.
- Engage family support.

PSYCHOTIC DISORDERS

A lack of a reality orientation and disorganized thinking are the hallmarks of psychosis. Psychotherapy is unproductive in the acute phase but profitable in the prodromal and residual phases, assisting the client to maintain the medication management program and discover a rewarding life.

- Establish the patient's current level of functioning.
- Encourage compliance with medication management program.
- Reduce stressors.
- Assist with acquiring basic necessities.
- Investigate drug and alcohol use.
- Consistently encourage a balanced life style.
- Discourage self-medication.
- Assist with enrollment in day hospital programs.
- Urge self-exploration of illness.
- Help establish boundaries.
- Assist with financial management.
- Build social skills.
- Teach patient to recognize psychotic features.
- Encourage personal hygiene.
- Teach listening skills.
- Always redirect when patient avoids.
- Enhance independent living skills.
- Prevent self-pity and despondency.
- Directly address noncompliance with treatment.

BIBLIOGRAPHY

American Psychiatric Association. (2013). *Diagnostic and statistical manual of mental disorders* (5th ed.). Arlington, VA: American Psychiatric Publishing.

American Psychotherapy Association. (2008). *Psychotherapist's oath*. Retrieved from http://www.americanpsychotherapy.com/about/oath/

Richmond, R. L. (2009a). *The psychotherapy process*. Retrieved from http://www.guidetopsychology.com/questions/questions.htm#process/

Richmond, R. L. (2009b). *Transference issues*. Retrieved from http://www.guidetopsychology.com/questions/questions.htm#trans/

Richmond, R. L. (2009c). *Termination issues*. Retrieved from http://www.guidetopsychology.com/questions/questions.htm#termin/

Zur, O. (2009). *The standard of care in psychotherapy and counseling: Bringing clarity to illusive relationships*. Retrieved from http://www.zurinstitute.com/standardofcare-therapy.html/

Chapter 3

Behavioral Therapy, Cognitive Behavioral Therapy, and Psychoanalysis

Behavioral Therapy and Cognitive Behavioral Therapy

DEFINITIONS

Behavioral Therapy

Behavioral therapy is any intervention or set of interventions that focuses on the patient behaviors as the primary focus of change. Maladaptive, self-defeating, self-destructive, or otherwise problematic behaviors can be replaced with more effective ones. Learning these new behaviors is a matter of education and reinforcement. Progressive muscle relaxation training and social skills training are the two examples.

Cognitive Therapy

Cognitive therapy includes interventions that target a patient's thinking process. The central principle in cognitive therapy (CT) is that thoughts produce feelings. That is, sadness and anxiety are, in part, the products of the thinking process. Faulty thinking precedes emotional distress. The thinking process is often fraught with faulty assumptions and unexamined tenets that often render the patient unnecessarily constrained and distressed. Through identification and examination of faulty or distorted thinking processes, patients are helped to consider themselves and their circumstances from an alternate perspective and thereby mitigate feelings of distress.

Cognitive Behavioral Therapy

Cognitive behavioral therapy (CBT) is a body of work in psychotherapy that draws from multiple theorists and focuses on the thoughts and behaviors that shape problematic emotional reactions and consequences.

- In the CBT framework, emotional distress is believed to be the result of faulty habits of thought that result in dysfunctional attitudes and behaviors.
- Maladaptive patterns of thinking create the emotional distress.

■ In order to alleviate that distress, new objective, evidence-based thought patterns have to be developed and new behavioral skills have to be adopted.
■ Through a systematic process of examining, labeling, and analyzing these cognitive errors, patients learn to replace them with more reality-based, self-enhancing ones.

BEHAVIORAL AND COGNITIVE BEHAVIORAL PROCESSES

Background

■ Behavioral therapy is based, in part, on work of B. F. Skinner and others who analyzed how operant conditioning determines behavioral responses and how these responses could be altered through effective environmental reinforcement.
■ Reward-based measures, such as token economies, are used to reinforce desired behaviors. Variations in specific theoretical frameworks and treatment techniques exist within behavioral therapy.
■ Thought leaders in CT include Albert Ellis (rational emotive therapy) and Aaron Beck (cognitive therapy), who through the 1960s advanced the notion that feelings or emotions were strongly influenced by the habitual patterns people used to make sense of their experiences.
■ These thought patterns were considered "automatic" in that they are an innate part of the "self-talk" that seems to be a universal human phenomenon.
■ These automatic thoughts are often based on misconceptions, deeply embedded erroneous assumptions (schema), and learned principles that confine the manner in which people respond to all kinds of life problems.
■ Although psychodynamically oriented approaches look to the origin of feelings in sometimes deeply conflicted psychosocial, developmental, and cognitive aspects, theorists propose that feelings originate from learned patterns of thinking that create unnecessarily confined mental structures that affect how people learn, grow, and solve problems.
■ These false, fixed notions of reality create mental prisons for those who live within them.

TERMS AND METHODS

Fundamental Features

CBT is a relatively short-term psychotherapy process (approximately, 6 to 18 sessions) that is structured and formalized. Attention to this structure is a hallmark of the approach. The steps of treatment usually include the following:

1. A thorough diagnostic interview
2. The partnering of patient and therapist forms an active collaborative team
3. The therapist–patient team works together to identify problematic areas in the patient's life by identifying cognitive distortions or errors that commonly impose a negative interpretation on everyday events.
4. The therapist–patient team adopts a step-by-step process to examine the underlying assumptions, fundamental beliefs, or "schemas" from which these self-defeating thought patterns and distortions originate. They are often outside the immediate conscious awareness of the patient.

5. The creating and maintaining of a written daily thought record includes the following:
   - Documenting specific events that evoke emotional distress
   - Identifying the specific cognitive distortions that are at work in many of these situations
   - Labeling and analyzing of cognitive distortions
   - Identifying alternative methods for thinking about these same events (cognitive correction process)
6. The assignment of carefully planned homework so that the patient remains actively engaged in the CBT process outside of the formal sessions
7. The therapist actively engages in coaching the patient through a systematic examination of the antecedents and consequences of these errors in thinking
8. The therapist–patient team designs strategies to examine evidence to determine the validity of these erroneous mental constructs
9. Prioritization and processing of these problems from a CBT framework
10. Recording the process of identification of goals in behavioral, measurable terminology
11. Trying on new behaviors that are outside the patient's usual pattern to explore potential results and sources of reinforcement
12. Ultimately, the patient becomes his or her own therapist, able to quickly identify erroneous thinking when it occurs and take steps to neutralize or counter it.
13. Coupled with the ability to initiate behavioral measures (relaxation and assertiveness), the patient can choose from a repertoire of skills to meet the demands of the emotionally charged situation and return to a state of emotional equilibrium.

Psychoeducation
- Psychoeducation is a major and ongoing component of the treatment and is usually woven into sessions throughout the course of treatment.
- Patients are introduced to a cognitive conceptualization of their problems and goals from the beginning.
- Psychoeducation teaches patients about the terms, strategies, and processes of CBT and is included in most of the sessions.

Cognitive Distortions
Cognitive distortions are automatic thoughts that are often irrational, illogical, or self-defeating. If occurring regularly, they can result in patterns of ineffective behavior. Although different theorists have developed somewhat idiosyncratic terminology to designate similar phenomena, the following are common to many of them:

- Emotional reasoning: the tendency to conclude that if a person feels awkward or uncomfortable after a social event, then the person must actually be socially awkward.
- Dichotomous thinking (all-or-nothing thinking): drawing absolute conclusions. A person whose marriage fails believes that he or she is a "complete loser."
- Discounting the positive: disqualifying all positive experiences or traits as being trivial or unimportant, especially when compared to a seemingly glaring error or shortcoming.
- Personalization: interpreting external data as being related to oneself without evidence for such a conclusion.

■ Arbitrary inference: drawing a conclusion without supporting evidence, or even in spite of contradictory evidence.
■ Minimization and magnification: overinflating the negative or underestimating the positive in the evaluation of the relative importance of events.
■ Catastrophizing: assuming that the worst possible outcome is the most likely.

Interactive Techniques
■ Setting an agenda: the agenda for each session is actively negotiated with the patient at the outset.
■ Feedback: the therapist deliberately requests feedback to ascertain patient's understanding of, and success with, process and methods. Eliciting and processing patient reactions to, concerns about, and impressions of both the therapy and the therapist are considered essential components of the CBT experience.
■ Socratic method: through a series of questions, the therapist gradually advances the nature of a discussion to lead the patient to first uncovering the distorted perspective, then drawing more accurate, self-affirming conclusions.
■ Guided discovery: examining evidence, weighing the value of alternatives, and exploring the advantages and disadvantages of various options. This is done in an integrated and accepting manner through discussion format.
■ Focused attentiveness: focusing on central ideas, relevant thoughts, assumptions, behaviors, and so on, that are germane to the problem being discussed.
■ Formulating a strategy for change: plan is actively negotiated with the patient and clearly outlines CBT strategies to be employed in the change process.

Qualities of the Therapist
■ CBT is a methodology that requires its practitioners to be well grounded in the essential skills of psychotherapy.
■ CBT does not replace basic psychotherapeutic practice. Rather, it builds from it.
■ The cognitive behavioral therapist must be well versed in conceptual and operational underpinnings of psychotherapeutic processes.
■ The therapist, while being specifically trained in CBT techniques, must possess and exhibit the fundamental features of any effective therapist, including:
  ● Graduate education in a mental health field (psychology, psychiatry, social work, nursing, professional counseling, etc.)
  ● Formal training in CBT
  ● Deeply embedded commitment to and demonstration of basic therapist skills and attributes like
    ● Expression of empathy
    ● Professionalism
    ● Sound, ethical practice
    ● Active listening
    ● Authenticity
    ● Understanding of complex psychological phenomena that influence human experiences
    ● Ability to understand the patient within the social, cultural, environmental context of that patient's lived experience

Evidence-Based Applications
■ Among psychotherapy methods, to its credit CBT has the largest body of empirical evidence to support its efficacy.

- Because of the formalized and structured nature of its tenets and interventions, CBT can be operationalized in a reproducible manner that creates sound reliability and validity.
- Common evidence-based applications include the following:
  - Anxiety disorders in adults and children
  - Depression
  - Addictions
  - Personality disorders (especially in the form of dialectical behavioral therapy)
- Examples of newer applications (some still under investigation) include the following:
  - Chronic pain
  - Chronic illness
  - Chronic fatigue syndrome
  - Tinnitus
  - Headache, especially with comorbid psychiatric symptoms
  - Schizophrenia
  - Child sexual abuse
  - Treatment of sex offenders
  - Somatoform disorders
  - Anxiety, depression, and insomnia in older adults
  - Psychological adjustment to breast cancer
  - Occupational stress

RELATED APPROACH: DIALECTICAL BEHAVIORAL THERAPY

- Mindfulness and radical acceptance are concepts that complement, draw from, or enhance a CBT.
- These concepts supplement or extend CBT methods and techniques to further target treatment-resistant emotional distress.
- Dialectical behavioral therapy (DBT), for example, provides a systematic and programmed method for dealing with the intense emotional distress that sometimes occurs in patients who struggle with borderline personality disorder.
- Mindful strategies and meditation help to decrease the emotional reactivity that may be, in part, physiologically activated, especially after prolonged periods of intense stress.
- Computer-based, program-driven CBT is now available and these programs claim to provide effective CBT in the absence of a psychotherapist.

Psychoanalysis

SIGMUND FREUD

Biographical Information
- Born in Moravia in 1856; died in London in 1939.
- Member of the Jewish faith, which had a significant influence on his worldview.
- Trained in neurology, he developed an interest in patients who exhibited neurological symptoms without any organic etiology.
- Studied with Jean Baptiste Charcot at the Salpetrière in Paris. This greatly affected his thinking about the influence of the unconscious on personality development and behavior.

■ After returning to Vienna, he developed the first comprehensive theory of personality.
■ His theory of personality led to the development of psychoanalysis.

FREUD'S PERSONALITY THEORY

Freud's ideas can be reviewed in two broad sections:

The Topographic Model (1900)
■ Saw personality as analogous to an iceberg with three distinct sections.
  ■ Conscious level: consists of current thoughts and perceptions.
  ■ Preconscious level: involves memories and stored knowledge that can be retrieved on demand.
  ■ Unconscious level: inaccessible feelings, urges, drives, desires, and demands. These are driven by a basic biological–sexual need for fulfillment.
■ The Topographic Model was represented in Freud's 1900 publication, *The Interpretation of Dreams*, in which he proposed that humans were guided by unconscious sexual energies that lead to conflicts in everyday life.

The Structural Model (ca. 1920)
■ As Freud's ideas matured, so did his conceptualization of personality structure.
■ While the topographical model was rigid with its three sections, the structural model remained fluid and offered interaction between the realms of one's personality.
■ The structural model has three semi-independent realms as follows:
  ■ The id
    ● The id is the only part of personality present at birth.
    ● The id operates on the pleasure principle.
    ● Wants instant gratification—"It wants, what it wants, when it wants it."
    ● No frustration tolerance.
    ● No empathy or compassion for others; completely egocentric.
    ● Goal of the id is to increase pleasure and decrease pain and anxiety.
    ● Inappropriate or psychotic behavior results when needs are delayed or denied.
    ● The id runs on libido energy (or life energy). The libido energy is a biological energy that drives an individual toward growth and development.
    ● Initially, because it is unconscious, the image of an object is just as rewarding as the object itself.
    ● The id is forced by the biological necessity to acknowledge the outside world and thus makes arrangements for some libido energy to act as a go-between.
  ■ The ego
    ● The ego begins as a fragile subsection of the id with the goal of satisfying id needs by any practical means.
    ● To satisfy id needs, the ego is in communication with reality and guides behavior.
    ● Gratifying the id's needs results in greater libido energy being shifted to the ego, which results in a stronger reality reorientation, socialization skills, and frustration tolerance.
    ● Failure to meet the id's needs leads to deteriorating ego influence and an increase in primitive, infantile, or psychotic behavior.

- The ego is in touch with reality and operates by the reality principle, which endorses delayed gratification.
- For most people, the ego continues to develop and becomes the executor of personality, balancing the other forces.

◈ The superego

- The last portion of personality to develop a relationship with both the unconscious and conscious.
- The superego begins to develop as the attitudes of authority figures are integrated into the personality structure and a sense of right and wrong is established.
- As the superego develops, it influences behavior by enhancing self-esteem for appropriate actions and punishing inappropriate behavior through guilt.
- In a healthy personality, there is a flow of energy among the three realms.
- If the libido energy becomes focused on the id, psychotic behaviors become prominent in the personality.
- If the libido energy should become focused on the superego, anxiety disorders become prominent.

In sum: The id is driven by inborn instincts such as anger and sex, while the superego is at the other extreme, urging social values and altruism. The ego is the executor and arbitrator, directing and balancing the demands of the id and the superego.

THE PSYCHOSEXUAL STAGES OF DEVELOPMENT

Freud adopted a stage theory of psychosexual personality development in his 1905 work, *Three Essays on the Theory of Sexuality* (see Table 3.1).

▨ The stages are invariant; they cannot be circumvented or skipped.
▨ The stages represent a shifting of libido energy to different areas of the body. These realms become the center of developmental psychosexual issues and attention.
▨ Each stage has a psychosexual crisis associated with it that must be successfully resolved before moving on to the next stage of development.
▨ Failure in resolving the psychosexual crisis associated with the stage results in fixation. Psychosexual energy remains stagnant and the individual (unconsciously) attempts to resolve the crisis. These attempts usually become socially inappropriate as the person ages.

Table 3.1   The Psychosexual Stages of Human Development

STAGE	AGE (YEAR[S])	EROGENOUS ZONE	PSYCHOSEXUAL CONFLICT
Oral	0–1	Mouth	Weaning, sucking, eating
Anal	1–3	Anus	Toilet training, feces
Phallic	3–5	Genitals	Oedipal conflict, sex
Latency	5–6	None	Period of calmness
Genital	Puberty	Mature sexual relationships	

The Oedipal Conflict
▦ In Greek mythology, Oedipus was the son of the King of Thebes, whose lover, unbeknownst to him, was his mother.
▦ When Oedipus became aware of the identity of his lover, he gouged out his eyes for violating a sexual taboo.
▦ The Oedipal conflict provides an explanation of gender orientation and operates unconsciously.
▦ During this phallic stage, libido energy builds, and the child begins to develop a sexual attraction for the opposite-sex parent.
▦ The course for boys and girls is different.
　▦ Boys
　　◦ The boy develops affection for his mother and jealously wishes to displace his father as the man in her life. As his psychosexual tension grows, he becomes fearful of reprisal, which leads to a belief that his father may remove him as a contender by removing his genitals, the castration complex.
　　◦ At this point, the anxiety is intolerable and the boy engages two defense mechanisms to reduce anxiety and resolve the psychosexual conflict. He represses his affection for his mother and identifies with his father, leading to a psychological male orientation that matches his physiology.
　　◦ A small proportion of boys fail to resolve this crisis and fail to establish a male identity. This concludes the phallic period and the child enters a period of psychosexual tranquility until puberty.
　▦ Girls
　　◦ A girl develops affection for her father and wishes to displace her mother who is now viewed as a rival.
　　◦ Eventually the conflict of losing her mother's love and having her mother separate her from the family becomes intolerable.
　　◦ Repressing her affection for her father and identifying with her mother successfully resolve the conflict.
　　◦ Her psychology now matches her physiology, and she now identifies herself as female.
　　◦ A small proportion of females fail to resolve the crisis and experience gender identity issues.

Defense Mechanisms
▦ The defense mechanisms serve as protective devices for the three mental structures (see Table 3.2).
▦ Their mission is to mitigate anxiety and stress and enhance stability in the personality structure.
▦ The defense mechanisms operate unconsciously.
▦ The implementation of defense mechanisms to manage a stressor is based on efficiency. If unsuccessful, less efficient mechanisms will be implemented and may, unfortunately, lead to a demonstration of age-inappropriate or pathological behavior.
▦ Psychotic individuals rely heavily on primitive defense mechanisms such as denial and projection.
▦ Healthy individuals use the most appropriate defense mechanism and can quickly select another when necessary.
▦ Individuals with personality disorders are unable to select appropriate mechanisms and rely heavily, even exclusively, on just one defense mechanism, such as paranoia.

Table 3.2　Defense Mechanisms

DEFENSE MECHANISM	ACTIVITY	EXAMPLE
Repression	Suppression of anxiety-laden material from consciousness.	A sailor cannot remember the attack on his ship.
Projection	Attributing repulsive attitudes and traits to another.	A student alleges faculty is out to get him.
Denial	Refusal to admit an obvious reality.	Following a divorce, the husband still says he's married.
Rationalization	Substituting a concocted reason rather than the real reason for an event.	Making an excuse using rationale. "If you had a wife like mine, you wouldn't go home either."
Reaction formation	Attesting to the opposite emotion of an impulse or desire.	After breaking up with Mary, Bob says he never really loved her.
Regression	Reverting to a more primitive behavior of an earlier developmental stage.	After losing an argument, Bob assaults his coworker.
Displacement	Substituting a less threatening object for the original object of hostility.	After being fired, Bob returns home and kicks his cat.
Sublimation	Substituting forbidden impulses for socially acceptable activities.	Bob plays tennis when he feels angry with his mother.

The Process of Psychoanalysis

⬛ Freud believed that patients would structure their own emotional resolution if allowed to explore the repressed conflicts that were impeding growth and development.

⬛ The unconscious is both an asset and an impediment to conflict resolution and development. It is, by its nature, protective of the structure by holding an aberrant impulse in abeyance and thus managing anxiety and pain. Simultaneously, it prevents resolution because of this material being inaccessible.

⬛ One of Freud's problems was to develop a mechanism that would prevent overwhelming anxiety to the conscious mind and slowly allow the patient to develop an understanding of unconscious conflicts and developmental failures.

⬛ To address the unconscious, Freud developed psychoanalysis, a procedure by which the client could address repressed issues at his or her own pace in an environment free of ridicule and condemnation.

⬛ The client would recline on a couch and engage in process of free association, a spontaneous discourse of whatever came to mind.

⬛ The psychoanalyst would position himself or herself out of the patient's line of sight and record the process and topics of discourse. Commentary by the psychoanalyst was held to a minimum.

⬛ Occasionally, patients were requested to recount dreams. Dream material was given special attention, as Freud believed defense mechanisms were less vigilant during sleep and repressed conflicts and desires would work their way toward consciousness or at least preconsciousness. Even in the sleep state, the repressed material was too anxiety-producing and had to be modified.

▦ Freud explained the matter as follows:

   ▦ The actual material and recollection of the dream consists of the manifest material. Thus, the content the patient remembers is a defensive modification of the repressed material. To the patient, the material may appear bizarre or nonsensical.

   ▦ The latent content is the underlying repressed conflicting material that has been distorted by the manifest content so as to prevent anxiety.

▦ Periodically, the analyst will interpret the latent content to the patient to facilitate resolution.

▦ As analysis continues, the client experiences the anxiety of the repressed conflicts. As conflict intensifies, the client will have a catharsis, an outpouring of emotion that facilitates resolution. The analyst's task is to facilitate a controlled release of emotion so the client is not overwhelmed by anxiety and does not suffer a regressive experience.

▦ The analyst must refrain from addressing specific behaviors or superficial material. Resolving a specific symptom without addressing the underlying conflict might predispose the patient to have symptom substitution, that is, the development of a new symptom to replace the old.

▦ The process of analysis may be impeded by the patient's unconscious, as the process of investigation will increase anxiety and conflict.

▦ Patients will develop resistance. They may become dissatisfied with the analyst, skip or be late for appointments, become silent, or fail to report important material.

▦ The analyst must address resistance as it occurs or it may (will) become self-defeating and prevent deeper understanding of conflict-laden material.

▦ The patient may develop transference (a specific type of projection), that is, the unconscious association of the analyst with someone of significance in the patient's past. This allows the patient to ascribe to the analyst feelings once attributed to that person.

▦ Because of the nature of psychoanalysis, the analyst may engage in the same phenomenon, a process known as countertransference.

▦ Repressed conflicts affect an individual's life in an adverse manner by persistent utilization of inappropriate defense mechanisms. The analyst must interpret and educate the patient about the self-destructiveness of defense mechanisms.

PROMINENT IDEAS OF FREUD

The role of the unconscious is paramount in personality development and daily behavior.

▦ Sex, or the enhancement of pleasure, is the driving force in development and behavior.

▦ Freud possessed a dark view of human nature. He theorized humans as driven by fantasies, conflicts, and sexual urges that were controlled by socialization, training, and religion.

▦ Freud put tremendous emphasis on early-life experiences. He proposed that most of our personality is formed by the age of 5.

▦ Freud outlined set stages of development. These were invariant and could not be circumvented. To obtain adequate psychological growth, the conflict at the end of each stage must be resolved so that libido energy can follow the appropriate developmental path.

THE FREUDIANS

Carl Jung, Analytical Psychology

▒ Jung was a Swiss colleague of Freud and a member of the inner circle until he developed his own theory of personality development.

▒ Jung believed that the personal unconscious could be understood by studying dreams, folklore, religion and mythology, and symbolism.

▒ As significant as the personal unconscious was the collective unconscious. He thought that there was a deeper level of the unconscious that was common to the entire species.

▒ Jung postulated the concept of archetype, a universal concept common to all humans. Many archetypes exist regarding behaviors such as motherhood and physical form. Archetypes are expressed in cultural and religious symbols.

▒ Mental health is the result of insight and self-realization. Mental illness is the consequence of conflicts that prevent self-exploration and self-realization.

Anna Freud, Ego Psychology

▒ Daughter of Sigmund Freud, Anna studied with her father and became an analyst in Vienna and London.

▒ Although a strong supporter of her father's theoretical positions, Anna came to believe that the ego should be the focus of attention.

▒ Anna Freud felt that the ego was the executor of personality and that analytical work should be directed at strengthening the ego to mitigate anxiety and stress.

▒ Anna Freud felt that the ego could become overwhelmed by conflicting demands of the id and the superego.

▒ Later in life, Anna Freud became a leader in child psychoanalysis and the psychological effects of depravation and poor nurturance.

Otto Rank, Humanistic Psychology

▒ Rank was Freud's closest associate for 20 years until publication of a paper advocating a different process of development and questioning the importance of early-life psychosexual growth.

▒ Over time, Rank moved further away from the classic tenets and eventually focused on the "here and now" in psychotherapy, rather than interpreting early-life experiences and repressed conflicts.

▒ Rank emphasized active learning and continued psychological growth throughout life. Psychotherapy concentrates on discovering give and take, separating and coming together. A patient must find a balance regarding all the forces in his or her environment to achieve mental health. The passiveness of the analysis was changed to an active dialogue with the patient.

▒ Rank had a profound effect on the professional development of Carl Rogers, Rollo May, and Erik Erikson. His writings are considered the foundation of humanistic and client-centered therapy.

Erik Erikson, Developmental Psychology

▒ Following his graduation from the Vienna Psychoanalytic Institute, Erikson moved to the United States where he taught at a number of universities and began to work with disadvantaged children and adolescents.

- Erikson revised Freud's five stages of psychosexual development into eight and said that human psychological development continues throughout life and that each stage has its individual challenges.
- Three stages were specific to adulthood and described challenges unique to that period.
- Like Anna Freud, Erikson was an ego psychologist who believed that the ego, not the id, was the focal point of personality.
- Social development, and not sexual development, was the underlying force behind growth.

Alfred Adler, Individual Psychology

- Along with Freud, Adler was one of the founders of psychoanalysis and the first colleague to break with Freud and establish his own school of thought.
- Adler believed in the unconscious and held that dream analysis was productive. However, he de-emphasized the role of psychosexual forces in favor of a conflict between inferiority and superiority.
- It was the work of the analyst to bring these two opposing forces into harmony.
- Central to Adler's technique was the concept of holistic treatment, which emphasized all psychological aspects of personal and social functioning of the patient.
- He abandoned the couch and had analyst and patient face each other in chairs. His therapeutic style utilized humor, historical incidents, and paradox.
- Adler's holistic approach led him to address how individuals integrate with society, and he became an advocate of prevention, democratic family structure, parent training, birth order, child psychology, organizational psychology, and women's rights.
- His work has been described as a precursor to modern CT.

Karen Horney, Feminine Psychology and Anxiety

- Psychoanalysis's first female practitioner, teacher, and theoretician, Horney broke with traditional Freudian teachings regarding psychosexual development and neurosis.
- Unlike Freud, who felt neurotic (anxiety) disturbance in mental functioning was the result of conflict, Horney viewed neurosis as a continuous process of managing stressors. All persons possessed some degree of "basic anxiety," which formed the foundation for a lifelong struggle.
- Because of adverse early experiences, some patients were more susceptible to periods of anxiety.
- The management of anxiety was the foundation of development. Horney developed 10 basic neurotic needs that were expressed in three categories: moving toward people, moving away from people, and moving against people.
- Horney suggested the "self" was at the core of personality. All persons possess a dual perception of the self: the real self, who we are; and the ideal self, who we wish to be.
- Anxiety is generated when the two selves are in conflict and disharmony.
- The job of the analyst is to resolve the conflict and enhance growth or self-actualization. This is a lifelong process.
- Horney felt Freud had overemphasized male sexual issues.
- She postulated that if women had "penis envy," then men must have "womb envy."

■ As such, women had a psychological advantage as self-actualization could be achieved by bearing children.

■ Men, unable to bear children, compensated for their feelings of inferiority by seeking self-actualization through external means, such as dominance and aggressiveness.

■ Horney felt cultural mores led women to be subservient to men, thereby preventing the attainment of self-actualization. She proposed that both genders had the ability to be productive and was an advocate for gender equality.

BIBLIOGRAPHY

American Psychological Association. (2002). *Ethical principles of psychologists and code of conduct.* Retrieved from http://www.apa.org/ethics/code2002.pdf.

American Psychotherapy Association. (2008). *Psychotherapist's oath.* Retrieved from http://www.americanpsychotherapy. com/about/oath/.

Beck, A. T., Rush, A. J., Shaw, B. F., & Emery, G. (1979). *Cognitive therapy of depression.* New York, NY: Guilford Press.

Beck, J. (1995). *Cognitive therapy: Basics and beyond.* New York, NY: Guilford Press.

Burns, D. (1999). *Feeling good: The new mood therapy.* New York, NY: HarperCollins.

Dimeff, L. A., & Koerner, K. (Eds.). (2007). *Dialectical behavioral therapy in clinical practice.* New York, NY: Guilford Press.

Freeman, A., Felgoise, S. H., Nezu, A. M., Nezu, C. M., & Reinecke, M. A. (Eds.). (2005). *Encyclopedia of cognitive behavioral therapy.* New York, NY: Springer Publishing Company.

Gosch, E. A., Flannery-Schroeder, E., Mauro, C. F., & Compton, S. N. (2006). Principles of cognitive-behavioral therapy for anxiety disorders in children. *Journal of Cognitive Psychotherapy, 20,* 247–262.

Hayes, S. C., Follette, V. M., & Linehan, M. (2004). *Mindfulness and acceptance: Expanding the cognitive-behavioral tradition.* New York, NY: Guilford Press.

Kenneth, H. K., Vessey, J., Lueger, R., & Schank, D. (1992). The psychotherapeutic delivery system. *Psychotherapy Research, 2,* 164–180.

Kuyken, W., Byford, S., Taylor, R. S., Watkins, E., Holden, E., White, K., . . . , Teasdale, J. D. (2008). Mindfulness-based cognitive therapy to prevent relapse in recurrent depression. *Journal of Consulting and Clinical Psychology, 76*(6), 966–978.

Linehan, M. (1993). *Cognitive-behavioral treatment of borderline personality disorder.* New York, NY: Guilford Press.

National Institute of Drug Abuse Treatment Manual for Cocaine Abuse. Available at http://www.nida.nih.gov/TXManuals/CBT/CBT1.html.

Richmond, R. L. (2009a). *The psychotherapy process.* Retrieved from http://www.guidetopsychology.com/questions/questions.htm#process.

Richmond, R. L. (2009b). *Transference issues.* Retrieved from http://www.guidetop sychology.com/questions/questions. htm#trans.

Richmond, R. L. (2009c). *Termination issues.* Retrieved from http://www.guidetop sychology.com/questions/questions. htm#termin.

Wheeler, K. (Ed.). (in press). *Psychotherapy for advanced practice nurses,* second edition. New York, NY: Springer Publishing Company.

Zur, O. (2009). *The standard of care in psychotherapy and counseling: Bringing clarity to an illusive standard*. Retrieved from http://www.zurinstitute.com/standardofcaretherapy .html.

WEB RESOURCES

■ Addiction Treatment and CBT: http://www.smartrecovery.org/resources/tool chest.htm/

■ Certification Information: Academy of Cognitive Therapy: http://www. acad-emyofct.org/

■ Commercial entities, including Computer-aided Cognitive Behavioral Therapy Ltd.: http://www.ccbt.co.uk/, a UK-based company that provides CBT online for panic and phobias, depression and stress, and obsessive-compulsive disorder.

■ Other sites that supply online assistance are educational rather than intervention based and are more research oriented. These provide materials at no cost with the user's agreement to participate in the research process. One such site is the Mood Gym, which operates from Centre for Mental Health Research (CMHR) at the Australian National University and is located at http://moodgym.anu.edu.au/

■ Overview of Cognitive Therapy of Depression: http://psychologyinfo.com / depression/cognitive.html/

■ Panic and Anxiety Treatment: http://www.paniccenter.net/

Part II

Principles of Clinical Psychopharmacology

Chapter 4

Clinical Neuroanatomy of the Brain

Clinical neuroanatomy is the method of studying lesions of the human nervous system as a tool to reinforce and amplify learning of the structure and organization of the central nervous system (CNS).

Clinical neuropharmacology is the study of drugs that alter processes controlled by the nervous system.

This chapter deals with the basic anatomy and physiology of the CNS, peripheral nervous system (PNS), somatic nervous system, blood–brain barrier, basal ganglia, hippocampus, hypothalamus, and neurotransmitters.

Nervous System

CENTRAL NERVOUS SYSTEM

- Composed of the brain and spinal cord, which are covered by protective membranes (meninges) and have fluid-filled spaces; weighs less than most desktop computers; receives and interprets sensory information and controls simple/complex motor behaviors

PERIPHERAL NERVOUS SYSTEM

- Composed of cranial and spinal nerves; the nerves contain nerve fibers, which conduct information to (afferent) and from (efferent) the CNS; efferent fibers are involved in motor function, such as contraction of muscles or activation of secretory glands; afferent fibers convey sensory stimuli from the skin, mucous membranes, and deeper structures.
- *Somatic nervous system*: part of PNS; innervates the structures of the body wall (muscles, skin, and mucous membranes)
- *Autonomic nervous system*: part of PNS; contains the sympathetic nervous system (SNS) ("fight or flight") and the parasympathetic nervous system (PSNS); controls activities of the smooth muscles, glands, and internal organs, including blood vessels, and returns sensory information to the brain.

CENTRAL NERVOUS SYSTEM

Brain and Spinal Cord

▨ CNS drugs are used medically to treat psychiatric disorders, seizures, and pain, and as anesthetics; nonmedically, they are used as stimulants, depressants, euphoriants, and mind-altering substances.

▨ The CNS drugs include at least 21 neurotransmitters:

▨ *Monoamines*: norepinephrine, epinephrine, dopamine, serotonin

▨ *Amino acids*: aspartate, glutamate, gamma-aminobutyric acid (GABA), glycine

▨ *Purines*: adenosine, adenosine monophosphate, adenosine triphosphate

▨ *Peptides*: dynorphins, endorphins, enkephalins, neurotensin, somatostatin, substance P, oxytocin, vasopressin

▨ *Others*: acetylcholine (ACh), histamine

Blood–Brain Barrier

The blood–brain barrier blocks the entry of some drugs and substances into the brain.

▨ *Elements*: supporting cells (neuralgia), particularly the astrocytes, and tight junctions between endothelial cells.

▨ *Function*: selectively inhibits certain substances in the blood from entering the interstitial spaces of the brain or cerebrospinal fluid. Certain metabolites, electrolytes, and chemicals have differing abilities to cross the blood–brain barrier. This has substantial implications for drug therapy because some antibiotics and chemotherapeutic drugs show a greater ability than others for crossing the barrier.

▨ *P-glycoprotein*: a protective element of the blood–brain barrier and a transport molecule that pumps various types of drugs out of cells. In capillaries of the CNS, P-glycoprotein pumps drugs back into the blood, thus limiting their access to the brain.

▨ Passage limited to lipid-soluble substances and drugs that cross by means of transport systems (protein-bound and highly ionized substances cannot cross).

▨ Protects brain from injury due to toxic substances but also acts as an obstacle to entry of therapeutic drugs.

THE BRAIN

▨ The brain is able to adapt to prolonged drug exposure, which can alter the therapeutic effects and side effects of some drugs (adaptive changes are often beneficial but can be harmful).

▨ Increased therapeutic effects, decreased side effects, tolerance, and physical dependences may occur.

▨ Acts as a control center by receiving, interpreting, and directing sensory information throughout the body.

▨ Composed of cerebrum (*telencephalon*—cerebral cortex, subcortical white matter, commissures, basal ganglia; *diencephalon*—thalamus, hypothalamus, epithalamus, subthalamus), brain stem (midbrain, pons, medulla oblongata), and cerebellum (cerebellar cortex, cerebellar nuclei). Cerebrum and cerebellum are organized into right and left hemispheres.

▨ There are *three major divisions* of the brain—the forebrain, the midbrain, and the hindbrain.

- The forebrain is responsible for receiving and processing sensory information, thinking, perceiving, producing and understanding language, and controlling motor function.
- The midbrain is responsible for auditory and visual responses and motor function.
- The hindbrain is responsible for maintaining balance and equilibrium, movement coordination, and the conduction of sensory information.
- *The limbic system* is often called the "pleasure center."
  - It is the group of structures that governs emotions and behavior.
  - It connects to all areas of the brain, especially the frontal cortex, which is the learning center.

PERIPHERAL NERVOUS SYSTEM

PNS is divided into the *somatic nervous system* (controls movement of skeletal muscles) and the *autonomic nervous system*. The autonomic nervous system is further divided into the PSNS and the SNS.

- *PSNS*—housekeeping chores of the body, and stimulation of these nerves slows heart rate, increases gastric secretions, empties bladder and bowel, focuses eye for near vision, constricts pupil, and contracts bronchial smooth muscle.
- *SNS*—three main functions: regulates the cardiovascular system, regulates body temperature, and implements the fight-or-flight response.
- The PNS uses three neurotransmitters to exert its actions: ACh (released by all preganglionic neurons of the PSNS and SNS, all postganglionic neurons of the PSNS, all motor neurons of the skeletal muscles, and most postganglionic neurons of the SNS that supply the sweat glands), norepinephrine (released by almost all postganglionic neurons of SNS with the exception of postganglionic neurons that supply sweat glands), and epinephrine (released by adrenal medulla).
- Two basic categories of PNS receptors and their subtypes (receptor subtypes make it possible for drugs to act selectively):
  - Cholinergic-mediated responses to ACh subtypes include the following:
    - Nicotinic$_N$ activation stimulates parasympathetic and sympathetic postganglionic nerves and causes release of epinephrine from adrenal medulla.
    - Nicotinic$_M$ activation causes contraction of skeletal muscle.
    - Muscarinic activation causes focus of lens for near vision, miosis, decreased heart rate, constriction of bronchi, promotion of secretions, increase in bladder pressure, urination, salivation, increased gastric secretions, increased intestinal tone and motility, sweating, erection, and vasodilation.
  - Adrenergic-mediated responses to epinephrine and norepinephrine subtypes include the following:
    - Alpha$_1$ activation by epinephrine, norepinephrine, or dopamine causes mydriasis, vasoconstriction, ejaculation, and prostate contraction.
    - Alpha$_2$ activation by epinephrine or norepinephrine causes *inhibition* of subsequent neurotransmitter release.
    - Beta$_1$ activation by epinephrine, norepinephrine, or dopamine causes increased heart rate, force of contraction, atrioventricular conduction, and increased renin release from the kidney.

- Beta$_2$ activation (only by epinephrine) causes vasodilation, bronchial dilation, uterine relaxation, glycogenolysis, and enhanced contraction of skeletal muscle.
- Dopamine (responds only to dopamine) activation causes dilation of kidney vasculature.

SOMATIC NERVOUS SYSTEM

- *Elements:* motor neurons arising from the spinal cord and brain and the neuromuscular junction.
- *Neuromuscular junction:* formed by the terminal of the motor neuron and the motor end plates (special sites on the muscle's membrane). Motor neurons release neurotransmitter ACh to the junction; subsequently, ACh activates its receptor (nicotinic$_M$ receptor) on the motor end plates and causes muscle contraction.
- *Drugs that target the neuromuscular junction:* cholinesterase inhibitors, nondepolarizing neuromuscular blockers, and depolarizing neuromuscular blockers.

Basal Ganglia (or Basal Nuclei)
It is a group of nuclei situated at the base of the forebrain and strongly connected to the cerebral cortex, thalamus, and other areas.

- *Elements:* striatum, pallidum, substantia nigra, and subthalamic nucleus.
- *Function:* they are associated with motor control and learning functions. The substantia nigra provides dopaminergic input to the striatum. The basal ganglia play a central role in a number of neurological conditions, including several movement disorders. The most notable are Parkinson's disease, which involves degeneration of the dopamine-producing cells in the substantia nigra, and Huntington's disease, which primarily involves damage to the striatum.
- Drugs are used for Parkinson's disease to increase the dopamine level at the striatum.

Hippocampus
The hippocampus belongs to the limbic system that forms the inner border of the cortex.

- *Function*: emotion, behavior, and long-term memory. Beta-amyloid, neuritic plaques and neurofibrillary tangles, and tau in the hippocampus and cerebral cortex are the prominent features of Alzheimer's disease (AD). Another characteristic of AD is that the level of ACh, an important neurotransmitter in the hippocampus and cerebral cortex, is significantly below normal.
- Drugs used to treat AD include cholinesterase inhibitors and N-methyl-D-aspartate (NMDA) receptor antagonist.

Hypothalamus
The hypothalamus is located below the thalamus and above the brainstem.

- The *pituitary gland* is located below the third ventricle of the brain and the hypothalamus, composed of anterior pituitary (adenohypophysis) and posterior pituitary (neurohypophysis). The pituitary stalk connects the hypothalamus to the pituitary gland.

▥ *Function:* The hypothalamus controls the anterior pituitary by hypothalamic-releasing factors, while it synthesizes oxytocin and antidiuretic hormone and projects its neuronal axon to the posterior pituitary. The hypothalamus controls body temperature, hunger, thirst, fatigue, and circadian cycles.

▥ Drugs that target the pituitary stimulate or inhibit the synthesis and release of hormones from the anterior pituitary gland. In addition, some drugs act as agonists or antagonists of pituitary gland hormone receptors.

Both in the PNS and CNS, neurons regulate physiological processes in the same way through two steps:

▥ *Axonal conduction*—an action potential is sent down the axon of a neuron.
  ▥ Drugs that influence axonal conduction are not selective, so they stop transmission in the axon of any neuron they reach.
  ▥ The only group of drugs that affects axonal conduction are local anesthetics.

▥ *Synaptic transmission*—a transmitter is released from the neuron carrying information across a synapse, or gap, to a postsynaptic cell receptor causing a change in that cell.
  ▥ Most drugs work by affecting synaptic transmission.
  ▥ Drugs that work by affecting synaptic transmission are very selective due to different types of transmitters and receptor sites.
  ▥ To work, drugs must have either a direct or an indirect effect on target cell receptors.

Synaptic transmission includes five steps:

▥ *Transmitter synthesis*—synthesis of the transmitter in the neuron
  ▥ Drugs work here by
    ◦ Increasing the amount of transmitter synthesized
    ◦ Decreasing the amount of transmitter synthesized
    ◦ Synthesizing a "super" transmitter that is more potent than the naturally occurring transmitter

▥ *Transmitter storage*—the transmitter is stored in vesicles in the axon terminal for later use.
  ▥ Drugs work here by
    ◦ Reducing the amount of transmitter stored

▥ *Transmitter release*—axonal conduction causes release of the transmitter into the synapse between the neuron and the target cell.
  ▥ Drugs work here by
    ◦ Increasing the amount of transmitter released
    ◦ Decreasing the amount of transmitter released

▥ *Receptor binding*—the transmitter binds to receptor sites on the postsynaptic, or target, cell causing a change in that cell.
  ▥ Drugs work here by
    ◦ Mimicking the natural transmitter and binding to additional target cell receptor sites to increase the effects on a target cell (agonist)
    ◦ Binding to target cell receptor sites to block the naturally occurring transmitter from binding to the target cell and decreasing the effect that the naturally occurring transmitter has on the target cell (antagonist)
    ◦ Binding to the same target cell receptor sites together with the naturally occurring transmitter to increase the target cell's response to the transmitter

■ *Termination of transmission*—the transmitter is depleted by reuptake, enzymatic degradation, or diffusion.
  ■ Drugs work here by
    ● Stopping the reuptake of the transmitter, allowing more transmitter to be available to bind to the target cell receptor sites
    ● Stopping the enzymatic degradation of the transmitter, allowing more transmitter to be available to bind to the target cell receptor sites

Neurotransmitters

Neurotransmitters are chemicals that account for the transmission of signals from one neuron to the next across a synapse. They are also found at the axon endings of motor neurons, where they stimulate the muscle fibers to contract.

■ Chemical substances stored in the terminal end of a neuron, released when the storing neuron "fires"; have the potential to influence the activity of a receiving cell (either increasing or decreasing likelihood of action).
■ Present in the synaptic terminal.
■ Action may be blocked by pharmacological agents.
■ Examples of CNS neurotransmitters include the following:
  ■ *ACh*—widely distributed throughout the CNS and the primary transmitter at the neuromuscular junction
  ■ *Dopamine*—involved in a wide variety of behaviors and emotions associated with parkinsonism and, perhaps, schizophrenia
  ■ *Serotonin*—involved in sleep regulation, dreaming, mood, eating, pain, and aggression and associated with depression (i.e., selective serotonin reuptake inhibitor)
  ■ *Glutamate*—an excitatory transmitter, associated in memory, arousal, and pain
  ■ *GABA*—widely distributed, largely an inhibitory transmitter

Neuropharmacology

Neuropharmacology is the study of drugs that alter processes regulated by the nervous system. The nervous system regulates almost all bodily processes and, therefore, almost all bodily processes can be influenced by drugs that alter neuron regulation. By blocking (antagonist) or mimicking (agonist) neuron regulation, neuropharmacological drugs can modify skeletal muscle contraction, cardiac output, vascular tone, respiration, gastrointestinal function, uterine motility, glandular secretion, and functions of the CNS, such as pain perception, ideation, and mood.

■ Neurons regulate physiological processes through a two-step process involving axonal conduction and synaptic transmission.
  ■ *Axonal conduction*—process of conducting an action potential down the axon of the neuron.
    ● Drugs (local anesthetics) that alter this conduction are not very selective, because the process of axonal conduction is almost the same in all neurons; therefore, a drug that alters conduction will alter conduction in all cells.

NEUROTRANSMITTER	FOCUSED AREAS

ACh	Neuromuscular junction, autonomic ganglia, parasympathetic neurons, motor nuclei of cranial nerves, caudate nucleus and putamen, basal nucleus of Meynert, portions of the limbic system
	Receptor: N, *action:* excitatory
	Receptor: M, *action:* excitatory or inhibitory
	Action: CNS—memory, sensory processing, motor coordination
	■ Muscarinic—found at postganglionic parasympathetic endings (heart, smooth muscle, glands); five subtypes of muscarinic receptors:
	  M_1 receptors found in ganglia and secretory glands
	  M_2 receptors predominate in myocardium and in smooth muscle
	  M_3 and M_4 receptors found in smooth muscle and secretory glands
	  M_5 receptors have been identified in the CNS along with the other four types
	■ Nicotinic receptors found in ganglia and at neuromuscular junction. Identified as:
	  N_M receptors found at the neuromuscular junction in skeletal muscle
	  N_G receptors found in autonomic ganglia, adrenal medulla, and CNS

Norepinephrine	SNS, locus coeruleus, lateral tegmentum *Action:* CNS—positive mood and reward, orienting and alerting responses, basic instincts (sex, eating, thirst) *C-receptors:* ■ $Alpha_1$ (postsynaptic) causes contraction of blood vessels, sphincters, radial muscle of eye ■ $Alpha_2$ (presynaptic): negative feedback loop inhibiting subsequent release of neurotransmitter; up regulation and downregulation occur in response to decreased or increased activation of receptors; present at extrasynaptic sites in blood vessels and the CNS; stimulation in the brain stem decreases sympathetic outflow; stimulation in the pancreas inhibits insulin release ■ $Beta_1$ (predominately cardiac) stimulation increases heart rate or strength of contraction ■ $Beta_2$ (predominately noncardiac) found on smooth muscle (bronchi; large blood vessels) causes relaxation and promotes insulin release, liver and muscle gluconeogenesis and glycogenolysis, and lipolysis in fat cells. ■ $Beta_3$ receptors are expressed in visceral adipocytes
Dopamine	Hypothalamus, midbrain nigrostriatal system *Receptors:* D1 and D2, action: inhibitory ■ $Dopamine_1$ (postsynaptic) receptors responsible for vasodilation in splanchnic and renal circulations; stimulation in chemoreceptor trigger zone causes nausea and vomiting. ■ $Dopamine_2$ (presynaptic) receptors initiate a negative feedback loop; Five forms are found in the brain. *Action:* Regulation of hormonal balance, voluntary movement, reward
Serotonin (5-HT)	Parasympathetic neurons in gut, pineal gland, nucleus raphe magnus of pons *Action:* CNS—sleep and emotional arousal, impulse control, cognition, pain processing, dreaming, homeostatic processes

(continued)

NEUROTRANSMITTER	FOCUSED AREAS
GABA	Cerebellum, hippocampus, cerebral cortex, striatonigral system *Receptor:* GABAa, *action:* inhibitory (postsynaptic) *Receptor:* GABAb, *action:* inhibitory (presynaptic)
Glycine	Spinal cord *Action:* inhibitory
Glutamic acid	Spinal cord, brainstem, cerebellum, hippocampus, cerebral cortex

ACh, acetylcholine; CNS, central nervous system; SNS, sympathetic nervous system; 5-HT, serotonin; GABA, gamma-aminobutyric acid.

- *Synaptic transmission*—process of carrying information across the synapse between the neuron and the postsynaptic cell and requires release of neurotransmitters and binding of these transmitters to receptors on the postsynaptic cell.
  - Most drugs act by altering this synaptic transmission because they are able to produce more selective effects by altering the following:
    – Transmitter synthesis and receptor activation can be increased; transmitter synthesis and receptor activation can be decreased; or transmitters that are more effective than the natural transmitter, which will cause receptor activation to increase, can be synthesized.
    – Transmitter storage can cause receptor activation to decrease by decreasing the amount of transmitter available.
    – Transmitter release can promote release and increase receptor activation or can inhibit release and reduce receptor activation.
    – Termination of transmitter action blocks transmitter reuptake or inhibition of transmitter degradation; both these actions will increase concentration of transmitter and cause receptor activation to increase.
  - In order for a drug to exert its effect, it must be able to directly or indirectly influence the receptor activity on the target cell. Drugs act on receptors by
    – Binding to them and causing activation (agonist)
    – Binding to them and blocking their activation by other agents (antagonists)
    – Binding to their components and indirectly enhancing their activation by the natural transmitter

CLINICAL NEUROANATOMY: RATIONALE FOR UNDERSTANDING

- Understanding neuroanatomy helps guide pharmacological approaches to treatment. A key goal of pharmacotherapy is to modify a patient's pathogenic nervous system activity.
  - The nervous system (CNS and PNS) regulates our bodily processes. Therefore, our body processes can be affected by the drugs that regulate neuronal activity. Understanding clinical neuroanatomy helps in the development of neuropharmacological drugs and treatment selection to modify a patient's pathogenic nervous system activity.

CLINICAL NEUROANATOMY: ASSOCIATION WITH DRUG ACTION

- Drug enters the body through various *routes of administration*—injection, oral, sublingual, inhalation, and transdermal
- What the body does to the drug (*pharmacokinetics*)
  - *Absorption* (transfer of drug from the site of application to the blood stream)
    - Affected by the rate of dissolution, surface area, blood flow, lipid solubility, and pH partitioning
    - Bioavailability (the fraction of unchanged drug that reaches site of action) affected by anything that alters absorption, distribution, or metabolism
  - *Distribution* (drug leaves blood stream → interstitial space of tissues → target cells responsible for therapeutic and adverse effects)
    - Determined by the blood flow to tissues, ability to exit the vascular system (capillary beds, blood–brain barrier, placental drug transfer, and protein binding), and ability to enter cells (lipid solubility and presence of transport system)
  - *Metabolism* (enzymatic alteration of drug structure or "bagging the trash," usually by liver)
    - Hepatic drug-metabolizing enzymes
  - *Excretion* (removal of drugs from body)
- What the drug does to the body (*pharmacodynamics*)
  - Dose–response relationship
    - Size of administered dose
    - Intensity of the response produced
  - *Drug–receptor interactions* (drugs interact with chemical)
    - *Receptor* (chemicals in the body to which the drug binds to produce effects)
      - Regulated by endogenous compounds or macromolecules (body's own receptors for hormones, neurotransmitters, and other regulatory molecules
      - Can be turned on or off
      - Turned on by interaction with other molecules
      - When the drug binds to receptors, it either mimics (*agonists*) or blocks (*antagonists*) the action of endogenous regulatory molecules such as neurotransmitters (supplied to receptors by neurons of the nervous system).
      - There are receptors for each neurotransmitter, each hormone, and all other regulatory molecules.
      - Drugs are selective to specific receptors (a receptor is analogous to a lock and a drug is analogous to a key for that lock), so only drugs with proper size, shape, and properties can bind to a receptor.

BIBLIOGRAPHY

Carter, R. (1999). *Mapping the mind*. Berkley, CA: University of California Press.

Haines, D. E. (1995). *Neuroanatomy: An atlas of structures, systems, sections, and systems* (4th ed.). Philadelphia, PA: Williams & Wilkins.

Kasschau, R. A. (2003). *Understanding psychology*. New York, NY: Glencoe McGraw-Hill.

Myers, D. G. (2004). *Psychology* (7th ed.). New York, NY: Worth Publishers.

Tortora, G. J., & Grabowski, S. R. (2003). *Principles of anatomy and physiology* (10th ed.). New York, NY: John Wiley and Sons Inc.

The Relationship of Psychopharmacology to Neurotransmitters, Receptors, Signal Transduction, and Second Messengers

The past 20 years have afforded scientists with a greater understanding of the brain. Extreme changes in psychopharmacology have produced newer medicines with fewer side effects and greater benefits than ever before. These changes translate into improved wellness for patients with mental health disorders.

This chapter presents the following:

- A basic outline of the currently understood processes by which the brain communicates
- Information to support an improved understanding of the inner brain mechanisms from synaptic and cellular viewpoints in regard to psychopharmacology
- The signaling pathways associated with the six neurotransmitters most commonly altered in modern psychopharmacological therapy
- A strong scientific background on which to base psychopharmacological prescribing practices

NEUROTRANSMITTERS

These are the molecules that mediate intracellular signaling of the brain.

- Neurotransmitters are chemicals that communicate their messages to the interior of the neurons
  - Through their release from the presynaptic terminal
  - By diffusing across the synaptic cleft
  - To further bind to receptors in the postsynaptic membrane

Table 5.1 Major Neurotransmitters in the Central Nervous System

NEUROTRANSMITTER	EFFECTS
Acetylcholine (ACh)	Cognition, learning, memory, alertness, muscle contraction
Dopamine	Pleasure, pain, movement control, emotional response
Gamma-aminobutyric acid	Psychomotor agitation/retardation, stress, anxiety
Glutamate	Memory, energy
Norepinephrine	Arousal, dreaming, depressed mood, suicide, apathy, psychomotor agitation/retardation, constricts blood vessels, increases heart rate and blood pressure, affects attention and the sleep—wake cycle
Serotonin	Mood control, temperature regulation, impulsiveness, aggression, cognitive problems, depressed mood, suicide, apathy, psychomotor agitation/retardation

■ There are more than several dozen known or suspected neurotransmitters in the brain.

■ Theoretically, there may be several hundred neurotransmitters based on the amount of genetic materials in the neurons.

■ Neurotransmitters are endogenous molecules; examples include various peptides and hormones (Table 5.1).

■ Psychoactive drugs act by increasing, decreasing, or otherwise modulating the actions of neurotransmitters at their receptor sites.

■ *Ligand* is a generic term referring to either endogenous or exogenous receptor binding partner proteins to which neurotransmitters bind, resulting in changes to downstream cellular processes.

■ The following six neurotransmitter systems are the major targets for psychotropic drugs:

   ■ **Serotonergic neurons** (neurotransmitter = serotonin) originating primarily in the raphe nuclei of the reticular formation extending from the medulla to the midbrain

   ■ **Noradrenergic neurons** (neurotransmitter = norepinephrine) originating in the locus coeruleus

   ■ **Dopaminergic neurons** (neurotransmitter = dopamine) originating primarily in the ventral tegmental area

   ■ **Muscarinic cholinergic neurons** (neurotransmitter = acetylcholine) one of the principal neurotransmitters in the autonomic nervous system

   ■ **Glutamatergic neurons** (neurotransmitter = glutamate) an amino acid transmitter synthesized by the brain from glucose and other nutrients for motor activity

   ■ **GABAergic neurons** (neurotransmitter = gamma-aminobutyric acid [GABA]) an inhibitory amino acid neurotransmitter, which is synthesized from glutamate in the brain and decreases activity in nerve cells

■ These six neurotransmitters are relatively low-molecular-weight amines or amino acids.

■ Multiple neurons that release more than one neurotransmitter may converge at a single synapse.

■ Cotransmission involves a monoamine coupled with a neuropeptide.

This natural combination of multiple signaling molecules at the synapse is the basis for the modern treatment rationale of prescribing drugs affecting multiple neuronal signaling pathways.

SIX NEUROTRANSMITTERS MOST COMMONLY AFFECTED BY PSYCHOPHARMACOLOGY TREATMENT REGIMENS*

Communication within the brain happens in three ways: *anterograde, retrograde,* or *nonsynaptic.* Chemical neurotransmission is the foundation of psychopharmacology.

- **Anterograde neurotransmission:**
  - Most predominant means of excitation-coupling and synapses.
  - Occurs in one direction (i.e., presynaptic to postsynaptic), from the cell body, down the axon, to the synaptic cleft.
  - Involves stimulation of a presynaptic neuron causing electrical impulses to be sent to its axon terminal (may be regarded as "classic" neurotransmission).
  - Electrical impulses are converted into chemical messengers, known as neurotransmitters.
  - Chemical messengers (neurotransmitters) are released to stimulate the receptors of the postsynaptic neuron.
  - Communication *within* a neuron is mediated by electrical conduction of an action potential from the cell body down the axon of the neuron where it ends at the synaptic cleft.
  - Communication *between* neurons is chemical and mediated by one of the several neurotransmitters described earlier.
  - Excitation–secretion coupling is the process by which an electrochemical signal in the first (i.e., presynaptic) neuron is converted from a chemical impulse into the release of a chemical signal at the synapse.
  - Electrical impulses result from the opening of *ion channels* in the neuronal cell membrane along the axon, causing a change in net charge of the neuron. The difference in charge between the inside of the cell and the outside of the cell is referred to as an *action potential.*
    - Voltage-sensitive sodium channels
    - Voltage-sensitive potassium channels
  - All this happens very quickly once the electrical impulse enters the presynaptic neuron.
  - Occurs predominately in one direction (from the cell body, down the axon, to the synaptic cleft).
- **Retrograde neurotransmission:**
  - Postsynaptic neurons can talk back directly and indirectly.
    - Indirectly through a long neuronal feedback loop
    - Directly through retrograde neurotransmission from postsynaptic to presynaptic
  - Examples of retrograde neurotransmitters synthesized in the postsynaptic neuron, released, and diffused into the presynaptic neuron are
    - Endocannabinoids (endogenous compounds similar to marijuana, also known as cannabis)
    - Nitric oxide

---

*Currently prescribed psychotropic medications are developed to target these neurotransmitter signaling pathways.

▪ **Nonsynaptic neurotransmission:**
  ▫ No neurotransmission across a synaptic cleft
  ▫ Chemical messengers sent by one neuron diffuse to compatible receptor sites distant to the synapse

RECEPTORS

These are proteins to which neurotransmitters bind, resulting in changes to downstream cellular processes.

▪ Found within plasma membranes and cytoplasm of a cell
▪ Affected by psychoactive drugs
▪ Located on cell membranes of neurons

Receptors Specific to Psychopharmacology
Psychotropic medications are developed to target these various receptor sites.

▪ *Serotonin:* binds to 5-HT1A, 5-HT1B, 5-HT1D, 5-HT1E, 5-HT1F, 5-HT2, 5-HT2A, 5-HT2B, 5-HT2C, 5-HT3, 5-HT4, and 5-HT5A receptors (Table 5.2)
▪ *Norepinephrine:* binds to $alpha_1$ and $alpha_2$, $beta_1$, $beta_2$, and $beta_3$ receptors (Table 5.3)
▪ *Dopamine:* binds to D1, D2, D3, D4, and D5 receptors (Table 5.4)
▪ *Acetylcholine:* binds to nicotinic (N) and muscarinic (M) receptors (Table 5.5)

Table 5.2   Serotonin

RECEPTOR TYPE	DISTRIBUTION	EFFECTS
5-HT1, 5-HT1A, 5-HT1B, 5-HT1D, 5-HT1E, 5-HT1F	Brain, blood vessels, intestinal nerves	*Inhibitory:* neuronal inhibition, cerebral vasoconstriction *Behavioral effects:* addiction, aggression, anxiety, appetite, impulsivity, learning, memory, mood, sexual behavior, sleep
5-HT2, 5-HT2A, 5-HT2B, 5-HT2C	Brain, blood vessels, heart, lungs, smooth muscle control, GI system, blood vessels, platelets	*Excitatory:* neuronal excitation, vasoconstriction *Behavioral effects:* addiction, anxiety, appetite, mood, sexual behavior, sleep
5-HT3	Limbic system, CNS, PNS, GI system	*Excitatory:* nausea *Behavioral effects:* addiction, anxiety, learning, memory
5-HT4	CNS, smooth muscle, GI system	*Excitatory:* neuronal excitation, GI *Behavioral effects:* anxiety, appetite, learning, memory, mood
5-HT5, 5-HT5A, 5-HT6, 5-HT7	Brain	*Inhibitory:* may be linked to BDNF *Behavioral effects:* sleep
5-HT6	CNS	*Excitatory:* may be linked to BDNF *Behavioral effects:* anxiety, cognition, learning, memory, mood
5-HT7	CNS, blood vessels GI system	*Excitatory:* may be linked to BDNF *Behavioral effects:* anxiety, memory, sleep, mood

BDNF, brain-derived neurotrophic factor; CNS, central nervous system; GI, gastrointestinal; PNS, peripheral nervous system.

Table 5.3   Norepinephrine

RECEPTOR TYPE	DISTRIBUTION	EFFECTS
Alpha$_1$	Brain, heart, smooth muscle	*Excitatory:* vasoconstriction, smooth muscle contraction
Alpha$_2$	Presynaptic neurons in brain, pancreas, smooth muscle	*Inhibitory:* vasoconstriction, gastrointestinal relaxation presynaptically
Beta$_1$	Heart, brain	*Excitatory:* increased heart rate
Beta$_2$	Lungs, brain, skeletal muscle	*Excitatory:* bronchial relaxation, vasodilation, smooth muscle relaxation
Beta$_3$	Adipose tissue	*Excitatory:* stimulation of effector cells

Table 5.4   Dopamine

RECEPTOR TYPE	DISTRIBUTION	EFFECTS
D1	Brain, smooth muscle	*Excitatory:* possible role in schizophrenia and Parkinson's
D2	Brain, cardiovascular system, presynaptic nerve terminals	*Inhibitory:* possible role in schizophrenia
D3	Brain, cardiovascular system, presynaptic nerve terminals	*Inhibitory:* possible role in schizophrenia
D4	Brain, cardiovascular system, presynaptic nerve terminals	*Inhibitory:* possible role in schizophrenia
D5	Brain, smooth muscle	*Excitatory:* possible role in schizophrenia and Parkinson's

Table 5.5   Acetylcholine

RECEPTOR TYPE	DISTRIBUTION	EFFECTS
M1	Ganglia, secretory glands	*Excitatory:* CNS excitation, gastric acid secretion
M2	Heart, nerves, smooth muscle	*Inhibitory:* cardiac inhibition, neural inhibition
M3	Glands, smooth muscle, endothelium, secretory glands	*Excitatory:* smooth muscle contraction, vasodilation
M4	CNS, PNS, smooth muscle, secretory glands	Inhibitory
M5	CNS	Inhibitory
N$_M$	Skeletal muscle, neuromuscular junction	*Excitatory:* neuromuscular transmission
N$_N$	Postganglionic cell body dendrites	*Excitatory:* ganglionic transmission

CNS, central nervous system; PNS, peripheral nervous system.

Table 5.6   GABA

RECEPTOR TYPE	DISTRIBUTION	EFFECTS
GABA$_A$	Central nervous system	Inhibitory
GABA$_B$	Autonomic nervous system	Excitatory

GABA, gamma-aminobutyric acid.

Table 5.7   Glutamate

RECEPTOR TYPE	DISTRIBUTION	EFFECTS
AMPA	CNS	Excitatory
Kainate	CNS	Excitatory
NMDA	CNS	Excitatory

AMPA, α-amino-3-hydroxy-5-methyl-4-isoxazolepropionic acid receptor; CNS, central nervous system; NMDA, N-methyl-D-aspartate receptor.

■ *GABA* binds to GABA$_A$ and GABA$_B$ receptors (Table 5.6)
■ *Glutamate* binds to AMPA, kainate, and NMDA receptors (Table 5.7)

SIGNAL TRANSDUCTION

Signal transduction is the movement of signals from the outside of a cell to the inside.

■ Signal → receptor → change in cell function
■ Plays a very specific role through messaging and activation of an inactive molecule
  ■ Starts a reaction that cascades through chemical neurotransmission via numerous molecules
    ● Long-term effects of late gene products and many more messages
    ● Can occur over the time course of minutes, hours, days, or weeks
    ● Effects may be temporary or permanent
■ Signal transduction translates into the following diverse biological responses:
  ■ Gene expression
  ■ Synaptogenesis

SECOND MESSENGERS

Second messengers are synthesized and activated by enzymes, and help mediate intracellular signaling in response to a ligand binding to its receptor.

■ Relay and amplify signals received by receptors such as cyclic adenosine monophosphate (cAMP), inositol trisphosphate (IP$_3$), used for signal transduction in biological cells and Ca^{2+}.

ENDOGENOUS NEUROTRANSMITTERS

■ See Table 5.8.

Table 5.8   Endogenous Neurotransmitters

NEUROTRANSMITTER	RECEPTOR	SIGNAL TRANSDUCTION	SECOND MESSENGER
Acetylcholine	Muscarinic	G-protein linked	cAMP or IP_3
	Nicotinic	Ion channel linked	Calcium
Dopamine	D1, D2, D3, D4, D5	G-protein linked	cAMP or IP_3
	$alpha_1$, $beta_2$	G-protein linked	cAMP or IP_3
GABA	$GABA_A$	Ion channel linked and ligand-gated ion channels	Calcium
	$GABA_B$	G-protein linked	cAMP or IP_3
Glutamate	AMPA, Kainate, and NMDA	Ion channel linked	Calcium
	Metabotropic	G-protein linked	cAMP or IP_3
Norepinephrine	$alpha_1$, $alpha_2$	G-protein linked	cAMP or IP_3
	$beta_1$	G-protein linked	cAMP or IP_3
Epinephrine	$alpha_1$, $alpha_2$	G-protein linked	cAMP or IP_3
	$beta_1$, $beta_2$	G-protein linked	cAMP or IP_3
Serotonin	5-HT1A, 5-HT1B, 5-HT1D, 5-HT1E, 5-HT1F	G-protein linked	cAMP or IP_3
	5-HT2, 5-HT2A, 5-HT2B, 5-HT2C	G-protein linked	cAMP or IP_3
	5-HT3	Ion channel linked	Calcium
	5-HT4	G-protein linked	cAMP or IP_3
	5-HT5A	G-protein linked	cAMP or IP_3

Principles of Pharmacokinetics and Pharmacodynamics

Pharmacokinetics and pharmacodynamics comprise the collective interactions between a drug and a patient.

■ *Pharmacokinetics* refers to the effects of the patient on the drug. The four primary pharmacokinetic processes are absorption, distribution, metabolism, and excretion.
■ *Pharmacodynamics* refers to the effects of the drug on the patient.

Pharmacokinetic Principles

■ The four pharmacokinetic processes of absorption, distribution, metabolism, and excretion describe the effects the patient's organ systems have on the drug from the time it enters until the time it leaves the body.
■ The extent to which a psychoactive drug will undergo each process is dependent on drug-specific and patient-specific variables.
  ■ Examples of drug-specific variables include the *chemical structure* and *route of administration*.
  ■ Examples of patient-specific variables include any *comorbidities*, overall *health*, the patient's *age*, and *concurrent pharmacotherapy*.

ABSORPTION

■ *Absorption* refers to the movement of a drug from its site of administration into the circulatory system.
■ Drug absorption is affected by the chemical properties of the drug as well as the route of drug administration.
  ■ Movement of drugs into the circulatory system most commonly requires drugs to pass across and through cellular compartments.
  ■ This movement occurs by active transport, passive diffusion, or direct penetration through the cell membranes.
  ■ Chemical properties of the drug, drug concentration, presence of drug-transporter molecules, and pH affect intercellular drug movement.
  ■ The dosage requirements for a drug may be noticeably different based on its route of administration.

■ Dosing differences are often necessary to ensure that *bioequivalence* is achieved when two different routes of administration of the same drug are employed.

■ Absorption following *oral administration*

■ Drugs enter the gastrointestinal (GI) tract and are absorbed through the stomach or small intestine. They travel via the portal vein first to the liver and then through the heart and into general circulation.

■ Oral administration results in more variable drug absorption and drug bioavailability than other administration routes.

■ *First-pass metabolism* (also known as the *first-pass effect*) refers to the inactivation of an orally administered drug by liver enzymes immediately following absorption from the GI tract and prior to the drug reaching general circulation. *Enterohepatic recirculation* refers to the cyclical movement of orally administered drugs from the GI tract to the liver, then packaged into bile and secreted into the small intestine, and then reabsorbed back into the liver.

■ Drug dissolution may be protracted up to approximately 8 hours by formulating sustained-release, extended-release, and controlled-release preparations. Sustained-release formulations (e.g., controlled-release paroxetine [*Paxil CR*]) may minimize GI distress, decrease the number of daily dosages, and provide more uniform drug absorption.

○ Many controlled release (CR) formulations are available only as brand name medications at a substantially increased price over standard-release formulations. CR formulations cannot be crushed or chewed. Only formulations that are scored can be split.

■ Drugs that are inactivated by gastric acid or that cause gastric irritation may be prepared with an *enteric coating*, which permits drug absorption to be delayed until the drug passes through the stomach and enters the intestine. Care should be exercised not to coadminister antacids with enteric-coated products, or the coating will dissolve in the higher pH.

■ Patients with GI distress may have impaired oral absorption.

Absorption following *transdermal administration*

■ Suitable formulation and route of administration for drugs able to permeate intact skin.

■ Toxic effects may occur during transdermal absorption if drugs are highly lipid soluble, or when applied to irritated or damaged skin, or if transdermal application is a patch and previous patch is not removed prior to next dose (or if patch is cut or divided prior to topical application). Exposure to heat can increase drug absorption and thus should be avoided (use of heating blankets, saunas, etc.).

■ Controlled-release transdermal formulations (e.g., nicotine patches) are becoming increasingly available for various medications.

■ Absorption following *intramuscular (IM) administration* and *subcutaneous (SC) administration*

■ Many similarities exist between IM and SC injections. Both provide relatively rapid absorption of aqueous solutions and relatively slow absorption of lipophilic solutions.

■ The rate of absorption and drug bioavailability following an IM or SC injection are dependent on the lipophilicity of the drug, fat content, and blood flow at the injection site.

■ Injections may provide even, prolonged absorption. A drug may be prepared in a depot formulation that is gradually absorbed over time. Coadministration of a vasoconstricting medication may prolong absorption.

■ SC injections may result in pain if irritant is present.

▪ Administration via *intravenous (IV) injection*
  ▪ Absorption is essentially instantaneous, as the drug is delivered directly into the circulatory system.
  ▪ It is useful when rapid drug effect is needed and allows for administration of poorly lipid-soluble drugs and irritants.
  ▪ Continued and repeated IV administration requires accessibility to patent veins.
▪ Absorption may involve passive diffusion or active transport.
  ▪ *Passive diffusion* is the movement of a drug across a cell membrane down its concentration gradient.
  ▪ Drugs that are smaller, less protein bound, and more lipophilic can be more readily absorbed via passive diffusion. Most psychotherapeutic drugs are absorbed via passive diffusion.
  ▪ *Active transport* is the facilitated movement of a drug across a cell membrane.
  ▪ Drugs unable to be absorbed via passive diffusion—either because of their chemical properties or the drug concentration gradient—require active transport in order to be absorbed.
  ▪ Active transport mechanisms include membrane-spanning proteins that facilitate the movement of drugs across cell membranes and into the circulatory system. Active transport of drugs is limited to those medications structurally related to endogenous compounds for which active transport mechanisms already exist (e.g., ions, amino acids, and simple carbohydrates).
▪ *Ion trapping* occurs when a drug classified as a weak acid transfers from a body compartment that is more acidic to one that is more alkaline (e.g., from the stomach to the plasma) or, conversely, when a weak base transfers from a more alkaline to a more basic compartment.
▪ Absorption-related *drug–drug* or *food–drug interactions* should be closely monitored. Antacids, for example, may impair the absorption of orally coadministered psychiatric drugs, leading to subtherapeutic concentrations of the coadministered drug.

DISTRIBUTION

▪ *Distribution* refers to the movement of a drug from the circulatory system to its site(s) of action. Drugs are distributed to sites in the body responsible for producing both therapeutic effects and adverse effects.
▪ The variables affecting drug distribution—and delivery of the drug to its site of action—include blood flow to the target tissue, lipid solubility, and plasma protein binding.
  ▪ Tissues of the body with *high blood flow* (e.g., the brain and muscle) will receive higher concentrations of a drug faster than tissues with low blood flow (e.g., adipose tissue).
  ▪ Drugs with *high lipid solubility* (e.g., nonpolar molecules) will more readily cross cell membranes, including the blood–brain barrier and placenta. These drugs will more readily localize in tissues with high lipid content (e.g., brain and adipose tissue).
  ▪ Drugs with a *low level of plasma protein binding* (e.g., lithium) have a less encumbered movement and have generally increased bioavailability than drugs with a high level of plasma protein binding (e.g., valproic acid). Table 6.1 identifies psychiatric drugs with high and low plasma protein binding.

Table 6.1   Relative Plasma Protein Binding

HIGH PROTEIN-BINDING PSYCHIATRIC DRUGS	LOW PROTEIN-BINDING PSYCHIATRIC DRUGS
Aripiprazole (>99%)	Lithium (0%)
Ziprasidone (>99%)	Gabapentin (3%)
Atomoxetine (99%)	Levetiracetam (10%)
Diazepam (99%)	Topiramate (15%)
Sertraline (98%)	Methylphenidate (15%)
Buspirone (95%)	Clonidine (20%)
Valproic acid (93%)	Venlafaxine (28%)

- The most abundant plasma protein is *albumin,* and the terms *plasma protein binding* and *albumin binding* are often used interchangeably.
- The biochemical properties that make a drug more readily absorbed into the circulatory system (e.g., high lipid solubility and low molecular weight) also make the drug more readily distributed throughout the body (Gupta, Hammarlund-Udenaes, Chatelain, Massingham, & Jonsson, 2006).
- The total accumulation of lipid-soluble drugs in *adipose tissue* is dependent on the fat content of an individual. Adipose tissue may serve as a drug reservoir, which may result in redistribution during instances of profound weight loss. This increase in adipose tissue is significant for the elderly—loss of muscle and increase in fat can put them at heightened risk.
- The *blood–brain barrier* results from brain capillary endothelial cells possessing continuous tight junctions, which impede drug movement from the circulatory system into the central nervous system (CNS). Drugs passing into the CNS require specific transporter proteins or high drug lipophilicity.
- Variables affecting *in utero drug distribution*
  - For women who are pregnant, special considerations should be given to the potential for maternal–fetal drug transfer via the *placenta.*
  - Similar properties dictate passive diffusion across the placenta as the blood–brain barrier. Often drugs are able to cross the placenta first.
  - Drugs that have a high degree of lipid solubility, low molecular weight, and low serum protein binding cross the placenta more readily than drugs with a low degree of lipid solubility, high molecular weight, and high serum protein binding.
  - Because fetal plasma is slightly more acidic than maternal plasma, ion trapping of alkaline drugs may result in the increased accumulation of drug in the placenta.
- Patients suffering from malnutrition or acute or chronic inflammatory responses may present with *hypoalbuminemia.* The decrease in serum protein caused by hypoalbuminemia may result in greater drug bioavailability, particularly for drugs that are highly protein bound, leading to potentially toxic effects.
- Distribution-related drug–drug or food–drug interactions should be closely monitored. Warfarin, for example, may compete for albumin binding with other highly protein-bound psychiatric drugs, leading to an *increased* bioavailable plasma concentration of either the psychiatric drug or warfarin. These increased drug levels

may be toxic and thus require dosage adjustments (Hisaka, Ohno, Yamamoto, & Suzuki, 2010).

METABOLISM

- *Metabolism* refers to the chemical modification of the administered drug by enzymes in the patient's body. Drug metabolism may take place before or after the drug reaches its site of action.
- Drugs may be metabolized (a) from active to inactive compounds, (b) from inactive to active compounds, or (c) from an active compound to a slightly less active compound (or vice versa).
  - Most commonly, drug metabolism leads to the *biotransformation* of a more lipophilic parent drug to a more hydrophilic metabolite, which is often essential to increase the rate of excretion from the body.
  - The chemically modified variant of the administered drug is referred to as a *metabolite.*
  - Metabolites of several commonly administered drugs are therapeutically active at the same sites as their parent drug (e.g., s-desmethylcitalopram, the metabolite of escitalopram).
  - Metabolites of other drugs produce effects different from their parent drug (e.g., desipramine, the metabolite of imipramine, blocks noradrenaline uptake, whereas imipramine itself inhibits serotonin reuptake).
- *Cytochrome P450 (CYP)* refers to the large family of enzymes, found primarily in the liver, responsible for facilitating the majority of drug metabolism in the body.
  - Each CYP family member has a unique collection of substrates (i.e., drugs and other exogenous compounds) that it metabolizes.
  - Metabolism of one psychotherapeutic drug may increase or decrease the metabolism of a second medication (Azzaro, Ziemniak, Kemper, Campbell, & VanDenBerg, 2007). This is often a consequence of alterations in CYP activity.
  - Identification of a drug's CYP metabolism is routinely established in preclinical and clinical testing. This information is generally included in the pharmacokinetics sections of printed drug guides or online/mobile device–based clinical management software (e.g., Lexi-Comp or ePocrates).
  - Individual drug effects on or by P450s may also be included as drug side effects or as drug–drug or food–drug interactions.
  - The standard nomenclature for specific CYP isozymes includes a three- to four-digit number–letter–number sequence, which identifies each isoform's sequence homologies.
  - The primary CYP isozymes present in humans and involved in metabolizing psychiatric drugs are CYP1A2, 2B6, 2C19, 2D6, and 3A4.
  - In addition to being substrates for specific CYPs, drugs may induce or inhibit P450 activity. Grapefruit juice, for example, specifically inhibits the drug metabolizing activity of CYP3A4. This leads to an increase in plasma concentration of other drugs that would have normally been metabolized by CYP3A4.
- The majority of drug metabolism occurs via P450s in the liver; however, in addition to hepatic P450s, notable amounts of drug metabolism also take place in the small intestine, kidney, and lungs.

■ Patients with impaired liver function, such as those suffering from hepatitis or cirrhosis, are at risk of having impaired drug metabolizing activity. This may lead to an increase in bioactive drug concentrations and require a decrease in dosing in order to avoid drug toxicity.

■ Metabolism-related drug–drug or food–drug interactions should be closely monitored. Grapefruit juice inhibits the metabolism of buspirone and other CYP 3A4 metabolites, leading to an *increased* plasma concentration of buspirone.

■ *Therapeutic drug monitoring* improves the quality and safety of psychiatric drug therapy. Valid specimens must be collected during a specific time window; for example, many psychiatric medications such as lithium and valproic acid are drawn as "trough" concentrations just prior to the next dose is due. Appropriate pharmacokinetic interpretation of monitoring data can decrease costs and improve therapeutic outcomes (Llorente Fernández, et al., 2010).

■ The term *half-life* ($t_{1/2}$) refers to the amount of time necessary to decrease the concentration of the drug in the patient by 50%. The term *plateau* refers to the steady-state drug levels achieved in the body with continual drug administration.

  ■ Due to the unique pharmacodynamic properties of psychiatric drugs (e.g., antidepressants), it is possible for there to be a significant delay in therapeutic response even after a plateau drug level has been reached.

  ■ Since psychoactive drugs often have delayed neurochemical effects (e.g., receptor remodeling), it is possible that physiological changes will be observed even after most of the medication has been removed from the body.

  ■ Drugs of the same pharmacological class may have very different half-lives (Table 6.2).

EXCRETION

■ *Excretion* refers to the removal of the drug and any drug metabolites from the patient's body. Of particular concern is the excretion of (a) a therapeutically active parent drug, (b) any bioactive metabolites, and (c) any toxic metabolites.

■ The primary organs facilitating drug excretion are the kidneys. Renal excretion includes (a) glomerular filtration, (b) active tubular secretion, and (c) passive tubular reabsorption.

Table 6.2 Comparison of Half-Lives of Commonly Administered SSRIs and Atypical Antipsychotics

SSRIs	ATYPICAL ANTIPSYCHOTICS
Paroxetine ($t_{1/2}$ = 17 hr)	Ziprasidone ($t_{1/2}$ = 3 hr)
Fluvoxamine ($t_{1/2}$ = 15 hr)	Risperidone ($t_{1/2}$ = 3 hr)
Sertraline ($t_{1/2}$ = 23 hr)	Quetiapine ($t_{1/2}$ =6 hr)
Citalopram ($t_{1/2}$ = 33 hr)	Clozapine ($t_{1/2}$ = 23 hr)
Escitalopram ($t_{1/2}$ = 33 hr)	Olanzapine ($t_{1/2}$ = 33 hr)
Fluoxetine ($t_{1/2}$ = 53 hr)	Aripiprazole ($t_{1/2}$ = 47 hr)

SSRIs, selective serotonin reuptake inhibitors.

■ Nonprotein-bound drug is filtered through the glomerulus. Transporter proteins facilitate active reabsorption.

■ Drugs may also be excreted through the *GI tract* via sequestration in bile or directly into the intestines. Drugs may also be excreted through the skin (e.g., sweat), oral mucosa (e.g., saliva), breast (e.g., lactation), and lungs (e.g., expiration).

■ Enterohepatic recirculation may impede excretion. Patients with impaired kidney function may have impaired drug excretion.

■ Although most drugs undergo hepatic metabolism, some drugs (e.g., lithium) are excreted in their active form.

Pharmacodynamic Principles

Pharmacodynamics refers to the effects of the drug on the patient. Pharmacodynamic effects can be observed at the molecular and cellular levels, as well as at the tissue and organ system levels.

MECHANISMS OF DRUG ACTION OR MOLECULAR DRUG TARGETS

■ Drugs most commonly produce their physiological effects through interactions with cellular drug targets, known as *receptors*. Receptors are most typically proteins and are expressed on a variety of tissues.

■ The term *ligand* refers to drugs and endogenous molecules (e.g., neurohormones).

■ Drug–receptor interactions account for the majority of *drug side effects* as well as *therapeutic effects*. A drug may interact with one or more receptors.

  ■ The drug–receptor interaction responsible for the therapeutic drug effect may be the same or different from the drug–receptor interaction responsible for specific drug side effects.

  ■ An example of therapeutic and adverse drug reactions being caused by the same drug–receptor interaction is illustrated by morphine: Both analgesia (therapeutic effect) and respiratory sedation (drug side effect) are caused by the binding of morphine to the mu opioid receptor.

  ■ An example of therapeutic and adverse drug reactions being caused by different drug–receptor interactions is illustrated by imipramine: The antidepressant effects result from interactions with serotonin and norepinephrine transporters and receptors; its side effects result from binding to cholinergic receptors (dry mouth, blurred vision, constipation) and histamine receptors (weight gain).

■ Drug receptors can be classified into five classes based on their cellular location and general function. The five classes are G protein-coupled receptors (GPCRs), ligand-gated ion channels, cell membrane–embedded enzymes and transporters, intracellular enzymes and signaling proteins, and nuclear transcription factors.

■ *GPCRs* comprise a superfamily of proteins, each containing seven membrane-spanning alpha helices and coupled to a guanosine triphosphate (GTP)-binding protein, which alters the activity of a cellular enzyme or ion channel.

■ Examples of GPCRs include muscarinic acetylcholine receptors, histamine receptors, serotonin receptors, and dopamine receptors.

■ *Ligand-gated ion channels* are located across cell membranes and permit a specific ion to cross into or out of a cell, down its concentration gradient.

■ Examples of ligand-gated ion channels include nicotinic acetylcholine receptors and gamma-aminobutyric acid receptors.

■ *Cell membrane–embedded enzymes and transporters* span the cell membrane and have catalytic activity. Examples include the insulin receptor and neurotransmitter reuptake pumps.

■ *Intracellular enzymes and signaling proteins,* such as monoamine oxidase, alter the cellular environment by catalyzing chemical reactions or conveying chemical messages.

■ *Nuclear transcription factors,* such as the glucocorticoid receptor and thyroid hormone receptor, bind to DNA and alter the transcription rates of specific gene families.

DRUG–RECEPTOR INTERACTIONS

■ A drug or endogenous chemical that activates a receptor is referred to as an *agonist.* Agonists may be classified as producing maximal receptor activation (full agonist) or less than that (partial agonist). A partial agonist may impede the actions of a full agonist, thus diminishing receptor activity.

■ A drug or endogenous chemical that inhibits a receptor from being activated is referred to as an *antagonist.* Antagonists block the actions of both drugs and endogenous chemicals (e.g., neurotransmitters).

　■ While the effects of *competitive antagonists* can be overcome by the increased concentration of an agonist, the effects of other antagonists, referred to as *noncompetitive antagonists,* will persist even if more agonist is present.

■ Drugs often act on more than one receptor, causing a multitude of both therapeutic and adverse drug effects.

■ The description of a drug binding to a receptor simply indicates a physical interaction. This may lead to either receptor agonism or antagonism.

■ Prolonged stimulation of a receptor may result in *desensitization,* in which the same concentration of a drug produces diminished therapeutic effects.

■ The amount of observed therapeutic effect produced by a drug is a measure of *efficacy.* Maximal efficacy is the greatest response produced.

■ The amount of effect a drug produces at a specific drug concentration is a measure of *potency.* High-potency drugs produce effects even when a small dose is given. Low-potency drugs may be nonetheless efficacious; however, they may require a greater dose to be administered.

■ The difference between high-potency and low-potency psychiatric drugs are exemplified by first-generation antipsychotics (FGAs), where high-potency FGAs such as haloperidol produce their therapeutic effects at 1/10 to 1/100 the dose of low-potency FGAs (e.g., chlorpromazine).

PHARMACODYNAMIC DRUG–DRUG INTERACTIONS AND SIDE EFFECTS

■ Pharmacodynamic drug–drug interactions occur when one drug affects the physiological activity of another drug unrelated to a direct chemical interaction or pharmacokinetic process. Most pharmacodynamic drug–drug interactions occur at the cellular or receptor level.

An example of a pharmacodynamic drug–drug interaction is serotonin syndrome, which is produced by the coadministration of a monoamine oxidase inhibitor (e.g., phenelzine) and a selective serotonin reuptake inhibitor (e.g., fluoxetine). Both drugs contribute to a toxic accumulation of serotonin because of their actions on their respective drug targets.

Interpatient Variability

PHARMACOKINETIC AND PHARMACODYNAMIC CHANGES ACROSS THE LIFE SPAN

▪ Life span considerations affect both pharmacokinetic and pharmacodynamic drug properties.

▪ In general, pediatric and geriatric patients are more at risk of experiencing increased sensitivity to therapeutic and adverse drug actions.

▪ Pregnancy causes alterations in the pharmacokinetic actions of certain drugs, primarily by altering the rates of drug absorption and excretion.

PHARMACOGENETIC IMPLICATIONS TO PHARMACOKINETICS AND PHARMACODYNAMICS

▪ *Pharmacogenetics* refers to the effect a patient's genetic profile has on the patient's response to drug therapy.

▪ Slight changes in the genetic code, referred to as *polymorphisms*, have been identified in DNA that direct the production of proteins that affect drug metabolism, leading to pharmacokinetic variability. Polymorphisms that direct the production of drug receptors have also been identified in DNA, leading to pharmacodynamic drug variability.

▪ An example of a genetic alteration affecting psychiatric drug pharmacokinetics is a polymorphism in CYP 3A4, leading to the rapid or delayed metabolism of CYP substrates.

▪ An example of a genetic alteration affecting pharmacodynamics is referred to as the short allele polymorphism of the serotonin (5-HT) transporter. Patients with short allele 5-HT transporter-experienced insomnia and agitation at higher rates during treatment with fluoxetine (Perlis et al., 2010).

REFERENCES

Azzaro, A. J., Ziemniak, J., Kemper, E., Campbell, B. J., & VanDenBerg, C. (2007). Selegiline transdermal system: An examination of the potential for CYP450-dependent pharmacokinetic interactions with 3 psychotropic medications. *Journal of Clinical Pharmacology, 47*, 146–158. doi: 10.1177/0091270006296151

Gupta, A., Hammarlund-Udenaes, M., Chatelain, P., Massingham, R., & Jonsson, E. N. (2006). Stereoselective pharmacokinetics of cetirizine in the guinea pig: Role of protein binding. *Biopharmaceutics & Drug Disposition, 27*, 291–297. DOI: 10.1002/bdd.509

Hisaka, A., Ohno, Y., Yamamoto, T., & Suzuki, H. (2010). Theoretical considerations on quantitative prediction of drug-drug interactions. *Drug Metabolism and Pharmacokinetics, 25*(1), 48–61.

Llorente Fernández, E., Parés, L., Ajuria, I., Bandres, F., Castanyer, B., Campos, F., ... To-Figueras, J. State of the art in therapeutic drug monitoring. *Clinical Chemistry and Laboratory Medicine: CCLM/FESCC, 48*(4), 437–446.

MacDonald, L., Foster, B. C., & Akhtar, M. H. (2009). Food and therapeutic product interactions: A therapeutic perspective. *Journal of Pharmacy & Pharmaceutical Sciences, 12*(3), 367–377.

Perlis, R. H., Smoller, J. W., Mysore, J., Sun, M., Gillis, T., Purcell, S., ... Gusella, J. (2010). Prevalence of incompletely penetrant Huntington's disease alleles among individuals with major depressive disorder. *The American Journal of Psychiatry, 167*(5), 574–579.

BIBLIOGRAPHY

Anon. Biosciences & Medicine—University of Surrey—Guildford. Available at: http://surrey.ac.uk/library/subject/mysubject/biosciences/

Birkett, D. J. (2002). *Pharmacokinetics made easy.* North Ryde, N.S.W.: McGraw-Hill.

Clark, B., & Smith, D. A. (1986). *An introduction to pharmacokinetics.* Oxford: Blackwell Science.

Gibson, G. G., & Skett, P., 2001. *Introduction to drug metabolism.* Cheltenham: Nelson Thornes. Retrieved from: http://lib.myilibrary.com/?id=23990&entityid=https://oala.surrey.ac.uk/oala/metadata

Jambhekar, S. S. (2012). *Basic pharmacokinetics.* London: Pharmaceutical Press.

MacDonald, L., Foster, B. C., & Akhtar, M. H. (2009). Food and therapeutic product interactions--A therapeutic perspective. *Journal of Pharmacy & Pharmaceutical Sciences, 12*(3), 367–377.

Principles and Management of Psychiatric Emergencies

DEFINITION

A psychiatric emergency is any disturbance in thoughts, feelings, or actions for which immediate therapeutic intervention is necessary.

- *Major emergencies:* suicidal patients; agitated and aggressive patients
- *Minor emergencies:* grief reaction; rape; disaster; panic attack
- *Medical emergencies:* delirium; neuroleptic malignant syndrome; serotonin syndrome, monoamine oxidase inhibitors (MAOI)/tyramine reactions; overdosages of common psychiatric medications; overdosages and withdrawal from addicting substances

ETIOLOGY/BACKGROUND

- Approximately 29% to 30% of psychiatric emergency patients are suicidal, approximately 10% are violent, and approximately 40% require hospitalization.
- Psychiatric emergencies peak between 6 p.m. and 10 p.m. when family members are home together and conflicts arise; substance use increases and aggravates disruptive behavior. Family physicians, pastors, counselors, and other resources are difficult to reach.
- Patients present with severe changes in mood, thoughts, or behavior; those experiencing severe drug adverse effects need urgent psychiatric assessment and treatment.
- Psychiatric emergencies often erupt suddenly. A person may curse, hit, throw objects, or brandish a weapon.
- Patients may neglect self-care, stop eating, exhibit confusion, wander into traffic, or appear unclothed in public.
- Because psychiatric emergencies can be concomitant with medical illnesses, it is imperative that the emergency department (ED) physician establish whether the patient's symptoms are caused or exacerbated by a medical disease, such as infection, metabolic abnormality, seizure, or diabetic crisis.
- Emergency psychiatry includes specialized problems such as substance abuse, child abuse, and spousal abuse, as well as violence (suicide, homicide, and rape) and

social issues (homelessness, aging, and competence). People with mental illness often lack a primary care physician and seek health care in crisis. Often uninsured, they have been denied coverage due to medical illness.

INCIDENCE

- Psychiatric emergencies from acute psychotic disturbances, manic episodes, major depression, bipolar disorder, and substance abuse are responsible for approximately 6% of all ED admissions in the United States.
- In bipolar mania, agitation occurs with a frequency of approximately 90%; in schizophrenia, agitation accounts for approximately 20% of psychiatric emergency visits.
- Drug and alcohol intoxication or withdrawal is the most common diagnosis in combative patients.
- In 2006, there were 1,742,887 drug-related ED visits nationwide.
  - Thirty-one percent involved illicit drugs only.
  - Twenty-eight percent involved misuse or abuse of pharmaceuticals (i.e., prescription or over-the-counter medications, dietary supplements) only.
  - Thirteen percent involved illicit drugs with alcohol.

SUICIDAL STATE

Suicidal ideation and behavior are the most serious and common psychiatric emergencies.

- Each year approximately 30,000 people in the United States and 1 million worldwide commit suicide; 650,000 receive emergency treatment after attempting suicide. It is the tenth leading cause of death worldwide.
- Suicide is highly prevalent in the adolescent population. Confounding comorbidities include depression, antisocial behavior, and alcohol abuse.
- A history of suicide attempts increases the odds of completing suicide more than any other risk factor.
- Most people who commit suicide reportedly never made a prior attempt and have never seen a mental health professional.
- People who attempt suicide more than once and later complete the act tend to be more anxious and socially withdrawn.
- In the United States, the majority of suicides are completed with firearms, followed by hanging among men and poisoning among women.
- Risk factors for suicide include the following:
  - Psychiatric illnesses
    - More than 90% of persons who attempt suicide have a major psychiatric disorder.
    - The most common mental health disorders leading to suicide include major depression, substance abuse, schizophrenia, and severe personality disorders.
  - Impulsivity and hopelessness
  - History of previous suicide attempts
  - Age, sex, and race
    - Risk increases with age.
    - Young adults attempt suicide more frequently, but successfully complete less frequently than the elderly.

- Elderly (above 85 years) White males have the highest suicide rate.
- Suicide rates have traditionally been higher among Whites compared with Blacks. The incidence of suicide attempts among young Blacks is rising.
- Marital status
  - Whatever the family structure, living alone increases risk of suicide.
- Occupation
  - Unemployed and unskilled persons are at higher risk.
- Health status
  - Risk increases with physical illness such as chronic or terminal illness, chronic pain, and recent surgery.

VIOLENT BEHAVIOR

Certain features can serve as warning signs that a patient may be escalating toward physically violent behavior. The following list is not exhaustive:

- Facial expressions are tense and angry
- Increased or prolonged restlessness, body tension, pacing
- General overarousal of body systems (increased breathing and heart rate, muscle twitching, dilating pupils)
- Increased volume of speech, erratic movements
- Prolonged eye contact
- Discontentment, refusal to communicate, withdrawal, fear, irritation
- Thought processes unclear, poor concentration
- Delusions or hallucinations with violent content
- Verbal threats or gestures
- Reporting anger or violent feelings
- Blocking escape routes

AGITATION AND AGGRESSION

- Aggressive, violent patients are often psychotic and diagnosed with schizophrenia, delusional disorder, delirium, acute mania, and dementia, but these behaviors can also result from intoxication with alcohol or other substances of abuse, such as cocaine, phencyclidine (PCP), and amphetamines.
- Medical disorders associated with violent behavior include (not all inclusive) the following:
  - *Neurological illnesses*—seizure disorders, hepatic encephalopathy, cerebral infarcts, encephalitis, Wilson's disease, Parkinson's disease, intracranial bleeds
  - *Endocrinopathies*—hypothyroidism, Cushing's syndrome, thyrotoxicosis, diabetic crisis
  - *Metabolic disorders*—hypoglycemia, hypoxia, electrolyte imbalance
  - *Infections*—AIDS, syphilis, tuberculosis
  - *Vitamin deficiencies*—folic acid, pyridoxine, vitamin B_{12}
  - *Temperature disturbances*—hypothermia, hyperthermia, vitamin D
  - *Poisoning*
- Behavioral signs of agitation include excessive motor restlessness, irritability, jitteriness, and purposeless and repetitive motor or verbal activity.

- Precautions should be taken to modify the environment to maximize safety.
  - Ensure that patient is physically comfortable and in an environment with low levels of stimulation.
  - Minimize waiting time.
  - Communicate in a safe, respectful attitude.
  - Remove all dangerous objects.
- Aggressive behavior is usually managed with some combination of seclusion, physical restraints, monitoring with constant observation by a sitter, and drug therapy.
  - Seclusion offers a decrease in external stimuli that may be enough to reduce aggressiveness.
  - Restraints may be needed to obtain a thorough assessment.
- Drug therapy such as tranquilization should target control of specific symptoms.
- Rapid calming or tranquilization of a patient is achieved with benzodiazepine or an antipsychotic given intramuscularly (IM) or intravenously (IV).
  - Typical or atypical antipsychotic may be used.
  - Benzodiazepines act more quickly but often have erratic IM absorption.
  - A combination of both drugs can be very effective.
- If oral medications are appropriate, orally disintegrating or liquid formulations are available for haloperidol, risperidone, olanzapine, and aripiprazole.

DRUG THERAPY FOR AGITATION IN PSYCHIATRIC EMERGENCIES

- It is better for a patient to take medication voluntarily and orally before the behavior escalates than to be involuntarily medicated after a crisis.
- The decision on which medication to use is often based on the underlying diagnosis. If the patient is known to be schizophrenic or bipolar and most likely is in a psychotic or manic state, then an antipsychotic should be used. If the diagnosis is unclear or the result of intoxication with drugs or alcohol, then lorazepam, a benzodiazepine, is most often administered.
- Medications discussed are those that have injectable dosage forms. There are other antipsychotics in liquids or disintegrating tablet forms that would work as well in the appropriate patient.

DIAGNOSTIC WORKUP

- Mental status examination to rule out contributing mental illness to psychiatric emergency
- Physical examination to rule out physical explanation for psychiatric emergency
- Laboratory evaluation:
  - *White blood cell count (WBC)*—to look for infectious contribution
  - *Serum electrolytes, creatinine, blood urea nitrogen (BUN)*—to rule out electrolyte abnormalities, such as hyponatremia, dehydration, and renal insufficiency, which can contribute to agitation
  - *Liver function tests*—hepatic encephalopathy and hyperammonemia can present with agitation and aggression
  - *Toxicological analysis of serum and urine*—substance abuse contribution to emergency
  - *Neuroimaging (CT/MRI)*—rule out stroke, tumor
  - *EEG*—if seizure disorder is suspected

MEDICAL/LEGAL PITFALLS

- Involuntary administration of psychotropic medications is allowed in emergencies that are considered life threatening. Wide variations exist in the legal definition of "life-threatening" and in the practice of administering involuntary medication.
- Timely documentation of the need for restraint and involuntary medication is essential.
- Informed consent: The most important element of informed consent is the assessment of decisional capacity, for example, through the use of the Mini-Mental State Examination.
- If the patient is suffering from either an organic or a functional acute change in mental status and is a danger to self or others, then the patient should undergo emergency medical evaluation. If the patient will not voluntarily submit to this evaluation, then a request for an emergency medical evaluation from a judge, justice of the peace, or police officer is obtained.
- Chemical or physical restraints may be necessary in the combative patient. Chemical restraints typically include benzodiazepines and/or antipsychotics. Physical restraints are a last resort and are used mostly by security with close observation.
  - Protocols for restraints will vary by community.
  - Physical restraints should be used in the least restrictive manner and for the least amount of time possible.

Drug Selection Table for Psychiatric Emergencies

CLASS	DRUG
Benzodiazepines (BZDs)	
	Lorazepam (*Ativan*)
	Midazolam (*Versed*)
First-generation (typical) antipsychotics	
	Haloperidol (*Haldol*)
	Fluphenazine HCl (*Prolixin*)
Second-generation (atypical) antipsychotics	
	Aripiprazole (*Abilify*)
	Olanzapine (*Zyprexa*)
	Ziprasidone (*Geodon*)
Antihistamine	
	Cyproheptadine (*Periactin* for supportive use during serotonin syndrome. Other antihistamines that are useful are benadryl/hydroxyzine, which can be used for anxiolysis and severe extrapyramidal symptom (EPS) resolution.)
Skeletal muscle relaxant	
	Dantrolene (*Dantrium*)
Dopamine agonist	
	Bromocriptine (*Parlodel*)

■ As required by the Joint Commission, institutions must have policies in place that deal with the use of restraints.
■ A person with capacity cannot be confined or restrained against his or her will. Doing so can lead to a legal charge of false imprisonment or battery.
■ Duty to warn:
    ■ Requires a clinician to warn a person who may be in danger from a combative patient
■ Failure to do so may make the clinician liable for injury to the third party.

EXPERT CONSENSUS GUIDELINES

Treatment of Behavioral Emergencies: Highlights of Treatment

■ Support the use of oral formulations (liquid concentrate, rapidly dissolving tablets) of atypical antipsychotics as first-line therapy for the initial management of agitation or aggression in the emergency setting. Provide faster times-to-peak concentration. Injection peaks faster; however, oral formulations are more legally preferred and patient-centered whenever possible.
■ Reserve IM injections for patients unable to cooperate with oral therapy.

Other Medical Emergencies in Psychiatry

DELIRIUM

Clinical Presentation: A condition of impaired attention, changes in behavior, and a clouded sensorium, which follows a waxing and waning course. The patient may be agitated, disoriented, and confused. Delirium is a disturbance of attention, not a disturbance of memory. It is acute in onset and may have concomitant neurological disturbances such as tremor, increased muscle tone, visual hallucinations, and impaired speech.

Etiology: Delirium is often caused by changes in acetylcholine balance. It can be caused by medications such as anticholinergics, narcotics, or steroids, or an underlying medical condition such as a urinary tract infection, liver failure, drug or alcohol abuse, or electrolyte/metabolic abnormalities. People with delirium need immediate medical attention.

Incidence: Delirium occurs in 30% of all elderly medical patients. The risk of delirium increases for people who are demented, dehydrated, and taking drugs that affect the nervous system.

Treatment: Treatment depends on the condition causing the delirium. The underlying medical condition should be treated first. Eliminate or change medications that can worsen confusion or that are unnecessary. Medications may be needed to control aggressive or agitated behaviors. These are usually started at very low doses and adjusted as needed. Most often antipsychotics and sedatives are selected but should be titrated slowly in the elderly and selected to target the symptom. It should be kept in mind that benzodiazepine usage in the elderly can worsen confusion and delirium.

Outcome: Delirium often lasts about 1 week although it may take several weeks for mental function to return to normal levels. Full recovery is common.

NEUROLEPTIC MALIGNANT SYNDROME (NMS)

Clinical Presentation: NMS is a rare but life-threatening neurological emergency associated with the use of antipsychotic agents and characterized by a clinical syndrome of mental status change, rigidity, fever, and dysautonomia. Mortality results from systemic complications and dysautonomia. The cardinal features include muscular rigidity, hyperthermia, autonomic dysfunction, and altered consciousness. Rigidity and akinesia usually develop initially or concomitantly with a temperature elevation as high as 41°C. Autonomic dysfunction includes tachycardia, labile blood pressure, diaphoresis, dyspnea, and urinary incontinence. Creatine kinase, complete blood count, and liver function testss are usually increased. Symptoms develop over 24 to 72 hours.

Etiology: The cause of NMS is unknown but is thought to be related to central dopamine blockade. The risk appears to be lower for the atypical antipsychotics than for the typical.

Incidence: It occurs in 0.2% to 3.2% of patients. Most patients are young adults, but the disease has been described in all age groups. It can occur hours to months after initial drug exposure.

Treatment: Discontinue any neuroleptic agent or precipitating drug. Maintain cardiorespiratory and euvolemic stability. Benzodiazepines can be used for agitation. Lower fever using cooling blankets.

SEROTONIN SYNDROME

Serotonin syndrome is a potential life-threatening syndrome associated with increased serotonergic activity in the central nervous system (CNS), such as from the combination of a selective serotonin reuptake inhibitor and a monoamine oxidase inhibitor (MAOI). It is associated with therapeutic use, drug interactions, or intentional self-poisoning. Classically, it is a triad of mental status changes, autonomic hyperactivity, and neuromuscular abnormalities. It is a clinical diagnosis; no laboratory test can confirm the diagnosis.

Clinical Presentation: Serotonin syndrome can manifest as a wide range of clinical symptoms from mild tremor to life-threatening hyperthermia and shock. Examination findings can include hyperthermia, agitation, ocular clonus, tremor, akathisia, deep tendon hyperreflexia, inducible or spontaneous clonus, muscle rigidity, dilated pupils, dry mucous membranes, increased bowel sounds, flushed skin, diaphoresis and increased heart rate, hypertension. Neuromuscular findings are typically more pronounced in the lower extremities.

Etiology: Serotonin syndrome occurs due to increased serotonin in the CNS. Postsynaptic 5-HT1A and 5-HT2A receptors are implicated. Occurs most commonly with the concomitant use of serotonergic drugs, with drugs that impair metabolism of serotonin, including MAOIs or with antipsychotics or other dopamine antagonists.

Treatment: Discontinue serotonergic agents. Provide supportive care such as IV fluids for hydration and benzodiazepines for agitation, myoclonus, hyperreflexia, and hyperthermia.

Specific Agents: Periactin (cyproheptadine) is an antihistamine with serotonergic antagonist properties. It should be considered in moderate to severe cases.

BIBLIOGRAPHY

Anderson, I. A., & Reid, I. C. (2006). *Fundamentals of clinical psychopharmacology: Third edition.* New York: Informa Healthcare.

Beitman, B. D., & Klerman, G. L. (Eds.) (1991). *Integrating pharmacotherapy and psychotherapy.* Washington, DC: American Psychiatric Press, Inc.

Bentley, K. J., & Walsh, J. F. (2001). *The social worker and psychotropic medication: Second edition.* Belmont, CA: Brooks/Cole.

Bezchlibnyk-Butler, K. Z., & Jeffries, J. J. (Eds.) (2003). *Clinical handbook of psychotropic drugs: Thirteenth revised edition.* Switzerland: Hogrefe & Huber.

Charney, D. S., & Nestler, E. J. (Eds.) (2004). *Neurobiology of mental illness: Second edition.* UK: Oxford University Press.

Cooper, J. R., Bloom, F. E., & Roth, R. H. (1996). *The biochemical basis of neuropharmacology: Seventh edition.* NY: Oxford University Press.

Curran, S., & Bullock, R. (Eds.) (2005). *Practical old age psychopharmacology: A multi-professional approach.* Oxford: Radcliffe Publishing.

Dziegielewski, S. F. (2006). *Psychopharmacology handbook: For the non-medically trained.* NY: W. W. Norton & Company.

Fisher, S., & Greenber, R. P. (Eds.) (1989). *The limits of biological treatments for psychological distress: Comparisons with psychotherapy and placebo.* Hillsdale, NJ: Lawrence Erlbaum Associates.

Freeman, L. (2004). *Mosby's complementary & alternative medicine: A research-based approach.* St. Louis, MO: Elsevier.

Hadad, P., Durson, S., & Deakin, B. (Eds.) (2004). *Adverse syndromes and psychiatric drugs: A clinical guide.* Oxford: Oxford University Press.

Healey, D. (1997). The *antidepressant era.* Cambridge, MA: Harvard University Press.

Healey, D. (2002). *The creation of psychopharmacology.* Cambridge, MA: Harvard University Press.

Healey, D. (2004). *Let them eat Prosac: The unhealthy relationship between the pharmaceutical industry and depression.* NY: New York University Press.

Hollander, E. (2001). *Professional's handbook of psychotropic drugs.* Springhouse, PA: Springhouse.

Hyman, S. E., & Nestler, E. J. (1993). *The molecular foundations of psychiatry.* Washington, DC: American Psychiatric Press, Inc.

Kelsey, J. E., Newport, D. J., & Nemeroff, C. B. (2006). *Principles of psychopharmacology for mental health professionals.* Hoboken, NJ: Wiley-Liss.

Keltner, N. L., & Folks, D. G. (2005). *Psychotropic drugs: Fourth edition.* St. Louis, MO: Elsevier Mosby.

Lewis, B. (2006). *Moving beyond Prozac, DSM, and the new psychiatry: The birth of postpsychiatry.* Ann Arbor, MI: The University of Michigan Press.

Meyer, J. S., & Quenzer, L. F. (2005). *Psychopharmacology: Drugs, the brain, and behavior.* Sunderland, MA: Sinauer Associates, Inc.

Nestler, E. J., Hyman, S. E., & Malenka, R. C. (2001). *Molecular neuropharmacology: A foundation for clinical neuroscience.* NY: The McGraw-Hill Companies, Inc.

Preston, J. D., O'Neal, J. H., & Talaga, M. C. (2005). *Handbook of clinical psychopharmacology for therapists: Fourth edition.* New Harbinger Publications, Inc.

Rose, S. (2005). *The future of the brain: The promise and perils of tomorrow's neuroscience.* Oxford: Oxford University Press.

Schachter, M. (Ed.) (1993). *Psychotherapy and medication: A dynamic integration.* Northvale, NJ: Jason Aronson.

Schatzberg, A., & Nemeroff, C. (Eds.) (2004). *Textbook of psychopharmacology: Third edition.* Washington, DC: American Psychiatric Publishing.

Spiegel, R. (2003). *Psychopharmacology: An introduction.* UK: Wiley.

Stahl, S. M. (2000). *Essential psychopharmacology: Neuroscientific basis and practical applications.* Second edition. Cambridge, UK: Cambridge University Press.

Stahl, S. M. (2005). *Essential psychopharmacology: The prescriber's guide.* New York: Cambridge University Press.

Stein, D., Lerer, B., & Stahl, S. (2005). *Evidence-based psychopharmacology.* NY: Cambridge University Press.

Walsh, B. T. (Ed.) (1998). *Child psychopharmacology.* Washington, DC: American Psychiatric Press, Inc.

Whitaker, R. (2002). *Mad in America: Bad science, bad medicine, and the enduring mistreatment of the mentally ill.* Cambridge, MA: Perseus.

WEB RESOURCE

http://www.icpsr.umich.edu/icpsrweb/SAMHDA/studies/34565

Part **III**

Syndromes and Treatments in Adult Psychiatry

Behavioral and Psychological Disorders in the Elderly

Delirium

BACKGROUND INFORMATION

Definition of Disorder
- Abnormality in cognitive processing affecting thinking, attention, awareness, memory, perception, and orientation to person, place, and time
- Onset is fairly rapid.
- Delirium is the direct result of an underlying medical condition, illness, or medication.
- Mimics dementia
- Often the first sign of illness in the elderly
- An acute confusional state
- Disturbed attention and lack of environmental awareness
- May involve visual illusions, hallucinations, and delusions

Etiology
- One theory is that delirium reflects neuronal dysfunction through excessive neurotransmitter release and abnormal signal conduction
- Medications—prescription or over-the-counter (OTC)—are the most common causes of delirium
- Anticholinergic toxicity from prescribed medications (diphenhydramine [Benadryl]), tricyclic antidepressants (TCAs; amitriptyline [Elavil], imipramine [Tofranil]), and antipsychotics (chlorpromazine [Thorazine], thioridazine [Mellaril])
- Benzodiazepines or alcohol
- Anti-inflammatory agents, including prednisone
- Cardiovascular (antihypertensives, digitalis)
- Diuretics, if dehydrated
- Gastrointestinal (cimetidine, ranitidine)
- Opioid analgesics (especially meperidine)
- Lithium

- Antipsychotic, sedative, or hypnotic drugs often used to treat confusion, agitation, or insomnia may precipitate an episode of delirium
- Infections: pneumonia, skin, urinary tract
- Metabolic acute blood loss, dehydration, electrolyte imbalance, organ failure, hyper- or hypoglycemia, hypoxia
- Heart: arrhythmia, congestive heart failure, myocardial infarction (MI), or shock
- Neurological: central nervous system infection, head trauma, seizures, stroke subdural hematoma, transient ischemic accidents, tumors
- Other: fecal impaction, postoperative recovery, sleep deprivation, urinary retention

Demographic
- Thirty to forty percent of hospitalized patients above the age of 65 years have experienced an episode of delirium.
- Forty to fifty percent of patients with delirium are recovering from surgery to repair a hip fracture.
- Thirty to forty percent of delirium patients have AIDS.
- Forty to seventy percent of delirium patients have cardiac problems.

Risk Factors
- Age: the very old and the very young are at risk for delirium.
- Persons with brain trauma, dementia, cerebrovascular disease, tumor, alcohol dependence, diabetes mellitus, cancer, blindness, or poor hearing are at risk for delirium.
- Persons on multiple medications
- Another mental health disorder, such as depression or substance abuse (alcoholism or drug abuse), increases the risk of developing delirium.
- Another physical disorder: infection, dehydration
- Metabolic, electrolyte, and endocrine disturbances

DIAGNOSIS

Differential Diagnosis
- Whether the patient has dementia is the most common issue in the differential diagnosis.
- Rule out the following:
  - Infection: urinary, pneumonia, skin
  - Diabetic-, hyper-, or hypoglycemia
  - Cardiac arrhythmias
  - Cerebral lesions
  - Alcohol withdrawal

ICD-10 Code
F03 (F03) (28 index entries)

Diagnostic Workup
- Assume reversibility
- Identify and correct underlying cause(s)
- Physical evaluation
- Blood sugar

■ Urinalysis (UA) for culture and sensitivity
■ Serum levels of medications
■ O$_2$ saturation
■ Arrhythmia
■ Vitamin B12
■ Brain imaging tests and measures of serum anticholinergic activity are experimental laboratory tests that show promise.

Initial Assessment

■ Delirium is often underrecognized by health care personnel, especially if the patient has hypoactive delirium, is 80 years of age or older, has vision impairment, or has dementia (Inouye, Foreman, Mion, Katz, & Cooney, 2001). Periodic application of simple cognitive tests, such as the Mini-Cog, the confusion assessment method for the intensive care unit (CAM-ICU), or the intensive care delirium screening checklist (ICDSC), may improve identification.
■ The clock face test is also a simple test of mental status.
■ White blood cell count, CBC (complete blood count), electrolytes (potassium, sodium, chloride, bicarbonate)
■ Interview.
■ Rule out infection and other medical causes.
■ Review prescriptions, especially recent ones and OTC medications for anticholinergic delirium.
■ History if drug and alcohol use.
■ Electrocardiogram—to identify any arrhythmias.

Clinical Presentation

■ Hypervigilance or inattention to the environment
■ Disorganized thinking or altered level of consciousness
■ Sleep–wake cycle disturbance
■ Progressing to anxiety, agitation, flight syndrome—tries to leave hospital
■ Perceptual disturbances (visual illusions, hallucinations, delusions)
■ Disorientation in regard to time, place, and person
■ Concomitant physical condition
■ Also may exhibit anxiety, fear, depression, irritability, and anger
■ Symptoms will fluctuate over a 24-hour period

DSM-5 Diagnostic Guidelines

■ Delirium is a disturbance in consciousness and/or a change in neurocognition that cannot be accounted for by a preexisting dementia.

TREATMENT OVERVIEW

Acute Treatment

See the American Psychiatric Association's *Practice Guideline for Treatment of Patients With Delirium.*

■ Identify the underlying cause.
■ Initiate psychiatric management through therapeutic interaction with the patient to reduce fear.

▦ Educate the family and other clinicians regarding the illness.
▦ Establish therapeutic trust when the patient is stable.
▦ Provide supportive measures.
▦ Modify the environment; ensure that the patient is oriented to the environment.
▦ Provide objects to orient patient to day and night (e.g., calendar, clock).
▦ Provide quiet and well-lit surroundings that dampen noise made by machines, overhead pagers, and equipment.
▦ Do not use physical restraints.
▦ Hydrate the patient.
▦ Provide familiar faces of family members or sitters.
▦ Stimulate daytime activity, mobilize the patient.
▦ Correct sensory deficits with eyeglasses, hearing aids, and portable amplification devices.
▦ Promote normal sleep with warm milk, massage, and nighttime noise reduction.
▦ Prevent dehydration (blood urea nitrogen [BUN] to creatinine ratio > 18) and fecal impaction.
▦ Review risk factors: use of physical restraints, dehydration, and bladder catheter.
▦ For acute agitation, use a high-potency low-anticholinergic, low-arrhythmogenic antipsychotic medication. If on antipsychotic medication (i.e., risperidone [Risperdal], olanzapine [Zyprexa], and quetiapine [Seroquel, Seroquel XR]), patients should have their electrocardiograms monitored. QTc interval greater than 450 msec or 25% over baseline warrants a cardiology consultation and reduction or discontinuation of the medication.
▦ Morphine (not meperidine) may be required if pain is a factor.

Chronic Treatment

▦ Most people respond well to treatment and can return to normal functioning in hours to days.
▦ Treatment can be complicated if the patient has another condition at the same time, such as substance abuse, depression, or other anxiety disorders.

Recurrence Rate

If the rate of recurrence is common, the patient needs to be monitored frequently.

PATIENT EDUCATION

▦ Information regarding delirium may be found in MD Consult: Delirium: Patient Education (http://www.mdconsult. com).
▦ Advise patients to avoid OTC medications for colds and sleep with high anticholinergic effect, including pseudophedrine or cimetidine.

MEDICAL/LEGAL PITFALLS

▦ Delirium is associated with significant morbidity and mortality. Estimated 3-month mortality rate of a patient with delirium ranges from 23% to 33%, 1-year mortality rate is as high as 50%.

- Persons with delirium are more likely to have a fall in the hospital or other events that will delay discharge and result in costlier hospital stays.
- Persons with delirium are more susceptible to dehydration or malnutrition because the lack of orientation delays satisfying the urge to eat or drink.
- Pain can also contribute to delirium.
- Alcohol use and withdrawal can cause delirium.

Dementia and Alzheimer's Disease

OVERVIEW

- More than 6 million people in the United States suffer from dementia and the disorder is under-diagnosed.
- Depression, anxiety, or other behavioral disturbances may accompany dementia.
- Cost of treating dementia in the elderly is estimated to be more than $148 billion annually.
- There are several types of dementia, including vascular, frontal, Lewy body, and Alzheimer's disease (AD).
- Reversible causes of dementia should be explored before initiating pharmacological therapy.
- In the United States, a patient is diagnosed with AD, a form of dementia, every 71 seconds.
- AD accounts for 70% of all dementias; the other 30% is due to other or multiple causes.

BACKGROUND INFORMATION

Definition of Disorder
- Noticeable decline in memory beginning with short-term memory loss
- Decline in other cognitive functions, including ability to perform familiar tasks (activities of daily living [ADLs]), language, orientation to time and place, poor or declining judgment, abstract thinking, misplacing objects in unusual places, changes in mood or behavior, loss of initiative sufficient to affect activities of daily living
- Insidious onset, progressive over months to years, and is rarely reversible.

Etiology
- A common denominator of all dementia disorders is that memory and cognitive function are impaired due to neuron death. Therefore, it is not reversible.

Demographic
- Approximately 1% of people aged 65 years or older and more than 50% of people aged 90 years or older have a dementia disorder.
- Worldwide, half of the demented persons (46%) live in Asia, 30% in Europe, and 12% in North America; 52% live in less-developed regions.
- Approximately 59% of women with dementia have AD.

Risk Factors
- Age: dementia increases with age
- Genetic changes: apolipoprotein E (ApoE and E4) allele is a strong risk factor.

▦ Probable risks: head trauma and genetics
▦ Evidence is moderate that low education has a moderate risk effect on dementia.
▦ Evidence is moderate at midlife that controlling high cholesterol levels and high blood pressure has a protective effect on dementia.
▦ Evidence is strong that antihypertensive drugs have a protective effect on dementia.
▦ Evidence is moderate that leisure activities/active lives have a protective effect.
▦ Evidence is insufficient that social network or personality type has a protective effect.
▦ Evidence is insufficient that obesity, high homocysteine levels, diet, folate/vitamin B_{12} deficiency, aluminum, and depression are risk factors for dementia.
▦ Evidence is insufficient that statins, hormone replacement therapy, and nonsteroidal anti-inflammatory drugs (NSAIDs) have a protective effect.
▦ Evidence is limited that moderate alcohol use has a protective effect on the risk of dementia.

Relationship to Other Diseases
▦ Dementia is unrelated to hypothyroidism or hyperthyroidism, but needs to be diagnosed and treated.
▦ Studies show variable results in regard to correlation between low vitamin B_{12} (cyanocobalamin) and dementia or Alzheimer's disease. There is a correlation between low folic acid levels and impaired cognitive function.

DIAGNOSIS

Differential Diagnosis
▦ Delirium
▦ Depression
▦ Thyroid disorders
▦ Diabetic: hyper- or hypoglycemia
▦ Cardiac arrhythmias
▦ Cerebral lesions
▦ Posttraumatic stress disorder (PTSD)
▦ Drug interactions or adverse effects
▦ Schizophrenia

ICD-10 Code
Alzheimer's disease (F30.9)
Progressive dementia (F03.90)
Vascular dementia (F01.51)

Diagnostic Workup
▦ Currently there is no simple, reliable test for diagnosing dementia at an early stage.
▦ A physical and neurological evaluation must be done.
▦ Evaluate mental status for short- and long-term memory, problem solving, and depression
▦ CBC with differential is done.
▦ Computed tomography (CT scan) and MRI scan can identify people who have AD.
▦ Electroencephalography brain mapping and apolipoprotein levels are currently not recommended for identifying AD.

Initial Assessment

▓ History from the family, friends, or caretaker close to the person will supplement the patient's account.

▓ Clock-drawing test or other simple exercises will allow selection for additional testing.

▓ Assess functional status.

▓ People with dementia are sometimes stigmatized. Understanding can lead to more compassion among patient, family, and friends.

Clinical Presentation

Early (1–3 years):

▓ Disorientation as to date

▓ Recall problems in relation to recent events

▓ Naming problems

▓ Mild language or decision-making problems

▓ Mild problem in copying figures (e.g., face of a clock)

▓ Social withdrawal

▓ Mood change

▓ Problems managing finances

Middle (2–8 years):

▓ Disorientation about date and place

▓ Getting lost in familiar areas

▓ Impaired new learning

▓ Impaired calculating skills

▓ Agitation and aggression

▓ Problems with cooking, shopping, dressing, or grooming

▓ Restlessness, anxiety, or depression

Late (6–12 years):

▓ Disoriented to time, place, or person

▓ Increasingly nonverbal

▓ Long-term memory gone

▓ Unable to copy or write

▓ Unable to groom or dress

▓ Incontinent

▓ Motor or verbal agitation end stage:
  ▓ Nonverbal
  ▓ Not eating or swallowing well
  ▓ Not ambulatory
  ▓ Incontinent of bowel and bladder

▓ Depression occurs in 50% of the patients and may cause rapid decline if not treated

DSM–5 Diagnostic Guidelines

▓ Dementia is a syndrome rather than an illness, with a set of signs and symptoms that includes a progressive decline in cognitive function due to damage or disease in the body beyond what might be expected from normal aging. Although dementia is far more common in the geriatric population, it may occur at any stage of adulthood.

▦ Symptoms of dementia can be classified as either reversible or irreversible, depending on the etiology of the disease. Fewer than 10% of cases of dementia are the result of causes that may presently be reversed with treatment. Without careful assessment of history, the short-term syndrome of delirium can easily be confused with dementia, because they have many symptoms in common. Some mental illnesses, including depression and psychosis, may also produce symptoms that mimic those of dementia.

TREATMENT OVERVIEW

Chronic Treatment

The focus of treatment is to improve the quality of life of the individual and the care provider by maintaining functional ability and by supporting remaining intellectual abilities, mood, behavior, and social support networks such as the Swedish Council on Technology Assessment in Health Care (http://www.sbu.se/en/).

▦ Treat comorbid physical illnesses, blood pressure, and diabetes.
▦ Support the family in setting realistic goals.
▦ Limit all medications, especially psychotropics or sedatives, to only essential medications.
▦ Maintain functional ability.

Nonpharmacological Approaches

▦ Care of the family member with dementia requires multilevel resources that increase the caregiver's burden over time.
▦ Behavior modification, including scheduled activities (e.g., toileting in late stages) and prompted activities (e.g., dressing in middle stages)
▦ Assistance provided only for what the elder cannot do.
▦ Familiar music
▦ Walking or light exercise
▦ Pet therapy
▦ Calm and slow approaches
▦ Well-lighted lit areas without shadows

Pharmacological Treatment

▦ Cholinesterase inhibitors such as Aricept, Reminyl, Exelon (benefit for 1–3 years)
▦ Record functional status and cognitive status.
▦ Treat agitation.

Support Caregiver

▦ Caregiver burden includes isolation and anxiety
▦ Arrange respite care to provide caregiver relief.

Recurrence Rate

Long-term chronic decline occurs.

PATIENT EDUCATION

▦ Alzheimer's Association: http://www.alz.org/index.asp
▦ Family caregiver alliance: http://www.caregiver.org/caregiver/jsp/home.jsp
▦ National caregiver alliance: http://www.caregiving.org/members/

Drug Selection Table for Dementia and Alzheimer's Disease

CLASS	DRUG
Cholinesterase inhibitors	**First-line drug therapy**
	Donepezil hydrochloride (*Aricept*)
	Rivastigimine tartrate (*Exelon and Exelon patch*)
	Galantamine (*Razadyne and Razadyne ER*)
N-methyl-d-aspartate (NMDA) receptor antagonist	
	Memantine (*Namenda*)

MEDICAL/LEGAL PITFALLS

- Dementia affects all areas of life, including physical, social, and financial aspects. The issues are complicated and require careful reflection on the human condition and the value of various interventions.
- Dementia affects the lives of family members in a way that requires treatment resources to support the caregiver.
- Legal resources are involved in drawing up living wills and wills before the patient is no longer able to make his or her wishes known.
- Protective services may be involved to protect the patient against financial or physical abuse.
- Judges and attorneys have few guidelines for amnesic cases.

Major Depressive Disorders (MDD) in the Elderly

OVERVIEW

- Prevalence of depression increases with aging.
- More than 30% of adults above 65 years of age have symptoms of depression.
- Symptoms may include decreased energy, sleep disturbances, weight changes, loss of interest, guilt, poor concentration, and thoughts of suicide.
- ICD-10 code **(F33)** depression, unspecified
- *DSM-5* criteria: Presence of two to four depressive symptoms of greater than 2 weeks duration
- Risk factors include acute stress, anxiety, and illness.
- Differential diagnoses include grief reaction, metabolic disorder, substance abuse, or medication-induced depression.

TREATMENT OVERVIEW

Acute Treatment
- Selective serotonin reuptake inhibitors (SSRIs) are indictated as first-line treatment for major depressive disorders (MDDs).
- Serotonin-norepinephrine reuptake inhibitors (SNRIs) may be considered if SSRIs do not achieve optimal results.

Drug Selection Table for Major Depressive Disorders

CLASS	DRUG
Selective serotonin reuptake inhibitors (SSRIs)	First-line drug therapy
	Fluoxetine (*Prozac*) Paroxetine (*Paxil*) Citalopram (*Celexa*) Escitalopram (*Lexapro*) Sertraline (*Zoloft*)
Serotonin and norepinephrine reuptake inhibitors (SNRIs)	
	Duloxetine (*Cymbalta*) Venlafaxine (*Effexor*) Desvenlafaxine (*Pristiq*)

Chronic Treatment
▩ SSRIs and SNRIs are also first-line options for persistent MDDs.

PSYCHOPHARMACOLOGY OF MDD IN THE ELDERLY

General Considerations
▩ Patients should avoid consuming alcohol while taking this medication.
▩ Use with caution in patients with history of seizure disorder and/or diabetes.
▩ Avoid abrupt withdrawal of this class of drug. Dosage should be tapered down prior to discontinuation.
▩ Monitor closely for clinical worsening and suicide risk.
▩ Monitor closely for serotonin syndrome.
▩ Contraindicated if patient has been on a monoamine oxidase inhibitor (MAOI) within 14 days or has taken thioridazine within weeks.

Generalized Anxiety Disorder (GAD) in the Elderly

OVERVIEW
▩ Prevalence of anxiety is not as common in older adults with the diagnosis of amnestic disorder.
▩ Anxiety may be associated with depression and/or dementia.
▩ Symptoms may include excessive worry, restlessness, poor concentration, irritability, or sleep disturbance typically for longer than 6 months. Typically, at least three symptoms are present.
▩ ICD-10 code.
▩ *DSM-5* criteria: 6 months of excessive worry about issues causing distress or impairment.
▩ Differential diagnoses include grief reaction, posttraumatic stress disorder, depression, metabolic disorder, cardiovascular disease, infection, or substance abuse.

Drug Selection Table for Generalized Anxiety Disorder

CLASS	DRUG
Serotonin 1A agonist	First-line drug therapy
	Buspirone (*BuSpar*)
Selective serotonin reuptake inhibitors	
	Paroxetine (*Paxil*)
	Escitalopram (*Lexapro*)
Selective norepinephrine reuptake inhibitors	
	Duloxetine (*Cymbalta*)
Benzodiazepines	Second-line drug therapy
	Lorazepam (*Ativan*)

TREATMENT OVERVIEW

Acute Treatment
▦ First-line drugs of choice for generalized anxiety disorder (GAD) are the SSRI antidepressants.
▦ Typical anxiolytics may be considered if atypical anxiolytics are ineffective.

Chronic Treatment
▦ Atypical or typical anxiolytics are also options for treatment of persistent generalized anxiety disorder.

PSYCHOPHARMACOLOGY OF GAD IN THE ELDERLY

General Considerations
▦ Atypical anxiolytics are the most commonly used medications for GAD in the elderly population.
▦ Typical anxiolytics are used with caution in the elderly.
▦ Patients should avoid consuming alcohol while taking any of these medications.
▦ Use with caution in patients with history of seizure disorders.
▦ Avoid abrupt withdrawal of this class of drug. Dosage should be tapered down prior to discontinuation.
▦ Monitor closely for clinical worsening and suicide risk.

REFERENCE

Inouye, S. K., Foreman, M. D., Mion, L. C., Katz, K. H., & Cooney, L. M. (2001). Nurses' recognition of delirium and its symptoms. *Archives of Internal Medicine, 161,* 2467–2473.

BIBLIOGRAPHY

American Psychiatric Association. (1999). Practice guideline for the treatment of patients with delirium. *American Journal of Psychiatry, 156*(5 Suppl), 1–20. Retrieved from http://www.psychiatryonline.com/pracGuide/loadGuidelinePdf.aspx?file = DeliriumPG05–15–06.

American Psychiatric Association (2000). *Diagnostic and statistical manual of mental disorders* (4th ed., text rev.). Washington, DC: American Psychiatric Press.

American Psychiatric Association. (2013). *Diagnostic and statistical manual of mental disorders* (5th ed.). Washington, DC: American Psychiatric Press.

Bourne, R. S., Tahir, T. A., Borthwick, M., & Sampson, E. L. (2008). Drug treatment of delirium: Past, present and future. *Journal of Psychosomatic Research, 65*(3), 273–282.

Chu, J. A., Frey, L. M., Ganzel, B. L., & Matthews, J. A. (1999). Memories of childhood abuse: Dissociation, amnesia, and corroboration. *American Journal of Psychiatry, 156*, 749–755.

Greenaway, M. C., Hanna, S. M., Lepore, S. W., & Smith, G. E. (2008). A behavioral rehabilitation intervention for amnesic mild cognitive impairment. *American Journal of Alzheimer's Disease and Other Dementias, 23*(5), 451–461.

Harrison, M., & Williams, M. (2007). The diagnosis and management of transient global amnesia in the emergency department. *Emergency Medicine Journal, 24*(6), 444–445.

Litaker, D., Locala, J., Franco, K., Bronson, D. L., & Tannous, Z. (2001). Preoperative risk factors for postoperative delirium. *General Hospital Psychiatry, 23*, 84–89.

Michaud, M., Bula, C., Berney, A., Camus, V., Voellinger, R., Stiefel, F., & Burnand, B. The Delirium Guidelines Development Group. (2007). Delirium: Guidelines for general hospitals. *Journal of Psychosomatic Research, 62*, 371–383.

Owen, D., Paranandi, B., Sivakumar, R., & Seevaratnam, M. (2007). Classical diseases revisited: Transient global amnesia. *Postgraduate Medical Journal, 83*(978), 236–239.

Pantoni, L., Bertini, E., Lamassa, M., Pracucci, G., & Inzitari, D. (2005). Clinical features, risk factors, and prognosis in transient global amnesia: A follow-up study. *European Journal of Neurology, 12*(5), 350–356.

Simeon, D., Guralnik, O., Knuntelska, M., & Schmeidler, J. (2002). Personality factors associated with dissociation: Temperament, defenses, and cognitive schemata. *American Journal of Psychiatry, 159*, 489–491.

Swedish Council on Technology Assessment in Health Care. (2008). *Dementia— Etiology and epidemiology: A systematic review* (Vol. 1). Stockholm, Sweden: Elanders Infologistics. Retrieved from http://www.sbu.se/en/.

Wilmo, A., Winblad, B., Aguero-Torres, H., & von Stauss, E. (2003). *The magnitude of dementia occurrence in the world*. Stockholm, Sweden: Aging Research Center.

WEB RESOURCES

- Alzheimer's Disease and Dementia/Alzheimer's Association: http://www.alz.org/index.asp/
- Family Caregiver Alliance: http://www.caregiver.org/caregiver/jsp/home.jsp/
- Family Caregiver Alliance: http://www.caregiving.org/members/
- American Psychiatric Association: http://www.psych.org/
- Freedom from Fear: http://www.freedomfromfear.org/

Chapter 9

Substance Use Disorders

Substance Use Disorder

BACKGROUND INFORMATION

Definition of Disorder
- Substance use disorder is a maladaptive pattern of substance use.
- The substance used poses a hazard to health.

Classes of Psychoactive Substances
- Alcohol
- Amphetamines/stimulants
- Caffeine
- Cannabis
- Cocaine
- Hallucinogens
- Inhalants
- Nicotine
- Opioids
- Phencyclidine (PCP)
- Sedatives, hypnotics, and anxiolytics

Etiology
- No single theory can explain the cause of substance abuse/dependence.
- Theoretical causes
  - Genetics
  - Biochemical
  - Psychopathological
    - Developmental influences
    - Personality traits
  - Social learning
    - Parental role modeling
    - Cultural and/or ethnic influences

Demographics

▪ Males are twice as likely to be affected than females.
▪ Young adults (aged 18–24 years) have high prevalence rates for use of all substances.
▪ More than 100 million Americans, aged 12 years or older, report illicit drug use at least once in their lives.
▪ Fifty to seventy-five percent of those with a mental health disorder struggle with substance addiction.
▪ More than 70% of the AIDS cases among women are drug related.
▪ Over 100,000 deaths in a year in the United States are caused by excessive alcohol consumption.
▪ Approximately 1 in 10 Americans has an alcohol problem.
▪ Marijuana is the most commonly abused illicit substance in the United States.

Risk Factors

▪ Unemployment
▪ Poor social coping skills
▪ History of emotional, physical, or sexual abuse
▪ Chaotic home environment
▪ History of mental illness
▪ Untreated physical pain
▪ Family history of addiction
▪ Peer pressure
▪ Educational level
▪ Economic status
▪ Recent incarceration

Common comorbidities: other substance use disorders, adolescent conduct disorder, adult antisocial personality disorder

DIAGNOSIS

Differential Diagnosis

Rule out medical problems that may mimic signs and symptoms of substance intoxication and/or withdrawal:

▪ Hypoglycemia
▪ Medication-induced intoxication
▪ Electrolyte (sodium, potassium, chloride, and sodium bicarbonate) imbalance
▪ Head injury/trauma
▪ Stroke
▪ Psychosis
▪ Neurological disorder

ICD-10 Code

Diagnostic codes for substance use are classified according to substance. The following code is for unknown substances: F19.99 = unspecified other (or unknown) substance-related disorder.

Diagnostic Workup
▩ Diagnosis of substance abuse/dependence is typically made by detailed subjective history.
▩ Blood, saliva, breath, or urine screening for substance(s).

Initial Assessment
▩ Medical history and examination
▩ Psychiatric history and examination
▩ Family and social history
▩ Cultural history related to substance use
▩ Detailed history of past and present substance use, tolerance, and withdrawal
▩ How do the substances affect the patient mentally and physically?
▩ How is the substance use affecting the patient's occupational, family, or social life?
    ▩ CAGE (cut down, annoyed, guilty, and eye opener) screening questionnaire to assess alcohol dependence
    ▩ SMAST (Short Michigan Alcoholism Screening Test), screening tool for alcohol use
    ▩ CIWA-Ar (Clinical Institute Withdrawal Assessment for Alcohol) is a validated 10-item assessment tool to evaluate alcohol withdrawal symptoms
    ▩ COWS (Clinical Opiate Withdrawal scale), assessment tool to evaluate opioid withdrawal symptoms

Clinical Presentation
Signs and symptoms will vary with individuals/substances used, but include

▩ Sudden weight loss/gain
▩ Periods of excessive sleep or inability to sleep
▩ Periods of excessive energy
▩ Chronic nosebleeds
▩ Chronic sinusitis
▩ Chronic cough or bronchitis
▩ Increased periods of agitation, irritability, or anger
▩ Depressed mood
▩ Temporary psychosis
▩ Interpersonal difficulties
▩ Inability to fulfill roles at work, home, or school

DSM-5 Diagnostic Guidelines
▩ Substance used in larger amounts and/or for a longer period of time than intended
▩ Persistent desire or unsuccessful attempts to cut down or control use of substance
▩ Much time is spent engaging in activities to obtain, use, or recover from the substance
▩ Presence of craving, or a strong desire or urge to use the substance
▩ Recurrent use of substance despite failure to fulfill role obligations at home, work, or school
▩ Recurrent use of the substance in situations in which use is physically hazardous
▩ Continued use despite persistent or recurrent social or interpersonal problems that are caused or worsened by the substance use
▩ Major social, recreational, or occupational activities are relinquished or reduced due to the substance use
▩ Continued use of substance despite awareness of psychological and/or physiological health problems that likely resulted from or are exacerbated by the substance use

TREATMENT OVERVIEW

Psychosocial Therapy
- Cognitive behavioral therapy (CBT)
- Motivational enhancement therapy (MET)
- Behavioral therapy
- Psychotherapy

Psychopharmacotherapy
- Treatment of withdrawal states
- Alcohol withdrawal symptoms cause clinically significant distress resulting from autonomic hyperactivity, anxiety, and gastrointestinal symptoms. Alcohol withdrawal is a life-threatening condition that can result in alcohol withdrawal delirium, tonic–clonic seizures, and in some cases, death.
- Medication to decrease reinforcing effects of substance(s)
- Maintenance medication management (agonist therapy)
- Medication for relapse prevention
- Treatment of comorbid conditions

Self-Help Groups
- Alcoholics Anonymous (AA)
- Narcotics Anonymous (NA)
- Cocaine Anonymous (CA)

Pharmacological Treatment for Use of Specific Substances
- Nicotine
  - Nicotine replacement: patch, gum, spray, lozenge, and inhaler
  - Bupropion (Wellbutrin)
  - Varenicline (Chantix)
- Alcohol
  - Symptoms of withdrawal may occur within 4 to 12 hours after cessation or reduction.
  - Thiamine replacement and fluids are given.
  - Electrolytes (and glucose—if indicated if symptoms of Wernicke's, only after thiamine is administered first), folic acid, and magnesium supplements may be given as well.
  - Benzodiazepine (BZD) is initiated using either "symptom triggered" dosing or "fixed dosing"—there are advantages to the first in that the dose is administered based on CIWA-Ar and patient receives an individualized dose. BZDs manage seizure risk and also minimize the withdrawal. Only specific BZDs are indicated—not all.
  - Clonidine (Catapres) may be given as needed for hypertensive episode due to withdrawal.
  - Naltrexone (Revia, Vivitrol, oral or intramuscular [IM]) or acamprosate (Campral) is given to decrease craving.
  - Disulfiram (Antabuse) is a deterrent to drinking.
- Marijuana
  - No recommended pharmacological treatment
- Cocaine
  - Pharmacological treatment is not indicated

Drug Selection Table for Managing Substance Abuse

CLASS	DRUG
Nicotinic receptor agonists	Nicotine, nicotine transdermal system, nicotine polacrilex *(Nicotrol NS, Nicotrol Inhaler, Commit, Habitrol, Nicoderm, Nicotrol ProStep, Nicorette Gum, Nicorette DS)*, varenicline (Chantix)
Opioid antagonists	Naltrexone hydrochloride *(Revia, Vivitrol)*
Substance abuse deterrents	Disulfiram *(Antabuse)* acamprosate calcium *(Campral)*
Vitamins	B-Complex *(Vitamin B₁/Thiamine)*
Norepinephrine/dopamine reuptake inhibitors (NDRIs)	Bupropion (Wellbutrin, Zyban)

- ▓ Opioids
  - ▓ Opioid overdose: naloxone is given to reverse respiratory depression.
  - ▓ Maintenance treatment: methadone (Dolophone Methadose) or buprenorphine (Subutex) is gradually tapered.
  - ▓ Alternative maintenance: naltrexone (Revia, Vivitrol)

Substance Dependence

In *DSM-5*, Substance Abuse and Substance Dependence are combined under Substance Use Disorder.

BACKGROUND INFORMATION

Definition of Disorder
- ▓ There is a distinction between abuse and dependence.
- ▓ Tolerance to substance is examined.
- ▓ Leads to withdrawal when substance is eliminated or significantly reduced.

Classes of Psychoactive Substances
- ▓ Alcohol
- ▓ Amphetamines
- ▓ Cannabis
- ▓ Cocaine
- ▓ Hallucinogens
- ▓ Inhalants
- ▓ Nicotine
- ▓ Opioids
- ▓ PCP
- ▓ Sedatives, hypnotics, and anxiolytics

Etiology
- ▓ No single theory can explain the cause of substance abuse/dependence
- ▓ Theoretical causes
  - ▓ Genetics

- Biochemical
- Psychopathological
  - Developmental influences
  - Personality traits
  - Social learning
- Parental role modeling
- Cultural and/or ethnic influences

Demographics
- Males are twice as likely to be affected than females.
- The use of illegal drugs is most common in young adults (aged 18–25 years).
- More than 100 million Americans, aged 12 years or older, report illicit drug use at least once in their lives.
- About 50% to 75% of people with a mental health disorder struggle with substance addiction.
- More than 70% of the AIDS cases among women are drug related.
- More than 100,000 deaths in the United States each year are caused by excessive alcohol consumption.
- Approximately, 1 in 10 Americans has an alcohol problem.
- Marijuana is the most commonly abused illicit substance in the United States.

Risk Factors
- Unemployment
- Poor social coping skills
- History of emotional, physical, or sexual abuse
- Chaotic home environment
- History of mental illness
- Untreated physical pain
- Family history of addiction
- Peer pressure
- Educational level
- Economic status
- Recent incarceration

DIAGNOSIS

Differential Diagnosis
Rule out medical problems that may mimic signs and symptoms of substance intoxication and/or withdrawal:

- Hypoglycemia
- Drug interactions
- Electrolyte imbalance (sodium, potassium, chloride, and bicarbonate);
- Head injury/trauma
- Stroke
- Psychosis
- Neurological disorder

ICD-10 Code
Diagnostic codes for substance use are classified according to the substance. The following codes are for unknown substances:

Substance Abuse (F19.18)

Substance Dependence (F19.28)
Substance Withdrawal (F10.30)
Substance Intoxication (F10)

Diagnostic Workup
▦ Diagnosis of substance abuse/dependence is typically made by detailed subjective history
▦ Blood, breath, or urine screening for substance(s)

Initial Assessment
▦ Medical history and examination
▦ Psychiatric history and examination
▦ Family and social history
▦ Cultural history related to substance use
▦ Detailed history of past and present substance use, tolerance, and withdrawal
▦ How do the substances affect the patient mentally and physically?
▦ How is the substance use affecting the patient's occupational, family, or social life?
▦ CAGE questionnaire or SMAST, a screening tool for alcohol use
▦ CIWA-Ar, an assessment tool to evaluate alcohol withdrawal symptoms
▦ COWS, an assessment tool to evaluate opioid withdrawal symptoms.

Clinical Presentation
Signs and symptoms will vary with individuals/substances used, but include
▦ Sudden weight loss/gain
▦ Periods of excessive sleep or inability to sleep
▦ Periods of excessive energy
▦ Chronic nosebleeds
▦ Chronic sinusitis
▦ Chronic cough or bronchitis
▦ Increased periods of agitation, irritability, or anger
▦ Depressed mood
▦ Temporary psychosis
▦ Inability to perform tasks at work, school, or home

DSM-5 Diagnostic Guidelines
▦ Maladaptive pattern of substance use may occur.
▦ Characterized by behavioral and physiological symptoms:
　▦ Physical dependence is due to tolerance to substance being used
　▦ Psychological dependence, overwhelming desire to repeat use of substance to achieve desired effect.

TREATMENT FOR SUBSTANCE DEPENDENCE

▦ Psychosocial therapy
　▦ CBT
　▦ MET
　▦ Behavioral therapy
　▦ Psychotherapy

▨ Psychopharmacotherapy
  ▨ Treat withdrawal states.
  ▨ Give medication to decrease reinforcing effects of substance(s).
  ▨ Maintenance medication management (agonist therapy)
  ▨ Give medication for relapse prevention.
  ▨ Treat comorbid conditions.
▨ Self-help group therapy

OVERVIEW OF PSYCHOPHARMACOTHERAPY FOR SPECIFIC SUBSTANCES

▨ Nicotine
  ▨ Nicotine replacement: patch, gum, spray, lozenge, and inhaler
  ▨ Bupropion (Wellbutrin)
  ▨ Varenicline (Chantix)
▨ Alcohol
  ▨ Symptoms of withdrawal may occur within 4 to 12 hours after cessation or reduction
  ▨ Thiamine replacement and fluids
  ▨ BZD tapered to prevent withdrawal
  ▨ Clonidine (Catapres) as needed for hypertensive episode due to withdrawal
  ▨ Naltrexone (Nalorex; oral or IM) or acamprosate (Campral) to decrease craving
  ▨ Disulfiram (Antabuse) as deterrent to drinking
▨ Marijuana
  ▨ No pharmacological treatment is recommended.
▨ Cocaine
  ▨ Pharmacological treatment is not indicated.
  ▨ Topiramate (Topamax), disulfiram (Antabuse), or modafinil (Provigil) with psychosocial treatment may be effective.
▨ Opioids
  ▨ Opioid overdose: naloxone is given to reverse respiratory depression.
  ▨ Maintenance treatment: methadone (Dolophone) or buprenorphine (Subutex) is gradually tapered.
  ▨ Alternative maintenance: naltrexone (Revia, Vivitrol, Nalorex).

Drug Selection Table for Substance Dependence

CLASS	DRUG
Nicotine replacement therapy	
	Nicotine, nicotine transdermal system, nicotine polacrilex (*Nicotrol NS, Nicotrol Inhaler, Commit, Habitrol, Nicoderm, Nicotrol ProStep, Nicorette Gum, Nicorette DS*)
Benzodiazepines (BZDs)	
	Chlordiazepoxide (*Librium*)
	Diazepam (*Valium*)
	Lorazepam (*Ativan*)

(continued)

Drug Selection Table for Substance Dependence (*continued*)

CLASS	DRUG
Partial opioid agonists	
	Buprenorphine HO (*Subutex*)
	Buprenorphine HCl and naloxone HCl dihydrate (*Suboxone*)
	Methadone HCl (*Methadose*)
Alpha-agonists	
	Clonidine (*Catapres, Catapres-TTS*)
Anticholinergic drugs	
	Dicyclomine (*Bentyl*)
NSAIDs	
	Ibuprofen (*Motrin*)
Antidiarrheal drugs	
	Loperamide (*Imodium*)
Opioid antagonists	
	Naltrexone (*Revia*)
Alcohol antagonists	
	Disulfiram (*Antabuse*)
Substance abuse deterrents	
	Acamprosate calcium (*Campral*)
Vitamins	
	B-Complex (*Vitamin B$_1$/Thiamine Hydrochloride*)
Antidepressants	
	Bupropion HCl (*Wellbutrin, Zyban*)
Nicotinic receptor agonists	
	Varenicline (*Chantix*)

NSAIDs, nonsteroidal anti-inflammatory drugs.

Recurrence Rate
▓ Rate of relapse, for those who have been in treatment, is approximately 90%.
▓ Majority of relapses take place within 3 months following treatment.

PATIENT EDUCATION

▓ Educate on importance of joining a support group. Information is available online for worldwide support groups, including NA, AA, and CA.
▓ Teach about relapse prevention. Encourage CBT to increase coping skills and individual therapy to enhance personal insight.

▨ Patients taking disulfiram (Antabuse) must be advised to avoid alcohol and any substances that contain alcohol. This includes mouthwash, colognes, cough syrups, and so forth.

MEDICAL/LEGAL PITFALLS

▨ Rates of suicide are three to four times more prevalent in those who abuse alcohol or drugs as compared to the general population.
▨ Individuals withdrawing from substances are at great risk for depression. When not properly treated, depression can lead to suicide.
▨ Individuals being treated for addiction may have a history of seeing multiple health care professionals to obtain medications ("doctor shopping"). Such practices may lead to accidental and/or intentional overdose.

Intoxication

BACKGROUND INFORMATION

Definition of Disorder
▨ An altered, reversible physical or mental state due to the use of substance
▨ A physical and mental state of euphoria, exhilaration, or excitement occurs

Classes of Psychoactive Substances
▨ Alcohol
▨ Amphetamines
▨ Cannabis
▨ Cocaine
▨ Hallucinogens
▨ Inhalants
▨ Opioids
▨ PCP
▨ Sedatives, hypnotics, and anxiolytics

DIAGNOSIS

Differential Diagnosis
Rule out medical problems that may mimic signs and symptoms of substance intoxication and/or withdrawal:

▨ Hypoglycemia
▨ Electrolyte (sodium, potassium, chloride, and sodium bicarbonate) imbalance
▨ Head injury/trauma
▨ Stroke
▨ Psychosis
▨ Neurological disorder

ICD-10 Codes

Note: Use the code that applies to the class of substances, but include name of specific substance. ICD-10 code for intoxication depends on whether or not there is a comorbid substance use disorder. If there is no comborbid substance use disorder, use F15.929.

Mental and behavioral disorders due to use of alcohol (F10.)
Mental and behavioral disorders due to use of opioids (F11.)
Mental and behavioral disorders due to use of cannabinoids (F12.)
Mental and behavioral disorders due to use of sedative hypnotics (F13.)
Mental and behavioral disorders due to use of cocaine (F14.)
Mental and behavioral disorders due to use of other stimulants, including caffeine
    (F15.)
Mental and behavioral disorders due to use of hallucinogens (F16.)
Mental and behavioral disorders due to use of tobacco (F17.)
Mental and behavioral disorders due to use of volatile solvents (F18.)
Mental and behavioral disorders due to multiple drug use and use of other psychoactive substances (F19.)

For substance intoxication for substances that are not included in any other class, use code for "other substance intoxication" 292.89 (F19.929) and include name of the substance.

If the substance is unknown, use the code for "other" or unknown (F19.929).

Diagnostic Workup

■ Diagnosis of substance abuse/dependence is typically made by detailed subjective history
■ Blood, breath, or urine screening for substance(s)

Initial Assessment

■ Medical history and examination
■ Psychiatric history and examination
■ Family and social history
■ Cultural history related to substance use
■ Detailed history of past and present substance use, tolerance, and withdrawal
■ How do the substances affect the patient mentally and physically?
■ How is the substance use affecting the patient's occupational, family, or social life?
■ CAGE questionnaire or SMAST, a screening tool for alcohol use
■ CIWA-Ar, an assessment tool to evaluate alcohol withdrawal symptoms
■ COWS, an assessment tool to evaluate opioid withdrawal symptoms

Clinical Presentation

Signs and symptoms will vary with individuals/substances used, but include

■ Slurred speech
■ Poor psychomotor coordination
■ Impairment in attention and concentration
■ Nystagmus
■ Stupor or coma
■ Pupil changes

DSM-5 Diagnostic Guidelines
- Reversible syndrome is due to recent exposure to the substance.
- Clinically significant and maladaptive psychological and behavioral changes occur, affecting the CNS.

TREATMENT OVERVIEW FOR SUBSTANCE USE

- Psychosocial
  - CBT
  - MET
  - Behavioral therapy
  - Psychotherapy
- Pharmacological
  - Treat withdrawal states.
  - Give medication to decrease reinforcing effects of substance(s).
  - Maintenance medication management (agonist therapy)
  - Give medication for relapse prevention.
  - Give treatment of comorbid conditions.
- Self-help groups
  - AA
  - NA
  - CA

Pharmacological Treatment for Use of Specific Substances
- Nicotine
  - Nicotine replacement: patch, gum, spray, lozenge, and inhaler
  - Bupropion (Wellbutrin)
  - Varenicline (Chantix)
- Alcohol
  - Symptoms of withdrawal may occur within 4 to 12 hours after cessation or reduction.
  - Thiamine replacement and fluids
  - BZD is tapered to prevent withdrawal.
  - Clonidine (Catapres) is used as needed for a hypertensive episode caused by withdrawal.
  - Naltrexone (Revia, Vivitrol, Nalorex; oral or IM) or acamprosate (Campral) is used to decrease craving.
  - Disulfiram (Antabuse) is a deterrent to drinking.
- Marijuana
  - No recommended pharmacological treatment
- Cocaine
  - Pharmacological treatment is not indicated.
  - Topiramate (Topamax), disulfiram (Antabuse), or modafinil (Provigil) with psychosocial treatment may be effective.
- Opioid
  - Opioid overdose: naloxone is used to reverse respiratory depression.
  - Maintenance treatment: methadone (Dolophone) or buprenorphine (Subutex) is gradually tapered.
  - Alternative maintenance: naltrexone (Revia, Vivitrol, Nalorex).

Recurrence Rate
- Rate of relapse for those who have been in treatment is approximately 90%.
- Majority of relapses take place within 3 months following treatment.

PATIENT EDUCATION

- Educate on importance of joining a support group. Information is available online for worldwide support groups, including NA, AA, and CA.
- Teach about relapse prevention. Encourage CBT to increase coping skills and individual therapy to enhance personal insight.
- Patients taking disulfiram (Antabuse) must be advised to avoid alcohol and any substances that contain alcohol. This includes mouthwash, colognes, cough syrups, and so forth.

MEDICAL/LEGAL PITFALLS

- Rates of suicide are three to four times more prevalent in those who abuse alcohol or drugs as compared to the general population.
- Individuals withdrawing from substances are at great risk for depression. When not properly treated, depression can lead to suicide.
- Individuals being treated for addiction may have a history of seeing multiple health care professionals to obtain medications ("doctor shopping"). Such practices may lead to accidental and/or intentional overdose.

Substance Withdrawal

BACKGROUND INFORMATION

Definition of Disorder
- Physiological and cognitive changes occur with cessation or reduction of substance. Follows period of heavy or prolonged drug use.

Classes of Psychoactive Substances
- Alcohol
- Amphetamines
- Caffeine
- Cannabis
- Cocaine
- Hallucinogens
- Inhalants
- Nicotine
- Opioids
- PCP

DIFFERENTIAL DIAGNOSIS FOR SEDATIVES, HYPNOTICS, AND ANXIOLYTICS

Rule out medical problems that may mimic signs and symptoms of substance intoxication and/or withdrawal:

- Hypoglycemia

- Drug interactions
- Electrolyte (sodium, chloride, potassium, sodium bicarbonate) imbalance
- Head injury/trauma
- Stroke
- Psychosis
- Neurological disorder

ICD-10 Codes
Mental and behavioral disorders due to use of alcohol (F10.)
Mental and behavioral disorders due to use of opioids (F11.)
Mental and behavioral disorders due to use of cannabinoids (F12.)
Mental and behavioral disorders due to use of sedative hypnotics (F13.)
Mental and behavioral disorders due to use of cocaine (F14.)
Mental and behavioral disorders due to use of other stimulants, including caffeine (F15.)
Mental and behavioral disorders due to use of hallucinogens (F16.)
Mental and behavioral disorders due to use of tobacco (F17.)
Mental and behavioral disorders due to use of volatile solvents (F18.)
Mental and behavioral disorders due to multiple drug use and use of other psychoactive substances (F19.)

Diagnostic Workup
- Diagnosis of substance abuse/dependence is typically made via a detailed subjective history.
- Blood, breath, or urine are screened for substance(s).

Initial Assessment
- Medical history and examination
- Psychiatric history and examination
- Family and social history
- Cultural history related to substance use
- Detailed history of past and present substance use, tolerance, and withdrawal
- How do the substances affect the patient mentally and physically?
- How is the substance use affecting the patient's occupational, family, or social life?
- CAGE questionnaire or SMAST, a screening tool for alcohol use
- CIWA-Ar, an assessment tool to evaluate alcohol withdrawal symptoms
- COWS, an assessment tool to evaluate opioid withdrawal symptoms

Clinical Presentation
Signs and symptoms will vary with individuals/substances used, but include

- CNS depressants:
  - Restlessness, anxiety
  - Sleep disturbances
  - Diaphoresis
  - Vital changes: increase in BP heart rate, and temperature
- CNS stimulants:
  - Depressed mood, fatigue
  - Anxiety
  - Intense cravings
- Opioids:
  - Runny nose

- Diaphoresis
- Yawning
- Anxiety
- Intense cravings
- Vital changes: increase in BP and pulse
- Muscle and bone pain
- Abdominal cramps
- Tremors
- Nausea, vomiting, and diarrhea

DIAGNOSIS

Definition of Substance Withdrawal
- Substance-specific syndrome is due to cessation or reduction of substance use that has been heavy and/or prolonged.
- Syndrome produces significant clinical distress or diminished functioning.

Treatment for Substance Abuse or Dependence
- Psychosocial
  - CBT
  - MET
  - Behavioral therapy
  - Psychotherapy
- Pharmacological
  - Treat withdrawal states.
  - Use medication to decrease reinforcing effects of substance(s).
  - Maintenance medication management (agonist therapy)
  - Use medication for relapse prevention.
  - Treat comorbid conditions.
- Self-help groups
  - AA
  - NA
  - CA

Pharmacological Treatment for Use of Specific Substances
- Nicotine
  - Nicotine replacement: patch, gum, spray, lozenge, and inhaler
  - Bupropion (Wellbutrin)
  - Varenicline
- Alcohol
  - Symptoms of withdrawal may occur within 4 to 12 hours after cessation or reduction.
  - Thiamine replacement and fluids
  - BZD is tapered to prevent withdrawal.
  - Clonidine (Catapres) is used as needed for a hypertensive episode caused by withdrawal.
  - Naltrexone (Revia, Vivitrol, Nalorex; oral or IM) or acamprosate (Campral) is used to decrease craving.
  - Disulfiram (Antabuse) is a deterrent to drinking.

▓ Marijuana
  ▓ No pharmacological treatment is recommended.
▓ Cocaine
  ▓ Pharmacological treatment is not indicated.
  ▓ Topiramate (Topamax), disulfiram (Antabuse), or modafinil (Provigil) with psychosocial treatment may be effective.
▓ Opioid
  ▓ Opioid overdose: naloxone is used to reverse respiratory depression.
  ▓ Maintenance treatment: methadone (Dolophone) or buprenorphine (Subutex) is gradually tapered.
  ▓ Alternative maintenance: naltrexone (Revia, Vivitrol, Nalorex).

Recurrence Rate
▓ Rate of relapse for those who have been in treatment is approximately 90%.
▓ Majority of relapses take place within 3 months following treatment.

PATIENT EDUCATION

▓ Educate on importance of joining a support group. Information is available online for worldwide support groups, including NA, AA, and CA.
▓ Teach about relapse prevention. Encourage CBT to increase coping skills and individual therapy to enhance personal insight.
▓ Patients taking disulfiram (Antabuse) must be advised to avoid alcohol and any substances that contain alcohol. This includes mouthwash, colognes, cough syrups, and so forth.

MEDICAL/LEGAL PITFALLS

▓ Rates of suicide are two to three times more prevalent in those who abuse alcohol or drugs as compared to the general population.
▓ Individuals withdrawing from substances are at greater risk for depression. When not properly treated, depression can lead to suicide.
▓ Individuals being treated for addiction may have a history of seeing multiple health care professionals to obtain medications ("doctor shopping"). Such practices may lead to accidental and/or intentional overdose.

Substance-/Medication-Induced Mental Disorders

Usually temporary, but can be severe CNS syndromes that develop as a result of substance use (both illicit and legal) and exposure to toxins.

May be induced by
▓ Alcohol
▓ Amphetamines
▓ Caffeine
▓ Cannabis
▓ Cocaine

▪ Hallucinogens
▪ Inhalants
▪ Nicotine
▪ Opioids
▪ PCP
▪ Sedatives, hypnotics, and anxiolytics

A variety of medications are used to treat medical and psychiatric conditions. Substance-induced mental disorders are described in relevant chapters.

Common characteristics of substance-induced mental disorders:

▪ Clinically significant presentation of a mental disorder, which (a) developed during or within 1 month of substance use, intoxication, or withdrawal *and* (b) substance/medication is capable of producing disorder
▪ Disorder not better explained by an independent mental disorder.
▪ Disorder does not occur only during delirium.
▪ Evidence of clinically significant impairment in social, occupational, or other areas of functioning

ICD-10 Codes

CM—single code combines substance-induced mental disorder with the substance use disorder.

Mental and behavioral disorders due to use of alcohol (F10.)
Mental and behavioral disorders due to use of opioids (F11.)
Mental and behavioral disorders due to use of cannabinoids (F12.)
Mental and behavioral disorders due to use of sedative hypnotics (F13.)
Mental and behavioral disorders due to use of cocaine (F14.)
Mental and behavioral disorders due to use of other stimulants, including caffeine (F15.)
Mental and behavioral disorders due to use of hallucinogens (F16.)
Mental and behavioral disorders due to use of tobacco (F17.)
Mental and behavioral disorders due to use of volatile solvents (F18.)
Mental and behavioral disorders due to multiple drug use and use of other psychoactive substances (F19.)

BIBLIOGRAPHY

American Psychiatric Association. (2006). *Practice guidelines for the treatment of patients with substance use disorders* (2nd ed.). Retrieved February 10, 2009, from http://www.Psychiatryonline.com/contenc.aspx?aID=14079

American Psychiatric Association. (2013). *Diagnostic and statistical manual of mental disorders* (5th ed.). Washington, DC: American Psychiatric Press.

Cleary, M., Hunt, G. E., Matheson, S. L., Siegfried, N., & Walter, G. (2008). Psychosocial interventions for people with both severe mental illness and substance misuse. *Cochrane Database of Systematic Reviews*, (1).

Ferri, M. M. F., Amato, L., & Davoli, M. (2006). Alcoholics Anonymous and other 12-step programmes for alcohol dependence. *Cochrane Database of Systematic Reviews*, (3).

Gowing, L., Ali, R., & White, J. M. (2006). Buprenorphine for the management of opioid withdrawal. *Cochrane Database of Systematic Reviews*, (2).

Naegle, M. (2008). Substance misuse and alcohol use disorders. In E. Capezuti, D. Zwicker, M. Mezey, & T. Fulmer (Eds.), *Evidence-based geriatric nursing protocols for best practice* (3rd ed., pp. 649–676). New York, NY: Springer Publishing Company.

Substance Abuse and Mental Health Services Administration. (2007). *2007 National survey on drug use & health: National results.* Retrieved February 13, 2009, from http://www.oas.samhsa.gov/nsduh/2k7nsduh/2k7Results.cfm#TOC

Vaz de Lima, F. B., da Silveira, D. X., & Andriolo, R. B. (2008). Effectiveness and safety of topiramate for drug dependents (Protocol). *Cochrane Database of Systematic Reviews*, (4), 431–435.

WEB RESOURCE

■ The Substance Abuse and Mental Health Services Administration: http://www.samhsa.gov/

Chapter 10

Psychotic Disorders

Brief Psychotic Disorder

BACKGROUND INFORMATION

Definition of Disorder
- Sudden onset of psychotic symptoms occurs.
- These include delusions, hallucinations, disorganized speech, or grossly disorganized or catatonic behavior.
- Episode lasts from 1 day to less than 1 month, with return to premorbid level of functioning.
- Symptoms may or may not meet the definition of schizophrenia.

Etiology
- Often precipitated by extremely stressful life events
- Cause is unknown.
- Patients with personality disorder may have predisposition toward development of psychotic symptoms.
- May have prevalence of mood disorders in family
- May have poor coping skills along with secondary gains for psychotic symptoms.
- May have defense against a prohibited fantasy, fulfillment of unattained wish, or escape from a distasteful situation.

Demographics
- Brief psychotic disorder is generally considered uncommon.
- More likely to occur in young rather than older patients
- It generally first occurs in early adulthood (ages: 20s and 30s) and is more common in women than in men.
- More frequent in lower socioeconomic classes
- Patient may have prior personality disorder.
- May predispose to survivors of disasters or major cultural changes.

Risk Factors
- Major life events that cause significant emotional stress
- Severity must be in relation to the patient's life.

Age
■ Young rather than old; most frequent in people in their 30s and 40s.

Gender
■ No differentiation, although women may be affected more than men.

Family History
More common in families with history of mood (bipolar) disorders. This suggests a genetic link.

Stressful Events in Susceptible People
■ Usually follows life-altering stressor
■ May present after series of less overtly stressful events
■ Stressor could be unrelated to the psychotic episode.
■ Paranoia is often predominant.

DIAGNOSIS

Differential Diagnosis
■ Factitious disorder with mainly psychological symptoms
■ Malingering
■ Psychotic disorder with medical causation
■ Substance-induced psychotic disorder
■ Seizure disorders
■ Delirium
■ Dissociative identity disorder
■ Borderline personality disorder symptoms
■ Schizotypal personality disorder symptoms

ICD-10 Codes
Brief Psychotic Disorder (F23)

Diagnostic Workup
■ Always includes at least one major symptom of psychosis
■ Delusions with rapidly changing delusional topics
■ Abrupt onset occurs
■ Affective symptoms, confusion, and impaired attention are presented
■ Emotional lability is observed.
■ Inappropriate dress or behavior is seen.
■ Patient is screaming or mute.
■ Impaired recent memory.
■ Organic workup includes complete blood count (CBC) with differentials; complete serum chemistry; thyroid function studies; and thyroid stimulating hormone, serum alcohol, and illegal substance levels (including anabolic steroids, cannabis, alcohol, tobacco, termazepam, opium, heroine/morphine, and methamphetamines).
■ No imaging studies are required to diagnose brief psychotic disorder.

Initial Assessment
- Medical history is obtained.
- Psychiatric history is obtained.
- In-depth mental status examination (a careful mental status examination can distinguish this disorder from delirium, dementia, or other organic brain syndromes, such as meningitis, transient ischemic attack, and epilepsy) is done.
- Family history is obtained.
- History may need to be obtained from significant others in acutely ill patients.
- Symptoms are observed.

Clinical Presentation
- Psychotic symptoms are seen, most likely paranoia.
- Sudden onset occurs.
- May not include entire spectrum of schizophrenia
- Mood variability occurs.
- Reactive confusion
- Reactive depression
- Impaired attention span
- Reactive excitation
- Screaming or silence
- Impaired short-term memory
- Changes in sleep or eating habits, energy level, or weight
- Inability to make decisions
- Garish style of dress

DSM-5 Diagnostic Guidelines
- Sudden onset of at least one psychotic symptom (i.e., delusions, hallucinations, disorganized speech, or grossly disorganized or catatonic behavior) occurs.
- Psychotic episodes *last less than 1 month and are followed by a full recovery*. This disorder can occur in the presence or absence of a major stressor.
- Diagnosis can only be made if other medical or psychiatric disorders have been excluded.

TREATMENT OVERVIEW

Acute Treatment
- In the acute phase, inpatient hospitalization may be necessary for safety and evaluation. This includes close monitoring of symptoms and assessment of danger to self and others.
- Mental status examination: patients usually present with severe psychotic agitation that may be associated with strange or bizarre behavior, uncooperativeness, physical or verbal aggression, disorganized speech, screaming or muteness, labile or depressed mood, suicidal and/or homicidal thoughts or behaviors, restlessness, hallucinations, delusions, disorientation, impaired attention, impaired concentration, impaired memory, poor insight, and poor judgment.
- A quiet, structured hospital setting may assist in regaining reality.

- Administration of antipsychotic medication as indicated, is most frequently a high-potency dopamine receptor antagonist. Conventional (typical) antipsychotic medications most commonly used in this disorder include haloperidol (Haldol) and chlorpromazine (Thorazine). Thorazine is used less frequently now due to the QTc risks.
- Newer medications, called atypical antipsychotic drugs, are used.
- Benzodiazepine medication may be given to patients who present or are at high risk for excitation, as they also are beneficial in the treatment of brief psychosis. Lorazepam (Ativan) or diazepam (Valium) may be used if the person has a very high level of anxiety or insomnia.
- While waiting for the pharmaceutical effects to take effect, one-to-one, seclusion, or physical restraint of the patient may be necessary for safety.
- If symptoms are only minimally impairing the patient's function and a specific stressor is identified, removing the stressor should suffice.
- Further inpatient care is unnecessary once the acute attack has ended.

Chronic Treatment

- Following the resolution of the episode, hypnotic medications may be useful.
- Long-term use of medications should be avoided. If maintenance medications are necessary, reevaluation of the diagnosis is indicated.
- Individual, family, and group psychotherapies are essential to integrate the experience psychologically into the lives of the patient and/or significant others.
- Therapies should include discussion of the precipitating stressors, the psychotic episode itself, and development of successful coping strategies. Sessions should be at least weekly, once the patient is discharged from the hospital, and last 6 to 8 weeks or longer.
- The length of acute and residual symptoms is usually less than a week.
- Depressive symptoms may present following cessation of psychosis.
- Risk for suicide can escalate in the postpsychotic depressive stage.

Recurrence Rate

Good prognosis can be predicted if:

- Prior good adjustment occurs
- Few premorbid schizoid tendencies occur
- The precipitating stressor is severe
- Onset of symptoms is sudden
- Affective symptoms are present
- During acute phase, manifestation of confusion and bewilderment is seen
- Minimal affective blunting occurs
- There is a short duration of symptoms
- There is an absence of schizophrenic relatives

In general, 50% to 80% of all patients have no further major psychiatric episodes.

PATIENT EDUCATION

- Information for patients and families is available in easy-to-understand language at www.webmd.com.
- Signs, symptoms, and treatment information can be obtained from www.healthline.com.

- Data on foundations and support groups are available at www.organizedwisdom .com.
- The National Alliance on Mental Illness—at www.nami.org—is the government-sponsored organization for information regarding mental illness.
- Specific information regarding this disorder is presented at www.medicinenet .com/brief psychotic disorder.

There is no known way to prevent brief psychotic disorder. However, early diagnosis and treatment can help decrease the disruption to the person's life, family, and friendships. Both the patient and the family must be educated about the illness and the potential adverse effects of the medications.

MEDICAL/LEGAL PITFALLS

Risk of suicide or harm to others may occur if no immediate safety measures are taken:

- Misdiagnosis may be the result of symptoms similar to those of other psychiatric/ medical disorders. General recommendations include serious consideration of medical causes in any acute-onset new psychosis. This does not necessarily mean ordering every possible test; but history and the physical examination often alert the clinician to the need for additional medical evaluation.
- Physical or chemical restraints may be necessary in cases of severe uncontrolled agitation to provide safety to self and/or others.

Delusional Disorder

BACKGROUND INFORMATION

Definition of Disorder
- Delusions can include paranoia, grandiosity, erotica, jealousy, somatic, and mixed responses.
- Incorrect inference about external reality persists despite the evidence to the contrary, and these beliefs are not ordinarily accepted by other members of the person's culture or subculture.

Etiology
- Cause is unknown.
- Distinction between schizophrenia and mood disorders is seen.
- Onset occurs later in life.
- Predominance varies depending on source reviewed.
- Increased prevalence occurs with personality traits of suspiciousness, jealousy, and secretiveness.
- Relatively stable diagnosis, with less than a quarter of delusional patients rediagnosed as schizophrenic and less than 10% as mood disordered, can be made.
- Delusional disorder may involve the limbic system or basal ganglia when intact cerebral cortical function is present.

Demographics
▨ Prevalence in the United States is estimated to be 0.025% to 0.03%.
▨ Annually, new cases account for one to three cases per 100,000 people.
▨ Four percent of all first admissions to psychiatric hospitals are for psychoses not due to a general medical condition or substance.
▨ Average age of onset is 40 years, with a range from 18 through the 90s.
▨ Slightly more females than men are affected.
▨ Many patients are married or employed.
▨ Some association with recent immigration or low socioeconomic status, celibacy among men, and widowhood among women is noted.
▨ Because of poor insight into their pathological experiences, patients with delusional disorder may rarely seek psychiatric help and often may present to internists, surgeons, dermatologists, police officers, and lawyers rather than to psychiatric professionals.
▨ Men are more likely than women to develop paranoid delusions; women are more likely than men to develop delusions of erotomania.
▨ Patients often do not present for treatment, and thus they do not commonly make themselves available for research studies.

Risk Factors
Age
▨ Eighteen to forty years

Gender
▨ Slightly more males than females

Family History
▨ A hostile family environment is observed, usually with an overcontrolling mother and a distant or sadistic father.

Stressful Events in Susceptible People
▨ Social isolation
▨ Less-than-expected levels of achievement
▨ Hypersensitivity
▨ Specific ego function, including reaction formation, projection, and denial
▨ Distrust in relationships evolving from hostility, abuse

Having Another Mental Health Disorder
▨ May have a mood component, but not severe enough to be classified as a mood disorder.

DIAGNOSIS

Differential Diagnosis
▨ Delusions can transpire simultaneously, with many medical and neurological illnesses.
▨ Most common sites for lesions are the basal ganglia and limbic system.
▨ Toxicology screening and routine lab studies, including CBC with differential, serum chemistries, and thyroid function, are done.

- Differs from malingering and factitious disorder
- Separated from schizophrenia by the absence of other schizophrenic symptoms and nonbizarre qualities of delusions, impairment of functioning
- Differs from depressive disorders in that somatic features are not pervasive
- Differences from somatoform disorders, due to which patients with delusional disorders cannot admit their symptoms, do not exist.
- In differentiating delusional disorder from paranoid personality disorder, it is necessary to determine the distinction between extreme suspiciousness and delusion. If in doubt that a symptom is a delusion, diagnosis of delusional disorder should not be made.

ICD-10 Code
Bipolar and Depressive Disorders (F22)

Diagnostic Workup
By psychiatric presentation:

- Olfactory or tactile hallucinations may be prominent but only if they are related to the content of the delusion.
- This disorder is unlike schizophrenia in that it has (a) no prominent auditory or visual hallucinations, (b) no thought disorder, (c) no significant flattening of affect, (d) psychosocial functioning is not markedly impaired, and (e) behavior is not obviously odd or bizarre.
- The delusions have lasted longer than any associated depression or mania.
- Laboratory studies: toxicology screening, CBC with differential, serum chemistries, and thyroid function studies (triiodothyronine [T3], thyroxine [T4], thyroid-stimulating hormone [TSH]).
- Computed tomography (CT) scan of the brain is done to visualize the lesions.

Initial Assessment
- Psychiatric history and presentation are assessed to establish whether pathology is present.
- Determining the presence or absence of important characteristics often associated with delusions is important.
- Delusional disorder should be seen as a diagnosis of exclusion.
- Medical history is obtained.
- Veracity of symptoms should be checked before automatically considering the content to be delusional.
- Assessment of homicidal or suicidal ideation is extremely important in evaluating patients with delusional disorder. The presence of homicidal or suicidal thoughts related to delusions should be actively screened for and the risk of carrying out violent plans should be carefully assessed.

Clinical Presentation
Mental status examination reveals patients as usually well-groomed and remarkably normal except for the specific delusional system:

- Patients may attempt to engage clinicians to agree with their delusions.
- Moods and affects are congruent with the delusions.

- No significant hallucinations occur unless strictly pertaining to the delusions presented.
- Disordered thought content is the primary symptom.
- Delusions are characterized as being possible and may be simple or complex.
- Sudden onset occurs.
- Below-average intelligence is seen.
- Intact memory and orientation
- No insight
- Poor impulse control

DSM-5 Diagnostic Guidelines
- No prominent auditory or visual hallucinations
- No thought disorder
- No significant flattening of affect
- Psychosocial functioning is not markedly impaired.
- Behavior is not obviously odd or bizarre.
- Delusions have lasted longer than any associated depression or mania.

TREATMENT OVERVIEW

Acute Treatment
- Hospitalization should be considered if a potential for harm or violence exists.
- A complete neurological and medical workup may be indicated to determine an organic cause for the symptoms.
- Delusional disorder is challenging to treat for various reasons, including patients' frequent denial that they have any problem, especially of a psychological nature, difficulties in developing a therapeutic alliance, and social/interpersonal conflicts.
- Avoiding direct confrontation of the delusional symptoms enhances the possibility of treatment compliance and response.
- Treatment of delusional disorder often involves both psychopharmacology and psychotherapy.
- Polypharmacy is common, most often including a combination of antipsychotic and antidepressant medications. No difference in response is noted between typical and atypical antipsychotic agents.
- Antidepressants, particularly the selective serotonin reuptake inhibitors (SSRIs), have been successfully used for the treatment of the somatic-type delusional disorder.
- Establishing a therapeutic alliance, establishing acceptable symptomatic treatment goals, and educating the patient's family are of paramount importance.
- Avoiding direct confrontation of the delusional symptoms enhances the possibility of treatment compliance and response.
- Outpatient treatment is preferred.

PSYCHOPHARMACOLOGY OF DELUSIONAL DISORDER

Atypical antipsychotic drugs are used as a first-line treatment of delusional disorder with success.

Owing to their more tolerable side effect profile, atypical antipsychotics are prescribed more frequently than conventional or typical antipsychotic medications. However, recent studies have not confirmed atypical drugs to be better than conventional antipsychotics in the treatment of delusional disorder. Lower doses of antipsychotic medications are used with delusional disorder than with schizophrenia. Most commonly used atypical antipsychotic drugs are all labeled by the Food and Drug Administration (FDA) with similar indications. Begin treatment usually in low doses. Clozapine (*Clozaril*) has also been used for treatment-resistant cases with some success but requires close monitoring owing to the potential side effect of agranulocytosis.

- *Typical (conventional) antipsychotic drugs that may be* used for the treatment of delusional disorder include the following:
  - Haloperidol (*Haldol*) and pimozide (*Orap*). Until recently, pimozide was touted as the drug of choice for delusional disorder; more recent evidence suggests no difference in improvement with pimozide and other antipsychotics. Also, the evidence suggests no difference in improvement between atypical and conventional antipsychotics in the treatment of patients with delusional disorder.
- If patients fail to respond to drug monotherapy, low-dose combination therapy using drugs from different pharmacological classes may be employed. Depressive symptoms, if present, may be treated with antidepressants. SSRIs have proven helpful with somatic-type delusions.
- Delusional disorder is difficult to treat due to the individual's frequent denial of any existing problem, difficulties in establishing a therapeutic alliance, and social/interpersonal conflicts. Nonetheless, recent evidence suggests that 50% of individuals who are adequately treated recover and 90% demonstrate at least some improvement.
- Somatic delusions seem to be more responsive to antipsychotic therapy than the other types of delusions and persecutory delusions respond less well (50% improvement rates with no reports of complete recovery).
- Psychotherapy or cognitive behavioral therapy (CBT) may be helpful, either as monotherapy or in combination with an antipsychotic agent.
  - Some form of supportive therapy is helpful with the goal of facilitating treatment adherence, providing education about the illness and treatment, providing social skills training, minimizing risk factors that increase symptoms, and providing realistic guidance in dealing with problems resulting from the illness.
  - CBT may be helpful to individuals with delusional disorder of the persecutory type by helping them to identify maladaptive thoughts and replacing them with alternative, more adaptive attributions.
  - Social skills training directed toward increasing the individual's control and promoting interpersonal competence has also been found to be helpful.
  - Insight-oriented therapy may be indicated rarely and even contraindicated according to the literature. Nonetheless, there are reports of successful treatment with the goals of the development of a therapeutic alliance, containment of projected negative feelings, and development of creative doubt in the internal perception of the negative worldview.

Drug Selection Table for Delusional Disorder

CLASS	DRUG
Antipsychotic drugs, atypical (second generation)	First-line drug therapy:
	Olanzapine (*Zyprexa, Relprevv long-acting formulation of zyprexa injection*)
	Risperidone (*Risperdal, Risperdal Consta*)
	Clozapine (*Clozaril, Fazaclo*)
Antipsychotic drugs, typical (first generation)	Second-line drug therapy:
	Haloperidol (*Haldol*)
	Pimozide (*Orap*)
Selective serotonin reuptake inhibitors	First-line drugs sometimes helpful for somatic delusions:
	Fluoxetine (*Prozac, Sarafem*)
	Sertraline (*Zoloft*)
	Escitalopram (*Lexapro*)

Chronic Treatment
- The chronic nature of delusional disorders suggests treatment strategies should be tailored to the individual needs of the patients and focus on maintaining social function and improving quality of life.
- For most patients with delusional disorder, some form of supportive therapy is helpful. The goals of supportive therapy include facilitating treatment adherence and providing education about the illness and its treatment.
- Educational and social interventions can include social skills training (e.g., not discussing delusional beliefs in social settings) and minimizing risk factors.
- Providing realistic guidance and assistance in coping with problems stemming from the delusional system may be very helpful.
- Cognitive therapeutic approaches may be useful for some patients by identifying delusional thoughts and then replacing them with alternative, more adaptive ones.
- It is important that goals be attainable, because a patient who feels pressured or repeatedly criticized by others will probably experience stress that may lead to a worsening of symptoms.
- Insight-oriented therapy is rarely indicated.

Recurrence Rate
- Delusional disorder has a relatively good prognosis when adequately treated: 52.6% of the patients recover, 28.2% achieve partial recovery, and 19.2% do not improve.
- Less than 25% of all cases are later diagnosed with schizophrenia.
- Less than 10% develop mood disorders.
- Good prognosis is predicted with high levels of occupational and social functioning, female gender, onset before age 30, sudden onset, and short duration of illness.

PATIENT EDUCATION

▨ Educating the family about the symptoms and course of the disorder is helpful. This is especially true as the family frequently feels the impact of the disorder the most.

▨ In addition to being involved with seeking help, family, friends, and peer groups can provide support and encourage the patient to regain his or her abilities.

MEDICAL/LEGAL PITFALLS

▨ Patients with delusional disorder are more susceptible to becoming dependent on alcohol, tobacco, and drugs.

▨ It is not uncommon for people with delusional disorder to make repeated complaints to legal authorities.

▨ Patients with delusional disorder may encounter legal or relationship problems as a result of acting on their delusions.

▨ In patients with delusional disorder who may be dangerous civil commitment focuses on preventing harm to self or others.

Schizoaffective Disorder

Definition of Disorder

▨ A diagnosis midway between the diagnosis of schizophrenia and bipolar I disorder.

▨ An individual has a mixture of psychotic and depressive/manic/mixed episode(s) that fail to meet the diagnostic criteria for either schizophrenia or bipolar I disorder.

▨ This disorder is not caused by a drug, medication, or general medical illness.

▨ The bipolar type of schizoaffective disorder is more common in younger patients, whereas the depressive type is more common in older patients.

▨ Individuals with this disorder have a better prognosis than individuals with schizophrenia but a worse prognosis than individuals with bipolar I disorder.

Etiology

▨ May either be a type of schizophrenia or a mood disorder, or both occurring at the same time, or not related to either

▨ May encompass bipolar and depressive types and may have a genetic component

▨ Relatives of the persons with the depressed type of schizoaffective disorder have a higher incidence of also having schizoaffective disorder.

▨ There is a tendency to respond to lithium and have a better course outcome.

▨ Balance of dopamine and serotonin in the brain may contribute to development of the disease. Other theories consider that it may be due to in utero exposure to viruses, malnutrition, or even birth complications.

▨ Abnormalities of the neurotransmitters serotonin, norepinephrine, and/or dopamine could all contribute to this disorder.

Demographics

▨ There is a lifetime prevalence rate of less than 1%.

▨ Diagnosis may be used when the clinician is unsure of the classification of symptoms.

▨ The prognosis for patients with schizoaffective disorder is thought to be between that of patients with schizophrenia and that of patients with a mood disorder, with the prognosis better for schizoaffective disorder than for schizophrenic disorder but worse than for a mood disorder alone.

▨ The incidence of suicide is estimated to be 10%. Whites have a higher rate of suicide than African Americans. Immigrants have higher suicide rates than natives.

▨ As in other psychiatric disorders, women attempt suicide more than men, but men complete suicide more often.

▨ Schizoaffective disorder affects more women than men, with more women in the depressive type as compared with the bipolar type.

▨ A poor prognosis in patients with schizoaffective disorder is generally associated with a poor premorbid history, an insidious onset, no precipitating factors, a predominant psychosis, negative symptoms, an early onset, an unremitting course, or having a family member with schizophrenia.

Risk Factors
Age

▨ Young people with schizoaffective disorder tend to have a diagnosis with the bipolar subtype, whereas older people tend to have the depressive subtype.

▨ Age of onset is later in women than in men.

Gender

▨ Prevalence is lower in men, and occurs less often in married women.

▨ Men with schizoaffective disorder may exhibit antisocial behavior and flat or inappropriate affect.

Family History

▨ Patients may have a genetic predisposition

▨ Inconsistent study results, although relatives with the depressed type may be at higher risk of acquiring the disorder; stressful events in the lives of susceptible people may trigger the disorder.

▨ No studies provide data on having another disorder.

▨ Not studied

DIAGNOSIS

Differential Diagnosis
Evaluate Medical Medications

▨ All mood and schizophrenic disorders should be considered in the differential diagnosis of schizoaffective disorder.

▨ Testing is done for use of amphetamines, phencyclidines (PCPs), hallucinogens, cocaine, alcohol, and steroids, as these can present with similar symptoms.

▨ Seizure disorders of the temporal lobe can mimic schizoaffective signs, as can HIV/ autoimmune deficiency syndrome, hyperthyroidism, neurosyphilis, delirium, metabolic syndrome, or narcolepsy.

ICD-10 Codes
Schizophrenia (F20.89)
Schizoeffective Disorder (F29.9)

Diagnostic Workup

▦ Schizoaffective disorder must meet *DSM-5* criteria for components of schizophrenia and mood disorders (depressed) concurrently.

▦ Delusions or hallucinations for at least 2 weeks may be seen in the absence of mood symptoms. Major mood episode must be present for a majority of the disorder's total duration.

▦ Laboratory studies include sequential multiple analysis, CBC, rapid plasma reagent, thyroid function, drug and alcohol screens, lipid panel, enzyme-linked immunosorbent assay (ELISA) test results, and the Western Blot test.

▦ If the patient's neurologic findings are abnormal, computed tomography or magnetic resonance imagery may be ordered to rule out any suspected intracranial pathology. Findings include decreased amounts of cortical gray matter and increased fluid-filled spaces.

Initial Assessment

▦ Medical workup, including neurological history and evaluation of laboratory data

▦ Psychiatric assessment, including mental status examination and history.

▦ Mental status examination may reveal appearances ranging from well groomed to disheveled; possible psychomotor agitation or retardation; euthymic, depressed, or manic mood; eye contact ranging from appropriate to flat affect; speech that ranges from poverty to flight of ideas or pressured; suicidal or homicidal ideation may or may not be present; presence of delusions and/or hallucinations.

▦ Psychological testing may assist with diagnosis and in rating the severity of the disease. These scales may be useful in assessing the patient's progress: Positive and Negative Symptoms Scale (PANSS), Hamilton Depression Scale, and Young Mania Scale. The CAGE questionnaire (cut down, annoyed, guilty, and eye opener) is helpful in determining alcohol consumption in patients with schizoaffective disorder.

Clinical Presentation: Symptoms

▦ All the signs and symptoms of schizophrenia, manic episodes, and depressive disorders occur.

▦ Symptoms can appear in concert or alternating.

▦ May be mood incongruent, which has a poor prognosis.

▦ Suicidal ideation or attempt(s) may occur.

DSM-5 Diagnostic Guidelines

▦ An uninterrupted period of illness occurs during which a major depressive episode, a manic episode, or a mixed episode occurs with symptoms that meet criteria for schizophrenia. The major depressive episode must include a depressed mood.

▦ Symptoms that meet the criteria for mood episodes are present for a substantial portion of the active and residual periods of the illness.

▦ The disturbance is not the direct physiologic effect of a substance (e.g., illicit drugs, medications) or a general medical condition.

▦ The bipolar type is diagnosed if the disturbance includes a manic or a mixed episode (or a manic or mixed episode and a major depressive episode).

▦ The depressive type is diagnosed if the disturbance includes only major depressive episodes.

TREATMENT OVERVIEW

Acute Treatment

▨ The major treatments include inpatient psychiatric hospitalization, medication, and psychosocial therapies. Inpatient treatment is mandatory for patients who are dangerous to themselves or others and for patients who cannot take care of themselves.

▨ Activity should be restricted if patients represent a danger to themselves or to others.

▨ Psychopharmacologic treatment involves use of antipsychotics to treat aggressive behavior and psychosis, along with antidepressants, and/or mood stabilizers. Agent selection depends on whether the depressive or manic subtype is present.

▨ In the depressive subtype, combinations of antidepressants plus an antipsychotic are used.

▨ In refractory cases, clozapine (Clozaril, FazaClo ODT) has been used as an antipsychotic agent. In the manic subtype, combinations of mood stabilizers plus an antipsychotic are used.

▨ Early treatment with medication along with good premorbid functioning often improves outcomes.

PSYCHOPHARMACOLOGY OF SCHIZOAFFECTIVE DISORDER

Overview

▨ *Second-generation (atypical) antipsychotics* are the first-line treatment for schizoaffective disorder.

▨ Consistent evidence has demonstrated that risperidone (*Risperdal*), olanzapine (*Zyprexa*), quetiapine (*Seroquel*), ziprasidone (*Geodon*), aripiprazole (*Abilify*), asenapine (*Saphris*), and paliperidone (*Invega*) are efficacious in the treatment of global psychopathology and the positive symptoms of the schizophrenic spectrum disorders, including schizoaffective disorder. Less consistent evidence has demonstrated that the negative symptoms improve as well.

▨ *Second-line treatment:* First-generation (typical or conventional) antipsychotics; although haloperidol (*Haldol*) was previously regarded as a first-line treatment for patients with schizoaffective disorder, it is now regarded as a second- or third-line treatment since atypical antipsychotics generally have a more tolerable side effect profile.

▨ In addition to an antipsychotic agent, antidepressant medications may be prescribed for the depressive symptoms. Mood stabilizers may be used to treat mixed symptoms occurring in schizoaffective disorder. Any of the SSRIs may be used for the depressive symptoms, but the most evidence available is for fluoxetine (*Prozac*).

▨ Lithium (*Eskalith, Lithobid*, lithium carbonate) has proven helpful as an adjunct to the antipsychotic agents. It has limited effectiveness as monotherapy in treating schizoaffective disorders. When combined with an antipsychotic agent, lithium augments the antipsychotic response in general, and negative symptoms specifically.

▨ Valproate (*Depakote*) studies have reported positive and negative results. Although the evidence base is limited because most studies have few patients, one study compared valproate (*Depakote*) with olanzapine (*Zyprexa*), valproate (*Depakote*) with risperidone (*Risperdal*), olanzapine (*Zyprexa*) with placebo, and risperidone (*Risperdal*) with placebo and concluded that the valproate (*Depakote*) groups improved significantly more rapidly over the first 2 weeks of treatment than the antipsychotic group alone.

- CBT, modified for this population, focuses on symptom management, symptom recovery in acute psychosis, relapse prevention, and early intervention. Patients are taught coping strategies, attention switching or attention narrowing, especially useful for dealing with hallucinations, modified self-statements and internal dialog, reattribution, awareness training, de-arousing techniques, increased activity levels, social engagement and disengagement, and reality-testing techniques.
- Electroconvulsive therapy (ECT) has been suggested as a treatment for resistant schizoaffective disorders; however, the evidence has been limited to case studies and uncontrolled studies. In general, antipsychotic treatment alone has produced better outcomes than ECT.
- Emphasis is being placed on early identification of any of the schizophrenic spectrum disorders, including schizoaffective disorders. Earlier identification allows for earlier intervention and not requiring patients and/or families to reach a high threshold of risk, disruption, or deterioration before accessing treatment. There is evidence that if symptoms are treated prior to the onset of a psychotic episode, full-blown consequences (such as schizoaffective disorder or schizophrenia) may be delayed or even prevented.

Drug Selection Table for Schizoaffective Disorder

CLASS	DRUG
Antipsychotic drugs, atypical (second generation)	First-line drug therapy:
	Aripiprazole (*Abilify, Abilify Discmelt ODT, Abilify Liquid, Abilify IM injection, long-acting Abilify once monthly injection*)
	Clozapine (*Clozaril, Fazaclo*)
	Olanzapine (*Zyprexa* Relprevv
	Risperidone (*Risperdal, Risperdal Consta*)
	Quetiapine (*Seroquel, Seroquel XR*)
	Ziprasidone (*Geodon, Geodon IM injection*)
	Paliperidone (*Invega*, Invega Sustenna long acting)
	Asenapine (*Saphris*)
Antipsychotic drugs, typical (first generation)	Second-line drug therapy:
	Haloperidol (*Haldol*)
	Fluphenazine (*Prolixin*)
Selective serotorin reuptake (SSRIs)	Adjunct treatment for mood or depression:
	Fluoxetine (*Prozac*)
	Paroxetine (*Paxil*)
	Sertraline (*Zoloft*)
Mood stabilizers	Adjunct treatment for mood; also approved for bipolar/mania, includes carbamazepine, lamotrigine—same as depakote:
	Lithium (*Eskalith, Lithobid, lithium carbonate*)
	Valproate (*Depakote*: divalproex = depakote ER tablets, and the regular delayed-release) tablet

IM, intramuscular.

Chronic Treatment

■ Patients who have schizoaffective disorder can benefit greatly from psychotherapy as well as psychoeducational programs and regularly scheduled outpatient medication management.

■ When making the transition to outpatient, stressing the importance of medication compliance is crucial.

■ If possible, select once-daily or long-acting medications to help with patient compliance.

■ Therapy is most effective if it involves their families, develops their social skills, and focuses on cognitive rehabilitation.

■ Psychotherapies should include supportive therapy and assertive community therapy in addition to individual and group forms of therapy and rehabilitation programs.

■ Family involvement is needed in the treatment of this particular disorder.

■ Treatment includes education about the disorder and its treatment, family assistance in compliance with medications and appointments, and maintenance of structured daily activities.

■ Otherwise, encourage patients who are schizoaffective to continue their normal routines and strengthen their social skills whenever possible.

Recurrence Rate

■ A good outcome is predicted in the presence of a good premorbid history, acute onset, a specific precipitating factor, few psychotic symptoms, a short course, and no family history of schizophrenia.

■ The prognosis for patients with schizoaffective disorder is thought to lie between that of patients with schizophrenia and that of patients with a mood disorder. Therefore, the prognosis is better with schizoaffective disorder than with a schizophrenic disorder but worse than with a mood disorder alone.

■ Individuals with the bipolar subtype are thought to have a prognosis similar to those with bipolar type I, whereas the prognosis of people with the depressive subtype is thought to be similar to that of people with schizophrenia.

■ Overall, determination of the prognosis is difficult.

PATIENT EDUCATION

■ Discuss compliance with patients as well as with family members. Always discuss all the risks, benefits, adverse effects, and alternatives of each medication.

■ Stress-reduction techniques are employed to prevent relapse and possible rehospitalization.

■ Education should also include social skills training and cognitive rehabilitation.

■ Family education should involve reducing of expressed emotions, criticism, hostility, or overprotection of the patient.

MEDICAL/LEGAL PITFALLS

■ Patients with schizoaffective disorder often lack judgment and insight into their illness. They commonly refuse to continue the medications started in the hospital after they are discharged. Noncompliance may also be the result of adverse effects of the medication, such as sedation and weight gain.

- Patients may begin to feel better as a result of their medications and believe that they no longer need to take them. This thinking leads to discontinuation of the medication and can result in rehospitalization.
- Be familiar with local mental health laws as patients with schizoaffective disorder, who represent a danger to self or others or are unwilling to seek help on a voluntary basis, may need to be committed for further evaluation and treatment.
- If nonadherence with medications is an issue, a court order may be necessary to "to treat the patient over his/her objection."
- Physical restraints may also be indicated for protection of self and/or others.

Schizophrenia

BACKGROUND INFORMATION

Definition of Disorder
- This is a chronic, severe, and disabling brain disorder characterized by disordered thoughts, delusions, hallucinations, and bizarre or catatonic behavior.

Etiology
- Several genes are found to be strongly associated with schizophrenia. However, genes alone are not sufficient to cause this disorder.
- Imbalance of the neurotransmitters dopamine and glutamate (and possibly others) are found to play a role in schizophrenia.
- Scientists believe that interactions between genes and the environment are necessary to develop schizophrenia. Environmental risk factors (e.g., exposure to viruses or malnutrition in the womb, problems during birth) and psychosocial factors (e.g., stressful conditions) are found to increase the risk of schizophrenia.
- Research shows that schizophrenia is hereditary. People who have first-degree relatives (a parent, sibling) or second-degree relatives (grandparents, aunts, uncles, cousins) with this disorder develop schizophrenia more often than the general population. The identical twin of a person with schizophrenia has the highest risk (40%–65%) of developing this disorder.

Demographics
- Schizophrenia occurs in 1% of the general population.
- Schizophrenia affects men and women equally and occurs at similar rates in all ethnic groups worldwide.
  - Patients with schizophrenia are found to abuse alcohol and/or drugs more often than the general population. Abusing a substance can reduce the effectiveness of treatment.
  - Patients with schizophrenia are more likely to be addicted to nicotine as compared with the general population (75%–90% vs. 25%–30%).
  - Patients may need higher doses of psychotropic medication if they smoke and dose reductions for some antipsychotics on cessation of smoking. Nicotine replacement does not mitigate the metabolic consequences of cessation.
  - Patients with schizophrenia attempt suicide much more often than people in the general population; approximately 10% succeed, especially among young adult males.

Risk Factors

Age

- In men, onset of symptoms typically emerges in the late teens and early 20s and in women, in the mid-20s to early 30s.
- Psychotic symptoms seldom occur after age 45 years and only rarely before puberty (although cases of schizophrenia in children as young as 5 years have been reported).

Gender

- The prevalence of schizophrenia among men and women is about the same.
- Pregnancy can worsen mental health in a subset of women with schizophrenia. Women are found to be especially susceptible for acute exacerbation of symptoms in the postpartum period.
- Compared to men, women tend to experience more pronounced mood symptoms.
- The gender differences in course and outcome are probably due to the effect of estrogen in women before menopause.

Family History

- Patients with immediate family members diagnosed as schizophrenic have approximately a 10% risk of developing the disorder.

Factors Associated With Birth

- Infants who experience a complication while in mothers' wombs or who experience trauma during delivery are at higher risk for developing schizophrenia.
- Intrauterine viral infection may occur in the womb.

Environmental Stressors

- Environmental stressors are found to be associated with the development of schizophrenia, including problems with interpersonal relationships, difficulties at school/work, and substance abuse.

Substance Abuse

- Most researchers do not believe that substance abuse causes schizophrenia; however, patients with schizophrenia abuse alcohol and/or drugs more often than the general population.

DIAGNOSIS

Differential Diagnosis

- Psychotic disorder due to a general medical condition, delirium, or dementia
- Substance-induced psychotic disorder, substance-induced delirium, substance-induced persisting dementia, and substance-related disorders may be seen
- Brief psychotic disorder
- Delusional disorder
- Schizophreniform disorder
- Psychotic disorder may not be otherwise specified
- Schizoaffective disorder
- Mood disorder with psychotic features
- Mood disorder with catatonic features

- Depressive disorder may not be otherwise specified
- Bipolar disorder may not be otherwise specified
- Pervasive developmental disorders (e.g., autistic disorder)
- Childhood presentations combining disorganized speech (from a communication disorder) and disorganized behavior (from attention-deficit/hyperactivity disorder)
- Schizotypal personality disorder
- Schizoid personality disorder
- Paranoid personality disorder

ICD-10 Codes
Schizophrenia (F20)
   Schizotypal disorders (033)
Schizotypal disorders (F21)
   Delusional disorders (034)
Persistent delusional disorders (F22)
Acute and transient psychotic disorders (F23)
   Schizoaffective disorders (036)
Induced delusional disorders (F24)
   Acute and transient psychotic disorders (035)
Schizoaffective disorders (F25)
   Other nonorganic psychotic disorders (037)

Diagnostic Workup
Check for Drug Interactions
- Physical and mental status examination
- CBC, including hemoglobin, hematocrit, red blood cell (RBC) count, white blood cell (WBC) count, WBC differential count, and platelet count
- Hepatic and renal function tests, including alanine transaminase (ALT), aspartate transaminase (AST), alkaline phosphatase (ALP), blood urea nitrogen (BUN), and creatinine
- Thyroid function tests (T3, T4, and TSH)
- Electrolytes (potassium, chloride, sodium, bicarbonate), glucose, B_{12}, folate, and calcium level
- For patients with a history of suspicion, check for HIV, syphillis, ceruloplasmin, antinuclear antibody test, urine for culture and sensitivity and/or drugs of abuse, and 24-hour urine collections for porphyrins, copper, or heavy metals
- Alcohol and drug screening
- Pregnancy test for female patients of childbearing age

Initial Assessment
- Current physical status and physical history
- Current mental status and mental health history, including symptoms patient experiences, how long patient has been having symptoms, when the symptoms started, how often the symptoms occur, when and where symptoms tend to occur, how long symptoms last, and what effect symptoms have on patient's ability to function
- Drug history including prescribed and over-the-counter drugs
- Safety needs

Clinical Presentation
■ Positive symptoms are extreme or exaggerated behaviors, including:
  ▪ Delusions (somatic, ideas of reference, thought broadcasting, thought insertion, and thought withdrawal)
  ▪ Hallucinations (visual, auditory, tactile, olfactory, and gustatory)
  ▪ Inappropriate or overreactive affect
■ Negative symptoms:
  ▪ Blunted or flat affect, unable to experience pleasure or express emotion (anhedonia)
  ▪ Inability to carry out goal-directed behavior (avolition)
  ▪ Limited speech (alogia)
  ▪ Lack of energy and initiative
  ▪ Poor coordination and self-care
■ Thought disorganization
  ▪ Abnormal thoughts
  ▪ Tangential, incoherent, or loosely associated speech.

DSM-5 Diagnostic Guidelines
■ The diagnosis is given if two Criterion A symptoms are present:
  ▪ Delusions
  ▪ Hallucinatons
  ▪ Disorganized speech
  ▪ Grossly disorganized or catatonic behavior
  ▪ Negative symptoms
    • The individual must have at least one of these three symptoms: delusions, hallucinations, and disorganized speech.
■ Continuous signs of the disturbance are exhibited for at least 6 months
■ Schizoaffective disorder and mood disorder have been excluded
■ Substance abuse and other general medical conditions have been excluded
■ Schizophrenia subtypes are defined by the predominant symptomatology at the time of evaluation. The five subtypes of schizophrenia are paranoid type, disorganized type, catatonic type, undifferentiated type, and residual type.
■ The first signs for the adolescent population may include drops in academic performance, changes of friends, sleep problems, or irritability. A diagnosis of schizophrenia can be difficult to make for members of this age group since many normal adolescents also exhibit these behaviors.

TREATMENT OVERVIEW

Acute Treatment
■ Inpatient treatment is necessary for patients with a serious suicidal or homicidal ideation and plan, whose behavior can unintentionally be harmful to self or others, who are incapable of providing self-care, or who are at risk for behavior that may lead to long-term negative consequences.
■ The goal of acute-phase treatment, usually lasting for 4 to 8 weeks, is to alleviate the most severe psychotic symptoms, such as agitation, frightening delusions, and hallucinations.

- Low-dose, high-potency antipsychotics have been found to be safe and effective in managing agitated psychiatric patients. For instance:
  - Haloperidol (Haldol) intramuscular (IM) is used to calm patients with moderately severe to very severe agitation. Subsequent doses may be needed within 1 hour depending on the responses.
  - Ziprasidone (Geodon) IM is recommended.
  - A low dose of a short-acting benzodiazepine (e.g., lorazepam [Ativan]) is also found to be effective in decreasing agitation during the acute phase and may reduce the amount of antipsychotic needed to control patients' psychotic symptoms.
  - Atypical (second generation) antipsychotic drugs are suggested to be used as a first-line treatment of schizophrenia because of their fewer side effects than conventional or typical antipsychotic medications.
  - ECT, in combination with antipsychotic medications, can be considered for patients with schizophrenia who do not respond to antipsychotic agents. The rate and number vary from patient to patient depending on clinical responses and side effects.
  - Substantial improvement of symptoms is seen in many patients by the 6th week of treatment. Providers may switch to other antipsychotic medications if patients are not responding to an adequate trial of a prescribed medication, are not able to tolerate a medication, or have poor medication adherence.

PSYCHOPHARMACOLOGY OF SCHIZOPHRENIA

- *Second-generation (atypical) antipsychotic drugs*: These are used as a first-line treatment of schizophrenia due to fewer side effects when compared to conventional or typical antipsychotic medications.
  - Commonly used *second-generation* atypical antipsychotic drugs include aripiprazole (*Abilify*), clozapine (*Clozaril*), olanzapine (*Zyprexa*), quetiapine (*Seroquel*), quetiapine fumarate (*Seroquel XR*), risperidone (*Risperdal*), long-acting risperidone (*Risperdal Consta*), ziprasidone (*Geodon*), and paliperidone (*Invega*). A newer atypical antipsychotic is asenapine (*Saphris* sublingual formulation) and is getting good reviews as effective for schizophrenia, especially if there is a mood component involved.
  - Clozapine (*Clozaril*) is the drug of choice for treatment-resistant schizophrenia (little or no symptomatic response to at least two antipsychotic trials of an adequate duration—at least 6 weeks—and at a therapeutic dose range) and it has a lower risk of tardive dyskinesia (TD). However, due to the potential side effect of agranulocytosis (loss of WBC), a blood test is required weekly for the first 6 months, and biweekly for the next 6 months. Monitoring can be done monthly if no hematological problems are found after 1 year of clozapine treatment.
- *First-generation (typical or conventional) antipsychotic drugs:*
  - Commonly used *first-generation* (typical or conventional) antipsychotic drugs: haloperidol (*Haldol*), fluphenazine (*Prolixin*), thioridazine (*Mellaril*), trifluoperazine (*Stelazine*).
  - Low-dose, high-potency antipsychotics such as haloperidol IM 2 to 5 mg have been found to be safe and effective in managing agitated psychiatric patients. Subsequent doses may be needed within 1 hr depending on responses.
- *Short-acting benzodiazepine*: A low dose of a short-acting benzodiazepine (e.g., lorazepam 0.5 to 2 mg every 1 hour IM or intravenous [IV] as needed no more than

2 mg every minute—maximum daily doses vary with diagnosis and condition;) is effective in decreasing agitation during the acute phase, and may reduce the amount of antipsychotic needed to control patients' psychotic symptoms.

▨ ECT in combination with antipsychotic medications can be considered for patients with schizophrenia who do not respond to antipsychotic agents. The rate and number of ECT varies from patient to patient depending on their clinical responses and side effects.

▨ Social skills training aimed to improve the way patients with schizophrenia interact with others (e.g., poor eye contact, odd facial expressions, inaccurate or lack of perceptions of emotions in other people) has been found to be effective in reducing relapse rate.

▨ CBT helps patients with schizophrenia acquire some insight into their illness and appears to be effective in reducing the severity of symptoms and decreasing the risk of relapse.

▨ Dialectical behavior therapy (DBT) combines cognitive and behavioral theories. Patients with schizophrenia may benefit from DBT to improve interpersonal skills.

▨ Individual psychotherapy focuses on forming a therapeutic alliance between therapists and patients with schizophrenia. A good therapeutic alliance is likely to help patients with schizophrenia remain in therapy, increase adherence to treatments, and have positive outcomes at 2-year follow-up evaluations.

▨ Personal therapy, a recently developed form of individual treatment, uses social skills and relaxation exercises, self-reflection, self-awareness, exploration of vulnerability and stress, and psychoeducation to enhance personal and social adjustment of patients with schizophrenia. Patients who receive personal therapy have shown better social adjustment and a lower rate of relapse after 3 years than those not receiving it.

▨ Many patients with schizophrenia benefit from art therapy because it helps them communicate with and share their inner word with others.

▨ Employment programs that include individualized job development, rapid placement, ongoing job supports, and integration of mental health and vocational services have been found to be effective in helping patients with schizophrenia to achieve employment (Table 10.3).

Chronic Treatment

▨ The treatment goals are to prevent relapse and to improve patient's level of functioning.

▨ It is estimated that 40% to 50% of patients are not adherent to treatment within 1 to 2 years. Long-acting medications are found to increase treatment adherence as compared to oral medications.

▨ It is important to monitor and manage side effects of antipsychotic medications, including extrapyramidal side effects (mostly common in patients treated with first-generation antipsychotics), tardive dyskinesia, sedation, postural hypotension, weight gain metabolic syndrome—including shifts in lipids and blood glucose—along with increased central adiposity, and disturbances in sexual function.

▨ If patients develop extrapyramidal symptoms, give benztropine or trihexyphenidyl or diphenhydramine as directed.

▨ For drug-induced dystonic reaction (especially of head and neck), give diphenhydramine (Benadryl) for pseudoparkinsonism reaction due to drug use, use trihexyphenidyl (Artane) or benztropine (Cogentin).

Drug Selection Table for Schizophrenia

CLASS	DRUG
Antipsychotic drugs, atypical (second generation)	**First-line drug therapy:** **Abilify Long Acting; Zyprexa Relprevv; Latuda** Aripiprazole (*Abilify, Abilify Discmelt ODT, Abilify Liquid, Abilify IM injection*) Clozapine (*Clozaril, Fazaclo*) Olanzapine (*Zyprexa*) Quetiapine (*Seroquel, Seroquel XR*) Risperidone (*Risperdal, Risperdal Consta*) Ziprasidone (*Geodon, Geodon IM injections*) Paliperidone (*Invega*) Asenapine (*Saphris*)
Antipsychotic drugs, typical (first generation)	**Second-line drug therapy:** Haloperidol (*Haldol*) Fluphenazine (*Prolixin*) Thioridazine (*Mellaril*) Trifluoperazine (*Stelazine*)
Benzodiazepines (BZDs)	**During acute phase:** Lorazepam (*Ativan*)

IM, intramuscular.

- The neuroleptic malignant syndrome (NMS), characterized by fever (hyperthermia), muscular rigidity, altered mental status, and autonomic dysfunction, is a rare but potentially fatal reaction to neuroleptic medications. If a parent has hyperthermia, or stops antipsychotic medications, give dantrolene and continue as needed until cumulative total dose is up to 10 mg/kg. After the acute phase, give dantrolene to prevent recurrence.
- Body mass index (BMI), fasting blood glucose, and lipid profiles are important health indicators to monitor since weight gain has occurred with most antipsychotic agents. It is recommended to weigh patients and check BMI for every visit for 6 months after a change in medications and abdominal girth.
- Clozapine (Clozaril, FazaClo ODT) is the drug of choice for treatment-resistant schizophrenia patients (little or no symptomatic response to at least two antipsychotic trials of an adequate duration [at least 6 weeks] and at a therapeutic dose range) and it has a lower risk of TD. However, due to the potential side effect of agranulocytosis (loss of WBCs), a blood test is required weekly for the first 6 months, and biweekly for the next 6 months. Monitoring can be done monthly if no hematological problems are found after 1 year of clozapine (Clozaril, FazaClo ODT) treatment.
- Social skills training, aimed at improving the way patients with schizophrenia interact with others (e.g., poor eye contact, odd facial expressions, inaccurate or lack of perceptions of emotions in other people), has been found to be effective in reducing the relapse rate.

■ CBT helps patients with schizophrenia to gain some insight into their illness and appears to be effective in reducing the severity of symptoms and decreasing the risk of relapse.

■ DBT combines cognitive and behavioral theories. Patients with schizophrenia may benefit from DBT to improve interpersonal skills.

■ Individual psychotherapy focuses on forming a therapeutic alliance between therapists and patients with schizophrenia. A good therapeutic alliance is likely to help patients with schizophrenia remain in therapy, increase adherence to treatments, and have positive outcomes at 2-year follow-up evaluations.

■ Personal therapy, a recently developed form of individual treatment, uses social skills and relaxation exercises, self-reflection, self-awareness, exploration of vulnerability and stress, and psychoeducation to enhance personal and social adjustment of patients with schizophrenia. Patients who receive personal therapy have shown better social adjustment and a lower rate of relapse after 3 years than those not receiving it.

■ Many patients with schizophrenia benefit from art therapy because it helps them communicate with and share their inner world with others.

■ Employment programs that include individualized job development, rapid placement, ongoing job supports, and integration of mental health and vocational services have been found to be effective in helping patients with schizophrenia to achieve employment.

■ Family-oriented therapies that help family and patients with schizophrenia understand the disorder and encourage discussions of psychotic episodes and events leading up to them may be effective in reducing relapses.

■ Treat patients for co-occurring substance abuse. Substance abuse is the most common co-occurring disorder in patients with schizophrenia. Integrated treatment programs for schizophrenia and substance use produce better outcomes.

■ Many studies show that integrating psychosocial and medication treatment produces the best results in patients with schizophrenia.

Recurrence Rate

The reported recurrence rates range from 10% to 60%; approximately 20% to 30% of patients with schizophrenia can have somewhat normal lives, 20% to 30% continue to experience moderate symptoms, and 40% to 60% of them remain significantly impaired for their entire lives.

PATIENT EDUCATION

■ Information regarding schizophrenia is available from the National Institutes for Mental Health website at http://www.nimh.nih.gov/health/ publications/schizophrenia/index.shtml.

■ Antipsychotic medications can produce dangerous side effects when taken with certain drugs. It is important for patients to tell health care providers about all medications, including over-the-counter medications, prescribed medications, vitamins, minerals, and herbal supplements that patients take. *Note*: Medications should be used with particular caution in children, pregnant/breastfeeding women, and older adults. *Note*: Black box warnings.

■ It is important to teach patients about the importance of medication adherence and to avoid using alcohol and other substances.

■ For excellent patient education resources, visit eMedicine's Mental Health and Behavior Center. See also eMedicine's patient education article on schizophrenia.

MEDICAL/LEGAL PITFALLS

■ Misdiagnosis
■ Patients with schizophrenia are addicted to nicotine at three times the rate of the general population (75%–90% vs. 25%–30%).
■ Approximately, 20% to 70% of patients with schizophrenia have a comorbid substance abuse problem, which is associated with increased violence, suicidality, nonadherence with treatment, hostility, crime, poor nutrition, and so forth.
■ Mental health providers should inform patients being treated with conventional antipsychotic medications about the risk of TD. AIMS (Abnormal Involuntary Movement Scale) is recommended for detecting TD early.
■ Patients with schizophrenia are found to have a higher risk for acquiring obesity, diabetes, cardiovascular disease, HIV, lung diseases, and rheumatoid arthritis. It is important for mental health care providers to monitor their physical conditions regularly.

Schizophreniform Disorder

BACKGROUND INFORMATION

Definition of Disorder
■ This is characterized by the presence of the principal symptoms of schizophrenia, including delusions, hallucinations, disorganized speech, disorganized or catatonic behavior, and negative symptoms.
■ An episode of the disorder (including prodromal, active, and residual phases) lasts at least 1 month but less than 6 months.

Etiology
■ The cause of schizophreniform disorder remains unknown.
■ Current biological and epidemiological data suggest that some of the schizophreniform patients are similar to those with schizophrenia, whereas others have a disorder similar to mood disorder.

Demographics
■ The lifetime prevalence rate of schizophreniform is 0.2%, and a 1-year prevalence rate is 0.1%.

Risk Factors
Age
■ Schizophreniform disorder is most common in adolescents and young adults.

Gender
■ The prevalence of schizophreniform disorder is equally distributed between men and women, with peak onset between the ages of 18 and 24 years in men and 24 and 35 years in women.

Family History
■ Studies show that relatives of individuals with schizophreniform disorder are at higher risk of having mood disorders than are relatives of individuals with schizophrenia.

▪ Relatives of individuals with schizophreniform disorder are more likely to have a psychotic mood disorder than are relatives of individuals with bipolar disorders.

DIAGNOSIS

Differential Diagnosis
▪ Schizophrenia
▪ Brief psychotic disorder
▪ Substance-induced psychotic disorder
▪ Bipolar disorder and major depression with mood-incongruent features

ICD-10 Codes
Sohizophreniform Disorder (F20.81)

Diagnostic Workup
Medical Medications (i.e., Steroids)
▪ Physical and mental status examination
▪ Electrolytes (potassium, chloride, and bicarbonate)
▪ Thyroid function tests (TSH, T3, and T4)
▪ Screen for alcohol and drugs, including amphetamines, methamphetamines, barbiturates, phenobarbital, benzodiazepines, cannabis, cocaine, codeine, cotinine, morphine, heroin, lysergic acid diethylamide (LSD), methadone, and PCP.

Initial Assessment
▪ Current physical status and physical history
▪ Current mental status and mental health history, including symptoms patient experiences, how long patient has been having symptoms, when the symptoms started, how often the symptoms occur, when and where symptoms tend to occur, how long symptoms last, and what effect symptoms have on patient's ability to function
▪ Drug history, including prescribed and over-the-counter drugs
▪ Safety needs

Clinical Presentation: Symptoms
▪ Delusions (somatic, ideas of reference, thought broadcasting, thought insertion, and thought withdrawal)
▪ Hallucinations (visual, auditory, tactile, olfactory, and gustatory)
▪ Disorganized speech (e.g., frequent derailment or incoherence)
▪ Grossly disorganized or catatonic behavior
▪ Negative symptoms (e.g., flat affect, lack of energy and initiative)

DSM-5 Diagnostic Guidelines
(a) Acute presentation of psychotic symptoms (2 weeks or less from a nonpsychotic to a clearly psychotic state); (b) symptoms present for the majority of the time since the establishment of an obviously psychotic clinical picture; and (c) acute polymorphic psychotic disorder ruled out.

Note: If the schizophrenic symptoms last for more than 1 month, the diagnosis should be changed to schizophrenia.

TREATMENT OVERVIEW

Acute Treatment

- Inpatient treatment is often necessary for patients with schizophreniform disorder for effective assessment and treatment. Patients who are at risk of harming themselves or others require hospitalization to allow comprehensive evaluation and to ensure their safety as well as others.
- The pharmacotherapy for schizophreniform disorder is similar to that for schizophrenia. Atypical (second generation) antipsychotics are mostly used at this time. See details in the schizophrenia discussion.
- Antidepressants may help reduce mood disturbances associated with schizophreniform disorder, but patients need to be monitored carefully for possible exacerbations of psychotic symptoms.

Chronic Treatment

- Long-acting medications are found to increase treatment adherence, including paliperidone (Invega Sustenna), a major active metabolite of risperidone (Risperdal Consta) and the first oral agent allowing once-daily dosing (6 mg PO in the morning).
- Ziprasidone (Geodon) and aripiprazole (Abilify) are available in injection form to help control acute psychotic symptoms. It is dose dependent and all second-generation antipsychotics (APS) are more likely to cause extrapyramidal symptoms extrapyramidal symptoms (EPS) for patients who are not antipsychotic-naive.
- Long-acting agents are made with aqueous vehicles—different from the typical injections that are sesame oil–based and can cause scarring and discomfort.
- It is critical to monitor and manage side effects of antipsychotic medications (e.g., extrapyramidal side effects, TD, sedation, postural hypotension, weight gain, disturbances in sexual function). See details in the schizophrenia section.
- Psychotherapeutic treatment modalities used in the treatment of patients with schizophrenia may be helpful in treating patients with schizophreniform disorder.

Drug Selection Table for Schizophreniform Disorders

CLASS	DRUG
Antipsychotic drugs, atypical	(Second generation) First-line drug therapy:
	Aripiprazole (*Abilify, Abilify Discmelt ODT, Abilify Liquid, Abilify IM injection*)
	Clozapine (*Clozaril, Fazaclo*)
	Olanzapine (*Zyprexa, Zyprexa Zydis*)
	Quetiapine (*Seroquel, Seroquel XR*)
	Risperidone (*Risperdal, Risperdal Consta*)
	Ziprasidone (*Geodon, Geodon IM injection*)
	Paliperidone (*Invega*)
	Asenapine (*Saphris*)

IM, intramuscular.

However, patients with schizophreniform disorder can become frightened in groups in which they are mixed with patients who have chronic schizophrenia.

■ Family therapy is proven to be appropriate for patients with schizophreniform disorder and their families.

■ In patients with schizophreniform disorder exhibiting impairments in social functioning, rehabilitative strategies similar to those described for patients with schizophrenia may be helpful.

It is estimated that 60% to 80% of patients with schizophreniform disorder will progress to full-blown schizophrenia despite treatment.

■ Nonadherence to the medications is a common cause of treatment failure. It is critical to monitor and manage side effects of antipsychotic medications.

■ Psychotherapy (e.g., CBT) is recommended; individual therapy has been found to be more effective than group therapy.

Recurrence Rate

It is estimated that 50% of patients with shared psychotic disorder recover at long-term follow-up, 20% show improved symptoms, and 30% have no change in symptoms.

PATIENT EDUCATION

■ Antipsychotic medications can produce dangerous side effects when taken with certain drugs. It is important for patients to tell health care providers about all medications, including over-the-counter medications, prescribed medications, vitamins, minerals, and herbal supplements that patients take.

■ It is important to teach patients about the importance of medication adherence and to avoid using alcohol and other substances.

Drug Selection Table for Delusional Disorder

CLASS	DRUG
Antipsychotic drugs, atypical (second generation)	First-line drug therapy: Olanzapine (*Zyprexa*, Zyprexa Relprevv Risperidone (*Risperdal, Risperdal Consta*) Clozapine (*Clozaril, Fazaclo*)
Antipsychotic drugs, typical (first generation)	Second-line drug therapy: Haloperidol (*Haldol* decanoate Pimozide (*Orap*)
Selective serotonin reuptake inhibitors	First-line drugs are sometimes helpful for somatic delusions: Fluoxetine (*Prozac, Sarafem*) Sertraline (*Zoloft*) Escitalopram (*Lexapro*)

▩ For excellent patient education resources, visit eMedicine's Mental Health and Behavior Center. See also eMedicine's patient education article, "Schizophrenia."

MEDICAL/LEGAL PITFALLS

▩ Misdiagnosis
▩ Mental health care providers should inform patients being treated with conventional antipsychotic medications about the risk of TD. AIMS is recommended for detecting TD early.
▩ Use medications with particular caution in children, pregnant/breastfeeding women, and older adults.

BIBLIOGRAPHY

American Psychiatric Association. (2006). *Practice guidelines for treatment: Compendium 2006.* Washington, DC: American Psychiatric Press.

American Psychiatric Association. (2013). *Diagnostic and statistical manual of mental disorders* (5th ed.). Washington, DC: American Psychiatric Press.

Azorin, J. M., Kaladjian, A., & Fakra, E. (2005). Current issues on schizoaffective disorder. *Encephale, 31*(3), 359–365.

Bond, G. R., & Drake, R. E. (2008). Predictors of competitive employment among patients with schizophrenia. *Current Opinions in Psychiatry, 21*(4), 362–369.

Cervini, P., Newman, D., Dorian, P., Edwards, J., Greene, M., & Bhalerao S. (2003). Folie a deux: An old diagnosis with a new technology. *Canadian Journal of Cardiology, 19*(13), 1539–1540.

Emsley, R., Oosthuizen, P., Koen, L., Niehaus, D. J., Medori, R., & Rabinowitz, J. (2008). Oral versus injectable antipsychotic treatment in early psychosis: Post hoc comparison of two studies. *Clinical Therapy, 30*(12), 2378–2386.

Etter, M., & Etter, J. F. (2004). Alcohol consumption and the CAGE test in outpatients with schizophrenia or schizoaffective disorder and in the general population. *Schizophrenia Bulletin, 30*(4), 947–956.

Fennig, S., Fochtmann, L. J., & Bromet, E. J. (2005). Delusional and shared psychotic disorder. In H. I. Kaplan & B. J. Sadock (Eds.), *Kaplan and Sadock's comprehensive textbook of psychiatry* (8th ed., pp. 1525–1533). New York, NY: Lippincott, Williams & Wilkins.

Fochtmann, L. J. (2005). Treatment of other psychotic disorders. In *Kaplan and Sadock's comprehensive textbook of psychiatry* (8th ed., pp. 1545–1550). New York, NY: Lippincott, Williams & Wilkins.

Harrow, M., Grossman, L. S., Herbener, E. S., & Davies, E. W. (2000). Ten-year outcome: Patients with schizoaffective disorders, schizophrenia, affective disorders and mood-incongruent psychotic symptoms. *British Psychiatry, 177,* 421–426.

Jones, R. T., & Benowitz, N. L. (2002). Therapeutics for nicotine addiction. In K. L. Davis, D. Charney, J. T. Coyle, & C. Nemeroff (Eds.), *Neuropsychopharmacology: The fifth generation of progress* (pp. 1533–1544). Nashville, TN: American College of Neuropsychopharmacology.

Kaplan, H. I., & Sadock, B. J. (Eds.). (2003). *Kaplan and Sadock's synopsis of psychiatry: Behavioral sciences/clinical psychiatry* (9th ed., pp. 508–511). New York, NY: Lippincott, Williams & Wilkins.

Kwon, J. S., Jang, J. H., Kang, D. H., Yoo, S. Y., Kim, Y. K., Cho, S. J.; APLUS Study Group. (2009). Long-term efficacy and safety of aripiprazole in patients with schizophrenia, schizophreniform disorder, or schizoaffective disorder: 26-week prospective study. *Psychiatry and Clinical Neuroscience, 63*(1), 73–81.

Marder, S. R. (2000). Integrating pharmacological and psychosocial treatments for schizophrenia. *Acta Psychiatrica Scandinavica Supplementum, 102*(407), 87–90.

Meltzer, H. Y., Alphs, L., Green, A. I., Altamura, A. C., Anand, R., Bertoldi, A., . . . Potkin, S.; International Suicide Prevention Trial Study Group. (2003). Clozapine treatment for suicidality in schizophrenia: International Suicide Prevention Trial (InterSePT). *Archives of General Psychiatry, 60*(1), 82–91.

Meltzer, H. Y., & Baldessarini, R. J. (2003). Reducing the risk for suicide in schizophrenia and affective disorders. *Journal of Clinical Psychiatry, 64*(9), 1122–1129.

Möller, H. J. (2005). Occurrence and treatment of depressive comorbidity/cosyndromality in schizophrenic psychoses: Conceptual and treatment issues. *World Journal of Biology and Psychiatry, 6*(4), 247–263.

Morken, G., Widen, J. H., & Grawe, R. W. (2008). Nonadherence to antipsychotic medication, relapse and rehospitalisation in recent-onset schizophrenia. *BMC Psychiatry, 8*, 32.

Mueser, K. T., & McGurk, S. R. (2004). Schizophrenia. *Lancet, 363*(9426), 2063–2072.

Pharoah, F. M., Mari, J. J., & Streiner, D. (2003). Family intervention for schizophrenia. *Cochrane Database of Systemic Reviews, 4*, CD000088.

Reif, A., & Pfuhlmann, B. (2004). Folie a deux versus genetically driven delusional disorder: Case reports and nosological considerations. *Comprehensive Psychiatry, 45*(2), 155–160.

Sadock, B. J., & Sadock, V. A. (2008a). Delusional disorder and shared psychotic disorder. In B. J., Sadock & V. A. Sadock (Eds.). *Kaplan and Sadock's concise textbook of clinical psychiatry* (3rd ed., pp. 182–190). Philadelphia, PA: Wolters Kluwer/Lippincott Williams &Wilkins.

Sadock, B. J., & Sadock, V. A. (2008b). Schizophrenia. In B. J. Sadock & V. A. Sadock (Eds.), *Kaplan and Sadock's concise textbook of clinical psychiatry* (3rd ed., pp. 156–177). Philadelphia, PA: Wolters Kluw/Lippincott, Williams & Wilkins.

Sadock, B. J., & Sadock, V. A. (2008c). Schizophreniform disorder. In B. J., Sadock & V. A. Sadock (Eds.). *Kaplan and Sadock's concise textbook of clinical psychiatry* (3rd ed., pp. 178–180). Philadelphia, PA: Wolters Kluwer/Lippincott Williams & Wilkins.

Shimizu, M., Kubota, Y., Toichi, M., & Baba, H. (2007). Folieà deux and shared psychotic disorder. *Current Psychiatry Report, 9*(3), 200–205.

Silveira, J. M., & Seeman, M. V. (1995). Shared psychotic disorder: A critical review of the literature. *Canadian Journal of Psychiatry, 40*(7), 389–395.

Solari, H., Dickson, K. E., & Miller, L. (2009). Understanding and treating women with schizophrenia during pregnancy and postpartum—Motherisk Update 2008. *Canadian Journal of Clinical Pharmacology, 16*(1), e23–32.

Suzuki, K., Awata, S., Takano, T., Ebina, Y., Takamatsu, K., Kajiwara, T.,...Matsuoka, H. (2006). Improvement of psychiatric symptoms after electroconvulsive therapy in young adults with intractable first-episode schizophrenia and schizophreniform disorder. *Tohoku Journal of Experimental Medicine, 210*(3), 213–220.

Wenning, M. T., Davy, L. E., Catalano, G., & Catalano, M. C. (2003). Atypical antipsychotics in the treatment of delusional parasitosis. *Annals of Clinical Psychiatry, 15*(3–4), 233–239.

WEB RESOURCES

- American Psychiatric Association: http://www.psych.org/
- Cleveland Clinic: http://www.ClevelandClinic.org/
- National Alliance on Mental Illness (NAMI): http://www.nami.org/
- National Mental Health Information Center: http://mentalhealth.samhsa.gov/
- Psych Central: http://psychcentral.com/

Chapter 11

Mood Disorders

Major Depressive Disorder (MDD)

BACKGROUND INFORMATION

Definition of Disorder

- Feelings of overwhelming sadness or lack of enjoyment, sometimes with anxiety and irritability, are the primary indicators.
- Hopelessness and a sense of feeling overwhelmed or helpless are common.
- Sense of worthlessness or low self-esteem are prominent features.
- Fatigue or somatic symptoms are also usually present.
- Often follows chronic stress or significant acute stressor(s).
- May complicate the treatment of other medical conditions such as stroke, diabetes, and so forth. For example, people with depression are four times more likely to develop a heart attack than those without a history of the illness. After a heart attack, they are at a significantly increased risk of death or a second heart attack.
- Negatively impacts social functioning, such as getting out of bed, going to work, and having positive relationships.
- Major depressive disorder (MDD) is a recurrent illness. Risk for relapse after one episode is 50%. After two episodes, risk for relapse is 80% to 90%. The average number of lifetime episodes is four.

Etiology

- Although heterogeneous in nature and poorly understood, the chronic stress response and the subsequent continuous activation of the hypothalamic–pituitary–adrenal axis results in chronic brain changes, such as a smaller hippocampus and changes in neurotransmitters.
- Corticotropin-releasing hormone (CRH) is a neuropeptide released by the hypothalamus to activate the pituitary in response to acute stress, but is hypersecreted in depression.
- Serotonin and norepinephrine are thought to be the primary neurotransmitters involved in depression, although dopamine can also be related to depression.
- Cognitive and personality factors, such as how people view their influence, their ability to change, and their interpretation of stressors, also play a role. The

depressive thinks that good things are temporary, limited in scope, and the result of sheer luck. Bad things are considered permanent, pervasive in impact, and his or her fault.

▤ MDD has been found to run in families, and this may mean that inheritance (genes) plays a strong role in determining who will get it. However, people who have no family history of the disorder also develop it.

▤ Often, depression occurs in the context of chronic illness or major life stressors.

Demographics

▤ Affects approximately 14.8 million American adults, or about 6.7% of the U.S. adult population

▤ Affects 17.6 million Americans annually

▤ Prevalence is 3% to 6% with a 2:1 female-to-male ratio.

▤ As many as 1 in 33 children and 1 in 8 adolescents have clinical depression.

▤ Individuals with MDD use two to three times the amount of health care services as nondepressed patients.

▤ MDD is the leading cause of disability in the United States for those aged 15 to 44 years and the leading cause of disability in the world for adolescents and adults.

▤ Suicide results in 32,000 deaths annually in the United States, and two thirds of these suicides are related to MDD.

▤ About 4.5 times more men than women die from suicide. White men complete more than 78% of all suicides and 56% of suicide deaths among men involve firearms. Poisoning is the predominant method among females.

▤ An estimated 8 to 25 attempted suicides occur for every completion. The majority of suicide attempts are expressions of extreme distress, not merely bids for attention.

▤ The rate of substance abuse (especially of stimulants, cocaine, and hallucinogens) in persons with MDD is 7% to 28%, a risk 4 to 14 times greater than that of the general population.

▤ Pregnant mothers with MDD are more likely to have infants of low birth weight for gestational age.

Risk Factors

Age

▤ First occurrence is often between the ages of 20 and 40 years

▤ The prevalence of major depression seems to be increasing in younger generations.

Gender

▤ Major depression is twice as common in women as in men.

▤ Pregnancy can either improve the condition or make it worse.

▤ The postpartum period is a time of especial susceptibility to major depression.

Family History

▤ Many studies have shown an increased incidence of major depression when there is a history of depression, alcoholism, or other psychiatric illnesses in first-degree relatives.

▤ The disorder is two times more common in first-degree relatives with MDD.

Past Medical History
▓ Comorbidities with chronic diseases are common, with conditions such as prior myocardial infarction, multiple sclerosis (MS), Parkinson's, and chronic pain having a greater than 40% prevalence.
▓ Current alcohol or substance abuse incidence during an MDD episode may have occurred.

Stressful Events in Susceptible People
▓ The initial appearance of MDD may follow a highly stressful event, such as being the victim of a crime, or the loss of a job, a loved one, or an important relationship.

Social History
▓ There is often a lack of social support
▓ Frequent use of medical resources in the absence of serious illness may be seen.
▓ Past or current history of abuse (childhood, sexual, or domestic violence) increases the incidence of MDD.

Having Another Mental Health Disorder
▓ A previous episode of depression may increase the risk of subsequent episodes of depression by as much as 90%.
▓ A history of dysthymic disorder precedes MDD in 10% to 25% of individuals.
▓ Having another mental health disorder, such as substance abuse (alcoholism or drug abuse), or a sleep disorder may increase the risk of developing MDD.
▓ Past history of suicide attempt

Risk Factors for Suicide
▓ Elderly
▓ Male gender
▓ Widows/widowers/unmarried people
▓ Unemployed
▓ People living alone
▓ History of previous psychiatric hospitalization
▓ Substance abuse
▓ Recent loss of significant relationship
▓ Recent loss of financial security
▓ Previous suicide attempt(s)

DIAGNOSIS

Differential Diagnosis
▓ More common:
  ▓ Thyroid disease
  ▓ Anemia
  ▓ Menopause
  ▓ Chronic fatigue syndrome
  ▓ If an underlying chronic health condition such as multiple sclerosis (MS) or stroke is the physiologic *cause* of the depressed mood, the diagnosis is mood disorder due to a general medical condition
  ▓ Bipolar disorder
  ▓ Bereavement

- ■ Adjustment disorder with depressed mood
- ■ Anxiety disorders
- ■ Dementia
- ■ Drug interactions or adverse effects
- ■ Infectious disease, such as autoimmune disorder, mononucleosis, or hepatitis C
- ■ Fibromyalgia
- ■ Personality disorder
- ■ Less common:
  - ■ Amphetamine or cocaine withdrawal
  - ■ Parathyroid disease
  - ■ Adrenal disease
  - ■ Cancer
  - ■ Neurological disease, such as cerebrovascular accident (CVA), MS, subdural hematoma, normal pressure hydrocephalus, or Alzheimer's disease
  - ■ Cardiovascular disease such as congestive heart failure (CHF) or cardiomyopathy
  - ■ Nutritional deficiency, such as B vitamin, folate, or iron deficiency
  - ■ Pulmonary disease, such as chronic obstructive pulmonary disorder (COPD)
  - ■ Heavy metal poisoning

ICD-10 Codes

MDD, single episode, unspecified degree (F32.3)
MDD, recurrent episodes, unspecified degree (F33.9)
Depressive Disorder (NOS, or not otherwise specified) (F32.9)

Diagnostic Workup

- ■ Physical and mental evaluation
- ■ Labs as needed to evaluate physical complaints
  - ■ Thyroid function studies (triiodothyronine [T_3], thyroxine [T_4], thyroid-stimulating hormone [TSH])
  - ■ Complete metabolic panel (CMP), including glucose, calcium, and albumin; total protein analysis; and levels of sodium, potassium, CO_2 (carbon dioxide, bicarbonate), chloride, blood urea nitrogen (BUN), creatinine, alkaline phosphatase (ALP), alanine aminotransferase (ALT, also called SGPT), aspartate aminotransferase (AST, also called SGOT), and bilirubin
  - ■ Complete blood count (CBC) with differentials: hemoglobin, hematocrit, red blood cells, white blood cells, white blood cell differential count, and platelet count
  - ■ Testing for infectious diseases, such as hepatitis C or HIV, if applicable.

Initial Assessment

- ■ Screening question: In the past month, have you felt down or depressed? In the past month, have you lost interest in the things you usually do?
- ■ Use of a standard screening tool, such as
  1. SIG E CAPS
     - ■ Depressed mood
     - ■ Decreased sleep (insomnia with 2 a.m. to 4 a.m. awakening)
     - ■ Interest decreased in activities (anhedonia)
     - ■ Guilt or worthlessness (not a major criterion)
     - ■ Energy decreased
     - ■ Concentration difficulties

      ▓ Appetite disturbance or weight loss
      ▓ Psychomotor retardation/agitation
      ▓ Suicidal thoughts
  2. Beck Depression Inventory: 21-question survey completed by patient
  3. Zung Self-Rating Scale: 20-question survey completed by patient, Likert-type scale format
  4. PHQ-9: The Patient Health Questionnaire, a brief survey completed by patient
▓ Past medical history
▓ Family medical history, with emphasis on psychiatric history
▓ Social history, including safety of relationships, family support, recent or ongoing stressors
▓ Past suicide attempts or past psychiatric hospitalizations
▓ Any prior manic/hypomanic episodes (*any* history suggests bipolar or cyclothymia diagnosis); Mood Disorder Questionnaire is a helpful tool
▓ What effect symptoms have had on ability to function (any missed work, etc.)?
▓ Assess for suicide ideation, suicide plan, and suicide intent

Clinical Presentation
▓ Somatization: often, presentation of depression is through complaints of (often multiple) physical symptoms that do not have clearly identifiable causes
▓ Sadness
▓ Lack of enjoyment of usual activities (anhedonia)
▓ Fatigue
▓ Sleep problems (early-morning awakening with difficulty or inability to fall back asleep is typical)
▓ Feelings of guilt
▓ Feeling overwhelmed
▓ Difficulty concentrating, focusing, or remembering
▓ Appetite disturbances (lack of appetite, or excessive eating)
▓ Irritability, agitation, or slowed movements
▓ Thoughts of suicide or wanting to "escape"
▓ Obsessive rumination about problems

Signs
▓ Flattened affect
▓ Slowed speech and movements, sighs, long pauses
▓ Tearfulness
▓ Lack of eye contact
▓ Memory loss, poor concentration, or poor abstract reasoning
▓ Sometimes irritability, belligerence, or defiance (more common in adolescence)

DSM-5 Diagnostic Guidelines
Diagnostic and Statistical Manual of Mental Disorders, fifth edition (DSM-5) distinguishes between MDD—single episode—and MDD—recurrent.
    For MDD—single episode:

▓ At least five of the following symptoms have been present for at least 2 weeks in duration: depressed mood, anhedonia, change in eating habits, sleep disturbance, psychomotor agitation or retardation, fatigue, excessive guilt or feelings of worth-lessness, difficulty concentrating, and recurrent thoughts of death or suicide (at least one of the symptoms being depressed mood or anhedonia).

- Symptoms must cause a significant social or occupational dysfunction or subjective distress.
- Symptoms cannot be caused by a medical condition, medications, drugs, or bereavement.

  For MDD—recurrent:

- Two or more major depressive episodes (MDEs) occur.
- Absence of manic, hypomanic, or "mixed" episodes

TREATMENT OVERVIEW

Acute Treatment

- Psychotropic medication should be selected based on relative efficacy, tolerability and anticipated side effects, co-occurring psychiatric or general medical conditions, half-life, cost, potential drug interactions, and the patient's preference and prior response to medication.
- The onset of benefit from pharmacological treatment may be more gradual in MDD than the onset of benefit in nonchronic depression.
- Treatment of nonresponsive patients should be re-evaluated for accuracy of diagnosis, unaddressed co-occurring medical or psychiatric disorders, such as substance abuse, the need for a change in treatment modalities, inadequate dose or duration of medical treatment, the need to augment medical treatment (with a second antidepressant from a different pharmacological class, or use of an adjunctive such as a second-generation atypical antipsychotic, anticonvulsant or thyroid hormone), inadequate frequency of psychotherapy, complicating psychosocial factors, nonadherence to treatment, and poor "fit" between patient and therapist.
- Common combinations of medications include a selective serotonin reuptake inhibitor (SSRI) with the addition of bupropion or the combination of mirtazapine and an SSRI or venlafaxine.
- Pharmacotherapy may increase the potential of suicidal ideation, particularly in patients younger than 25 years of age. General guidelines include:
  - Patients initiated on any psychiatric medication intervention should be monitored carefully for changes in mood or suicidal behavior or ideation.
  - Depressed patients with suicidal ideation, plan, and intent should be hospitalized, especially if they have current psychosocial stressors and access to lethal means.
  - Depressed patients with suicidal ideation and a plan but without intent may be treated on an outpatient basis with close follow-up, especially when they have good social support and no access to lethal means.
  - Depressed patients who express suicidal ideation but deny a plan should be assessed carefully for psychosocial stressors. Remove weapons from the environment.
  - Pay careful attention in the first 1 to 4 weeks of treatment to a sudden lift of depression or to worsening mood as initial response to antidepressant therapy as these could be signs of increased risk for suicide.
  - Pharmacotherapy for MDD should begin at the lowest dosage and gradually be increased, if needed, following a 4-week evaluation for therapeutic response. Patients should be observed 1 to 2 weeks after initiation of therapy for evaluation of adverse drug effects. Frequency of monitoring should be determined based on symptom severity, co-occurring disorders, availability of social support, patient cooperation with treatment, and side effects of medication.

▪ The combination of pharmacological therapy and cognitive behavioral therapy (CBT), individually or in combination, is effective in more than 85% of cases.

Chronic Treatment

▪ Pharmacotherapy with or without individual counseling, particularly CBT, is the treatment of choice, and should be considered for patients.

▪ Cognitive restructuring involves substituting positive perceptions for negative perceptions and assistance with problem solving and stress management.

▪ Once the patient has reached remission of symptoms, the patient is monitored for an additional 4 to 9 months prior to tapering the medication, or, in the case of three or more episodes, the patient is placed on maintenance treatment.

▪ In cases in which medication loses its effectiveness, alternative regimens and diagnoses should be explored.

▪ Electroconvulsive therapy (ECT) is recommended as the treatment of choice for patients with severe MDD that is not responsive to pharmacologic treatment and psychotherapy.

▪ Pharmacologic education should include:
  ▪ Frequency of dosing
  ▪ The likelihood that side effects will occur prior to improvement of symptoms
  ▪ Expectations that it will take 2 to 4 weeks prior to beneficial effects and 4 to 8 weeks prior to full effects of the dosage
  ▪ The importance of taking medication even after feeling better
  ▪ Consulting with the health care provider before discontinuing medication
  ▪ Correcting misconceptions about medication use, and explaining what to do if side effects, questions, or worsening symptoms arise.

▪ Nonpharmacologic recommendations should also be made such as:
  ▪ Proper sleep hygiene
  ▪ Decreased use or elimination of caffeine, tobacco, and alcohol
  ▪ Light therapy
  ▪ Regular exercise.

▪ Consider long-term treatment in patients with two or more episodes. A history of three or more episodes of depression indicates a very high risk for recurrence and the need for continuous treatment.

▪ Also may increase the risk of bleeding for patients on NSAIDs/ASA and anticoagulation therapy.

▪ Stress management and lifestyle changes, such as regular exercise, which have been found to decrease depression, are essential for ongoing prevention.

▪ Behavioral therapy involves various relaxation techniques, self-care strategies, and cognitive and dialectical therapy may also be helpful. Studies suggest that augmentation of antidepressant effect occurs with adjunct use of omega-3 fish oil supplements, 1,000 mg twice daily. B vitamin supplementation has also been used in some studies, with equivocal results.

▪ Treatment can be complicated by having another condition at the same time, such as substance abuse, depression, or other anxiety disorders.

NOTES ON SSRIs AS FIRST LINE OF DRUG THERAPY

▪ SSRIs are one of the more commonly used medications for MDD.

▪ SSRI medications typically display fewer side effects than tricyclic antidepressants (TCAs) and monoamine oxidase inhibitors (MAOIs), with minimal risk of death in

Drug Selection Table for Major Depressive Disorder

CLASS	DRUG
Selective serotonin reuptake inhibitors (SSRIs)	First-line drug therapy: Fluoxetine (*Prozac*) Sertraline (*Zoloft*) Paroxetine (*Paxil, Paxil CR*) Citalopram (*Celexa*) Escitalopram (*Lexapro*) Fluvoxamine (*Luvox*) Fluoxetine (*Sarafem*)
Serotonin–norepinephrine reuptake inhibitors (SNRIs)	Venlafaxine (*Effexor*); Venlafaxine XR (*Effexor XR*) Duloxetine (*Cymbalta*) Desvenlafaxine (*Pristiq*)
Serotonin-2 antagonist/reuptake inhibitors (SARIs)	Second-line drug therapy: Nefazodone (*Serzone*) Trazodone (*Desyrel*)
Noradrenergic and specific serotonergic antidepressants (NaSSAs)	Alternative therapy option: Mirtazapine (*Remeron*)
Norepinephrine/dopamine reuptake inhibitors (NDRIs)	Alternative therapy option: Bupropion (*Wellbutrin, Zyban*), bupropion SR (*Wellbutrin SR*), and bupropion XL (*Wellbutrin XL*)
Tricyclic antidepressants (TCAs)	Amitriptyline (*Elavil*) Clomipramine (*Anafranil*) Desipramine (*Norpramin*) Imipramine (*Tofranil*) Nortriptyline (*Pamelor*)
Monoamine oxidase inhibitors (MAOIs)	Phenelzine (*Nardil*) Isocarboxazid (*Marplan*) Tranylcypromine (*Parnate*)

an intentional overdose. Treatment decisions should take into consideration patient symptoms and medication side effect profile.
■ They also may increase the risk of bleeding for patients on NSAIDs/ASA and anti-coagulation therapy.
■ SSRI medications may not be preferred for patients with sexual dysfunction or who find sexual dysfunction as an intolerable side effect.
■ Limited or no cholinergic, histaminergic, dopaminergic, or adrenergic receptor activity (i.e., they do not cause hypotension or anticholinergic response)
■ May be of benefit to perimenopausal women experiencing hot flashes
■ Patients reporting intolerable side effects from one SSRI may benefit from switching to another SSRI.
■ SSRIs inhibit serotonin 2A receptors and serotonin reuptake
■ Receptor inhibition produces a sedating effect.

Recurrence Rate
Rate of recurrence is 50% after one episode, 80% after two episodes, and greater than 90% after three episodes.

PATIENT EDUCATION

- Information regarding MDD and support groups can be obtained from the National Institute for Mental Health (see further outpatient care).
- Advise patients with MDD to avoid nicotine and excess alcohol intake (no more than 1 svg/day for a woman, 2 svg/day for a man).
- Thirty minutes of daily exercise has been found to be beneficial for MDD patients, and daily exposure to outdoor light may also be beneficial.

MEDICAL/LEGAL PITFALLS

- Failure to monitor for suicide risk
- Failure to screen for bipolar disorder (any history of mania/hypomania)
- Pay careful attention in the first 1 to 4 weeks of treatment to a sudden lift of depression or to worsening mood as initial response to antidepressant therapy, as these could be signs of increased risk for suicide.
- When initiating treatment, see patients on a more frequent basis until response to antidepressant is clear.
- Have a follow-up system to ensure that there are calls to patients who fail to schedule follow-up appointments or fail to show up for scheduled appointments.
- Patients with MDDs are more likely than the general population to use alternative therapies. Use of dietary supplements (e.g., herbs) should be discussed to avoid drug interactions.

Bipolar Disorder

BACKGROUND INFORMATION

Definition of Disorder
- Historically, it has been referred to as manic depression or manic-depressive illness.
- Neurobiological psychiatric disorder is characterized by sustained extreme mood swings from extremely low (depression) to extremely high (mania) and an abnormal increase in energy and activity.
- Both phases of this disorder are deleterious in that they adversely affect thoughts, behaviors, judgment, and relationships.
- Patients with bipolar I disorder have episodes of sustained mania and often experience depressive episodes.
- Patients with bipolar II disorder have one or more MDEs, with at least one hypomanic episode.
- Extreme mood swings that occur hourly or daily are very rarely associated with this disorder, and other medical and/or psychiatric diagnoses should be considered and ruled out first.

▦ An age of onset of mania after the age of 40 years alerts the practitioner that the symptoms are most likely due to a medical condition or substance use, and newly diagnosed mania is uncommon in children and adults older than 65 years.

▦ It is not uncommon for bipolar disorder to go undetected.

▦ Patients in the manic phase of the disorder often do not seek psychiatric or medical attention.

▦ Patients experiencing the depressive phase of the disorder often present initially to a primary care setting due to an increase in health issues, somatic complaints, or chronic pain that does not appear to have an objective or identifiable etiology. This is often erroneously diagnosed with unipolar depression which can then be treated with unopposed antidepressant therapy (and may cause switch to mania).

Etiology

▦ The exact cause of bipolar disorder is not known.

▦ The "kindling theory" is the current predominant theory, meaning the disorder is likely caused by multiple factors that potentially interact and lower the threshold at which mood changes occur. Eventually, a mood episode can start itself and thus become recurrent.

  ▩ Environmental factors:
    ◦ Sleep deprivation can trigger episodes of mania while hypersomnia can trigger MDEs.
    ◦ Traumatic and/or abusive events in childhood.
    ◦ Approximately, one fifth of individuals with bipolar disorder, mostly those with bipolar II, have mood symptoms that wax and wane with the seasons. It is hypothesized that those with a diurnal pattern are affected mostly by both fluctuating light and temperature.

  ▩ Biological perspectives:
    ◦ Genetics:
      – Twin studies consistently show that identical twins (40%–70%) are far more concordant for mood disorders than fraternal twins (0%–10%).
      – The overall heritability of bipolar spectrum disorders has been put at 0.71.
      – Between 4% and 24% of first-degree relatives of individuals with bipolar I disorder are also diagnosed with bipolar I disorder.
    ◦ Neural processes:
      – Hypersensitivity of melatonin receptors
      – Structural abnormalities in the amygdala, hippocampus, and prefrontal cortex
      – Larger lateral ventricles
  ▩ White matter hyperintensities
    ◦ Endocrine models:
      – Hypothyroidism can cause depression and/or mood instability.
      – Abnormalities have also been found in the hypothalamic–pituitary axis due to repeated stress.

Demographics

▦ True prevalence is not known due to misdiagnosis or undetected episodes of mania.

▦ Bipolar disorder affects approximately 2.3 million American adults annually.

▦ Lifetime prevalence is 1% for bipolar I and between 0.5% and 1% for bipolar II.

▦ First-degree biological relatives of individuals with bipolar I disorder are more likely to have an earlier onset of bipolar spectrum disorders.

- Forty percent or more of patients with this disorder experience mixed episodes (MDE + manic episode).
- The World Health Organization identified bipolar disorder as the sixth leading cause of disability-adjusted life years worldwide among people aged 15 to 44 years.
- Cardiovascular disease, obesity, type 2 diabetes mellitus, and other endocrine disorders occur more often in patients with bipolar spectrum disorders.
- Patients with bipolar disorder have higher rates of comorbid neurological disorders and migraine headaches.

Risk Factors

Age

- The average age of onset is 20 years.
- Late adolescence and early adulthood are peak years for the onset of bipolar disorder.
- Approximately, 10% to 15% of adolescents with recurrent MDEs are more likely to develop bipolar I disorder.
- Mixed episodes appear more likely in adolescents and young adults than in older adults.
- Often, the cycling between depression and mania accelerates with age.

Gender

- Men and women are affected equally.
  - Men:
    - The first episode in males is most likely to be a manic episode.
    - Early-onset bipolar disorder tends to occur more frequently in men and it is associated with a more severe condition.
    - Men with bipolar spectrum disorders tend to have higher rates of substance abuse (drugs, alcohol).
    - The number of manic episodes equals or exceeds the number of MDEs in men.
  - Women:
    - The first episode in females is most likely to be an MDE.
    - There is a higher incidence of rapid cycling and mixed mood episodes among women.
    - Women have higher incidences of bipolar II disorder.
    - The number of MDEs exceeds the number of manic episodes in women.
    - Women with bipolar I disorder appear to have an increased risk of developing mood episodes in the immediate postpartum period.
    - Women in the premenstrual period may have worsening of ongoing major depressive, manic, mixed, or hypomanic episodes.

Family History

- Genetic factors account for 60% of the cases of bipolar disorder.
- The approximate lifetime risk in relatives of a bipolar proband is 40% to 70% for a monozygotic twin and 5% to 10% for a first-degree relative.
- Family members of patients with bipolar disorder also have a higher-than-average incidence of other psychiatric problems.
- Schizophrenia
- Schizoaffective disorder
- Anxiety disorders
- Attention deficit hyperactivity disorder
- Major depression
- Obsessive-compulsive disorder

Stressful Events in Susceptible People

▨ There have been repeated findings that about one third to one half of adults diagnosed with bipolar disorder report traumatic/abusive experiences in child-hood, particularly events stemming from a harsh environment rather than from the child's own behavior. This is generally associated with earlier onset, a worse course, and more co-occurring mental health disorders such as posttraumatic stress disorder (PTSD) or other anxiety-related disorders.

▨ Ongoing psychosocial stressors have been shown to destabilize moods in patients with bipolar spectrum disorders.

Having Another Mental Health Disorder

▨ Anxiety disorders
   ▨ There is a greater than 50% lifetime comorbidity of anxiety disorders with bipolar illness and these patients appear to have a more difficult course of illness.
   ▨ Decreased likelihood of recovery
   ▨ Poorer role functioning and quality of life
   ▨ Greater likelihood of suicide attempts
▨ Substance-use disorders
   ▨ Sixty-one percent of patients diagnosed with bipolar I disorder and 48% of patients diagnosed with bipolar II disorder also have coexisting substance-use disorders.
   ▨ The most common substance-use disorder appears to be alcohol abuse/dependence.
   ▨ Lifetime prevalence of alcohol abuse/dependence is 49% of men and 29% of women diagnosed with bipolar spectrum disorders.
   ▨ Attention deficit hyperactivity disorder; a diagnosis of attention deficit hyperactivity disorder as a child may be a marker for a bipolar spectrum diagnosis as an adult.
▨ Personality disorders
   ▨ Approximately one third of patients with bipolar disorder also have a cluster B (borderline, narcissistic, antisocial, and histrionic) personality disorder.
   ▨ Marked personality disorder symptoms negatively influence treatment-related outcomes in patients with bipolar disorder.

Risk Factors for Suicidal Behavior in Bipolar Spectrum Disorders

▨ Completed suicide occurs in 10% to 15% of individuals with bipolar I disorder.
▨ Personal or family history of suicidal behavior
▨ Severity and number of depressive episodes or mixed mood states
▨ Alcohol or substance abuse/dependence
▨ Level of pessimism and hopelessness
▨ Level of impulsivity and/or aggression
▨ Younger age of onset of the disorder
▨ A concomitant personality disorder diagnosis
▨ Patients with remitting depressive symptoms are thought to be at increased risk for suicide.

Risk Factors for Harm to Others in Bipolar Spectrum Disorders

▨ A history of violent behavior has consistently been shown to be the best single predictor of future violence.

▓ The presence of symptoms that increase the risk of violence in the absence of overt threats includes presenting as guarded and/or paranoid, psychosis, command hallucinations, cognitive disorders, and substance use. Child abuse, spouse abuse, or other violent behavior may occur during severe manic episodes or during mood episodes with psychotic features.

▓ Younger age

▓ Gender is not a factor and the rates of violence among the genders are equal in patients who are acutely mentally ill.

▓ A history of victimization as a child or witnessing or experiencing violence after the age of 16 years

▓ Level of impulsivity

▓ More than half of victims of violence by persons with mental health disorders are family members

▓ The availability of firearms and/or weapons

DIAGNOSIS

Differential Diagnosis

There is a broad differential diagnosis for bipolar spectrum disorders that includes ruling out the following:

▓ Thyroid or other metabolic disorders
▓ Epilepsy (partial complex seizures)
▓ Diabetes mellitus
▓ Sleep apnea
▓ Brain lesions
▓ MS
▓ Systemic infection
▓ Tertiary syphilis
▓ Systemic lupus erythematosus
▓ Cerebral vascular accident
▓ HIV
▓ Steroid-induced mood symptoms
▓ Vitamin B_{12} deficiency
▓ Vitamin D deficiency
▓ Posttraumatic stress disorder (PTSD)
▓ Attention deficit hyperactivity disorder
▓ Cyclothymic disorder
▓ MDD
▓ Dysthymic disorder
▓ Schizoaffective disorder
▓ Schizophrenia
▓ Personality disorders
▓ Eating disorder
▓ Drug interactions or adverse effects that can cause mood symptoms (e.g., baclofen, bromide, bromocriptine, captopril, cimetidine, corticosteroids, cyclosporine, disulfiram [Antabuse], hydralazine, isoniazid, levodopa, methylphenidate [Ritalin], metrizamide, procarbazine, procyclidine [Kemadrin])
▓ Drug or alcohol intoxication or withdrawal

ICD-10 Code

Bipolar disorder not otherwise specified (NOS) (F31.9)
Bipolar I disorder, single manic episode, unspecified degree (F31.10)
Bipolar I disorder, most recent episode manic (F31.73)
Bipolar I disorder, most recent episode depressed (F31.75)
Bipolar II disorder (specify if most recent episode is hypomanic/depressed) (F31.82)

Diagnostic Workup

▨ There are no biological tests that confirm bipolar disorder. Rather, tests are carried out to rule in/out medical issues that may be mimicking a mood disorder.
  ▨ Antinuclear antibody (ANA): ANAs are found in patients whose immune systems may be predisposed to cause inflammation against their own body tissues. Antibodies that are directed against one's own tissues are referred to as autoantibodies.
  ▨ Thyroid and other metabolic function studies suggest hyperexcitability or hypoexcitability symptoms.
  ▨ Blood glucose level rules out diabetes
  ▨ Serum proteins
  ▨ Lithium levels are measured if patient has history of diagnosis and is taking this medication.
  ▨ CBC with differential is performed to rule out anemia or other blood dyscrasias.
  ▨ Urine toxicology screening for drugs and alcohol (see previous data)
  ▨ Urine copper level is measured.
  ▨ Venereal disease research lab VDRL text random plasma glucose (RPG) is performed.
  ▨ HIV testing (enzyme-linked immunosorbent assay [ELISA] and Western Blot test);
  ▨ Electrocardiogram
  ▨ Electroencephalography to exclude epilepsy
  ▨ Sleep study
  ▨ Magnetic resonance imagery
  ▨ Computed tomography scan of head
▨ Clinical history
▨ Collateral information from close friends and family

Initial Assessment

▨ It is important to gain a complete history and carefully assess for historical and/or current episodes of mania and/or hypomania as well as depression.
▨ Physical examination with a focus on neurological and endocrine systems and infectious diseases
▨ Ask specific screening questions to assess for manic episodes, mixed episodes, or hypomanic episodes:
  ▨ Have you ever experienced periods of feeling uncharacteristically energetic?
  ▨ Have you had periods of not sleeping but not feeling tired?
  ▨ Have you ever felt that your thoughts were racing and that there was nothing you could do to slow them down?
  ▨ Have you ever experienced periods during which you were participating in risky activities, more interested in sex than usual, or spending more money than you usually would?
▨ Use standardized screening tools:
  ▨ Bipolar Spectrum Diagnostic Scale (BSDS)

■ Mood Disorder Questionnaire (MDQ)
■ Violence Screening Checklist (VSC): reliably indicates the level of risk during the next 24-hour period
■ The short-term assessment of risk and treatability (START): assesses risk and guides treatment for violence, suicide, self-neglect, substance use, and victimization
■ Psychiatric assessment with a focus on current symptoms, date of onset, potential precipitating factors, and perpetuating factors (e.g., drug or alcohol use), traumatic events in childhood, and substance use
■ Family history with an emphasis on psychiatric history and suicide attempts and completed suicides
■ Social history with an emphasis on current social support and safety issues in relationships, recent psychosocial stressors, ability to maintain employment, and financial concerns
■ Assessment of safety risk with an emphasis on history of harm to self or others, history of childhood abuse or victimization, plan and intent, and access to firearms and/or weapons
■ Level of functional impairment and need for hospitalization (e.g., assess ability to work, engage in self-care activities, ability to conduct activities of daily living, and ability to get along with others)

Clinical Presentation
■ Manic episode:
  ■ Affect/moods:
    ● Euphorically elevated, overly happy, outgoing
    ● Irritable mood, agitation, jumpy, "wired"
    ● Inappropriately joyous
  ■ Behaviors:
    ● Increased goal-directed activity
    ● Excessive involvement in high-risk activities
    ● Impulsivity
    ● Restlessness
    ● Energized behavior
    ● Clothing may look disorganized or disheveled
    ● Increased psychomotor changes
    ● Religiosity
    ● Decreased need for sleep
    ● Behavior may become aggressive, intrusive, or combative.
    ● No patience or tolerance for others
    ● Increased talkativeness or rapid, pressured speech
  ■ Thoughts:
    ● Inflated self-worth
    ● Expansive and optimistic thinking
    ● Flight of ideas and/or loose associations
    ● Racing thoughts and feeling that their minds are active
  ■ Perceptions:
    ● Approximately, three fourths have delusions
    ● Manic delusions reflect perceptions of power, prestige, position, self-worth, and glory
    ● Some have auditory hallucinations and delusions of persecution.

- Hypomanic episode:
  - Affect/moods:
    - Up
    - Expansive
    - Irritable
  - Behaviors:
    - Busy
    - Active
    - Overinvolved
    - Increased energy
    - Increase in planning and doing things
    - Others notice the increase in his or her activity but the patient often denies that anything about him or her has changed
  - Thoughts:
    - Optimistic
    - Future focused
    - Positive attitude
  - Perceptions:
    - Patients with hypomania typically do not experience perceptual changes.
- MDE:
  - Affect/moods:
    - Sadness dominates affect and is often blunted or flattened
    - Feeling sad, depressed, empty, and isolated
    - Hopelessness
    - Helplessness
    - Worthlessness
    - Easily overwhelmed
  - Behaviors:
    - Poor grooming
    - Increased tearfulness
    - Poor eye contact or no eye contact
    - Psychomotor changes: moves slowly or moves very little, with psychomotor retardation
    - Social withdrawal, shyness, or increase in social anxiety
    - Decreased interest in sexual activity and/or difficulty enjoying sexual activity
    - Somatization (e.g., increase in physical or somatic complaints without objective, identified able cause)
    - Difficulty with attention and concentration
    - Appetite disturbances (increase or decrease)
    - Sleep disturbance
    - Decrease in energy and increase in fatigue regardless of amount of sleep
    - Attempts at suicide
  - Thoughts:
    - Increased thoughts of death or morbid thoughts, and/or suicidal thoughts or specific plans for committing suicide
    - Thoughts that reflect their sadness (negative thoughts about self, world, and future)
    - Nihilistic concerns
    - Short-term memory deficits
    - Increase in worry and rumination; also referred to as brooding
    - Inappropriate guilt

- Perceptions:
  - In severe episodes, psychotic symptoms may be present (e.g., auditory hallucinations).
  - Delusions, for example, that they have sinned
- Mixed features (includes depressive signs and symptoms within manic or hypomanic phases of the illness):
  - Affect/moods:
    - Marked irritability
    - Agitation
    - Anxiety
    - Rage
  - Behaviors:
    - Aggressiveness
    - Belligerence
    - Impulsiveness
    - Sleep disturbance
    - Rapid and pressured speech
    - Psychomotor agitation
    - Fatigue
  - Thoughts:
    - Confusion
    - Morbid thoughts and/or suicidal ideation
    - Paranoia and/or persecutory delusions
    - Racing thoughts
    - Increased worry and rumination
  - Perceptions:
    - Patients may exhibit hallucinations and/or delusions congruent with either depression or mania or both.

DSM-5 Diagnostic Guidelines
Manic Episode
- The patient's mood is disturbed and characterized as high, irritable, or expansive, with an increase in overall energy for at least 1 week.
- The patient exhibits three or more of the following:
  - Grandiose thinking
  - Diminished sleep
  - Volubility, or rapid and pressured speech
  - Racing thoughts
  - Distractibility, trouble concentrating
  - Increased goal-directed activity
  - Expanded pleasurable activities that have potential for adverse outcomes (e.g., spending sprees)
  - Psychomotor agitation
  - Psychotic features (e.g., delusions of grandeur, hallucinations)
- Symptom severity results in one or both of the following:
  - Reduced social functioning (social, marital, occupational)
  - Hospitalization (owing to the presence of safety risk)
- The symptoms are not more easily ascribed to other medical diagnoses, other medical conditions, substance use, or withdrawal from prescription medications.

Major Depressive Episode
■ The patient has experienced five or more of the following in a 2-week period:
  ■ Depressed mood
  ■ Anhedonia
  ■ Change in eating habits, weight loss, or weight gain
  ■ Psychomotor agitation or retardation
  ■ Fatigue
  ■ Feelings of guilt, feelings of worthlessness
  ■ Problems with concentration, short-term memory deficits
  ■ Suicidal ideation

  Note: Depressed mood or anhedonia must be one of the five.

■ Symptom severity results in one or both of the following:
  ■ Reduced social functioning (social, marital, occupational)
  ■ Hospitalization (owing to the presence of safety risk)
■ The symptoms cannot be more easily ascribed to other medical diagnoses, other medical conditions, substance use, or withdrawal from prescription medication.

Hypomanic Episode
■ Elevated, expansive, or irritable mood for at least 4 days
■ During this same period the patient has had three or more of the following:
  ■ Grandiose thinking, inflated self-esteem
  ■ Diminished sleep
  ■ Volubility
  ■ Racing thoughts
  ■ Problems with concentration
  ■ Psychomotor agitation
  ■ A focus on goal-directed activities
  ■ Poor judgment and increased engagement in activities that have potential for adverse consequences (e.g., spending sprees)
■ Psychotic features are absent.
■ Social functioning is not impeded.
■ Hospitalization is not required.
■ The symptoms are not more easily ascribed to other medical diagnoses, other medical conditions, substance use, or withdrawal from prescription medication.

Bipolar I
■ Criteria for one manic episode have been met.
■ If the patient is experiencing a hypomanic episode, he or she must have had at least one prior manic episode.
■ Markedly reduced social or occupational functioning
■ For a majority of patients, depression is present more often than mania.
■ The symptoms cannot be ascribed to other medical diagnoses, other medical conditions, substance use, or withdrawal from prescription medication.

Bipolar II
■ The patient has had one or more MDEs.
■ The patient has had one or more hypomanic episodes.
■ A history of manic episodes is absent.
■ The symptoms cause significant distress or significantly reduced functioning in the patient.

■ The symptoms cannot be more easily ascribed to other medical diagnoses (including other psychiatric diagnoses), other medical conditions, substance abuse, or withdrawal from prescription medication.

Rapid Cycling (Can Be Applied to Both Bipolar I or Bipolar II Disorder)
■ The patient has experienced four or more of the following: MDEs, manic episodes, or hypomanic episodes (any combination) within a 12-month period.
■ Episodes are generally separated by periods of at least 2 months of full or partial remission, or there is a switch to an episode of the opposite polarity.

TREATMENT OVERVIEW

Acute Treatment
■ The primary goal of the acute phase is to manage acute mania, hypomania, or depressive episodes, and associated safety-risk issues.
■ Diagnostic tests should be performed to rule out potential medical etiologies for mood symptoms, especially if this is the first episode of mania, hypomania, mixed mood symptoms, or depression.
■ How to handle suicidal ideation?
　■ A patient with suicidal ideation with plan and intent should be hospitalized (voluntarily or involuntarily) due to acute safety risk.
　■ A patient with suicidal ideation with plan but no intent may be treated on an outpatient basis with close follow-up if he or she does not have access to the means to carry out the plan and does not have adequate social support.
　■ A patient with suicidal ideation without plan and no intent requires careful assessment of current psychosocial stressors, access to weapons and other lethal means, substance use, and impulse-control issues. Any lethal means should be removed.
■ How to handle aggression and potential harm to others?
　■ If patients have access to firearms and or weapons, they should be removed.
　■ Those with thoughts of harming others with plan and intent should be hospitalized (voluntarily or involuntarily).
　■ Antipsychotics are often used for management in emergent situations, which the patient presents as possibly psychotic, agitated, and making overt threats.
　■ Those with thoughts of harming others with plan but no intent can be treated on an outpatient basis, with increased intensity of treatment with an established provider, depending on risk factors.
　■ Those with thoughts of harming others without plan or intent do require increased intensity of treatment and perhaps increased dosages of medications.
■ Acute manic episode with or without mixed features:
　■ Hospitalization is necessary in patients who present with significant suicide risk, increased aggressiveness, and significant risk of violence against others, the potential for serious alcohol withdrawal symptoms, or when the differential includes other medical disorders that warrant admission.
　■ Antidepressants, if they have been prescribed, should be discontinued if the patient is presenting with an acute manic episode with or without mixed features.
　■ Patient should be advised to decrease alcohol, caffeine, and nicotine use.
　■ Most patients are started on long-term mood stabilizers and also are given antipsychotic medications if agitated and/or experiencing psychotic symptoms.

- Medications in the acute phase are commonly used to induce remission in acute mania or hypomania.
- Acute hypomanic episode:
  - Treatment for hypomania, which can lead to either a manic or depressive episode, may decrease symptom progression
- Acute MDE:
  - Hospitalization is necessary if patient presents with a significant suicide risk, if there is potential for serious withdrawal symptoms, or when the differential includes other medical disorders that warrant admission.
  - Antidepressant medications have not been shown to be an effective adjunctive therapy and, as a monotherapy, they can precipitate mania in individuals with bipolar disorder.
  - Be alert to sudden decreases of depressed mood or to worsening mood as initial response to antidepressant therapy, as these could be signs of increased risk for suicide.
- Medication noncompliance is common because mania and hypomania may be a desired state for many individuals with bipolar disorder, and many are reluctant to take medications to eliminate these states.
- Because bipolar disorder is a lifelong and recurrent illness, long-term treatment is needed to manage and control mood symptoms.
- Cardiovascular mortality is almost twice as high in patients with bipolar disorder. The risk of sudden death may also theoretically be increased due to reduced heart-rate variability.

Chronic Treatment
- The continuation phase of treatment lasts weeks to months and the primary goal is to reach full remission of symptoms and restoration of functioning.
- The primary goal of the maintenance phase of treatment is to achieve full and sustained symptom remission for at least 1 year after resolution of symptoms.
- Long-term life maintenance is recommended for patients who have suffered three or more manic episodes.
- Study results from a large-scale National Institute of Mental Health–funded clinical trial found patients treated with both medications and intensive psychotherapy (30 sessions over 9 months of therapy) demonstrated the following:
  - Fewer relapses
  - Lower hospitalization rates
  - Better ability to stick to treatment plans
  - More likely to get well faster and stay well longer
- Medications:
  - Long-term management of bipolar disorder should be treated with a mood stabilizer
  - Patients who fail to respond to one mood stabilizer may need to be switched to another, or the addition of another mood stabilizer or an atypical antipsychotic may be required.
  - Risk of suicide is reduced 13-fold with long-term maintenance therapy with lithium.
  - There is limited research on all of the atypical antipsychotics in the maintenance phase of treatment; however, any of the atypical antipsychotics may be considered when other treatments are unsuccessful.

▪ ECT is used only as a last resort if the patient does not adequately respond to medications and/or psychotherapy.
  ▪ Psychotherapy
  ▪ CBT: helps individuals with bipolar disorder learn to change harmful and negative thought patterns and behaviors, as well as learn coping skills, such as stress management, identifying triggers for mood symptoms, and relaxation techniques.
  ▪ Family therapy: this therapy includes family members. By doing so, it helps family members enhance coping strategies, such as recognizing new episodes and knowing how to help their loved one. Therapy also focuses on communication skills and problem solving.
  ▪ Interpersonal therapy: helps people with bipolar disorder improve their relationships with others.
  ▪ Social rhythm therapy: therapy focuses on maintaining and managing daily routines, such as regular sleep/wake cycles, eating patterns, and social routines.
  ▪ Psychoeducation: focuses on teaching individuals with bipolar disorder about the illness and its treatment. This form of treatment helps people realize signs of relapse so that they can access treatment early before a full episode occurs. This usually occurs in a group format and may also be helpful for family members and caregivers.
▪ Follow-up care by a chemical dependence treatment specialist is recommended when indicated.
▪ Patients with cardiac comorbidity, abnormal findings on cardiac examination, or significant risk factors for heart disease should be referred to a cardiologist.
▪ Patients with endocrine dysfunction, such as hyperthyroidism or hypothyroidism, should be referred to an endocrinologist.
▪ Treatment can be complicated or have a poorer course by having another condition at the same time, such as substance abuse, depression, anxiety disorders, or a personality disorder.
▪ Concomitant substance abuse/dependence is correlated with increased hospitalizations and a worse illness course coupled with increased safety risk.

PSYCHOPHARMACOLOGY OF BIPOLAR DISORDER

Overview of Psychopharmacology of Bipolar Disorder
▪ *Mood stabilizers,* including mood-stabilizing anticonvulsants and lithium, are identified as first-line treatment approaches. Lithium is recommended for bipolar depression. Mood-stabilizing anticonvulsants (e.g., valproate) are preferred for rapid-cycling disorders.
▪ Hypomanic episodes and mild depressive episodes are generally managed with a single mood stabilizer. Acute manic and severe depressive episodes often require two or three medications.
▪ A benzodiazepine (e.g., diazepam or lorazepam) may be considered as an adjunct short-term treatment for reducing insomnia or agitation.
▪ Use of antidepressants by primary care providers for treating bipolar patients should be avoided. Antidepressant monotherapy may precipitate mania or induce rapid-cycling disorders between mania and depression.
▪ Dosage adjustments may be required if the patient experiences a partial response or breakthrough symptoms.

Drug Selection Table for Bipolar Disorders

CLASS	DRUG
Mood-stabilizing anticonvulsants	**First-line drug therapy:**
	Valproate sodium, valproic acid, divalproex sodium (Depacon, Depakene, *Depakote, Depakote ER, Depakote* Sprinkle)
	Carbamazepine *(Tegretol, Equetro, Tegretol XR)*
	Topiramate (*Topamax*)
	Lamotrigine (*Lamictal, Lamictal XR*)
Nonanticonvulsant mood stabilizer	**First-line drug therapy for bipolar depression:**
	Lithium (*Eskalith, Lithobid*)
Atypical antipsychotics (second generation)	**Aripiprazole (*Abilify*)**
	Olanzapine (*Zyprexa*)
	Risperidone (*Risperdal, Risperdal Consta*)
	Quetiapine (*Seroquel, Seroquel XR*)
	Ziprasidone (*Geodon*)

■ ECT may be considered for treatment-resistant or severe mania. In general, mood stabilizer treatment has produced better outcomes than ECT.

Recurrence Rate
■ Bipolar I disorder
  ■ The course of bipolar I disorder is marked by relapses and remissions, often alternating manic with depressive episodes.
  ■ Ninety percent of individuals who have a single manic episode go on to have future manic or hypomanic episodes within another 5 years.
  ■ Approximately 60% to 70% of manic episodes occur immediately before or after an MDE.
  ■ The majority of individuals with bipolar I disorder experience symptom reduction among episodes; however, between 20% and 30% continue to have mood lability and other symptoms.
  ■ Sixty percent of sufferers experience chronic interpersonal and occupational difficulties among acute episodes.
  ■ Patients with bipolar I fare worse than patients with a major depression. Within the first 2 years after the initial episode, 40% to 50% of patients experience another manic episode.
  ■ Psychotic symptoms can develop days or weeks after a previous nonpsychotic manic or mixed episode.
  ■ Individuals who have manic episodes with psychotic features are more likely to have subsequent manic episodes with psychotic features.
  ■ Ninety percent of individuals with bipolar I disorder have at least one psychiatric hospitalization and two thirds have two or more hospitalizations in their lifetime.

- Bipolar II disorder
  - This disorder is studied less and the course is less well understood.
- Patient behaviors that can lead to a recurrence of depressive or manic symptoms:
  - Discontinuing or lowering one's dose of medication.
  - An inconsistent sleep schedule can destabilize the illness. Too much sleep can lead to depression, whereas too little sleep can lead to mixed states or mania.
  - Inadequate stress management and poor lifestyle choices. Medication raises the stress threshold somewhat, but too much stress still causes relapse.
  - Using drugs or alcohol can either trigger or prolong mood symptoms.

PATIENT EDUCATION

- Advise patients that it is important to deal with mania early in the episode, and thus recognizing the early warning signs is the key so that more intensive treatment can be administered before symptoms escalate.
- Advise patient to stay on all medications and to not decrease or stop any medications without medical supervision. This is especially important when experiencing mania or hypomania.
- Also advise patients that sometimes several medication trials are needed to find ones that will be efficacious in controlling mood symptoms.
- Advise patients that symptoms will improve gradually, not immediately, as they begin to remit.
- In general, there is little research about herbal or natural supplements for bipolar spectrum disorders and not much is known about their efficacy; however, St. John's wort may cause a switch to mania and can make other medications less effective (e.g., antidepressants and anticonvulsants). Additionally, the effects of Sam-E or omega-3 fatty acids are not known. All herbal and natural remedies for mood symptoms should be discussed with a medical provider.
- The best approach to treatment is a combination of psychotherapy and medications. This helps prevent relapses, reduces hospitalizations, and helps the patient get well faster and stay well longer.
- If patients plan extensive travel into other time zones, advise them to call their doctor before leaving to determine whether any changes in their medicines should be made and what to do if they have a manic or depressive episode while away.
- Women who are pregnant or would like to become pregnant and have been diagnosed with a bipolar spectrum disorder should speak with their doctors about the risks and benefits of all treatments during pregnancy. Mood-stabilizing medications used today can cause harm to the developing fetus or a nursing infant. Additionally, stopping or reducing medications during pregnancy can cause a recurrence of mood symptoms.
- Helping the individual identify and modify stressors provides a critical aspect of patient and family awareness.
- Changes in sleep patterns can sometimes trigger a manic or depressive episode. Advise patients to keep a regular routine such as eating meals at the same time every day and going to sleep at the same time nightly and waking up at the same time daily.
- Patients should be encouraged to keep a chart of daily mood symptoms, treatments, sleep patterns, and life events to both help themselves and their providers treat the illness most effectively. This is often referred to as a "life chart."

▨ Advise patients with bipolar spectrum disorders to avoid nicotine, sympathomimetic or anticholinergic drugs, caffeine, alcohol, or illicit drugs.

▨ For excellent patient education resources, visit eMedicine's Mental Health and Behavior Center and Bipolar Center. See also eMedicine's patient education articles on bipolar disorder.

MEDICAL/LEGAL PITFALLS

▨ Failure to assess, monitor, and treat safety risk issues

▨ Failure to assess for history of manic or hypomanic episodes when patient presents with depressive symptoms

▨ Failure to assess for coexisting substance-use disorders

▨ Failure to discontinue antidepressants if individual presents with acute mania or mixed mood symptoms

▨ Failure to monitor for toxicity or metabolic changes associated with prescribed lithium and atypical antipsychotics

▨ Prescribing an antidepressant during a MDE and not also prescribing a mood-stabilizing agent in patients with known bipolar spectrum disorders is a mistake. Only taking an antidepressant increases the risk of switching one's mood to either mania or hypomania, or developing rapid-cycling symptoms.

Cyclothymic Disorder

BACKGROUND INFORMATION

Definition of Disorder

▨ Cyclothymia is considered a mild, subthreshold form of bipolar disorder and is often referred to as a "soft" bipolar spectrum disorder.

▨ The main difference between cyclothymic disorder and bipolar I disorder is the severity of the mania in that the symptoms do not meet the criteria for a manic episode in cyclothymia.

▨ The main difference between cyclothymic disorder and bipolar II disorder is the severity of the depressive symptoms in that the depressive symptoms do not meet the full criteria for an MDE.

▨ Mood changes in cyclothymic disorder can be abrupt and unpredictable, of short duration, and with infrequent euthymic episodes.

▨ Both phases of the disorder appear deleterious to psychosocial functioning; however, they can also have high levels of achievement and creativity, which can be socially advantageous due to hypomania.

▨ Hypomania or subthreshold depressive symptoms can last for weeks or days. In between up and down moods, a person may have normal moods or may continue to cycle continuously from hypomanic to depressed with no normal periods in between.

▨ The mood swings in this disorder appear to be biphasic.

▨ Cyclothymia symptoms are typically chronic, often do not appear to be related to life events, and appear to an observer as a personality trait.

■ Although the mood symptoms are milder than those of bipolar I and bipolar II disorders, they can be disabling due to unstable moods and the unpredictability of the mood pattern can cause significant distress.

■ Some patients with cyclothymic disorder were characterized as being interpersonally sensitive, hyperactive, or moody as young children.

■ Onset of cyclothymic disorder after the age of 65 years is rare and alerts the practitioner to rule out organic reasons for the mood fluctuations.

■ It is not uncommon for cyclothymic disorder to go undetected.

■ Patients rarely seek treatment during the periods of hypomania because it is often considered a desired state.

Etiology

■ The exact cause of cyclothymic disorder is not known.

■ The "kindling theory" is the current predominant theory, meaning that the disorder is likely to be caused by multiple factors that potentially interact and lower the threshold at which mood changes occur. Eventually, a mood episode can start itself and thus become recurrent.

  ▨ Environmental factors:
    ● Irregular sleep/wake patterns have been shown to trigger mood symptoms.
  ▨ Biological perspectives:
    ● Genetics:
      – Cyclothymic disorder appears more common in first-degree biological relatives of individuals with bipolar disorder.
      – An individual appears two to three times more likely to have cyclothymic disorder if first-degree biological relatives also have the disorder.
    ● Neural processes:
      – There does not appear to be research investigating the underlying molecular or neurotomical etiology for cyclothymic disorder.
      – The disorder appears to have a circadian component. Some patients state, for example, that they can go to bed in a good mood and wake up with sub-threshold depressive symptoms.
      – Declines in rapid eye movement (REM) period latency during the sleep cycle have been noted in patients with cyclothymia.
      – Reduced skin conductance has been found in patients with cyclothymic disorder.
    ● Endocrine models:
      – Endocrine studies in cyclothymia are very limited.
      – Hypothyroidism can cause depression and/or mood instability.
      – Cortisol hypersecretion and poor regulation of cortisol have been noted in patients with cyclothymia when faced with an experimental stressor.

Demographics

■ True prevalence is not known due to misdiagnosis or undetected episodes of hypomania.

■ At this time, it does not appear that epidemiological studies have been specifically conducted for cyclothymic disorder; however, lifetime prevalence of cyclothymic disorder is estimated to range from 0.3% to 6%, depending on the criteria used.

■ Women and men are affected equally, but women typically present for treatment more often than do men.

▧ Medically, research has shown the following related to dysthymia, the subthreshold depression associated with this disorder:
  ▧ Due to the subthreshold depression, patients with this disorder are approximately 2.6 times more likely to suffer a cerebral vascular accident and are at greater risk for cardiovascular disorders.
    ◉ The presence of depressive symptoms in the absence of MDEs is associated with greater risk for cardiac events.
    ◉ The aspect of depression, hopelessness, has been linked to sudden death.
    ◉ The presence of vital exhaustion (fatigue, irritability, and demoralized feelings) has been reported to predict progression of coronary artery disease and/or cardiac events.
    ◉ Cardiovascular mortality is almost elevated for individuals who have dysthymia. The risk of sudden death may also theoretically be increased due to reduced heart-rate variability.
  ▧ Overall, 28% of patients who have mild depressive symptoms suffer from incapacitating medical conditions.
    ◉ Forty-five percent of patients have chronic insomnia.
    ◉ Four percent to eighteen percent have comorbid diabetes mellitus.
    ◉ Fourteen percent to twenty percent have HIV infection.
    ◉ Three percent to thirty-one percent have significant premenstrual syndrome.
    ◉ Fourteen percent have Parkinson's disease.
    ◉ Twenty-eight percent experience chronic pain.
  ▧ Individuals with dysthymia use medical treatment to a higher degree than the general population.

Risk Factors
Age
▧ Cyclothymic disorder usually begins in adolescence or in early adulthood.
▧ True age of onset is typically difficult to ascertain due to the insidious nature of the mood symptoms and its chronic course.
▧ Incidence rates are rare before puberty, and hypomanic episodes are not known in children.
▧ Cyclothymia and dysthymia appear common in adolescents, when the depressive onsets outnumber the nondepressive onsets.
▧ Often, the cycling between moods accelerates with age.

Gender
▧ Some studies indicate that men and women are affected equally and others state that women are affected more than men.
▧ Women in the premenstrual period may have worsening of ongoing hypomanic episodes or depressive symptoms.

Family History
▧ Individuals who have first-degree relatives diagnosed with bipolar disorder are at greater risk of cyclothymic disorder.

Stressful Events in Susceptible People
▧ Often patients with cyclothymic disorder cannot identify an environmental precipitant to their moods.
▧ Ongoing psychosocial stressors have been shown to destabilize moods.
▧ Major life changes have also been shown to destabilize moods.

Having Another Mental Health Disorder
- Substance-use disorders
  - Individuals with cyclothymia are at heightened risk for substance abuse issues due to the high frequency of their mood symptoms.
  - Substance abuse is common in cyclothymic disorder and it is hypothesized that the individual is attempting to self-medicate the dysthymic mood symptoms and/or sleep disturbance or to precipitate and sustain hypomania.
- Bipolar I or bipolar II disorder
  - This disorder has a 15% to 50% risk that the individual will eventually develop bipolar I or bipolar II disorder.
- A diagnosis of attention deficit hyperactivity disorder
  - The diagnosis for a child may be a marker for a bipolar spectrum diagnosis as an adult.
- Personality disorders
  - Differentiating between individuals with cyclothymic disorder and particularly cluster B personality disorders (borderline personality disorder, histrionic personality disorder, and antisocial personality disorder) is difficult because the affective instability is similar.
  - Mood symptoms from cyclothymic disorder can be so flagrant that a personality disorder may be erroneously diagnosed.
  - Marked personality disorder symptoms negatively influence treatment-related outcomes in patients with bipolar disorder.

Risk Factors for Suicidal Behavior in Bipolar Spectrum Disorders
- Patients with cyclothymic disorder are at higher risk for suicide due to frequently changing mood episodes.
- Personal or family history of suicidal behavior
- Severity and number of depressive episodes
- Alcohol or substance abuse/dependence
- Level of pessimism and hopelessness
- Level of impulsivity and/or aggression
- Younger age of onset of the disorder
- A concomitant personality disorder diagnosis
- Patients with remitting depressive symptoms are thought to be at an increased risk for suicide.

Risk Factors for Harm to Others in Bipolar Spectrum Disorders
- A history of violent behavior has consistently been shown to be the best single predictor of future violence.
- The presence of symptoms that increase the risk of violence in the absence of overt threats includes presenting as guarded and suspicious.
- Younger age
- Gender is not a factor and the rates of violence among genders are equal in patients who are acutely mentally ill.
- A history of victimization as a child or witnessing or experiencing violence after the age of 16 years.
- Level of impulsivity
- More than a half of victims of violence by persons with mental health disorders are family members.
- The availability of firearms and/or weapons.

DIAGNOSIS

Differential Diagnosis

There is a broad differential diagnosis for bipolar spectrum disorders that includes the following:

- Thyroid or other metabolic disorders
- Epilepsy (partial complex seizures)
- MS
- Diabetes mellitus
- Sleep apnea
- Brain lesions
- Systemic infection
- Systemic lupus erythematosus
- Cerebral vascular accident
- HIV
- Steroid-induced mood symptoms
- Vitamin B_{12} deficiency
- Vitamin D deficiency
- PTSD
- Attention deficit hyperactivity disorder
- Bipolar I or II disorder with rapid cycling
- MDD
- Dysthymic disorder
- Borderline personality disorder
- Eating disorder
- Drug interactions or adverse effects that can cause mood symptoms (e.g., baclofen, bromide, bromocriptine, captopril, cimetidine, corticosteroids, cyclosporine, disulfiram [Antabuse], hydralazine, isoniazid, levodopa, methylphenidate [Ritalin], metrizamide, procarbazine, procyclidine [Kemadrin])
- Drug or alcohol intoxication or withdrawal

ICD Code

Cyclothymic disorder (F34.0)

Diagnostic Workup

- There are no biological tests that confirm cyclothymic disorder. Rather, tests are carried out to rule in/out medical issues that may be mimicking a mood disorder.
  - ANA: ANAs are found in patients whose immune system may be predisposed to cause inflammation against their own body tissues. Antibodies that are directed against one's own tissues are referred to as autoantibodies.
  - Thyroid and other metabolic function studies suggest hyperexcitability or hypoexcitability symptoms.
  - Blood glucose level rules out diabetes
  - Serum proteins
  - Lithium levels should be measured if patient has a history of diagnosis and is taking this medication.
  - CBC with differential is used to rule out anemia or other blood dyscrasias.
  - Urine toxicology screening for drug and alcohol screening (see previous data)
  - Urine copper level; high levels indicate toxic exposure

- Venereal disease research lab test
- HIV testing (ELISA and Western Blot test)
- EKG determines cardiac anomolities.
- Electroencephalogram may exclude epilepsy.
- Sleep study: sleep apnea
- Magnetic resonance imagery determines presence of aneurysms, past head trauma, brain tumors.
- Computed tomography scan of head is used to rule out head injury.
- Clinical history
- Diagnosis is difficult to establish without a prolonged period of observation or obtaining an account from others about their moods and functioning across their life span. Thus, collateral information from close friends and family is important.

Initial Assessment

- It is important to gain a complete history and carefully assess for historical and/ or current episodes of mania and/or hypomania as well as major depression and episodes of subclinical depression.
- Physical examination with a focus on neurological and endocrine systems and infectious diseases
- Differentiation of cyclothymic disorder from personality disorders:
  - Periods of elevation and depression that typify affective disorders tend to be endogenous in cyclothymic disorder. This means that the mood symptoms come out of the blue with little external provocation.
  - Diurnal variations with worsening symptoms in the morning are typical in cyclothymic disorder.
  - The disturbances in cyclothymia are biphasic.
- Specific screening questions to assess for and rule out manic episodes, mixed episodes, or hypomanic episodes:
  - Have you ever experienced periods of feeling uncharacteristically energetic?
  - Have you had periods of not sleeping but not feeling tired?
  - Have you ever felt that your thoughts were racing and that there was nothing you could do to slow them down?
  - Have you ever experienced periods during which you did riskier things, were, more interested in sex than usual, or were spending more money than you usually would?
- Uses of standardized screening tools:
  - Bipolar Spectrum Diagnostic Scale (BSDS)
  - Mood Disorder Questionnaire (MDQ)
  - The START: assesses risk and guides treatment for violence, suicide, self-neglect, substance use, and victimization.
- Psychiatric assessment with a focus on current symptoms, date of onset, potential precipitating factors, and perpetuating factors (e.g., drug or alcohol use), traumatic events in childhood, and substance use
- Family history with an emphasis on psychiatric history and suicide attempts and completed suicides
- Social history with an emphasis on current social support and safety issues in relationships, recent psychosocial stressors, ability to maintain employment, and financial concerns

■ Assessment of safety risk with an emphasis on history of harm to self or others, history of childhood abuse or victimization, plan and intent, and access to firearms and/or weapons
■ Level of functional impairment and need for hospitalization (e.g., ability to work, engage in self-care activities, ability to conduct activities of daily living, and ability to get along with others)

Clinical Presentation

Hypomanic Episode

■ Affect/moods:
  ■ Up
  ■ Expansive
  ■ Irritable
  ■ Moody
■ Behaviors:
  ■ Busy
  ■ Active
  ■ Overinvolved
  ■ Increased energy
  ■ Increase in planning and doing things
  ■ Social warmth
  ■ Increased creativity and productivity
  ■ Can be hypersexual
  ■ Others notice their increase in activity but the patient often denies anything about him or her has changed.
■ Thoughts:
  ■ Optimistic
  ■ Future focused
  ■ Positive attitude
■ Perceptions
  ■ Patients with hypomania typically do not experience perceptual changes.

Dysthymia

■ Vegetative symptoms usually seen in MDEs are not as common.
■ Affect/moods:
  ■ Continuously feeling sad
  ■ Gloomy
  ■ Irritable
  ■ Excessive anger
■ Behavior:
  ■ Poor appetite
  ■ Sleep disturbance
  ■ Apathy
  ■ Lack of motivation
  ■ Introversion
  ■ Social withdrawal
  ■ Quiet and less talkative
  ■ Generalized loss of interest or pleasure and incapable of fun
  ■ Passive

- Somatization (e.g., increase in physical or somatic complaints without objective, identifiable cause)
  - Conscientious and self-disciplining
- Thoughts:
  - Self-critical, self-reproaching, and self-derogatory
  - Pessimistic
  - Poor concentration and indecisiveness
  - Worry and rumination (brooding)
  - Preoccupied with their inadequacy, failures, or negative life events
  - Hopelessness
  - Helplessness
- Perceptions:
  - Patients with dysthymia typically do not experience perceptual changes.
  - Biphasic characteristics of cyclothymic disorder
- Lethargy alternates with good moods.
- Unexplained tearfulness alternates with excessive wit and humor.
- Introversion and self-absorption alternate with uninhibited seeking of people.
- Mental confusion alternates with sharpened thinking.
- Shaky self-esteem alternates between low self-confidence and overconfidence.

DSM-5 Diagnostic Guidelines
Cyclothymic Disorder
- For at least 2 years the patient has had multiple periods in which hypomanic symptoms have been present, and multiple periods of low mood that have not fulfilled the criteria for a MDE or hypomanic episode.
- The longest period in which the patient has been free of mood swings is 2 months.
- During the first 2 years of the disorder, the patient had not had periods of mood disturbance in which the criteria for a manic episode, a mixed episode, or a MDE were also met.
- The symptoms are not more easily ascribed to other medical diagnoses, other medical conditions, substance use, or drug withdrawal.
- The disturbances in mood engender significant distress for the individual and/or a reduction in social or other important areas of functioning.

Hypomanic
- For at least 4 days, the patient manifests a mood that is elevated, expansive, or irritable, and representing a distinct departure from the patient's nondepressed baseline mood.
- During this period, the patient has three or more of the following:
  - Grandiose thoughts, inflated self-esteem
  - Diminished sleep
  - Volubility
  - Racing thoughts
  - Increased levels of distractibility
  - Psychomotor agitation
  - A focus on goal-directed activities
  - Poor judgment; activities that have potential for adverse outcomes (e.g., spending sprees)
- Psychotic features are absent.
- Appropriate social and occupational functioning are maintained.

■ Hospitalization is not required.
■ The symptoms are not more easily ascribed to other medical diagnoses, other medical conditions, substance use, or withdrawal from prescription medication.

TREATMENT OVERVIEW

Acute Treatment

■ The primary goal of the acute phase is to manage acute hypomania episodes and subclinical depression and associated safety risk issues.
■ Specific treatment studies for cyclothymic disorder separate from other bipolar spectrum disorders are minimal.
■ Diagnostic tests should be performed to rule out potential medical etiologies for mood symptoms, especially if this is the first episode of mania, hypomania, mixed mood symptoms, or depression.
■ How to handle suicidal ideation:
  ■ With suicidal ideation with plan and intent patient should be hospitalized (voluntarily or involuntarily) due to acute safety risk.
  ■ With suicidal ideation with plan but no intent patients may be treated on an outpatient basis with close follow-up if they do not have access to the means to carry out their plan and adequate social support.
  ■ With suicidal ideation without plan and no intent, the patient requires careful assessment of current psychosocial stressors, access to weapons, and other lethal means, substance use, and impulse control issues. Any lethal means should be removed.
■ How to handle aggression and potential harm to others:
  ■ If patients have access to firearms and/or weapons, they should be removed.
  ■ Those with thoughts of harming others with plan and intent should be hospitalized (voluntarily or involuntarily).
  ■ Those with thoughts of harming others with plan but no intent can be treated on an outpatient basis, with increased intensity of treatment with an established provider, depending on risk factors.
  ■ Those with thoughts of harming others without plan or intent do require increased intensity of treatment and perhaps increased dosages of medications.
■ Acute hypomanic episode
  ■ Treatment for hypomania, which can lead to either a manic or depressive episode, may decrease symptom progression.
■ Medication noncompliance is common because hypomania may be a desired state for many individuals with cyclothymic disorder, and many are reluctant to take medications.
■ Because this disorder is considered a chronic and lifelong illness, long-term treatment is needed to manage and control mood symptoms.

Chronic Treatment

■ The primary goal of long-term treatment is to prevent cyclothymia from worsening and progressing to full-blown manic episodes.
■ Specific treatment studies for cyclothymia as distinct from other bipolar spectrum disorders are minimal.
■ Study results from a large-scale National Institute of Mental Health–funded clinical trial found patients treated with both medications and intensive psychotherapy (30 sessions over 9 months of therapy) for bipolar spectrum disorders demonstrated:

- ▩ Fewer relapses
- ▩ Lower hospitalization rates
- ▩ Better ability to stick to treatment plans
- ▩ More likely to get well faster and stay well longer
- ▩ Medications:
  - ▩ Long-term management of cyclothymic disorder should be treated with a mood stabilizer.
  - ▩ Antidepressant medications have not been shown to be an effective adjunctive therapy, and as a monotherapy they can precipitate mania, mixed mood symptoms, or hypomania.

Overview of Pharmacotherapy for Cyclothymic Disorder

- ▩ *Mood stabilizers*, including mood-stabilizing anticonvulsants, atypical antipsychotic agents, and lithium, are identified as first-line treatment approaches. Lithium and Lamictal are recommended for bipolar depression. Mood-stabilizing anticonvulsants (e.g., valproate and lamotrigine) are preferred for rapid-cycling disorders.
- ▩ For patients unresponsive to monotherapy, a combination of lithium plus mood-stabilizing anticonvulsant or mood stabilizer plus atypical antipsychotic may be considered.
- ▩ Hypomanic episodes and mild depressive episodes are generally managed with a single mood stabilizer. Acute manic and severe depressive episodes often require two or three medications.
- ▩ A benzodiazepine (e.g., diazepam or lorazepam) may be considered as an adjunct short-term treatment for reducing insomnia or agitation.
- ▩ Use of antidepressants by primary care providers for treating bipolar patients should be avoided. Antidepressant monotherapy may precipitate mania or induce rapid-cycling disorders between mania and depression.
- ▩ Dosage adjustments may be required if the patient experiences a partial response or breakthrough symptoms.

Drug Selection Table for Cyclothymic Disorder

CLASS	DRUG
Mood-stabilizing anticonvulsants	First-line drug therapy:
	Valproate sodium, valproic acid, divalproex sodium (Depacon, Depakene, *Depakote, Depakote ER, Depakote* Sprinkle)
	Carbamazepine (*Tegretol, Carbatrol, Tegretol XR*)
	Topiramate (*Topamax*)
	Lamotrigine (*Lamictal, Lamictal XR*)
Nonanticonvulsant mood stabilizer	First-line drug therapy for bipolar depression:
	Lithium (*Eskalith, Lithobid*)
Atypical antipsychotics (second generation)	Aripiprazole (*Abilify*)
	Olanzapine (*Zyprexa*)
	Risperidone (*Risperdal, Risperdal Consta*)
	Quetiapine (*Seroquel, Seroquel XR*)
	Ziprasidone (*Geodon*)

■ ECT may be considered for treatment-resistant or severe mania. In general, mood-stabilizer treatment has produced better outcomes than ECT.
■ ECT is used only as a last resort if the patient does not adequately respond to medications and/or psychotherapy.
■ Psychotherapy:
    ■ CBT: helps individuals with bipolar disorder learn to change harmful and negative thought patterns and behaviors, as well as learn coping skills such as stress management, identifying triggers for mood symptoms, and relaxation techniques.
    ■ Family therapy: this therapy includes family members. By doing so, it helps family members enhance coping strategies, such as recognizing new episodes and how to help their loved one. Therapy also focuses on communication skills and problem solving.
        ■ Interpersonal therapy: helps people with bipolar disorder improve their relationships with others.
    ■ Social rhythm therapy: this therapy focuses on maintaining and managing their daily routines such as regular sleep/wake cycles, eating patterns, and social routines.
    ■ Psychoeducation: focuses on teaching individuals with bipolar disorder about the illness and its treatment. This form of treatment helps people realize signs of relapse so that they can access treatment early before a full episode occurs. This is usually in a group format and it may also be helpful for family members and caregivers.
    ■ Psychodynamic and psychoanalytic therapies do not appear to have an effect in patients with this disorder.
    ■ Follow-up care by a chemical dependence treatment specialist is recommended when indicated.
    ■ Patients with cardiac comorbidity, abnormal findings on cardiac examination, or significant risk factors for heart disease should be referred to a cardiologist.
    ■ Patients with endocrine dysfunction, such as hyperthyroidism or hypothyroidism, should be referred to an endocrinologist.
    ■ Treatment can be complicated or have a poorer course by having another condition at the same time, such as substance abuse, depression, anxiety disorders, or a personality disorder.
    ■ Concomitant substance abuse/dependence is correlated with increased hospitalizations and a worse course of the illness and increases safety risk.

Recurrence Rate
■ Approximately one third of all patients diagnosed with cyclothymic disorder will develop a major mood disorder during their lifetime, and it is usually bipolar II disorder.
■ Retrospective studies of patients with cyclothymia, taking lithium over a 2-year period, indicated the following:
    ■ Only 26% to 36% were free of depression symptoms as compared to 42% to 55% for patients with bipolar II and 31% to 42% of patients with a unipolar designation.
    ■ The probability rate for hospitalization due to severity of depression symptoms was 69% for patients with cyclothymia vs. 51% for patients with bipolar II and 64% for patients with a unipolar designation.

▦ Patients diagnosed with cyclothymia and treated with Valproate required lower doses and serum concentrations to achieve mood stabilization as compared to patients with BP disorder.

▦ Patient behaviors that can lead to a recurrence of depressive or manic symptoms:

   ▦ Discontinuing or lowering one's dose of medication

   ▦ An inconsistent sleep schedule can destabilize the illness. Too much sleep can lead to depression, whereas too little sleep can trigger and sustain hypomania.

   ▦ Inadequate stress management and poor lifestyle choices

   ▦ Medication raises the stress threshold somewhat, but too much stress still causes relapse.

   ▦ Using drugs or alcohol can either trigger or prolong mood symptoms.

PATIENT EDUCATION

▦ Advise patients that it is important to deal with mania early in the episode, and thus recognizing the early-warning signs is the key so that more intensive treatment can be administered before symptoms escalate.

▦ Advise patient to stay on all medications and to not decrease or stop any medications without medical supervision. This is especially important when experiencing mania or hypomania.

▦ Also advise patients that sometimes several medication trials are needed to find ones that will be efficacious in controlling mood symptoms.

▦ Advise patients that symptoms will improve gradually, not immediately, as they begin to remit.

▦ In general, there is little research about herbal or natural supplements for bipolar spectrum disorders and not much is known about their efficacy; however, St. John's wort may cause a switch to mania and can make other medications less effective (e.g., antidepressants and anticonvulsants). May cause serious drug interactions and serotonin syndrome--as this is a natural SSRI and people don't realize that. Additionally, the effects of Sam-E or omega-3 fatty acids are not known. All herbal and natural remedies for mood symptoms should be discussed with a medical care provider.

▦ The best approach to treatment is a combination of psychotherapy and medications. This helps prevent relapses, reduces hospitalizations, and helps the patient get well faster and stay well longer.

▦ If patients plan extensive travel into other time zones, advise them to call their doctors before leaving to determine whether any changes in their medicines should be made and what to do if they have mood episode while away.

▦ Women who are pregnant or would like to become pregnant and have been diagnosed with a cyclothymic disorder should speak with their doctors about the risks and benefits of all treatments during pregnancy. Mood-stabilizing medications used today can cause harm to the developing fetus or a nursing infant. Additionally, stopping or reducing medications during pregnancy can cause a recurrence of mood symptoms.

▦ Helping the individual identify and modify stressors provides a critical aspect of patient and family awareness.

▦ Changes in sleep patterns can sometimes trigger a manic or depressive episode. Advise patients to keep a regular routine such as eating meals at the same time every day and going to sleep at the same time nightly and waking up at the same time daily.

- Patients should be encouraged to keep a chart of daily mood symptoms, treatments, sleep patterns, and life events to help both themselves and their providers treat the illness most effectively. This is often referred to as a "life chart."
- Advise patients with cyclothymia to avoid nicotine, sympathomimetic or anticholinergic drugs, caffeine, alcohol, or illicit drugs.
- For excellent patient education resources, visit eMedicine's Mental Health and Behavior Center and Bipolar Center. See also eMedicine's patient education articles on bipolar disorder.

MEDICAL/LEGAL PITFALLS

- Failure to assess, monitor, and treat safety-risk issues
- Failure to assess for history of manic or hypomanic episodes when patient presents with depressive symptoms
- Failure to assess for coexisting substance-use disorders
- Failure to monitor for toxicity or metabolic changes associated with prescribed lithium
- Prescribing and not properly monitoring divalproex (Depakote) and valproic acid (Depakene) for women younger than 20 years is problematic. This medication may increase the levels of testosterone, which can lead to polycystic ovary syndrome (PCOS). Most PCOS symptoms begin after stopping treatment with valproic acid (Depakene).
- Prescribing an antidepressant for depressive symptoms and not also prescribing a mood-stabilizing agent in patients with known bipolar spectrum disorders is risky. Only taking an antidepressant increased the risk of switching the patient's mood to either mania or hypomania, or developing rapid-cycling symptoms.

Persistent Depressive Disorder (Dysthymic Disorder)

BACKGROUND INFORMATION

Definition of Disorder
- This is a chronic mood disorder characterized by depressed mood more days than not, indicated by the individual or by others.
- Dysthymic disorder is associated with increased morbidity from physical disease.
- Patients often possess a negative, gloomy outlook on life with ruminative coping strategies.
- Tendency toward self-criticism and a sense of inadequacy
- Tend to spend limited time in leisure activities

Persistent depressive disorder is characterized by long-term (2 years or longer) but less severe symptoms that may not disable a person but that prevents normal functioning or feeling well. People with dysthymia may also experience one or more episodes of major depression during their lifetimes.

Etiology
- It is thought to be a result of an interplay between genetic factors, chronic stress, and personality factors.

■ Biological factors such as alterations in neurotransmitters, endocrine, and inflammatory mediators are also thought to play a role.

■ Cognitive and personality factors, such as how people view their influence, their ability to change, and their interpretation of stressors, play a role.

■ Cases are very likely to have a family history of mood disorders, particularly dysthymia and MDD.

Demographics

■ Data suggest that the disorder affects 3% to 6% of the U.S. general population and 5% to 15% of the primary care population. It affects approximately 36% of patients in outpatient mental health treatment centers.

■ Women are twice as likely to present with dysthymic disorder than men.

■ It often starts at childhood or adolescence with an early sense of unhappiness without clear cause.

■ One large study showed it to be more common in African Americans and Mexican Americans than in Whites (the opposite pattern from MDD).

■ One study showed a 77% of lifetime risk of developing MDD and a higher risk of suicide attempts among patients with dysthymic disorder than patients with MDD.

■ The prevalence rate of dysthymic disorder is 0.6% to 1.7% in children and 1.6% to 8% in adolescents.

■ Patients with dysthymic disorder should not be seen as simply having a "mild form of depression." They are at high risk for developing MDD and often have MDD, which is harder to treat.

■ Patients with dysthymic disorder should be evaluated for suicide risk.

Risk Factors

Gender

■ Like other depressive disorders, dysthymic disorder is approximately two times more common in women than men.

Family History

■ Studies have shown an increased incidence of dysthymic disorder when there is a history of depression, bipolar disorder, or dysthymia in first-degree relatives.

■ There are learned or genetic personality factors such as poor coping skills, particularly ruminative, rather than problem-solving or cognitive-restructuring strategies.

Past Medical History

■ Chronic medical illness

■ History of MDD

Social History

■ Lack of social support

■ Multiple relationship losses

Having Another Mental Health Disorder

■ Diagnosis with a personality disorder (antisocial, borderline, dependent, depressive, histrionic, or schizotypal), in particular, places a patient at higher risk for dysthymia.

▦ Alcohol abuse or substance abuse places a patient at higher risk of dysthymic disorder.

Approximately, 15% of patients with DD have comorbid substance dependence.

DIAGNOSIS

Differential Diagnosis

▦ Common:
  ▦ MDD
  ▦ Recurrent brief depressive disorder
  ▦ Alcoholism or substance abuse
  ▦ Thyroid disease
  ▦ Anemia
  ▦ Chronic fatigue syndrome
  ▦ If an underlying chronic health condition such as MS or stroke is the physiologic *cause* of the depressed mood, the diagnosis is mood disorder due to a general medical condition.
  ▦ Anxiety disorders, such as PTSD or obsessive-compulsive disorder
  ▦ Dementia
  ▦ Drug interactions or adverse effects
  ▦ Sleep apnea
  ▦ Personality disorder
▦ Less common:
  ▦ Bipolar disorder
  ▦ Amphetamine or cocaine withdrawal
  ▦ Infectious disease, such as autoimmune disorder, mononucleosis, or hepatitis C
  ▦ Parathyroid disease
  ▦ Adrenal disease
  ▦ Fibromyalgia
  ▦ Cancer
  ▦ Neurologic disease, such as cerebral vascular accident, MS, subdural hematoma, normal pressure hydrocephalus, or Alzheimer's disease
  ▦ Cardiovascular disease such as CHF or cardiomyopathy
  ▦ Nutritional deficiency, such as B vitamin, folate, or iron deficiency
  ▦ Pulmonary disease, such as COPD
  ▦ Heavy metal poisoning

ICD-10 Code

Persistent depressive disorder (dysthymia) (F34.1)

Diagnostic Workup

▦ Physical and mental evaluation:
  ▦ Thyroid function studies (T3, T4, TSH levels)
  ▦ CMP
  ▦ CBC with differential
  ▦ Vitamin D level
  ▦ Testing for infectious diseases such as hepatitis C or HIV, if applicable

Initial Assessment

▪ Mental status examination often shows slowed speech, decreased eye contact, diminished range of facial expression with self-doubt, sadness, guilt, hopelessness, and/or negative outlook. Thought will be organized without disruption of intellect, memory, abstraction, or significant abnormalities (such as delusions).

▪ Use of a standard depression screening tool such as Beck Depression Inventory, or Zung Self-Rating Scale, to rule out MDD

▪ Past medical history: If any MDD in the past 2 years, the patient does not have dysthymic disorder

▪ Family medical history, with emphasis on psychiatric history

▪ Social history, including safety of relationships, family support, and recent or ongoing stressors

▪ Past suicide attempts or past psychiatric hospitalizations

▪ Any prior manic/hypomanic episodes (*any* history suggests bipolar or cyclothymia diagnosis)

▪ What effect have symptoms had on ability to function, particularly participation in nonoccupational activities?

▪ Assess for suicide ideation, suicide plan, and suicide intent

Clinical Presentation

▪ Low self-esteem
▪ Difficulties with sleep
▪ Low energy or fatigue
▪ Difficulty in decision making
▪ Feeling hopeless
▪ Changes in eating habits, either decrease or increase in appetite
▪ Decreased facial expression
▪ Slowed speech or movements
▪ Decreased eye contact
▪ Poor concentration

DSM-5 Diagnostic Guidelines

▪ Persistent, long-term depressed mood and/or anhedonia (2 years or more in adults, 1 year or more in children and adolescents) in combination with at least 2 of the following:
  ▪ Changes in eating habits
  ▪ Changes in sleep habits
  ▪ Fatigue, low energy
  ▪ Lowered self-esteem
  ▪ Distractibility, problems with concentration
  ▪ Hopelessness
▪ Periods of remission have not been greater than 2 months
▪ There has been no MDE during the same period
▪ Psychotic features are absent
▪ Absence of manic or hypomanic episodes
▪ Evidence for cyclothymia is absent
▪ The symptoms engender distress in the individual and/or a reduction in social functioning.

TREATMENT OVERVIEW

Therapies

▦ Studies support the pharmacological approach as the first-line treatment for dysthymic disorder. Approximately, 55% of patients with DD will respond to pharmacologic therapy. Doses are the same as for major depression.

▦ Both psychological and pharmacological therapies are effective in the treatment of dysthymic disorder and each has its own merits. The combination of antidepressant and psychotherapy, such as talk therapy, is recommended for dysthymic disorder patients for long-term treatment.

▦ Pay careful attention in the first 1 to 4 weeks of antidepressant treatment to a sudden lift of depression or to worsening mood as initial response to antidepressant therapy, as these could be signs of increased risk for suicide.

▦ Be aware of the Federal Drug Administration black box warning regarding antidepressant treatment in children and younger adults and use appropriate caution in these patients.

▦ Regular follow-up for medication management, assistance for overcoming treatment resistance through augmentation therapy, and so forth, tracking patient progress in individual psychotherapy, monitoring for MDD, and reinforcement of patient self-efficacy are all important to care.

▦ Stress management and lifestyle changes, such as regular exercise, are essential to ongoing care.

▦ Studies suggest that augmentation of antidepressant effect occurs with adjunct use of omega-3 fish oil supplements, 1,000 mg twice daily. B vitamin supplementation has also been used in some studies, with equivocal results.

▦ Psychodynamic therapy, addressing an understanding of maladaptive interpersonal responses, CBT, and interpersonal therapy—which involves addressing interpersonal conflicts through improved strategies—have all been found beneficial in the treatment of patients with dysthymic disorder. Group therapy may also be helpful.

▦ Treatment may be complicated by having another condition at the same time, such as substance abuse, personality disorders, or other anxiety disorders, and these should also be addressed.

Drug Selection Table for Dysthymic Disorders

CLASS	DRUG
Selective serotonin reuptake inhibitors (SSRIs)	First-line drug therapy:
	Fluoxetine (*Prozac*)
	Sertraline (*Zoloft*)
	Paroxetine (*Paxil, Paxil CR*)
	Citalopram (*Celexa*)
	Escitalopram (*Lexapro*)
	Fluvoxamine (*Luvox*)

(continued)

Drug Selection Table for Dysthymic Disorders (*continued*)

CLASS	DRUG
Serotonin/norepinephrine reuptake inhibitors (SNRIs)	Venlafaxine (*Effexor*)
	Venlafaxine XR (*Effexor XR*)
	Duloxetine (*Cymbalta*)
	Desvenlafaxine (*Pristiq*)
Serotonin-2 antagonist/reuptake inhibitors (SARIs)	Second-line drug therapy:
	Nefazodone (*Serzone*)
	Trazodone (*Desyrel*)
Noradrenergic and specific serotonergic antidepressants (NaSSAs)	Alternative therapy option
	Mirtazapine (*Remeron*)
Norepinephrine/dopamine reuptake inhibitors (NDRIs)	Alternative therapy option:
	Bupropion (*Wellbutrin, Zyban*)
	Bupropion SR (*Wellbutrin SR*)
Tricyclic antidepressants (TCAs)	Bupropion XL (*Wellbutrin XL*)
	Amitriptyline (*Elavil*)
	Clomipramine (*Anafranil*)
	Desipramine (*Norpramin*)
	Imipramine (*Tofranil*)
Monoamine oxidase inhibitors	Nortriptyline (*Pamelor*)
	Phenelzine (*Nardil*)
	Isocarboxazid (*Marplan*)
	Tranylcypromine (*Parnaite*)

Recurrence Rate

■ In one study, there was a 53% estimated 5-year recovery rate from dysthymic disorder, but a very high risk of relapse.

PATIENT EDUCATION

■ Advise patients with dysthymic disorder to avoid nicotine and to avoid alcohol.
■ Thirty minutes of daily exercise have been found to be beneficial for dysthymic disorder patients and daily exposure to outdoor light may be beneficial.
■ For excellent patient education resources, visit eMedicine's Mental Health and Behavior Center and Depression Center. See also eMedicine's patient education articles on Dysthymic Disorder.

MEDICAL/LEGAL PITFALLS

■ Failure to monitor for suicidal thoughts
■ Failure to screen for bipolar disorder (any history of mania/hypomania)
■ Pay careful attention, in the first 1 to 4 weeks of treatment, to a sudden lift of depression or to worsening mood as an initial response to antidepressant therapy, as these could be signs of increased risk for suicide.

■ It is important that patients with dysthymic disorder be viewed as having a severe and chronic condition, which must be monitored and managed.

■ When initiating treatment, see patients on a more frequent basis until response to antidepressant is clear.

■ Have a follow-up system to ensure that there are calls to patients who fail to schedule follow-up appointments or fail to show up for scheduled appointments.

■ Patients with dysthymic disorder are more likely than the general population to use alternative therapies. Use of dietary supplements (e.g., herbs) should be discussed to avoid drug interactions.

BIBLIOGRAPHY

Akiskal, H. S. (2001). Dysthymia and cyclothymia in psychiatric practice a century after Kraepelin. *Journal of Affective Disorders, 62*(1–2), 17–31.

American Psychiatric Association. (2013). *Diagnostic and statistical manual of mental disorders* (5th ed.). Washington, DC: American Psychiatric Press.

Bauer, M., Beaulieu, S., Dunner, D. L., Lafer, B., & Kupka, R. (2008). Rapid cycling bipolar disorder–diagnostic concepts. *Bipolar Disorders, 10*(1 Pt 2), 153–162.

Ghaemi, S. N., Hsu, D. J., Thase, M. E., Wisniewski, S. R., Nierenberg, A. A., Miyahara, S., & Sachs, G. (2006). Pharmacological treatment patterns at study entry for the first 500 STEP-BD participants. *Psychiatric Services, 57*(5), 660–665.

Goldberg, J. F., Allen, M. H., Miklowitz, D. A., Bowden, C. L., Endick, C. J., Chessick, C. A.,…Sachs, G. S. (2005). Suicidal ideation and pharmacotherapy among STEP-BD patients. *Psychiatric Services, 56*(12), 1534–1540.

Goldberg, J. F., Perlis, R. H., Ghaemi, S. N., Calabrese, J. R., Bowden, C. L., Wisniewski, S.,…Thase, M. E. (2007). Adjunctive antidepressant use and symptomatic recovery among bipolar depressed patients with concomitant manic symptoms: Findings from the STEP-BD. *American Journal of Psychiatry, 164*(9), 1348–1355.

Harel, E. V., & Levkovitz, Y. (2008). Effectiveness and safety of adjunctive antidepressants in the treatment of bipolar depression: a review. *Israel Journal of Psychiatry and Related Sciences, 45*(2), 121–128.

Hirshfeld, R. M. (2002). The mood disorder questionnaire: A simple, patient-related screening instrument for bipolar disorder. *Primary Care Companion for the Journal of Psychiatry, 4*(1), 9–11.

Manning, J. S., Ahmed, S., McGuire, H. C., & Hay, D. P. (2002). Mood disorders in family practice: Beyond unipolarity to bipolarity. *Primary Care Companion to the Journal of Clinical Psychiatry, 4*(4), 142–150.

Martinez, J. M., Marangell, L. B., Simon, N. M., Miyahara, S., Wisniewski, S. R., Harrington, J.,…Thase, M. E. (2005). Baseline predictors of serious adverse events at one year among patients with bipolar disorder in STEP-BD. *Psychiatric Services, 56*(12), 1541–1548.

Miklowitz, D. J., Otto, M. W., Frank, E., Reilly-Harrington, N. A., Kogan, J. N., Sachs, G. S.,…Wisniewski, S. R. (2007). Intensive psychosocial intervention enhances functioning in patients with bipolar depression: results from a 9-month randomized controlled trial. *American Journal of Psychiatry, 164*(9), 1340–1347.

Miklowitz, D. J., Otto, M. W., Wisniewski, S. R., Araga, M., Frank, E., Reilly-Harrington, N. A.,…Sachs, G. S. (2006). Psychotherapy, symptom outcomes, and role functioning over one year among patients with bipolar disorder. *Psychiatric Services, 57*(7), 959–965.

National Mental Health. (n.d.) *A report of the surgeon general.* Retrieved from http://www.surgeongeneral.gov/library/mentalhealth/home.html.

Perlis, R. H., Ostacher, M. J., Patel, J. K., Marangell, L. B., Zhang, H., Wisniewski, S. R.,…Thase, M. E. (2006). Predictors of recurrence in bipolar disorder: primary outcomes from the Systematic Treatment Enhancement Program for Bipolar Disorder (STEP-BD). *American Journal of Psychiatry, 163*(2), 217–224.

President's New Freedom Commission on Mental Health. (2003). Retrieved from http://www.mentalhealthcommission.gov/reports/Finalreport/toc exec.html.

Schneck, C. D., Miklowitz, D. J., Miyahara, S., Araga, M., Wisniewski, S., Gyulai, L., Allen, M. H.,…Sachs, G. S. (2008). The prospective course of rapid-cycling bipolar disorder: Findings from the STEP-BD. *American Journal of Psychiatry, 165*(3), 370–377; quiz 410.

WEB RESOURCES

- American Psychiatric Association: http://www.psych.org/
- American Psychological Association: www.apa.org/
- Depression and Bipolar Support Alliance (DBSA): www.dbsalliance.org/
- Mac Arthur Initiative on Depression and Primary Care: http://www.depression-primarycare.org/
- National Alliance of the Mentally Ill (NAMI): http://www.nami.org/
- National Institute of Mental Health: www.nimh.gov/
- National Suicide Prevention Lifeline: http://www.suicidepreventionlifeline.org/
- Systematic Enhancement Program for Bipolar Disorder (STEP-BD): http://www.stepbd.org/

Anxiety Disorders

OVERVIEW

- Anxiety disorders are the most common type of psychiatric disorders, with an incidence of 18.1% and a lifetime prevalence of 28.8%.
- They account for an annual cost of $42.3 billion in the United States, with more than 50% of the total sum directed toward nonpsychiatric medical treatment costs.
- Patients with anxiety disorders also have a high comorbidity with mood disorders.
- Types of anxiety disorders: separation anxiety disorder, selective mutism, specific phobia, social anxiety disorder (social phobia), panic disorder (PD), agoraphobia, generalized anxiety disorder (GAD), substance/medication-induced anxiety disorder, anxiety disorder due to another medical condition, other specified anxiety disorder, and unspecified anxiety disorder.

Separation Anxiety Disorder

BACKGROUND INFORMATION

Definition of Disorder

The primary trait of separation anxiety disorder is a disproportionate fear or anxiety pertaining to separation from home or an attachment figure. The anxiety level exceeds what would be considered expected in relation to the individual's developmental level. To meet the diagnostic criteria for separation, anxiety disorder symptoms must persist for a period of at least 4 weeks for children and adolescents younger than 18 years and persist for a period of 6 months or longer for adults. In relation to adult separation anxiety, there is some degree of flexibility regarding the time frame and thus the criterion of symptoms over a period of 6 months is provided as a general guide. A key feature is that the symptoms result in significant distress or impairment in important areas of social functioning.

Etiology

Anxiety and overprotection by a parent may be associated with separation anxiety disorder. Separation anxiety may also be heritable to some degree. Separation anxiety often develops in response to life stress, especially related to a significant loss.

Demographics
In adults, in the United States, there is 0.9% to 1.9% prevalence for a 12-month period, whereas for children, a 6- to 12-month prevalence is 1.6%.

Risk Factors

Age
■ More prevalent in children younger than 12 years but can occur at any age.

Gender
■ Equally prevalent in males and females. Girls may exhibit more avoidance behavior than boys, such as reluctance to go to school. The expression of separation anxiety disorder in boys may be more indirect, such as a reluctance to be away from home.

Family History
■ Parental overprotection and anxiety may be associated with separation anxiety disorder.

Stressful Events in Susceptible People
■ Stressful life events and significant loss are often related to the development of separation anxiety disorder.

DIAGNOSIS

Differential Diagnosis
■ GAD
■ PD
■ Agoraphobia
■ Conduct disorder
■ Social anxiety disorder
■ Posttraumatic stress disorder
■ Illness anxiety disorder
■ Bereavement
■ Depressive and bipolar disorders
■ Oppositional defiant disorder
■ Psychotic disorders
■ Personality disorders

ICD-10 Code
Separation anxiety disorder (F93.0)

Diagnostic Workup
■ Physical and mental evaluation

Initial Assessment
■ Full history and physical (H&P) examination
■ Developmental history and family history
■ Assessment of trauma or past event/stressor
■ Symptoms: emotional, cognitive, and physical

▓ Labs as needed to evaluate anxiety symptoms and physical symptoms
▓ Thyroid function, complete metabolic panel, B_{12} level, and complete blood count (CBC)

Clinical Presentation

Excess worry and anxiety related to actual or potential separation from home or attachment figures and avoidance of activities that would require being away from home or attachment figures.

Children may exhibit clinging behavior.

DSM-5 Diagnostic Guidelines

Diagnostic Criteria Include the Following:

A. Excessive fear or anxiety related to separation from an attachment figure that is developmentally excessive, which includes at least one of the following criteria:
   1. The distress experienced is recurrent in nature related to experiencing a separation from home or from attachment figures.
   2. Ongoing worry related to losing an attachment figure
   3. Excessive fears related to an anticipated event such as getting lost, being kidnapped, or other event that would result in a separation from the attachment figure.
   4. Fear of separation leads to a reluctance to leave home.
   5. Fear of being alone without the presence of the attachment figure
   6. Reluctance to sleep away from home or go to sleep without the presence of the attachment figure
   7. Recurrent nightmares with the theme of separation
   8. Physical complaints with anticipation of separation from the attachment figure
B. Fear and anxiety lasting a period of 4 weeks in children and adolescents, and at least 6 months for adults; symptoms are persistent in nature.
C. There is marked distress along with impairment in social functioning in areas that are significant to the individual.
D. The symptoms are not better explained by another mental disorder, health problem, or concerns about significant others.

TREATMENT OVERVIEW

▓ Cognitive behavioral therapy (CBT)
▓ Relaxation exercises
▓ Family therapy when young children or adolescents are experiencing separation anxiety disorder
▓ Stress reduction techniques (systematic desensitization)

PSYCHOPHARMACOLOGY

▓ Selective-serotonin reuptake inhibitors (SSRIs)

PATIENT EDUCATION

▓ Education regarding the development of separation anxiety disorder related to a significant loss; individual therapy for adults and adolescents

MEDICAL/LEGAL PITFALLS

■ Screen for a medical condition that mimics anxiety disorders.

Selective Mutism

BACKGROUND INFORMATION

Definition of Disorder

Children with selective mutism demonstrate a lack of speech in social situations. In such situations, they do not initiate speech or respond with speech. Children with selective mutism will speak in their homes with immediate family members but tend not to speak with extended family or friends. They often refuse to speak at school, leading to academic problems. Shyness, anxiety, clinging behavior, withdrawal, and social isolation are common associated features. Some children may exhibit mild oppositional behavior or temper tantrums. Children with selective mutism generally have normal language skills; however, at times there may be a communication disorder.

Etiology

Selective mutism is a rare disorder with a prevalence between 0.03% and 1%.

Demographics

The prevalence of selective mutism does not vary by gender, race, or ethnicity.

Risk Factors

The disorder occurs in young children rather than adolescents and adults. Risk factors have not been well identified. Shyness and a parental history of shyness may play a significant role. Children with language difficulties may be more predisposed as compared to young children without language difficulties. There may be a genetic component given that there is a significant co-occurrence between social anxiety disorder and selective mutism.

Age

■ Onset of selective mutism is usually before the age of 5 years. Social mutism may be detected when the child begins school, when there is an increase in social interaction.

Gender

■ There has been no difference identified between girls and boys.

Family History

■ There may be a genetic component given that there is a significant co-occurrence between social anxiety and selective mutism. Parental history of shyness may also be a contributing factor.

Stressful Events in Susceptible People

■ Environmental factors that may contribute to selective mutism in children may include parents who themselves demonstrate social inhibition and who also are overprotective.

Diagnosis
■ Differential diagnosis
■ Communication disorders
■ Neurodevelopmental disorders
■ Schizophrenia and other psychotic disorders
■ Social anxiety disorder (social phobia)

ICD-10 Code
Selective mutism (F94.0)

Diagnostic Workup
■ There are no particular laboratory tests.

Initial Assessment
■ Assess for communication disorders
■ Psychiatric assessment and developmental history
■ Family history
■ Comprehensive medical H&P examination

Clinical Presentation: Symptoms
Children are reluctant to speak in social situations outside their immediate family. Children with selective mutism exhibit anxiety in situations where they are expected to speak, such as in class.

DSM-5 Diagnostic Guidelines
A. Failure to speak in social situations where there is an expectation for speaking despite the ability to speak
B. The failure to speak significantly interferes with education and/or occupational development.
C. The disturbance lasts at least 1 month.
D. The failure to speak is not due to a lack of language development or inability to use spoken language that would be required in a social situation.
E. Failure to speak is not related to a communication disorder.

TREATMENT OVERVIEW

■ CBT
■ Family education and family therapy
■ Stress reduction techniques such as relaxation exercises, imagery, role play, and progressive desensitization
■ Consultation with the school and teachers

PSYCHOPHARMACOLOGY

Treating symptoms of anxiety related to selective mutism may include SSRIs.

PATIENT EDUCATION

■ Family education
■ Stress reduction techniques

MEDICAL/LEGAL PITFALLS

- Rule out biological bases of selective mutism.
- Rule out neurodevelopmental disorders and psychotic disorder.

Phobias (Including Social Phobia)

OTHER NAMES

- Simple phobia
- Specific phobia
- Social phobia
- Social anxiety disorder

BACKGROUND INFORMATION

Definition of Disorder

- There are two types of phobias: specific and social
- To be diagnosed with a phobia, the person must have a marked, persistent fear of specific objects or situations, social situations, or performance situations.
- The fear may be manifested in a panic attack or resemble a panic attack.
- The phobic stimulus is avoided or dreaded.
- An immediate anxiety response is provoked by exposure to the phobic object or situation.
- Adults recognize that the fear is unreasonable or excessive.
- The avoidance, fear, and panic attacks must significantly interfere with the person's daily routine, occupation, or social life, or else the phobia causes marked distress to the person.
- The anxiety, panic attacks, and avoidance must not be caused by another mental condition, a general medical condition, or a drug.

Etiology

- Specific phobia
  - Phobias are usually objects or situations that may be threatening or have been threatening in the past.
  - Persons may be predisposed to phobia onset by:
    - Personal traumatic experiences or viewing others' traumatic experiences
    - Being attacked by an animal or viewing another being attacked by an animal
    - Observing others fearing an object or situation
    - Informational transmission of things to be feared
    - Unexpected panic attacks in a to-be-feared situation
  - Phobias secondary to trauma or unexpected panic attacks tend to be acute and have no characteristic age of onset.
  - Phobias continuing into adulthood remit in about 20% of cases.
- Social phobia
  - May emerge in a child with social inhibition and shyness
  - Onset may be abrupt or secondary to stressful or humiliating experience.
  - Onset may be insidious.

- Duration is frequently lifelong with remission or attenuation in adulthood.
- Social phobia severity may wax and wane depending on stressors and life events.

Demographics
- Prevalence for specific phobia in the community is 4% to 8.8%.
- Lifetime prevalence for specific phobia is 7.2% to 11.3%, with a decline in older adults.
- Prevalence estimates for social phobias vary depending on the threshold used to determine distress and impairment in each study.
- Prevalence estimates have been as high as 20% in those with anxiety disorders but as low as 2% in the general population.
- Lifetime prevalence for social phobia is 3% to 13%.

Risk Factors
Age
- Specific phobia
  - Onset depends on type of phobia
  - Usually occurs in childhood/early adolescence
- Social phobia
  - Usually occurs in midteens
  - Childhood onset may occur if a child has social inhibition and shyness.

Gender
- Specific phobia
  - Women are affected more than men (2:1).
  - About 90% of animal and natural environment phobias and situational phobias affect women.
- Social phobia
  - Women are affected more than men in the general population.
  - Men are affected more than women or are equal in the clinical setting.

Family History
- Family members of those with a specific phobia have increased risk for a specific phobia, especially if the phobia is animal type, situational type, or fear of blood or injury.
- Especially in the generalized type of social phobia, first-degree biological relatives are more likely to have this phobia than the general population.

Stressful Events in Susceptible People
- Specific phobia
  - Traumatic events may trigger phobias.
  - Stressful events may cause reemergence of a phobia.
- Social phobia
  - May be caused by stressful experience.
  - Stress may cause resurgence of a phobia after remission or attenuation.

Having Another Mental Health Disorder
- Having one specific phobia does not predispose a person to having another phobia unless the phobia developed in adolescence.

▪ Having any specific phobia does not predispose or increase risk for another mental health disorder.
▪ Those with a social phobia are more likely also to have anxiety disorders, depression, substance abuse, and dependence.

TREATMENT OVERVIEW

Acute Treatment
Specific Phobia
▪ Cognitive behavioral interventions are the most studied and most efficacious for this disorder.
▪ Multiple exposure treatments, in vivo or virtual reality, work very well in extinguishing the phobia.
▪ Applied relaxation and tension treatments have shown promise but need more studies to show efficacy.
▪ Cognitive restructuring treatments and psychodynamic psychotherapy may also be useful but more studies need to be done.

Social Phobia
▪ CBTs
  ▪ These therapies work on the belief that dysfunctional beliefs and biased information processing strategies are responsible for the social phobia.
  ▪ The therapies focus on the patients' beliefs and avoidance.
  ▪ Therapies used include exposure treatments alone, exposure treatments plus cognitive restructuring treatments (either in a group session or an individual session), social skills training, and relaxation strategies.
  ▪ Exposure treatments with cognitive restructuring treatments are most effective.
  ▪ Social skills training and relaxation strategies are less effective alone but have increased efficacy when either is combined with exposure treatments and cognitive restructuring treatments in a group setting.
▪ Various medications have been used to improve patients with a social phobia, including phenelzine (Nardil) and sertraline (Zoloft).
▪ SSRIs are the treatment of choice—but Zoloft is the American version of sertraline (not sercerin). Also, Nardil is a monoamine oxidase (MAO) inhibitor and is reserved as the last line of treatment due to the dietary interactions and side effects. Drug therapy should be continued for 6–12 months.
  ▪ Medication use alone was associated with a high relapse rate despite an earlier initial benefit.
  ▪ Relapse rate was decreased when medication use was combined with cognitive behavioral group therapy.
  ▪ More studies need to be done to determine better treatment guidelines.
▪ Psychodynamic therapy, interpersonal psychotherapy, and acceptance and commitment therapy are used clinically but should be studied more to determine efficacy as compared to CBTs and medication use.

Chronic Treatment
Specific Phobia
▪ Long-term therapy may be needed if exposure therapy does not work.
▪ More research needs to be done on therapy for the specific phobia.

Drug Selection Table for Phobias

CLASS	DRUG
Beta-blockers	Drugs used for short-term treatment. Treatment of physical symptoms—does not treat the root of the problem. Helps control heart rate.
	Propranolol (*Inderal*)
Benzodiazepines (BZDs)	Drugs used for short-term treatments:
	Alprazolam (*Xanax/Xanax XR/Niravam*)
	Lorazepam (*Ativan*)
	Diazepam (*Valium*)
	Chlordiazepoxide (*Librium*)
Selective-serotonin reuptake inhibitors (SSRIs)	First-line drug therapy:
	Sertraline (*Zoloft*)
	Fluoxetine (*Prozac*)
	Paroxetine (*Paxil*)
	Fluvoxamine (*Luvox*)
	Citalopram (*Celexa*)
	Escitalopram (*Lexapro*)
Serotonin and norepinephrine reuptake inhibitors (SNRIs)	First-line drug therapy: Venlafaxine (*Effexor, Effexor XR*)
Tricyclic antidepressants (TCAs)	Drugs for treatment-resistant cases:
	Imipramine (*Tofranil*)
	Desipramine (*Norpramin*)
	Clomipramine (*Anafranil*)

Social Phobia
▦ Long-term therapy may be needed if the patient is refractory to acute treatment.
▦ Therapy may include cognitive behavioral, medication, or another type of therapy.

Recurrence Rate
▦ Rate of recurrence is variable. It depends on life stressors, attenuation, and remission of phobia.

PATIENT EDUCATION

▦ Both MD Consult and e-Medicine have patient education articles on phobias.
▦ Many support groups can be found online, including www.dailystrength.org.
▦ Advise patients to avoid self-medication with alcohol or other drugs.

MEDICAL/LEGAL PITFALLS

▨ Patients with some phobias may abuse alcohol or illicit drugs as a coping mechanism. Health care workers should screen for this during the H&P examination.

DIAGNOSIS

Differential Diagnosis
▨ Specific phobia:
- ▨ Social phobia
- ▨ PD with agoraphobia
- ▨ PD without agoraphobia
- ▨ Posttraumatic stress disorder symptoms
- ▨ Separation anxiety disorder
- ▨ Obsessive–compulsive disorder (OCD)
- ▨ Hypochondriasis
- ▨ Anorexia nervosa
- ▨ Bulimia nervosa
- ▨ Schizophrenia or another psychotic disorder

▨ Social phobia:
- ▨ Specific phobia
- ▨ PD without agoraphobia
- ▨ Agoraphobia without history of PD
- ▨ Separation anxiety disorder
- ▨ GAD
- ▨ Pervasive development disorder
- ▨ Schizoid personality disorder
- ▨ Avoidant personality disorder

ICD-10 Codes
Specific phobia: (F40.298)

Social phobia: (F40.10)

Diagnostic Workup
▨ Physical and mental evaluations are done.

Initial Assessment
▨ Full history and physical examinations are included.
▨ Past medical history including psychiatric history
▨ Traumatic or past event/stressor is determined.
▨ Symptoms you experience (emotional or physical symptoms)
▨ Physical and mental evaluations are included.
▨ Thyroid function studies (thyroid-stimulating hormone [TSH], triiodothyronine [T3], and thyroxine [T4]) are done.
▨ Complete metabolic panel (CMP) includes glucose, calcium, albumin, total protein count, levels of sodium, potassium, CO_2 (carbon dioxide and bicarbonate), chloride, blood urea nitrogen (BUN), creatinine, alkaline phosphatase (ALP), alanine amino transferase (ALT, also called SGPT), aspartate amino transferase (AST, also called SGOT), and bilirubin.

▦ Complete blood count (CBC) with differentials: hemoglobin, hematocrit, red blood cell (RBC) count, white blood cell (WBC) count, WBC differential count, and platelet count.

Clinical Presentation
▦ Panic (or panic-like) attacks
▦ Extreme anxiety and/or fear
▦ Extreme avoidance of the phobia

Specific Phobia

DIAGNOSIS

Differential Diagnosis
▦ Agoraphobia
▦ Social anxiety disorder
▦ Separation anxiety disorder
▦ PD
▦ OCD
▦ Trauma- and stressor-related disorders
▦ Eating disorders
▦ Schizophrenia spectrum and other psychotic disorders

DSM-5 Diagnostic Guidelines
A. Excessive fear about a distinct item or situation, such as the fear of flying, medical procedures, or a type of animal, among others. In children, the clinician may see the anxiety manifested as tearfulness, temper tantrums, or clingy behavior.
B. When the individual is exposed to the item or situation, fear or anxiety is triggered and the individual will actively seek to avoid the item or situation.
C. The fear or anxiety is in excess to the real danger presented by a situation or item.
D. The avoidant behavior or fear and anxiety lasts for at least 6 months and results in work and social impairment.
E. The symptoms are not related to another medical condition.

Social Anxiety Disorder (Social Phobia)

BACKGROUND INFORMATION

Social anxiety disorder's (social phobia) key characteristic is an intense fear or anxiety in social situations when an individual believes he or she is being negatively evaluated by others. The anxiety and fear occurs in most social situations. Individuals who occasionally experience fear and anxiety in social situations would not meet the criteria of social anxiety disorder. The fear and anxiety is out of proportion to the actual risk of being negatively evaluated. To distinguish social anxiety from a transient social fear, the disturbance usually spans at least 6 months. The disturbance significantly interferes with social functioning or occupational functioning.

A specific subtype of social anxiety disorder deals with a fear-of-performance type of social anxiety disorder. Individuals with performance fears experience impairment in their professional lives but do not experience fear or avoidance in nonperformance social situations.

Diagnostic Criteria

A. Intense fear or anxiety experienced by an individual in one or more social situations.

    The individual believes he or she is being viewed negatively. Examples of such situations include meeting unfamiliar people, being observed, or performing in front of others.

    Note: To meet criteria, children with social anxiety disorder need to experience fear and anxiety in peer settings and not just in situations with adults.

B. The individual fears that he or she will exhibit symptoms of anxiety that will result in being negatively evaluated. He or she experiences feelings of being humiliated or embarrassed with the belief that he or she will be rejected and/or that the behavior has offended others.

C. Fear and anxiety occur in most social situations.

    Note: In children, behaviors such as crying, tantrums, freezing, clinging, shrinking, or failing to speak in social situations may occur reflective of social anxiety and fear.

D. Individuals attempt to avoid social situations. When they cannot avoid social situations, they experience significant anxiety and fear.

E. The fear or anxiety experienced by the individual is disproportionate to the actual threat.

F. Symptoms of fear, anxiety, and avoidance are persistent, lasting most times for 6 months or more.

G. The individual experiences significant impairment and/or distress in social, occupational, or other significant areas of functioning.

H. Symptoms of fear, anxiety, or avoidance are not attributable to the physiological effects of a substance (drugs or medications) or a medical condition.

I. Symptoms of fear, anxiety, or avoidance are not better explained by another mental disorder.

J. If there is a co-occurring medical condition (e.g., Parkinson's disease, obesity, disfigurement from burns or injury), the fear, anxiety, or avoidance is unrelated or is excessive.

Differential Diagnosis

▦ Normative shyness
▦ Agoraphobia
▦ PD
▦ GAD
▦ Separation anxiety disorder
▦ Specific phobias
▦ Selective mutism
▦ Major depressive disorder
▦ Body dysmorphic disorder
▦ Autism spectrum disorder
▦ Personality disorders
▦ Other mental disorders

▦ Other medical conditions
▦ Oppositional defiant disorder

ICD-10 Code
Social anxiety disorder (social phobia) (F40.10)

Etiology
May emerge in a child with social inhibition and shyness.

▦ Onset may be abrupt or secondary to stressful or humiliating experience.
▦ Onset may be insidious.
▦ Duration is frequently lifelong with remission or attenuation in adulthood.
▦ Social phobia severity may wax and wane depending on stressors and life events.
▦ First onset of social anxiety disorder is rare but is more likely to occur following a stressful or humiliating event.

Demographics
In the United States, the 12-month prevalence rate is higher than in much of the world. The comparison based on the same diagnostic instrument is as follows: United States, approximately 7%; Europe, approximately 2.3%; and worldwide, approximately 0.5% to 2.0%.

Risk Factors
▦ Age: The onset of social anxiety in the United States is between the ages of 8 and 15 years, with a median age of 13 years.
▦ Gender: Higher rates of social anxiety disorder occur in females than in males, with ratios ranging from 1.5% to 2.2%.
▦ Family history: There is a two to six times greater chance of developing social anxiety disorder among first-degree relatives. Genetic and environmental factors contribute to the increased predisposition.
▦ Stressful events in susceptible people: Persons who exhibit traits such as behavioral inhibition and fears of being negatively evaluated may be at greater risk.
▦ Environmental factors that contribute to increased risk include stressful events that lead to a feeling of being humiliated or significantly embarrassed.

Diagnostic Workup
▦ There are no specific laboratory studies for social anxiety disorder (social phobia).

Initial Assessment
▦ Comprehensive physical examination
▦ Comprehensive psychiatric evaluation

Clinical Presentation
The major presentation is extreme anxiety or fear related to social situations. The person has an intense fear of being evaluated negatively by others. Persons who occasionally experience anxiety or fear in social situations would not meet the criteria for social anxiety disorder.

PSYCHOPHARMACOLOGY

Treating symptoms of anxiety related to social anxiety disorder (social phobia) may include SSRIs.

Panic Disorder

BACKGROUND INFORMATION

- Sudden feelings of terror that strike without warning
- Can occur at any time, even during sleep
- Mimics a heart attack or feeling that death is imminent
- Panic disorder (PD) is defined as recurrent, unexpected panic attacks followed by at least 1 month of persistent concern about having another attack, worry about the consequences of panic attacks, and a change in behavior as a result of the attacks.
- Diagnostic workup includes physical and mental evaluation.
- Often, the first attacks are triggered by physical illnesses, a major life stress, or medications that increase activity in the part of the brain involved in fear reactions.

Risk Factors

- Age: PD typically strikes in the late teen years or young adulthood.
- Gender: Women are twice as likely as men to develop PD.
- Family history: PD has been found to run in families; this may mean that inheritance (genes) plays a strong role in determining who will get it. However, many people who have no family history of the disorder develop it.

DIAGNOSIS

Differential Diagnosis

- Thyroid disorders
- Diabetic hyper- or hypoglycemia
- Cardiac arrhythmias
- Cerebral lesions
- Substance-induced anxiety disorder

PSYCHOPHARMACOLOGY

Overview

- SSRIs are the most commonly used medications for PD.
  - They include fluoxetine (Prozac), sertraline (Zoloft), paroxetine (Paxil), fluvoxamine (Luvox), citalopram (Celexa), and escitalopram (Lexapro).
  - They take up to 8 to 12 weeks to reach maximum therapeutic efficacy.
  - If these do not help or if more immediate symptomatic relief is necessary, use of BZDs may be considered if the person does not have a history of drug dependence.
- SNRIs are also used as first-line therapy for PD.
- BZDs are associated with dependence and addiction.
  - They are used on a temporary basis and for immediate relief.
- MAOIs, such as phenelzine (Nardil), tranylcypromine (Parnate), and isocarboxazid (Marplan), are only used when all other drugs do not work.
  - MAOIs are the most effective medications for PD, but they have serious side effects and interactions with other drugs and foods (recommend initiation of this type of treatment to be conducted with a mental health provider).

▦ Behavioral therapies should be used together with drug therapy. These include CBT, exposure therapy, relaxation techniques, pleasant mental imagery, and cognitive restructuring (learning to recognize and replace panic-inducing thoughts). Behavioral treatment appears to have long-lasting benefits.

▦ Regular exercise, adequate sleep, and regularly scheduled meals may help reduce the frequency of the attacks. Caffeine and other stimulants should be reduced or eliminated.

PATIENT EDUCATION

▦ Individuals with PD have a suicide rate 18 times higher than the general population.

▦ The rate of substance abuse (especially stimulants, cocaine, and hallucinogens) in persons with PD is 7% to 28%, 4 to 14 times greater than that of the general population.

Drug Selection Table for Panic Disorder

CLASS	DRUG
Selective-serotonin reuptake inhibitors (SSRIs)	First-line drug therapy:
	Sertraline (*Zoloft*)
	Fluoxetine (*Prozac*)
	Paroxetine (*Paxil, Paxil CR*); paroxetine mesylate (*Pexeva*)
	Fluvoxamine (*Luvox CR*)
	Citalopram (*Celexa*)
	Escitalopram (*Lexapro*)
Serotonin-norepinephrine reuptake inhibitors (SNRIs)	First-line drug therapy:
	Venlafaxine (*Effexor, Effexor XR*)
	Desvenlafaxine (*Pristiq*)
	Duloxetine (*Cymbalta*)
Tricyclic antidepressants (TCAs)	Drugs for treatment-resistant cases:
	Imipramine (*Tofranil*)
	Desipramine (*Norpramin*)
	Nortriptyline (*Pamelor*)
Benzodiazepines (BZDs)	Drugs used only in first weeks while establishing levels of SSRIs or SNRIs:
	Alprazolam (*Xanax/Xanax XR/Niravam*)
	Lorazepam (*Ativan*)
	Clonazepam (*Klonopin*)
Serotonin 1A agonist	Drug for augmentation:
	Buspirone (*BuSpar*)

MEDICAL/LEGAL PITFALLS

▣ Pregnant mothers with PD are more likely to have infants of smaller birth weight for gestational age.

▣ PD patients are nearly twice as likely to develop coronary artery disease, and those with known coronary disease can experience myocardial ischemia during their panic episodes.

Agoraphobia

BACKGROUND INFORMATION

Definition of Disorder

▣ The disorder is associated with significant anxiety or fear with an anticipated or actual exposure to place or situation with concurrent fear that one cannot escape the place.

▣ To meet criteria for agoraphobia, two of the following situations need to cause the person significant anxiety or fear: (a) using public transportation, (b) being in open spaces, (c) being in enclosed spaces, (d) being in a crowd, or (e) being outside one's home alone.

▣ The level of fear and anxiety may vary in relation to the anticipation or presence of the agoraphobic situation.

▣ A key feature is that the fear or anxiety is persistent in relation to the situation and occurs consistently.

▣ Individuals with agoraphobia experience fear, anxiety, and avoidance in relation to the situation that is disproportionate to the actual threat.

Etiology

▣ Individuals who are behaviorally inhibited and are more anxious are more predisposed to agoraphobia but they are also more predisposed to a range of anxiety disorders (phobias, PD).

▣ Individuals who have experienced a negative or stressful event may have an increased risk of developing agoraphobia.

Demographics

▣ Initial onset for agoraphobia is typically before the age of 35 years in two thirds of individuals with agoraphobia.

▣ The mean age of onset for agoraphobia is 17 years.

▣ Although the greatest risk for agoraphobia is during adolescence and early adulthood, there is also an increased risk phase after the age of 40 years.

▣ Agoraphobia tends to present as chronic. The prevalence of agoraphobia does not vary in relation to culture or race.

Risk Factors

▣ Age: Low prevalence in children. Although the initial onset is most often seen in adolescents and young adults, agoraphobia does present across the life span.

▣ Gender: Males present with a higher rate of comorbid substance abuse disorders.

▣ Family history: Of the phobias, agoraphobia has the strongest association with heritability.

▓ Stressful events in susceptible people: Many individuals with agoraphobia have experienced anxiety symptoms in the past. Common comorbid diagnoses include specific phobias, PD, and social anxiety disorder.

DIAGNOSIS

▓ Extreme fear and anxiety in two or more of the following situations: (a) Anxiety related to the use of public transportation; (b) fear of open spaces; (c) fear of being in enclosed spaces; (d) anxiety and fear related to being in a crowd; and (e) fear of being outside one's home alone.
▓ Avoidance of situation when an individual fears that he or she cannot escape readily in the event of increased anxiety and potential panic-like symptoms
▓ The agoraphobic situations consistently result in fear and anxiety.
▓ The agoraphobic situations are avoided or are not avoided if accompanied by another or if the person in the agoraphobic situation experiences extreme fear and/or anxiety.
▓ The fear or anxiety is disproportionate to the actual situation.
▓ Avoidance of the feared situation has existed for at least 6 months.
▓ The fear and anxiety related to the feared situation has caused significant impairment in the person's social functioning.
▓ If the fear, anxiety, and avoidance are related to a medication condition, the symptoms are considered extreme and excessive.
▓ The fear, anxiety, and avoidance are not better explained by another anxiety disorder, OCD or posttraumatic stress disorder.

Note: The diagnosis of agoraphobia need not be accompanied by symptoms of panic. If the individual experiences panic with agoraphobia, both diagnoses would be given.

ICD10-Code
Agoraphobia (F40.0)

Diagnostic Workup
There are no specific laboratory studies for agoraphobias.

Initial Assessment
▓ Comprehensive physical examination.
▓ Comprehensive psychiatric evaluation.

Clinical Presentation: Symptoms
Apart from anxiety and fear, the individual may have panic-like symptoms when exposed or potentially exposed to feared situations, as described in the diagnostic criteria.

TREATMENT OVERVIEW

▓ CBT includes systematic desensitization.
▓ Supportive therapy
▓ Stress reduction techniques
▓ Exposure therapy
▓ Thought stopping

PSYCHOPHARMACOLOGY

■ Anxiety may be treated with SSRIs.
■ In the case of panic or panic-like symptoms, a benzodiazepine (BZD) may help to reduce the intensity of the fear and/or anxiety; in the case of panic or panic-like attacks, BZD may decrease the number and intensity of the attacks.

PATIENT EDUCATION

■ Coping skills training and stress reduction techniques may help decrease the severity of symptoms.

MEDICAL/LEGAL PITFALLS

■ Rule out potential medical conditions that may be an underlying cause of anxiety.

Generalized Anxiety Disorder (GAD)

BACKGROUND INFORMATION

Definition of Disorder
■ The most common anxiety disorder is seen by primary care physicians.
■ Patients have chronic anxiety, worry, and tension, which is without, or out of proportion to, any provocation or stimulus.
■ Symptoms are not situational or limited to certain events.
■ Patients are unable to assure themselves that their anxiety is greatly exaggerated in comparison to the situation.

Etiology
■ Exact cause of GAD is unknown.
■ Some research suggests that environmental and genetic factors may play a role.
■ GAD may be caused by an imbalance between dopamine and serotonin.

Demographics
■ Prevalence 5.9% among adolescents and 2.9% among adults in the United States
■ Prevalence rates in other countries range from 0.4% to 3.6%
■ Females are twice as likely as males to experience GAD.
■ The diagnosis peaks during middle age and declines as the individual ages.

Family History
■ There is some evidence that anxiety disorders, including GAD, tend to run in families.
■ Studies of twins suggest that there may be a genetic factor.

Stressful Events in Susceptible People
■ Stressful events can exacerbate symptoms in patients with GAD.

Having Another Mental Health Disorder
■ The comorbidities that accompany GAD include other anxiety disorders (PD, social phobia), substance abuse, and mood disorders (dysthymic disorder, major depressive disorder). These comorbidities should be treated along with GAD.

DIAGNOSIS

Differential Diagnosis
■ Anxiety disorder due to another medical condition
■ Substance-/medication-induced anxiety disorder
■ Social anxiety disorder
■ OCD
■ Posttraumatic stress disorder and adjustment disorders
■ Depressive, bipolar, and psychotic disorders.

ICD-Code
Generalized anxiety disorder (F41.1)

Diagnostic Workup
■ There are no particular laboratory tests that diagnose GAD, but tests can be done to rule out other organic causes (e.g., thyroid function test, CBCs, basic metabolic panels, urinalysis).
■ Diagnosis of PD can be difficult because several other physical and mental health disorders may be confused with GAD.
■ Physical and mental evaluations are done.
■ Two scales are used to evaluate for GAD (GAD 2 and GAD 7 scales).

Initial Assessment
■ Medical history
■ Symptoms:
  ■ How long has patient been having symptoms?
  ■ When did the symptoms start?
  ■ How often do they occur?
  ■ When and where do they tend to occur?
  ■ How long do they last?
  ■ What effect do they have on the patient's ability to function?

Clinical Presentation
■ Worry is excessive and typically interferes with psychosocial functioning.
■ Worry is pervasive, pronounced, and distressing to the individual.
■ Restlessness
■ Feeling keyed up
■ Easily fatigued
■ Difficulty in concentrating
■ Irritability
■ Muscle tension
■ Sleep disturbances with difficulty falling or staying asleep or restless, unsatisfying sleep
■ Trembling

- ▦ Twitching
- ▦ Feeling shaky
- ▦ Sweating
- ▦ Nausea
- ▦ Diarrhea
- ▦ Accelerated heart rate
- ▦ Shortness of breath
- ▦ Irritable bowel syndrome
- ▦ Headaches.

DSM-5 Diagnostic Guidelines

A. Extreme anxiety or worry that occurs for 6 months or more and creates impairment in school or work requirements. It may also cause problems with social relationships.
B. The patient has difficulty controlling the worry or anxiety.
C. The anxiety or worry may also accompany restlessness, complaints of being tired, problems concentrating, irritability, and difficulty with sleep. Children may only have one of the previous symptoms.

TREATMENT OVERVIEW

In the treatment of GADs, the main focus of treatment is to reduce the agent that is causing the anxiety. In the event the anxiety cannot be controlled or eliminated and is considered acute, psychopharmacology is the standard of care. Once the anxiety is under control, psychotheraphy is the next step in treatment.

PSYCHOPHARMACOLOGY

- ▦ SSRIs are the most common first-line agents used with GAD.
- ▦ TCAs can be effective in treating GADs; however, the initial side effects of the drugs when first initiated (jitteriness and insomnia) can reduce patient adherence to therapy. These medications are generally reserved for GAD resistant to treatment with SSRIs and SNRIs.
- ▦ Serotonin–norepinephrine reuptake inhibitor (SNRI) has Food and Drug Administration (FDA) approval for treatment of GAD.
- ▦ The non-BZD anxiolytic agent buspirone can be efficacious for the anxiety component, but it has no effect on depression and should not be used if concomitant depression is present.
- ▦ BZDs are generally the most efficacious in patients who only have anxiety symptoms; however, the health care provider needs to be cautious while using these agents for treating the elderly. Additionally, patients may become physically dependent with long-term use. These drugs may be used as part of an initial treatment regimen and then discontinued when a long-term treatment plan has been developed.

Chronic Treatment

- ▦ Follow-up care by a chemical dependence treatment specialist is recommended when indicated.

Drug Selection Table for Generalized Anxiety Disorder

CLASS	DRUG
Selective-serotonin reuptake inhibitors (SSRIs)	First-line drug therapy: Escitalopram (*Lexapro*) Sertraline (*Zoloft*) Paroxetine (*Paxil, Paxil PR*) Paroxetine mesylate (*Pexeva*)
Serotonin and norepinephrine reuptake inhibitors (SNRIs)	First-line drug therapy: Venlafaxine (*Effexor, Effexor XR*) Duloxetine (*Cymbalta*)
Calcium channel moderator	Drug augmentation Pregabalin (*Lyrica*)
Tricyclic antidepressants (TCAs)	Drugs for treatment-resistant cases: Imipramine (*Tofranil, Tofranil PM*) Desipramine (*Norpramin*)
Benzodiazepines (BZDs)	Drugs used only in first weeks while establishing levels of SSRI or SNRI: Alprazolam (*Xanax/Xanax XR/Niravam*) Clonazepam (*Klonopin*) Lorazepam (*Ativan*) Diazepam (*Valium*)
Antihistamines	Drug augmentation: Hydroxyzine (*Vistaril*)
Anxiolytics	Drug augmentation: Buspirone (*BuSpar*)

▓ Psychiatric referral should be considered in patients who do not improve with medical treatment or those with suicidal ideations.

Psychotherapy
▓ Complementary and alternative medicine (CAM):
  ▫ Acupuncture
  ▫ Aromatherapy

PATIENT EDUCATION

▓ Patients should continue to take all medications as prescribed and never stop any medicines before discussing this with their physician.
▓ For excellent patient education resources, visit eMedicine's Mental Health and Behavior Center and Anxiety Center.

MEDICAL/LEGAL PITFALLS

▓ Persons with GAD are more likely to have other anxiety disorders (e.g., PD).

- Anxiety disorders are more frequently seen in patients with chronic medical illness (chronic obstructive pulmonary disease [COPD], irritable bowel syndrome [IBS], hypertension) than in the general population.
- Patients are more likely to present to their primary care physicians frequently with multiple complaints over time.
- Patients with GAD tend to smoke cigarettes and abuse other substances (alcohol, prescription or illicit drugs).

Substance-/Medication-Induced Anxiety Disorder

BACKGROUND INFORMATION

Definition of Disorder

The signs and symptoms of the anxiety are related to a specific substance the patient ingested. The substance creates the anxiety symptoms rather than an underlying disorder.

Etiology

Substances that may cause the anxiety disorder include alcohol, caffeine, cannabis, phencyclidine, inhalants, opioids, sedatives, hypnotics, anxiolytics, stimulants, cocaine, hallucinogens, or an unknown substance.

Demographics

The disorder is rare, with a 12-month prevalence of around 0.002% of the general population. In the clinical population, the numbers may be higher.

Risk Factors

- Age: unknown
- Gender: unknown
- Family history: unknown

DIAGNOSIS

Differential Diagnosis

- Substance intoxication and substance withdrawal
- Anxiety disorder (i.e., not induced by a substance/medication)
- Delirium
- Anxiety disorder due to another medical condition

Diagnostic Workup

- Urine drug screen

DSM-5 Diagnostic Guidelines

- Anxiety or panic attacks are the main feature of the disorder. Also obsessions or compulsions.
- The symptoms occur right after the substance has been ingested or occur when the substance is discontinued.

▥ The anxiety or panic attacks are not exclusive to delirium.
▥ The anxiety or panic attacks affect personal relationships and/or school or work.

TREATMENT OVERVIEW

Once the identified substance that created the anxiety or panic attacks is discontinued, the symptoms should resolve within several days, weeks, or a month. If the symptoms were present prior to the ingestion or discontinuation of the substance, other causes should be explored.

PATIENT EDUCATION

Anxiety or panic attacks can occur from the discontinuation of alcohol, opioids, sedatives, or cocaine. Medications that could create anxiety or panic attacks include anesthesia, antihistamines, antiparkinsonian drugs, corticosteroids, antihypertensive medications, bronchodilators, or birth control pills. Carbon monoxide, gasoline, paint, and other heavy metals can cause anxiety or panic attacks.

Anxiety Disorder Due to Another Medical Condition

BACKGROUND INFORMATION

Definition of Disorder
▥ The individual who exhibits an anxiety disorder due to a medical condition presents with symptoms of anxiety and/or panic that are not related to another anxiety disorder.
▥ The symptoms are best explained as a physiological response to the medical condition, and there is supporting evidence from a comprehensive history/physical examination, psychiatric evaluation, and laboratory findings indicating that the symptoms are a consequence of a medical condition.
▥ Anxiety due to another medical condition is the appropriate diagnosis when (a) the medical condition is known to be associated with symptoms of anxiety and (b) when the medical condition precedes the onset of the anxiety and/or panic symptoms.

Etiology
▥ Symptoms of anxiety and/or panic coincide with the medical condition and have not been present previously.
▥ The emergence of the anxiety and/or panic symptoms demonstrates a clear temporal association with the occurrence of a medical condition.

Risk Factors
▥ There are several medical diagnoses that are associated with the development of anxiety symptoms, including endocrine disease, cardiac disease, respiratory disease, metabolic disturbances, neurological diseases, and various cancers.

Stressful Events in Susceptible People
▥ Individuals who have medical conditions that have been associated with the development of anxiety as a manifestation of the medical condition.

DIAGNOSIS

- Anxiety and/or panic symptom
- Findings from the history, physical examination, and laboratory tests support that the symptoms have a direct physiological basis
- The symptoms are not related to another mental disorder.
- Anxiety and/or panic are not due to delirium.
- There is significant distress and impairment in important areas of social functioning.

Differential Diagnosis
- Delirium
- Mixed presentation of symptoms such as mood symptoms and anxiety symptoms
- Substance/medication-induced anxiety disorder

ICD-Code
Anxiety Disorder Due to Another Medical Condition (F06.4)

Diagnostic Workup
- Comprehensive history and physical examination
- Laboratory studies relevant to medical diagnosis
- Psychiatric history and psychiatric assessment

Initial Assessment
- Rule out psychiatric history and existing psychiatric diagnosis.

Clinical Presentation: Symptoms
- Anxiety and/or panic symptoms that emerge as a consequence of a medical condition

TREATMENT OVERVIEW

- Treatment of the medication condition:
  - Relaxation exercises
  - Supportive therapy

PSYCHOPHARMACOLOGY

- SSRIs may be helpful.

PATIENT EDUCATION

- Patient education regarding anxiety symptoms and the relationship to the medical condition

MEDICAL/LEGAL PITFALLS

- Careful assessment regarding any co-occurring substance use or abuse
- Assessment of comorbid psychiatric disorders

Other Specified Anxiety Disorder

BACKGROUND INFORMATION

■ An individual would meet the criteria for "other specified anxiety disorder" when his or her symptoms do not meet the full criteria for an anxiety disorder but he or she is experiencing symptoms that cause significant distress.

■ There may also be significant impairment in social functioning.

■ When this diagnosis is used, there needs to be a rationale for how it does not meet the criteria for a specific anxiety disorder using the diagnostic criteria for the justification. For example, in a case when the individual experiences significant anxiety that occurs some days but not the majority of days in a week, the rationale would be listed as "General anxiety does not occur more days than not."

Unspecified Anxiety Disorder

■ Individuals who meet the criteria for unspecified anxiety disorder experience significant anxiety symptoms and may also experience impairment in social functioning but do not meet the full criteria for any of the anxiety disorders.

■ The clinician does not specify the reason why the criteria are not met but rather may include that there is insufficient evidence to make a specific diagnosis.

Obsessive–Compulsive Disorder

DEFINITION OF DISORDER

■ This disorder is characterized by obsessions and compulsions.

■ Obsessions: recurrent and persistent thoughts, urges, or images; experienced as intrusive and unwanted.

■ Compulsions: repetitive behaviors or mental acts that an individual feels compelled to perform in response to obsessions or rules (American Psychiatric Association, 2013).

■ Level of insight occurs on a continuum from good or fair, to poor, to absent/delusional.

Etiology

■ Neuropsychiatric disorder

■ Multiple theories of causation
  ■ Structural and functional brain dysfunction
  ■ Hyperactivity of frontal–subcortical neuronal circuit
    ● Hyperactivity in orbitofrontal cortex
    ● Subcortical frontal gyrus
    ● Hyperactivity in anterior cingulate cortex
    ● Deficient volume, thickness and surface area of right anterior cingulate gyrus (ACG)
    ● Hyperactivity in striatum
  ■ Decreased right lingual gyrus surface area
  ■ Significant increase in the right inferior parietal cortical thickness
  ■ Significant increases in gyrification in the left insula, left middle frontal and left lateral occipital regions extending to the precuneus and right supramarginal gyrus

- Dysfunction in caudate nucleus; decreased volume but increased neurotransmission
- Dysfunction of thalamus
- Genetics: specific markers have been identified
- Cognitive and behavioral factors

Demographics
- There is a 2.5% lifetime prevalence.
- There is a 1.2% 12-month prevalence of OCD in the United States.
- Mean age of onset is 19.5 years; 6 to 15 years of age for males and 20 to 29 years for females. Females are affected at a slightly higher rate than males in adulthood, but males are more commonly affected in childhood.
- Similar prevalence rates appear around the world.
- No difference exists across socioeconomic backgrounds.
- Ranked by the World Health Organization as one of the 10 most disabling disorders.

Temperament
- Greater internalizing symptoms, higher negative emotionality, and behavioral inhibition in childhood are possible temperamental risk factors.

Environment
- Head injury infection

Genetics and Physiology
- Pregnancy and perinatal period
- Family members with an OCD

DIAGNOSIS

ICD-10 Codes
Obsessive–compulsive disorder (F42)

OCD Prevalence With Other Disorders

Depressive disorders: 19% to 90%

Bipolar disorder: Varying rates depending on source: 15% to 35%

Schizophrenia: 10% to 60%

    Anxiety disorders: 76%
    22% for specific phobia
    18% for social anxiety disorder (social phobia)
    12% for PD
    30% for generalized anxiety disorder

Tic disorders: 30%

Personality disorders: 23% to 32%

OCD, obsessive–compulsive disorder; PD, panic disorder.

Diagnostic Workup

▓ Screening can be accomplished with a brief instrument, such as the Zohar-Fineburg Obsessive–Compulsive Screen, which can be administered in less than 1 minute.

▓ Neuropsychological/psychological testing may be helpful for a differential diagnosis.

▓ Yale–Brown obsessive–compulsive scale (Y-BOCS) is used to determine severity.

▓ Assess symptoms against Y-BOCS symptom checklist.

▓ Children's version of Y-BOCS (CY-BOCS) is available for pediatric population.

▓ Vancouver Obsessional Compulsive Inventory assesses symptoms.

▓ Pandua Inventory—Washington State University Revision assesses symptoms.

▓ Level 1—Crosscutting symptom measures

▓ Level 2—Repetitive thoughts and behaviors

▓ Assess medical needs due to lack of medical care in severe cases.

Initial Assessment

▓ Family psychiatric history

▓ Onset of symptoms

▓ Severity of symptoms

▓ Functioning at home and school

▓ Level of insight

▓ Impact on patient/family

▓ How much time is the patient spending ritualizing/obsessing?

▓ How much time is family spending accommodating (obliging/responding to, or otherwise engaging/coping with ill relative's OCD symptoms)?

Clinical Presentation

▓ Severe anxiety, worry, or distress

▓ Avoidant behavior

▓ Excessive time spent on parts of daily routine, that is, showering, cleaning

▓ Obsessions and compulsions

▓ Odd or excessive behaviors

▓ Significant impairment (i.e., patient is unable to work/attend school or participate in social activities).

DSM-5 Diagnostic Guidelines

▓ Either obsessions or compulsions

▓ Obsessions are defined by the following:

  ▓ Recurrent thoughts, urges, or images are experienced as intrusive and unwanted, and in most people cause marked distress or anxiety.

  ▓ The individual makes attempts to ignore or suppress the offending thoughts, urges, or images, or to neutralize them with other thoughts and/or activities.

- ■ Compulsions are defined by
  - Repetitive behaviors (e.g., handwashing) or repetitive mental activities (e.g., counting items, repeating words silently)
  - The individual feels driven to perform these repetitive behaviors or mental activities (often according to rules that, he or she believes, must be stringently adhered to)
- ■ Children may or may not be able to explain their behaviors or mental activities.
- ■ The obsessions or compulsions cause distress for the individual, are time consuming, or significantly interfere with daily routine.
- ■ The obsessive–compulsive symptoms are not characteristic of the physiological effects of a substance (e.g., a drug of abuse, a medication) or another medical condition.
- ■ If another psychiatric disorder is present, the content of the obsessions or compulsions does not center on that disorder (e.g., preoccupation with food in the presence of an eating disorder, or excessive worrying about everyday events as seen in GAD.
- ■ Specify level of insight
- ■ Specify if tic-related

TREATMENT OVERVIEW

- ■ OCD is usually a chronic (persistent) condition; therefore, treatment and support are offered indefinitely.
- ■ OCD treatment can help bring symptoms under control so that they do not control the person's life. The two main treatments for OCD include psychotherapy and medication.
- ■ For mild to moderate cases of OCD, psychotherapy may be offered without medication, while severe cases warrant medications and psychotherapy treatments.
- ■ Exposure and response prevention (ERP) and CBT offer the greatest benefits, or efficacy and specificity, in treating the symptoms.
- ■ ERP involves gradually exposing person to a feared object or obsession, such as something dirty, while teaching the patient ways to cope with the resulting anxiety.
- ■ CBT involves retraining thought patterns and routines so that compulsive behaviors are no longer needed to relieve anxiety.

PSYCHOPHARMACOLOGY OVERVIEW FOR OCD

- ■ It is not unusual to try several medications before finding one that works. To control symptoms, medications from different pharmacologic categories may be combined. Consult with a specialist as necessary.
- ■ Behavioral therapies should be used together with drug therapy. These include ERP, CBT, relaxation techniques, pleasant mental imagery, and cognitive restructuring (learning to recognize and replace panic-inducing thoughts). Behavioral treatment appears to have long-lasting benefits.
- ■ Regular exercise, adequate sleep, and regularly scheduled meals may help reduce the frequency of the attacks. Caffeine and other stimulants should be reduced or eliminated.

Drug Selection Table for OCD

CLASS	DRUG
Selective-serotonin reuptake inhibitors (SSRIs)	First-line drug therapy:
	Fluoxetine (*Prozac*)
	Sertraline (*Zoloft*)
	Paroxetine (*Paxil, Paxil CR*)
	Paroxetine mesylate (*Pexeva*)
	Fluvoxamine (*Luvox CR*)
	Citalopram (*Celexa*)
Tricyclic antidepressants (TCAs)	Drugs for treatment-resistant cases:
	Clomipramine (*Anafranil*)

- SSRIs. These are considered first-line treatments. As a guideline, upper end of dosing limits should be used to achieve best outcomes.
  - Sertraline (Zoloft). Starting dosage: 50 mg/day. Increase to maximum dosage of 200 mg/day (Fluoxetine [Prozac] starting dosage: 40 mg. Increase to maximum dosage of 60 mg/day).
  - Fluvoxamine (Luvox). Starting dosage: 50 mg. Increase to maximum dosage of 200 mg/day.
  - Citalopram (Celexa). Starting dosage 20 mg. Increase to maximum dosage of 40 mg/day. Beware of patients with preexisting heart disease; use caution with hepatic impairment, those on Cimetidine, and those who are CYP 2 C 19 poor metabolizers. Additional FDA safety announcements issued in 2011, revised 2012. Patients older than 60 years of age should not take doses exceeding 20 mg/day.
  - Escitalopram (Lexapro). Starting dosage 10 mg. Increase to maximum 20 mg/day.
  - Paroxetine (Paxil). Starting dosage 20 mg. Increase to maximum 40 mg/day.
- Tricyclic antidepressants, including, clomipramine (Anafranil), Starting dosage 25 mg. Increase to 100 to 250 mg/day.
  - Pediatric dosing. (See also "Practice Parameter," 2012). Fluvoxamine (Luvox), Fluoxetine (Prozac), Sertraline (Zoloft), and Clomipramine (Anafranil) have FDA approval for use in pediatric populations with OCD; start low and go slow.
- Selective-serotonin reuptake inhibitors (SSRIs) have a black box warning for their potential to increase suicidal thoughts in children, adolescents, and young adults, although new analysis of data reveal conflicting information about this risk.
- Monitor antidepressants for nausea, agitation, sleep disturbance, suicidal thoughts, changes in appetite, and drowsiness; in paroxetine (Paxil) and clomipramine (Anafranil), also monitor for seizures. Medication should not be abruptly stopped.
- Augmentation with an atypical antipsychotic, such as risperidone (Risperdal), quetiapine (Seroquel), aripiprazole (Abilify), may be warranted after weighing the risk/benefits.

PATIENT EDUCATION

- About diagnosis/prognosis—treatable, but has no cure.
- Available treatment is discussed, with side effects carefully explained.

MEDICAL/LEGAL PITFALLS

- Patient may present with life-threatening medical conditions but refuse treatment.
- Physician may have to determine whether patient needs commitment, based on symptoms.

REFERENCE

American Psychiatric Association (APA). (2013). *Diagnostic and statistical manual of mental disorders* (5th ed.). Washington, DC: American Psychiatric Press.

BIBLIOGRAPHY

Ahmari, S. E., Spellman, T., Douglass, N. L., Kheirbek, M. A., Simpson, H. B., Deisseroth, K., & Hen, R. (2013). Repeated cortico-striatal stimulation generates persistent OCD-like behavior. *Science, 340*(6137), 1234–1239.

American Psychiatric Association. (2000). *Diagnostic and statistical manual of mental disorders* (4th ed., text revi.). Washington, DC: American Psychiatric Association.

American Psychiatric Association. (2007). *Practice guideline for the treatment of patients with obsessive-compulsive disorder*. Arlington, VA: American Psychiatric Press.

Angoa-Perez, M., Kane, M. J., Briggs, D. I., Sykes, C. E., Shah, M. M., Francescutti, D. M., & Kuhn, D. M. (2012). Genetic depletion of brain 5HT reveals a common molecular pathway mediating compulsivity and impulsivity. *Journal of Neurochemistry, 121*(6), 974–984.

Bjorgvinsson, T., Hart, J., & Heffelfinger, S. (2007). Obsessive-compulsive disorder: Update on assessment and treatment. *Journal of Psychiatric Practice, 13*, 362–372.

Beucke, J. C., Sepulcre, J., Talukdar, T., Linnman, C., Zschenderlein, K., Endrass, T., . . . Kathmann, N. (2013). ABnormally high degree connectivity of the orbitofrontal cortex in obsessive-compulsive disorder. *JAMA Psychiatry, 70*(6), 619–629. doi: 10.1001/jamapsychiatry.2013.173

Bloch, M. H., Green, C., Kichuk, S. A., Dombrowski, P. A., Wasylink, S., Billingslea, E., & Pittenger, C. (2013). Long-term outcome in adults with obsessive-compulsive disorder. *Depress Anxiety, 30*(8), 716–722.

Bloch, M. H., Landeros-Weisenberger, A., Kelmendi, B., Coric, V., Bracken, M. B., & Leckman, J. F. (2006). A systematic review: Antipsychotic augmentation with treatment refractory obsessive-compulsive disorder. *Molecular Psychiatry, 11*(7), 622–632.

Bloch, M. H., Sukhodolsky, D. G., Dombrowski, P. A., Panza, K. E., Craiglow, B. G., Landeros-Weisenberger, A., & Schultz, R. T. (2011). Poor fine-motor and visuospatial skills predict persistence of pediatric-onset obsessive-compulsive disorder into adulthood. *Journal of Child Psychology and Psychiatry, and Allied Disciplines, 52*(9), 974–983.

Burns, G. L., Keortge, S. G., Formea, G. M., & Sternberger, L. G. (1996). Revision of the Padua inventory of obsessive compulsive disorder symptoms: Distinctions between worry, obsessions, and compulsions. *Behavior Research and Therapy, 24*, 163–173.

Clomipramine Collaborative Study Group. (1991). Clomipramine in the treatment of patient with obsessive-compulsive disorder. *Archives of General Psychiatry, 48*, 730–738.

Dougherty, D. D., Rauch, S. L., & Jenike, M. A. (2004). Pharmacotherapy for obsessive-compulsive disorder. *Journal of Clinical Psychology, 60*, 1195–1202.

Fan, Q., Palaniyappan, L., Tan, L., Wang, J., Wang, X., Li, C., & Liddle, P. F. (2013). Surface anatomical profile of the cerebral cortex in obsessive-compulsive disorder: A study of cortical thickness, folding and surface area. *Psychology Medicine, 43*(5), 1081–1091.

Gibbons, R. D., Brown, C. H., Hur, K., Davis, J., & Mann, J. J. (2012). Suicidal thoughts and behavior with antidepressant treatment: Reanalysis of the randomized placebo-controlled studies of fluoxetine and venlafaxine. *Archives of General Psychiatry, 69*(6), 580–587.

Goodman, W. K., Price, L. H., Rasmussen, S. A., Mazure, C., Fleischmann, R. L., Hill, C. L.,...Charney, D. S. (1989). The Yale-Brown obsessive compulsive scale: Pt. I. Development, use, and reliability. *Archives of General Psychiatry, 46*, 1006–1011.

Hachiya, Y., Miyata, R., Tanuma, N., Hongou, K., Tanaka, K., Shimoda, K., & Hayashi, M. (2013). Autoimmune neurological disorders associated with group-A beta-hemolytic streptococcal infection. *Brain & Development, 35*(7), 670–674. doi: 10.1016/j.braindev.2012.10.003

Mavrogiorgou, P., Nalato, F., Meves, S., Luksnat, S., Norra, C., Gold, R., & Krogias, C. (2013). Transcranial sonography in obsessive–compulsive disorder. *Journal of Psychiatric Research, 47*(11), 1642–1648.

Ponniah, K., Magiati, I., & Hollon, S. D. (2013). An update on the efficacy of psychological therapies in the treatment of obsessive-compulsive disorder in adults. *Journal of Obsessive-Compulsive and Related Disorders, 2*(2), 207–218.

Posner, J., Marsh, R., Maia, T. V., Peterson, B. S., Gruber, A., & Simpson, H. B. (2013). Reduced functional connectivity within the limbic cortico-striato-thalamo-cortical loop in unmedicated adults with obsessive compulsive disorder. *Human Brain Mapping* (e-pub ahead of print).

Practice parameter for the assessment and treatment of children and adolescents with obsessive-compulsive disorder. (2012). *Journal of the American Academy of Child and Adolescent Psychiatry, 51*(1), 98–113. doi: 10.1016/j.jaac.2011.09.019

Rauch, S. L., & Carlezon, W. A., Jr. (2013). Neuroscience. Illuminating the neural circuitry of compulsive behaviors. *Science, 340*(6137), 1174–1175.

Russell, E. J., Fawcett, J. M., & Mazmanian, D. (2013). Risk of obsessive-compulsive disorder in pregnant and postpartum women: A meta-analysis. *Journal of Clinical Psychiatry, 74*(4), 377–385.

Stein, D. J., Koen, N., Fineberg, N., Fontenelle, L. F., Matsunaga, H., Osser, D., & Simpson, H. B. (2012). A 2012 evidence-based algorithm for the pharmacotherapy for obsessive-compulsive disorder. *Current Psychiatry Reports, 14*(3), 211–219. doi: 10.1007/s11920-012-0268-9

Thordarson, D. S., Radomsky, A. S., Rachman, S., Shafran, R., Sawchuk, C. N., & Ralph Hakstian, A. (2004). The Vancouver obsessional compulsive inventory (VOCI). *Behavior Research and Therapy, 42*, 1289–1314.

Venkatasubramanian, G., Zutshi, A., Jindal, S., Srikanth, S. G., Kovoor, J. M., Kumar, J. K., & Janardhan Reddy, Y. C. (2012). Comprehensive evaluation of cortical structure abnormalities in drug-naive, adult patients with obsessive-compulsive disorder: A surface-based morphometry study. *Journal of Psychiatric Research, 46*(9), 1161–1168.

Weissman, M. M., Bland. R. C., Canino, G. J., Greenwald, S., Hwu, H. G., Lee, C. K., ... Wickramaratne, P. J. (1994). The cross national epidemiology of obsessive compulsive disorder (The Cross National Collaborative Group). *Journal of Clinical Psychiatry, 55*, 5–10.

World Health Organization. (2001). *The World Health report 2001—Mental health: New understanding, new hope.* Geneva, Switzerland: Author.

Wu, K., Hanna, G. L., Rosenberg, D. R., & Arnold, P. D. (2012). The role of glutamate signaling in the pathogenesis and treatment of obsessive-compulsive disorder. *Pharmacology, Biochemistry, and Behavior, 100*(4), 726–735. doi: 10.1016/j.pbb.2011.10.007

Zhang, T., Wang, J., Yang, Y., Wu, Q., Li, B., Chen, L., &Gong, Q. (2011). Abnormal small-world architecture of top-down control networks in obsessive-compulsive disorder. *Journal of Psychiatry Neuroscience, 36*(1), 23–31.

WEB RESOURCES

- American Anxiety Disorders Association: http://www.adaa.org/
- Obsessive Compulsive Foundation: http://www.ocfoundation.org/
- Peace of Mind Foundation: http://www.peaceofmind.co/

Chapter 13

Somatic Symptom and Related Disorders

Somatic Symptom and Related Disorders

Somatic symptom and related disorders are presented as one disorder with many components.

BACKGROUND INFORMATION

Definition of Disorder

- These are individuals who present to a health care provider with somatic symptoms that are either very distressing or produce significant disruption of functioning. The individuals have extreme and unbalanced thoughts, feelings, and behaviors regarding those symptoms.
- The symptoms are typically persistent for at least 6 months. Pain is often a factor.
- All of the somatic symptoms and related disorders focus on somatic symptoms and their initial presentations are mainly in medical rather than mental health care settings.
- The diagnosis is made based on distressing somatic symptoms and the negative thoughts, feelings, and behaviors associated with the symptoms and *is not* due to the absence of a medical explanation for the symptoms.
- The somatic symptom and related disorders include illness, anxiety disorder, conversion disorder (functional neurological symptom disorder), psychological factors affecting other medical conditions, factitious disorder, other specified somatic symptom and related disorders, and unspecified somatic symptoms and related disorders.

Etiology

- Somatic symptoms may be present by themselves or along with a medical condition. It is the individual's distressing response to the symptoms that indicates the diagnosis.
- The cause or origin of somatic symptoms is linked to the notion of a mind–body dualism and the fact that these patients do experience their symptoms.

Drug Selection Table for Somatic Symptom and Related Disorders

CLASS	DRUG
Selective serotonin reuptake inhibitors (SSRIs)	First-line drugs for treatment: Mood instability and anxiety:
	Sertraline (*Zoloft*)
	Paroxetine hydrochloride (*Paxil, Paxil CR*)
	Fluoxetine (*Prozac, Prozac Weekly, Sarafem*)
	Escitalopram (*Lexapro*)
	Vilazodone (*Viibryd*)
Serotonin and norepinephrine reuptake inhibitors (SNRIs)	First-line drugs for treatment: Mood instability and anxiety
	Duloxetine (*Cymbalta*)
	Venlafaxine (*Effexor*)
	Desvenlafaxine (*Pristiq*)
Serotonin and norepinephrine reuptake inhibitors (SNRIs) aka dual-acting antidepressants	First-line drugs for treatment: Bodily pain relief
	Venlafaxine (*Effexor*)
	Duloxetine (*Cymbalta*)
Second-generation (atypical) antipsychotics	For treatment of dissociation, psychosis, severe anxiety:
	Aripiprazole (*Abilify*)
	Olanzapine (*Zyprexa*)
	Ziprasidone (*Geodon*)

■ Somatic symptoms may be influenced by the patients' sociocultural heritage, their personality, their level of anxiety, and perceived locus of control.
■ Research has linked the symptoms of somatic symptom disorders to a past history of abuse and/or trauma, parental neglect, maltreatment, and/or abandonment.
■ Medically unexplained symptoms remain a key feature in conversion disorder and pseudocyesis because symptoms are not consistent with medical pathophysiology.

Demographics
■ It has been estimated that between 3% and 7% of the adult population experience these disorders; females generally tend to have more reported symptoms with a likely higher occurrence.
■ Individuals have a high level of medical care utilization, seek care from multiple providers, and are often unresponsive to interventions.

Risk Factors

■ Individuals with personality traits that manifest in negative emotions
■ Individuals with existing anxiety and depression may have worse symptoms and impairment
■ Individuals with less education, lower socioeconomic status, and more stressors
■ Past history of trauma, abuse, neglect, or maltreatment
■ Individuals with concurrent chronic physical and psychiatric illnesses
■ There is no known genetic heritability among somatic symptom disorders
■ There is some suggestion that somatic symptoms may be precipitated by major life stress or learned behavior (American Psychiatric Association, 2013).

DIAGNOSIS

Differential Diagnosis

■ Somatic symptoms, medical symptoms, and amplification of medical symptoms can all coexist in the same patient. Diagnoses that need to be ruled out include neurological diseases, panic disorder, generalized anxiety disorder, depressive disorders, delusional disorder, body dysmorphic disorder, obsessive-compulsive disorder, adjustment disorder, neurological disease, and borderline personality disorder. This complicates the assessment and treatment but, most important, the real possibility of a medical illness.
■ A thorough diagnostic workup is necessary. It is useful and therapeutic for patients to trust that you *believe* them and will work toward an end to their suffering.

ICD-10 Codes

Somatic symptom disorder (F45.1)
Illness anxiety disorder (F45.21)
(Depends on symptom type) Conversion disorder (functional neurological symptom disorder) (F44.4–F44.7)
Psychological factors affecting other medical conditions (F54)
Factitious disorder (F68.10)
Other specified somatic symptom and related disorder (F45.8)
Unspecified somatic symptom and related disorder (F45.9)

Screening Question

■ A screening question useful for the interview is as follows:
    ■ "Do you worry about your physical health more than most people? Do you get sick more often than most people?"
    ■ If yes, ask "Do these experiences significantly affect your daily life?"
    ■ If yes, ask "Which is worse for you, worrying about the symptoms you experience or worrying about your health and the possibility that you are sick"?

Diagnostic Workup

- Complete history and physical examination with consideration of previous neurological trauma; past illnesses, surgeries, and health care seeking for their symptoms
- Psychiatric evaluation should specifically include a thorough focus on personal and social history to illuminate any past abuse, trauma, conflicted relationships, unstable living situations, and/or parental neglect or absence in their childhood and adolescence.
- Patients with histories of abuse are unlikely to report this unless specifically asked about abuse in the medical or psychiatric history.
- Lab as needed to evaluate physical complaints
- Thyroid function studies (triiodothyronine [T3], thyroxine [T4], thyroid-stimulating hormone [TSH])
- Complete metabolic panel (CMP), including glucose, calcium, albumin; total protein count; levels of sodium, potassium, CO_2 (carbon dioxide and bicarbonate), chloride, blood urea nitrogen (BUN), creatinine, alkaline phosphatase (ALP), alanine aminotransferase (ALT, also called serum glutamic pyruvic transaminase [SGPT]), aspartate aminotransferase (AST, also called serum glutamic oxaloacetic transaminase [SGOT]), and bilirubin
- Complete blood count (CBC) with differentials: hemoglobin, hematocrit, red blood cell (RBC) count, white blood cell (WBC) count, WBC differential count, and platelet count

Clinical Presentation: Symptoms

- Patient may present with one symptom or multiple symptoms crossing over multiple systems within the body.
- Each diagnostic category has specifiers to assist in determining the diagnosis.

DSM-5 Diagnostic Guidelines

Illness Anxiety Disorder

- There is a preoccupation with having or acquiring a serious illness and individuals are encountered more often in medical than mental health settings. (This disorder is similar to the previous diagnosis of hypochondriasis.)
- Somatic symptoms do not exist or, if they do, are mild in intensity.
- The individual has an abnormal level of anxiety about health and easily gets distressed about his or her own health status. He or she often consults multiple providers for the same problem.
- The individual performs unwarranted behaviors related to health such as checking the body for signs of illness or evades appointments and doctor visits.
- The preoccupation has been present for at least 6 months or greater.

Conversion Disorder (Functional Neurological Symptom Disorder)

- Presence of one or more symptoms of altered voluntary motor or sensory functioning, which causes clinically significant distress or impairment in areas of functioning, such as social or occupational functioning
- Symptoms may include motor or movement disorders; altered, reduced, or absent sensory disorders; limb shaking (psychogenic seizures); unresponsiveness; speech issues; or lump in the throat. Specific symptoms types are coded separately.
- The severity of the illness is comparable to medical diseases.
- Another medical (neurological) or mental explanation does not exist.

▪ The symptom or deficit does not comprise or represent a culturally sanctioned behavior.

Psychological Factors Affecting Other Medical Conditions
▪ A medical condition must be present besides the mental disorder.
▪ The psychological or behavioral issues clinically interfere with, delay, or exacerbate the medical condition requiring medical attention.
▪ The psychological or behavioral issues create firm health risks for the person.
▪ The deceptive behavior is evident even in the absence of obvious external rewards.
▪ These can occur across the life span.

Factitious Disorder (Imposed on Self or Imposed on Another)
▪ The individual falsifies symptoms, both physical or psychological. He or she may also induce injury or disease *in himself or herself or another.*
▪ The individual presents himself or herself *or* another (victim) to others as ill or harmed.
▪ The individual takes secretive or sly actions to misrepresent, simulate, or cause signs or symptoms of illness or injury in the absence of obvious external rewards.
▪ The psychological or behavioral issues are not explained by another mental disorder.

TREATMENT OVERVIEW

Acute Treatment
▪ The clinician's most important initial task is to develop a relationship with these patients and to help clarify the biopsychosocial components of their symptoms.
▪ The clinician may also act as an intermediary for the patient vis-à-vis the medical care system. In essence, the clinician becomes the advocate and joins with the patient in a therapeutic relationship.
▪ This relationship, grounded in psychotherapy, can begin to form an alliance in which, the clinician endeavor to educate the patient about the pitfalls, challenges, and problems of evaluating and managing somatic symptoms.
▪ Symptoms must be understood and conveyed to the patient as (a) real, (b) the cause of suffering in the patient, and (c) frequently disabling.
▪ *Pharmacological management* needs to focus on symptom relief from antidepressants (selective serotonin reuptake inhibitors [SSRIs] and serotonin-norepinephrine reuptake inhibitors [SNRIs]) for mood instability and anxiety; dual-acting antidepressants may be useful for bodily pain relief; and atypical antipsychotics for bizarre, mood-congruent symptoms, such as dissociation, psychosis, or severe anxiety.

Chronic Treatment
▪ It is essential that the clinician, who manages the patient with this disorder, work in tandem with a primary care team, a psychiatric and mental health nurse practitioner (PMHNP), a psychiatrist, and/or all other members involved in the treatment. The patient needs the communication to be maintained among all members of the health care team.
▪ Psychotherapy for patients with chronic somatic symptoms is usually more successful if the patient is encouraged to be an active participant in the treatment. Cognitive behavioral therapy (CBT) has been found to be useful. Psychodynamic

psychotherapy is indicated for the patient who is insightful and willing to understand how the past influences the current experience of life, living, and interacting with others.

▨ It is essential that the patients be offered the opportunity to enter into psychotherapy with a clinician whom they trust and also are able to see on a regular basis. Referral to a skilled therapist/clinician is also essential.

▨ *Pharmacological management* needs to be monitored and titrated to manage the symptoms.

Recurrence Rate

▨ These diagnoses can be defined as severe and persistent psychiatric and medical illnesses that require ongoing assessment, treatment, management, and communication among the entire treatment team. These are seen more commonly in medical settings than in psychiatric settings. Recurrence may be attributed to a failure or lack of communication between health care systems and providers.

Medication should be prescribed to treat the significant symptoms of depression, anxiety, mood disturbances, and/or delusions as determined by a thorough evaluation of the patient. Dual-acting antidepressants may be effective when a combination of symptoms occurs; randomized controlled trials have found antidepressants effective at times.

PATIENT EDUCATION

▨ *Psychoeducation* in the form of individual therapy or group work can assist the patient in understanding the cognitive patterns, behaviors, and how they interrelate with the way the body feels and responds.

▨ It will be important for the patient to learn new ways of interacting and trusting those who assist and manage their care.

▨ The patients can be guided to utilize alternative ways to relate to the health care system, deal with past and current family dynamics, and resolve excessive worry about their symptoms.

MEDICAL/LEGAL PITFALLS

▨ It is essential that, if a clinician agrees to manage a patient with a somatic symptom disorder, the clinician be prepared to be work with the patient over a long period of time. If this is outside of the clinician's scope of practice, it is best that the patient be referred to a more skilled and able clinician.

▨ Often patients who are suffering from somatic symptom disorders may have comorbidity of other illnesses, such as mood and anxiety disorders, as well as personality disorders. This complexity often leads to a complex treatment plan, which must be adhered to and be maintained by all members of the treatment team.

▨ These patients may have concurrent medical conditions or develop significant medical problems; therefore, it is essential to provide ongoing assessment, diagnosis, and management in the form of a team-based treatment plan.

▨ Medical neglect and/or abandonment, whether perceived or a reality, are certainly litigious and can be a major pitfall for the clinician.

REFERENCE

American Psychiatric Association. (2013). *Diagnostic and statistical manual of mental disorders* (5th ed.). Washington, DC: American Psychiatric Press.

BIBLIOGRAPHY

De Gucht, V., & Fischler, B. (2002). Somatization: A critical review of conceptual and methodological issues. *Psychosomatics, 43*, 1–9.

Dimsdale, J., & Creed, F. (2009). The proposed diagnosis of somatic symptom disorders in *DSM-V* to replace somatoform disorders in *DSM-IV*—A preliminary report. *Journal of Psychosomatic Research, 66*(6), 473–476.

Dimsdale, J., Creed, R., Escobar, J., Sharpe, M., Wulsin, L., Barsky, A.,...Levenson, J. (2013). Somatic symptom disorder: An important change in DSM. *Journal of Psychosomatic Research, 75*(3), 223–228.

Fallon, B. (2004). Pharmacotherapy of somatoform disorders. *Journal of Psychosomatic Research, 56*, 455–460.

Ford, C. V. (1983). *The somatizing disorders: Illness as a way of life.* New York, NY: Elsevier Biomedical.

Konijnenberg, A. Y., de Graeff-Meeder, E. R., van der Hoeven, J., Kimpen, J. L., Buitelaar, J. K., & Uiterwaal, C. (2006). Psychiatric morbidity in children with medically unexplained chronic pain: Diagnosis from the pediatrician's perspective. *Pediatrics, 117*(3), 889–897.

Kroenke, K. (2007). Efficacy of treatment for somatoform disorders: A review of randomized controlled trials. *Psychosomatic Medicine, 69*(9), 881–888.

Loewenstein, R. J. (1990). Somatic form disorders in victims of incest and child abuse. In R. P. Kluft (Ed.), *Incest-related disorders of adult psychopathology* (pp. 75–113). Washington, DC: American Psychiatric Press.

Nussbaum, A. (2013a, September). *Of dictionaries and disorders: DSM-5 and the treatment of persons with psychotic and bipolar disorders.* Paper presented at the Colorado Society of Clinical Nurse Specialists in Psychiatric Nursing, Breckenridge, CO.

Nussbaum, A. (2013b). *The pocket guide to DSM-V diagnostic exam.* Washington, DC: American Psychiatric Press.

Sadock, B. J., & Sadock, V. A. (2008). *Synopsis of psychiatry* (10th ed.). Philadelphia, PA: Lippincott, Williams & Williams.

Sar, V., Akyüz, G., Kundakçi, T., Kızıltan, E., & Dogan, O. (2004). Childhood trauma, dissociation, and psychiatric comorbidity in patients with conversion disorder. *American Journal of Psychiatry, 161*, 2271–2276.

Soltis-Jarrett, V. (2004). Interactionality: Willfully extending the boundaries of participatory research in psychiatric mental health nursing. *Advances in Nursing Science, 27*(4), 316–329.

Sumathipala, A. (2007).What is the evidence for the efficacy of treatments for somatoform disorders? A critical review of previous intervention studies. *Psychosomatic Medicine, 69*(9), 889–890.

Tylee, A., & Gandhi, P. (2005). The importance of somatic symptoms in depression in primary care. *Journal of Clinical Psychiatry, 7*, 167–176.

van der Kolk, B., Pelcovitz, D., Roth, S., Mandel, E. S., McFarlane, A., & Herman, J. L. (1996). Dissociation, somatization, and affect dysregulation: The complexity of adaptation to trauma. *American Journal of Psychiatry, Festschrift Supplement, 153*, 83–93.

WEB RESOURCES

- http://www.webmd.com/mental-health/somatoform-disorders-symptoms-types-treatment/
- http://psycnet.apa.org/psycinfo/2009–07668-004/
- http://familydoctor.org/online/famdocen/home/common/pain/disorders/162.html/
- http://www.medscape.com/viewarticle/781189/

Chapter 14

Dissociative Disorders

Adjustment Disorder With Anxiety

BACKGROUND INFORMATION

Definition of Disorder
- Patient displays excessive emotional or behavioral symptoms due to a psychosocial stressor.
- The symptoms occur within 3 months of the onset of the stressor.
- The emotional reaction is greater than what would normally be expected for the situation or causes social or occupational impairment.
- This subtype of adjustment disorder (AD) has primary symptoms of nervousness, fears, and/or worry.

Etiology
- AD classifications provide a way of classifying mental health symptoms that are significant enough to require treatment but not sufficient enough to meet the specific criteria *for diagnosis of a mental illness.*
- ADs have no specific symptoms.
- Any combination of maladaptive responses may qualify if they cause distress, impairment in functioning, are a result of a stressor, and develop within 3 months of the stressor.
- Frequently occurs in patients with physical diagnoses (e.g., myocardial infarction [MI], cerebrovascular accident [CVA], HIV, diabetes mellitus [DM], cancer, head and neck surgery).
- May be a maladaptive response to multiple, relatively minor stressors, not just one large stressor.
- Stressors more likely to be chronic in adolescents than adults.
- Conclusions from a twin study suggest a genetic link.
- The development of AD is partially determined by the meaning of the stressor to the individual, the strength of the person's "sense of self," his or her history of successfully dealing with stressors, and his or her support network.

Demographics
- Equally affects both men and women
- Can occur in any age group
- Consider the patient's cultural context when making the clinical judgment of maladaptive behavior.

Risk Factors
▪ There is a history of poor adaptive behaviors
▪ In children, there is the lack of a warm and supportive primary caregiver.
▪ Medical illness
▪ Existing mental illness
▪ Disadvantaged life circumstances

DIAGNOSIS

Differential Diagnosis
▪ Axis I disorders of depression, anxiety, posttraumatic stress disorder (PTSD), acute stress disorder
▪ Bereavement
▪ Other subtypes of AD
▪ Medication noncompliance
▪ Psychosocial stressors

ICD-10 Code
AD with anxiety (F43-43.9)

Diagnostic Workup
▪ Physical examination
▪ Medical and psychiatric history
▪ Lab as needed to evaluate physical complaints
  ▫ Thyroid function studies (triiodothyronine [T3], thyroxine [T4], thyroid-stimulating hormone [TSH])
  ▫ Complete metabolic panel (CMP), including glucose, calcium, albumin; total protein count; levels of sodium, potassium, CO_2 (carbon dioxide and bicarbonate), chloride, blood urea nitrogen (BUN), creatinine, alkaline phosphatase (ALP), alanine amino transferase (ALT, also called SGPT), aspartate amino transferase (AST, also called SGOT), and bilirubin
  ▫ Complete blood count (CBC) with differentials: hemoglobin, hematocrit, red blood cell (RBC) count, white blood cell (WBC) count, WBC differential count, and platelet count

Initial Assessment
▪ When did symptoms begin?
▪ What was going on in your life?
▪ Any recent major health concerns?
▪ Have you ever had anything like this before?
▪ How have these symptoms interfered in your life?
▪ Any thoughts of harm to yourself or another?

Clinical Presentation Symptoms
▪ Physical complaints, may be vague
▪ Avoidance of work or school
▪ Avoidance of social life
▪ Emotional distress, feeling overwhelmed, restless, fearful
▪ In children, fear may be of separation from parents or major attachment figure

▪ Symptoms developed after an identifiable stressor or multiple stressors
▪ Eleven percent may have a suicidal ideation.

DSM-5 Diagnostic Guidelines
▪ A psychological response to an identifiable psychosocial stressor that includes the development of clinically significant emotional or behavioral symptoms
▪ The symptoms develop within 3 months of the onset of the stressor.
▪ The individual's distress is in excess of what would be expected on the basis of the level or magnitude of the stressor.
▪ The symptoms cannot be better accounted for by another psychiatric disorder or the exacerbation of a preexisting psychiatric disorder.
▪ Diagnosis does apply in the case of bereavement greater than 60 days (the maladaptive reactions are not better ascribed to AD with depressed mood, AD with mixed anxiety and depressed mood, AD with disturbance of conduct, AD with mixed disturbance of emotions and conduct).
▪ Symptoms are likely to include jitteriness, worry, nervousness, or fear.
▪ Duration is as follows: Acute—lasting for less than 6 months; chronic—lasting for more than 6 months.

TREATMENT OVERVIEW

Acute Treatment
▪ Identify, limit, or reduce the stressor if possible. ADs secondary to a physical illness often remit after the patient becomes well or learns how to adapt to a chronic illness.
  ▪ Psychotherapy is first-line treatment.
    ○ Cognitive behavioral, interpersonal, or psychodynamic therapy
    ○ Some areas of therapy: Identification of the meaning of the stressor, putting feelings into words, understanding existing strengths and capacities, and developing a support network
  ▪ Psychopharmacology is used when psychotherapy has not been effective. Most often, selective serotonin reuptake inhibitors (SSRIs) or anxiolytics can be effective for anxiety/depressive symptoms of disorder but they are not Food and Drug Administration (FDA) indicated for core disorder of adjustment.

Chronic Treatment
▪ Short-term therapy is often sufficient. Ongoing therapy is used if there were preexisting symptoms or to help the individual identify reasons for poor stress tolerance.
▪ Group therapy can be helpful for individuals with similar stressors (e.g., postmastectomy groups).

Recurrence Rate
▪ A study looking at hospital readmission rates among patients with ADs and major depressive disorder concluded that the readmission rates are reduced for ADs.

PATIENT EDUCATION

▪ Encourage basic self-care: healthy diet, exercise, plenty of sleep.
▪ Avoid alcohol, drugs, caffeine, and any stimulating herbal preparation.

- Keep in contact with friends and family. Enlist their support.
- Learn ways to relax with breathing and muscle relaxation techniques.

MEDICAL/LEGAL PITFALLS

- Suicide attempts and completions occur with ADs as well as other psychiatric disorders.
- The interval from the start of symptoms to the suicide attempt is shorter in ADs as compared to major depressive disorder.
- Suicide attempts tend to be more impulsive with ADs than other mood disorders.
- There is more deliberate self-harm than with other disorders.

Adjustment Disorder With Depressed Mood

BACKGROUND INFORMATION

Definition of Disorder

Patient exhibits excessive emotional or behavioral symptoms due to a psychosocial stressor. The symptoms occur within 3 months of the onset of the stressor. The emotional reaction is excessive as compared with what would normally be expected for the situation or causes social or occupational impairment. This subtype of AD has primary symptoms of depressed mood, frequent tearfulness, and/or a loss of interest in activities.

Etiology

- AD classifications provide a way of classifying mental health symptoms that are significant enough to require treatment but insufficient to meet the specific criteria for another Axis I disorder.
- ADs have no specific symptoms. Any combination of maladaptive responses may qualify if they cause distress, impairment in functioning, are a result of a stressor, and develop within 3 months of the stressor.
- Frequently occurs in patients with physical diagnoses (e.g., MI, CVA, HIV, DM, cancer, head and neck surgery)
- May be a maladaptive response to multiple, relatively minor stressors, not just one large stressor
- Stressors are more likely to be chronic in adolescents than adults.
- Conclusions from a twin study suggest a genetic link.
- The development of AD is partially determined by the meaning of the stressor to the individual, the strength of the person's "sense of self," the history of successfully dealing with stressors, and the support network.

Demographics

- Equally affects both men and women
- Can occur in any age group
- Consider the patient's cultural context when making the clinical judgment of maladaptive behavior.

Risk Factors
■ Patient has a history of poor adaptive behaviors.
■ In children, there is the lack of a warm and supportive primary caregiver.
■ Medical illness
■ Existing Axis I diagnosis
■ Disadvantaged life circumstances

DIAGNOSIS

Differential Diagnosis
■ Axis I disorders of depression, anxiety, PTSD, acute stress disorder
■ Bereavement
■ Other subtypes of AD
■ Medication noncompliance
■ Psychosocial stressors (V codes).

ICD-10 Code
Adjustment reaction with adjustment disorder with depressed mood (F43.21)

Diagnostic Workup
■ Physical examination
■ Medical and psychiatric history
■ Lab as needed to evaluate physical complaints
    ▨ CBC with differentials
    ▨ Chemistry panel
    ▨ Thyroid studies

Initial Assessment
■ When did symptoms begin?
■ What was going on in your life?
■ Any recent major health concerns?
■ Have you ever had anything like this before?
■ How have these symptoms interfered in your life?
■ Any thoughts of harm to yourself or another?

Clinical Presentation
■ Physical complaints, patient may be vague
■ Avoidance of work or school
■ Avoidance of social life
■ Emotional distress, sadness, lack of enjoyment in previously enjoyed activities
■ Symptoms developed after an identifiable stressor or multiple stressors.
■ Eleven percent may have a suicidal ideation.

DSM-5 Diagnostic Guidelines
■ A psychological response to an identifiable psychosocial stressor that includes the development of clinically significant emotional or behavioral symptoms
■ The symptoms develop within 3 months of the onset of the stressor.
■ The individual's distress is in excess of what would be expected on the basis of the level of magnitude of the stressor.

▦ The symptoms cannot be more easily ascribed to another psychiatric disorder or the exacerbation of a preexisting psychiatric disorder.
▦ The maladaptive reactions are not better classified as AD with anxiety, AD with disturbance of conduct, or AD with mixed disturbance of emotions and conduct.
▦ Primary symptoms are depressed mood, tearfulness, and/or hopelessness.
▦ The acute illness lasts less than 6 months. The chronic illness lasts more than 6 months.

TREATMENT OVERVIEW

Acute Treatment
▦ Identify, limit, or reduce the stressor if possible. ADs secondary to a physical illness often remit after the patient becomes well or learns how to adapt to a chronic illness.
▦ Psychotherapy is first-line treatment.
▦ Cognitive behavioral, interpersonal, or psychodynamic therapy
▦ Some areas of therapy: identification of the meaning of the stressor, putting feelings into words, understanding existing strengths and capacities, and developing a support network.
▦ Psychopharmacology is used when psychotherapy has not been effective. Most often, SSRIs or anxiolytics are used judiciously.

Chronic Treatment
▦ Short-term therapy is often sufficient. Ongoing therapy is used if there were preexisting symptoms or to help the individual identify reasons for poor stress tolerance.
▦ Group therapy can be helpful for individuals with similar stressors (e.g., postmastectomy groups).

Recurrence Rate
▦ A study looking at hospital readmission rates among patients with ADs and major depressive disorder concluded that the readmission rates are fewer for ADs.

PATIENT EDUCATION

▦ Encourage the basics. Have patient eat a healthy diet, get moderate exercise, and get plenty of sleep.
▦ Avoid alcohol, drugs, and caffeine.
▦ Keep in contact with family and friends. Ask for their support.
▦ Notify physician of any changes in mood.
▦ Monitor for suicidal ideation.

MEDICAL/LEGAL PITFALLS

▦ Suicide attempts and completions occur with ADs as well as other psychiatric disorders.
▦ The interval from the start of symptoms to the suicide attempt is shorter with ADs as compared to major depressive disorder.
▦ Suicide attempts tend to be more impulsive with ADs than other mood disorders.
▦ There is more deliberate self-harm than with other disorders.

Adjustment Disorder, Unspecified

BACKGROUND INFORMATION

Definition of Disorder
Patient exhibits excessive emotional or behavioral symptoms due to a psychosocial stressor. The symptoms occur within 3 months of the onset of the stressor. The emotional reaction is excessive as compared to what would normally be expected for the situation or causes social or occupational impairment. This subtype of AD would not have *primary* symptoms of depressed mood, anxiety, or disturbance in conduct. It would be possible to see physical complaints, social withdrawal, or avoidance of work or school.

Etiology
- AD classifications provide a way of classifying mental health symptoms that are significant enough to require treatment but insufficient to meet the specific criteria for another Axis I disorder.
- ADs have no specific symptoms. Any combination of maladaptive responses may qualify if they cause distress, impairment in functioning, are a result of a stressor, and develop within 3 months of the stressor.
- Frequently occurs in patients with physical diagnoses (e.g., MI, CVA, HIV, DM, cancer, head and neck surgery)
- May be a maladaptive response to multiple, relatively minor stressors, not just one large stressor
- Stressors are more likely to be chronic in adolescents than adults.
- Conclusions from a twin study suggest a genetic link.
- The development of AD is partially determined by the meaning of the stressor to the individual, the strength of the person's "sense of self," the history of successfully dealing with stressors, and the support network.

Demographics
- Equally affects both men and women
- Can occur in any age group
- Consider the patient's cultural context when making the clinical judgment of maladaptive behavior.

Risk Factors
- There is a history of poor adaptive behaviors.
- In children, there is the lack of a warm and supportive primary caregiver.
- Medical illness
- Existing Axis I diagnosis
- Disadvantaged life circumstances

DIAGNOSIS

Differential Diagnosis
- Axis I disorders of depression, anxiety, PTSD, acute stress disorder
- Bereavement if over 60 days

- Other subtypes of AD
- Medication noncompliance
- Psychosocial stressors (V codes)

ICD-10 Code
Unspecified adjustment reaction (F43.20)

Diagnostic Workup
- Physical examination
- Medical and psychiatric history
- Lab as needed to evaluate physical complaints
  - Thyroid function studies (T3, T4, TSH)
  - CMP, including glucose, calcium, albumin; total protein count; levels of sodium, potassium, CO_2 (carbon dioxide and bicarbonate), chloride, BUN, creatinine, ALP, ALT, AST, and bilirubin
  - CBC with differentials: hemoglobin, hematocrit, RBC count, WBC count, WBC differential count, and platelet count

Initial Assessment
- When did symptoms begin?
- What was going on in your life?
- Any recent major health concerns?
- Have you ever had anything like this before?
- How have these symptoms interfered in your life?
- Any thoughts of harm to yourself or another?

Clinical Presentation
- Physical complaints, patient may be vague.
- Avoidance of work or school
- Avoidance of social life
- Emotional distress
- Symptoms developed after an identifiable stressor or multiple stressors
- Eleven percent may have a suicidal ideation.

DSM-5 Diagnostic Guidelines
- There is a psychological response to an identifiable psychosocial stressor that includes the development of clinically significant emotional or behavioral symptoms.
- The symptoms develop within 3 months of the onset of the stressor.
- The individual's distress is in excess of what would be expected on the basis of the level of magnitude of the stressor.
- The symptoms cannot be more easily ascribed to another psychiatric disorder or the exacerbation of a preexisting psychiatric disorder.
- Diagnosis does apply in the case of bereavement if longer than 60 days.
- The maladaptive reactions are not better classified as AD with anxiety, AD with mixed anxiety and depressed mood, AD with disturbance of conduct, or AD with mixed disturbance of emotions and conduct.
- Symptoms for the unspecified subtype are likely to include physical complaints, social withdrawal, and impairment in work or academic performance.

TREATMENT OVERVIEW

Acute Treatment
■ Identify, limit, or reduce the stressor if possible. ADs secondary to a physical illness often remit after the patient becomes well or learns how to adapt to a chronic illness.
  ■ Psychotherapy is first-line treatment.
  ■ Cognitive behavioral, interpersonal, or psychodynamic
■ Some areas of therapy: identification of the meaning of the stressor, putting feelings into words, understanding existing strengths and capacities, and developing a support network
■ Psychopharmacology is used when psychotherapy has not been effective. Most often, SSRIs or anxiolytics are used judiciously for depressive/anxiety symptoms. They are not FDA approved for the core disorder.

Chronic Treatment
■ Short-term therapy is often sufficient. Ongoing therapy is used if there were preexisting symptoms or to help the individual identify reasons for poor stress tolerance.
■ Group therapy can be helpful for individuals with similar stressors (e.g., postmastectomy groups).

Recurrence Rate
■ A study looking at hospital readmission rates among patients with ADs and major depressive disorder concluded that the readmission rates are fewer for ADs.

PATIENT EDUCATION

■ Encourage the basics: healthy diet, exercise, plenty of sleep.
■ Have patient avoid alcohol, drugs, and caffeine.
■ Ask friends and family for support. Keep in contact with them.
■ Stress the importance of following up with mental health treatment.

MEDICAL/LEGAL PITFALLS

■ Suicide attempts and completions occur with ADs as well as other psychiatric disorders.
■ The interval from the start of symptoms to the suicide attempt is shorter with ADs as compared to major depressive disorder.
■ Suicide attempts tend to be more impulsive with ADs than other mood disorders.
■ There is more deliberate self-harm than with other disorders.

Dissociative Amnesia

BACKGROUND INFORMATION

Definition of Disorder
■ Inability to remember personal information
■ Information lost is important and too extensive to be caused by forgetfulness
■ Gaps in recall occur usually about traumatic events or stressful information

▪ Is not caused by illness, substance use, or injury to the brain
▪ Memories are stored in the brain and not retrievable, but lack of recall is reversible.

Etiology

▪ Can occur at any age
▪ Onset can be gradual or sudden.
▪ Time lost can be from minutes to years. One episode of lost time is most common, but multiple time periods may be lost.
▪ Different types of memory loss may occur.
▪ Localized amnesia—inability to remember specific events like an earthquake
▪ Systematized amnesia—inability to remember categories of information, such as friends
▪ General amnesia—patients are unable to remember anything about their lives, including their own identity
▪ Continuous amnesia—inability to remember events in the past and up to the current time
▪ Frequency increases during wartime or natural disasters

Demographics

▪ Occurs more frequently in women than men
▪ Can occur at any age past infancy
▪ Occurs most frequently at ages 30 to 50 years
▪ Approximately 2% to 7% of the population is affected.
▪ Controversial as a scientific diagnosis; difference in how American and Canadian psychiatrists view dissociative amnesia. Only 13% of Canadian psychiatrists think there is strong scientific validity to include it as a mental health diagnosis.

Risk Factors

▪ Victims of sexual abuse, domestic violence, trauma, or combat
▪ Difficult to diagnose prior to puberty because inability to remember events prior to age 4 years is normal
▪ Appears to occur also in other family members, suggesting a possible genetic link
▪ Comorbidities: conversion disorders, bulimia nervosa, alcohol abuse, depression, personality disorders (borderline, dependent, histrionic)

DIAGNOSIS

Differential Diagnosis

▪ Seizure disorder
▪ Head injury
▪ Alcohol or substance intoxication
▪ Korsakoff's disease
▪ Medication side effect
▪ Sleep deprivation
▪ Brain disease
▪ Delirium or dementia
▪ Other dissociative disorders
▪ Malingering factitious disorder

ICD-10 Code
Dissociative amnesia (F44.0)

Diagnostic Workup
- Diagnosis of exclusion
- Medical and psychiatric history
- Labs as needed to evaluate physical complaints:
  - Thyroid function studies (T3, T4, TSH)
  - CMP, including glucose, calcium, albumin; total protein count; levels of sodium, potassium, CO_2 (carbon dioxide and bicarbonate), chloride, BUN, creatinine, ALP, ALT, AST, and bilirubin
  - CBC with differentials: hemoglobin, hematocrit, RBC count, WBC count, WBC differential count, and platelet count
- Psychological examination to include possible screening:
  - The Dissociative Experiences Scale (DES): this is a self-report screen.
  - The Structured Clinical Interview for *DSM-4* Dissociative Disorders (SCID-D): this is a guided interview; it is the "gold standard" in diagnosis of dissociative disorders, but time consuming.

Initial Assessment
- Is the amnesia transient or persistent?
- Has there been a recent blow to the head?
- Is there fever?
- Is recent memory intact?
- Any recent medication or substance?
- Functional limitations?

Clinical Presentation
- Loss of memory of important life events is usually retrograde (traumatic event is prior to amnesia)
- The unconscious memories influence the conscious state.
  - A rape victim may not remember being raped, but may act like a victim of a violent crime;
  - Demoralization and detachment
  - Mild depression and/or anxiety
  - Agitation at stimuli related to the unrecalled traumatic event

DSM-5 Diagnostic Guidelines
- One or more episodes of the inability to recall important personal information (often though not necessarily of stressful or threatening import)
- The deficit is too extensive to be ascribed to ordinary forgetfulness.
- The disturbance does not occur concurrently with dissociative identity disorder, dissociative fugue, somatization disorder, or PTSD.
- The disturbance is not the direct physiological effect of substance use or a neurological or other condition;
- The symptoms engender distress in the individual and impairment of social functioning.

TREATMENT OVERVIEW

Acute Treatment
▦ Initially, supportive therapy and creation of a safe environment may restore past memories.
▦ Hypnosis
⬧ Age regression may help patients access previously unavailable memories.
⬧ Screen technique—the patient recalls the traumatic event on an imaginary movie screen, which allows the patient to separate the psychological from the somatic aspects of the memory, to make it more bearable. Assists with the cognitive restructuring of the trauma. Patients who are not highly hypnotizable may benefit from this technique.
▦ Medication, if there is depression and/or anxiety:
⬧ Usually SSRIs, SNRIs, anxiolytics, or atypical antipsychotics; antipsychotics are not used as monotherapy for anxiety or depression; SSRI/SNRI can be used with augmentation with anxiolytics or atypical antipsychotics for severe symptoms.

Chronic Treatment
▦ Psychotherapy is used to strengthen the ego, find new ways to cope, improve relationships, and optimize functioning.

Drug Selection Table for Dissociative Amnesia

CLASS	DRUG
Selective serotonin reuptake inhibitors (SSRIs)	First-line drug therapy:
	Escitalopram (*Lexapro*) Sertraline (*Zoloft*) Paroxetine (*Paxil, Paxil PR*) Paroxetine mesylate (*Pexeva*)
Serotonin and norepinephrine reuptake inhibitors (SNRIs)	First-line drug therapy:
	Venlafaxine (*Effexor, Effexor XR*) Duloxetine (*Cymbalta*)
Calcium channel moderator	Drug augmentation:
	Pregabalin (*Lyrica*)
Tricyclic antidepressants (TCAs)	Drugs for treatment-resistant cases:
	Imipramine (Tofranil, Tofranil PM) Desipramine (*Norpramin*)
Benzodiazepines (BZDs)	Use benzodiazepines during first few weeks of initiating SSRI/SNRI until full therapeutic effects are observed/reported.
	Alprazolam (*Xanax/Xanax XR/Niravam*) Clonazepam (*Klonopin*) Lorazepam (*Ativan*) Diazepam (*Valium*)
Antihistamines	Drug augmentation:
	Hydroxyzine (*Vistaril*)
Anxiolytics	Drug augmentation:
	Buspirone (*BuSpar*)

Recurrence Rate
- Rarely recurs

PATIENT EDUCATION

- Advise patients to avoid alcohol and drugs
- Encourage healthy lifestyle and treatment follow-up
- Online resources: Cleveland Clinic, National Alliance on Mental Health (NAMI), Psychcentral.org (also support group information).

MEDICAL/LEGAL PITFALLS

- Criminal cases have involved the recall of previously "repressed" memories of abuse. It is not completely accepted that recovery of repressed memories exists. Some argue that false memories can occur through the power of suggestion during therapy. The position of the American Psychological Association is that a recovered memory cannot be distinguished from a false memory without corroborating information.

BIBLIOGRAPHY

American Psychiatric Association. (2013). *Diagnostic and statistical manual of mental disorders* (5th ed.).Washington, DC: American Psychiatric Press.

Collins, R. D. (2003). *Algorithmic diagnosis of symptoms and signs.* Philadelphia, PA: Lippincott, Williams & Wilkins.

Jones, R. (2002). Readmission rates for adjustment disorders: Comparison with other mood disorders. *Journal of Affective Disorders, 71*(1), 199–203.

Kay, J., & Tasman, A. (2006). *Essentials of psychiatry.* West Sussex, England: John Wiley & Sons.

Sadock, B., & Sadock, V. (2000). *Kaplan & Sadock's comprehensive textbook of psychiatry* (7th ed.). Philadelphia, PA: Lippincott, Williams &Wilkins.

Steinberg, M., Barr, D., Sholomskas, D., & Hall, P. (2005). SCL-90 symptom patterns: Indicators of dissociative disorders. *Bulletin of the Menninger Clinic, 69*(3), 237–249.

WEB RESOURCES

- www.psychcentral.com/
- Freedom from Fear: www.freedomfromfear.org/; nformation on anxiety and mental health treatment, not specifically adjustment disorders.
- www.icd10data.com/
- International Society for the Study of Dissociation: www.issd.org/
- National Institute of Mental Health: www.nimh.nih.gov/
- WebMD: www.webmd.com/

Chapter 15

Sexual Dysfunction

Female Sexual Interest/Arousal Disorder

BACKGROUND INFORMATION

Definition of Disorder
In the *Diagnostic and Statistical Manual of Mental Disorders,* fifth edition *(DSM-5;* American Psychiatric Association, 2013), disorders of sexual desire and sexual arousal were combined into female sexual interest/arousal disorder.

- The disorder is defined as a lack of, or significantly reduced, sexual interest/ arousal characterized by at least three of the following: (a) absent or reduced interest in sexual activity; (b) absent or reduced sexual or erotic thoughts or fantasies; (c) absent or reduced initiation of sexual activity along with a lack of receptivity to initiation by a partner; (d) absent or reduced sexual excitement or pleasure during sexual activity in almost all or all sexual encounters either in identified situational or all contexts; absent or reduced sexual interest/arousal in response to any external or internal written, verbal, or visual sexual cues; and (e) absent or reduced genital or nongenital sensations during sexual activity in almost all or all identified situations or all contexts.
- Symptoms have persisted for at least 6 months.
- Symptoms cause clinically significant distress in the individual.
- Symptoms cannot be attributed to a nonsexual mental disorder, or as a consequence of severe relational distress or other stressors, or the effects of a substance or medication or a medical condition.

  The disorder is specified as lifelong or acquired and generalized or situational. The severity of the symptoms are specified as mild, moderate, or severe.

Etiology
- Sexual response is not necessarily a linear process. Rather, phases of the sexual response cycle may occur in a variety of patterns. For example, some women have reported that desire precedes arousal, whereas others have experienced arousal prior to desire.

▓ Problems related to sexual response may be due to psychological factors, organic factors, or a combination of both. An understanding of interpersonal contexts is important.

▓ Examples of psychological factors include relationship issues/discord, cognitive and affective factors, and cultural and societal factors. For example, communication difficulties between partners, both inside and outside of the bedroom, can be the sole causative factor behind arousal dysfunction.

▓ Depression and anxiety often affect arousal. In fact, women who experience anxiety just prior to erotic stimuli often experience decreased subjective arousal.

▓ Other psychological factors include worry, stress, low self-esteem, negative attitudes toward sex, and unhappiness with one's body.

▓ Relationship factors such as longer relationship duration, low partner attractiveness, having a partner with a sexual dysfunction, and low outcome expectancy may decrease sexual desire. A history of sexual abuse can also impact arousal.

▓ Low sexual desire has not been linked with illicit drug or alcohol use.

▓ Organic causes include endocrine dysfunction, autonomic nervous system (ANS) dysfunction, and cardiovascular/medical issues.

▓ As women age, production of androgens, hormones linked to sexual desire, decreases. This occurs independent of menopause.

▓ Oral contraceptives may increase the sex hormone binding globulin, leading to a decrease in free testosterone.

▓ Low sexual desire has been correlated with hyperprolactinemia, however, not all patients with chronic hyperprolactinemia have low sexual desire.

▓ For sexual arousal to occur in women, normal amounts of estrogens and androgens must be present along with a normal, functioning sympathetic nervous system.

▓ Women with decreased or absent estrogen production have reduced tissue sensitivity of the vagina and vulva and decreased or absent vaginal lubrication.

▓ ANS dysfunction includes spinal cord lesions.

▓ Cardiovascular issues include vascular disease and hypertension.

▓ Female sexual arousal disorder may be lifelong or acquired and situational or generalized.

Demographics

Consistently higher rates of sexual dysfunction have been reported in women with commonly identified decreased or absent desire.

▓ Although sexual desire may decrease with age, some older women report less distress about low sexual desire compared to their younger counterparts.

▓ Prevalence statistics differ depending on the population sampled, sample size, and the instruments used in the study.

▓ Literature reports vary on prevalence statistics due to nonstandardized approaches in studying female sexual disorders.

▓ It is fairly uncommon for a premenopausal woman to have an arousal problem without a decreased libido.

▓ Antidepressants and antipsychotics are two common classes of drugs that may interfere with orgasm.

Risk Factors

▓ Age: can develop at any age and may be present for the woman's entire sexual life.

▓ Family history: there is no evidence that this disorder is familial.

- Stressful events in susceptible people: stressful events in one's life and stressful situations between couples may be the sole cause of this disorder.
- Having another mental health problem, such as a mood or anxiety disorder
- The presence of another sexual function disorder
- Negative thoughts and/or attitudes about sexuality
- Environmental factors, such as developmental difficulties, childhood relationships, and stressors
- Medical conditions, such as diabetes or thyroid dysfunction
- It has been suggested that genetic factors may increase vulnerability to sexual problems in women.

DIAGNOSIS

Differential Diagnosis
- Sexual dysfunction due to a general medical disorder
- Substance-induced sexual disorder
- Another Axis I disorder (major depressive disorder, etc.)
- Occasional problems with sexual arousal
- History of rape, physical, and/or sexual abuse
- Current rape, physical, and/or sexual abuse
- Relationship conflict
- Significant stress
- Other interpersonal factors
- Menopause

ICD-10 Codes
Psychosexual dysfunction, sexual excitement (F52.22)

Diagnostic Workup
- Complete history, physical examination, and psychiatric assessment or evaluation
- This sexual dysfunction may be due to a general medical condition (female androgen insufficiency, chronic renal failure, hyperprolactinemia, pregnancy, and lactation).
- The patient should complete one of the following to aid in diagnosis and treatment: the Sexual Interest and Desire Inventory—Female, Hurlbert Index of Sexual Desire, or Sexual Desire Inventory Questionnaire.
- Laboratories as needed to evaluate physical complaints:
  - Thyroid function studies (triiodothyronine [T3], thyroxine [T4], thyroid-stimulating hormone [TSH])
  - CMP, including glucose, calcium, albumin; total protein count; levels of sodium, potassium, CO_2 (carbon dioxide and bicarbonate), chloride, blood urea nitrogen (BUN), creatinine, alkaline phosphatase (ALP), alanine amino transferase (ALT, also called SGPT), aspartate amino transferase (AST, also called SGOT), and bilirubin
  - Complete blood count (CBC) with differentials: hemoglobin, hematocrit, red blood cell (RBC) count, white blood cell (WBC) count, WBC differential count, and platelet count

Initial Assessment

There may be different symptom profiles in how the disorder is expressed. It is important to note that a woman who has a lower desire for sexual activity than her partner does not meet the criteria for this disorder.

In addition to the listed subtypes, the following five areas must be considered in assessing and diagnosing the disorder: (a) partner factors, (b) relationship factors, (c) individual vulnerability factors, (d) cultural/religious factors, and (e) medical factors.

- Medical history with detailed social history
- Psychiatric history
- Traumatic history (including any form of abuse)
- Sexual history
- Current medication use
- Any recent changes in medication?
- Have you ever had problems with low or absent sexual desire?
- For how long have you had low or absent sexual desire?
- Does this problem only occur in a certain situation or with a certain partner?
- Do you have decreased desire to masturbate or use a vibrator?
- What effect is this having in your relationship?
- Did any emotional or other stressful life event occur when you began to have decreased or absent sexual desire?
- What effect is this decreased/absent sexual desire having on your daily functioning?
- Is there anything you do not like or do not feel comfortable with in your sexual encounters?
- Do you feel like your partner pushes you or is upset with your decreased desire?
- Have you ever had problems with attaining arousal? If so, for how long?
- Have you ever had a problem with lubrication? If so, for how long?
- Do you ever have problems attaining orgasm?
- Do you have pain during sex?
- Does this problem occur only in a certain situation or with a certain partner?
- Do you have difficulty with arousal only while masturbating or using a vibrator?
- How long does it take to become aroused now, compared with the past?
- What effect is this having in your relationship?
- Did any emotional or other life stress occur when the problems with arousal began?
- When did you undergo menopause?
- Have you ever had your ovaries removed?
- Have you ever taken hormone replacement therapy?
- What brought you to seek treatment now?
- What effect is this problem having on your daily functioning?
- Do you feel safe with your partner?
- Have you ever been threatened or harmed by him in any way?

Clinical Presentation

- No specific physical symptoms
- Patients may be in distress if treatment has not worked or if this disorder recurs after treatment.

TREATMENT OVERVIEW

Acute Treatment
- Interventions include psychologic and biologic interventions.
- Psychologic therapy consists of marital therapy, explorations of emotions from abuse, psychotherapy for trust and intimacy issues, and cognitive behavioral therapy (CBT).
  - There is limited evidence of effectiveness of CBT therapy for this disorder.
  - CBT consists of identifying and correcting dysfunctional attitudes toward sexual pleasure, masturbation, and sensate focus.
  - Emphasis is also on couple communication.
- Biologic therapy includes
  - For decreased lubrication, there are lubricants, and estrogen-related products
    - In postmenopausal patients, be cautious using estrogen-related products
    - Estrogen-related products may increase risk of breast cancer as well as endometrial cancer in women with an intact uterus.
  - Eros
    - Clitoral vacuum device approved by Food and Drug Administration (FDA)
  - Zestra
    - Botanical massage, oil is applied to vulva
    - Investigation for efficacy is ongoing.
  - Phosphodiesterase inhibitors and alprostadil
    - Only one study with unreplicated results showed any promise of these medications helping women with sexual arousal disorder and normal libido.
    - Sildenafil and nitric oxide do increase the physical arousal stage but do not affect the subjective arousal feelings in women with this disorder.

Chronic Treatment
- Continue psychologic therapy to completion.
- Continue medication with regular follow-up.
- Patients should be aware that this condition may recur and treatment may not be permanent.

Recurrence Rate
More research needs to be done on this subject with more studies using standardized instruments.

PATIENT EDUCATION

Information regarding this disorder can be found at the Merck website under the subject of sexual dysfunction in women.

- For more patient education resources, visit eMedicine's website under the topic of female sexual problems and visit familydoctor.org under "sexual dysfunction in women"
- Patient education on disease process

MEDICAL/LEGAL PITFALLS

- Patients may become very frustrated if treatments do not work.
- In some cases, therapy will not work unless the patient's partner agrees with therapy.

■ Patients may try herbal supplements in attempts to increase arousal.
■ Patient should be counseled on side effects and interactions of supplements with other medications.
■ Arousal difficulties may be due to cardiovascular issues; patients should be screened for hypertension and vascular disease.

Gender Dysphoria

BACKGROUND INFORMATION

Definition of Disorder
The diagnosis of gender dysphoria replaces the prior diagnosis of "gender identity disorder," which emphasized cross-gender identification. Gender dysphoria is not considered to be a sexual dysfunction or a paraphilia, but rather, a condition resulting from experienced gender incongruence with resulting gender dysphoria.

Separate criteria are provided for children, adolescents, and adults.

Gender Dysphoria in Children
■ In children, there is a marked incongruence between assigned gender and experienced/expressed gender manifested by at least six of the following: (a) a desire to be the other gender or insistence that one is the other gender; (b) a strong preference for cross-dressing as the opposite gender of one's assigned gender; (c) a strong preference for cross-gender roles; (d) a strong preference for toys, games, or activities typically engaged in by the opposite gender; (e) a strong preference for playmates of the opposite gender; (f) a strong rejection of typically masculine games and activities when the assigned gender is male, and a strong rejection of typically feminine games and activities when the assigned gender is female; (g) a strong dislike of one's sexual anatomy; and (h) a strong desire for the primary or secondary sex characteristics matching the experienced gender.
■ Associated with clinically significant distress or impairment in social, school, or other important areas of functioning.
■ Must specify whether this occurs with a disorder of sex development.

Gender Dysphoria in Adults and Adolescents
■ A marked incongruence between one's expressed/experienced gender and assigned gender of at least 6 months' duration and characterized by at least two of the following: (a) a marked incongruence between one's experienced/expressed gender and actual or anticipated primary and/or secondary sexual characteristics; (b) a strong desire to be rid of one's actual or anticipated primary and/or secondary sexual characteristics; (c) a strong preference for the primary or secondary sexual characteristics of the other gender; (d) a strong desire to be the other gender, or an alternative gender from assigned gender; (e) a strong desire to be treated as the other gender, or an alternative gender from assigned gender; and (f) a strong conviction that one has the typical feelings and reactions of the other gender, or an alternative gender from assigned gender.
■ Associated with clinically significant distress or impairment in social, school, occupational, or other important areas of functioning.

■ Must specify whether this occurs with a disorder of sex development.
■ Must specify whether the individual has transitioned to full-time living in the desired gender with or without a legal change and has either undergone or is preparing to have at least one cross-sex medical procedure or treatment regimen (posttransition).

Early onset: Starts in childhood and continues into adolescence and adulthood. May have a period where dysphoria remits and individual identifies self as gay.
Late onset: Starts near puberty or later.

Gender Dysphoria Associated With a Disorder of Sex Development
■ For many, issues of gender assignment already raised by health care providers or parents
■ Frequently associated with early-onset gender atypical behavior
■ Individuals with a disorder of sex development may not develop gender dysphoria but may experience uncertainty about their gender.
■ For females there may be associated infertility.

Other Specified Gender Dysphoria
■ Applies to individuals who present with symptoms characteristic of gender dysphoria that (a) cause clinically significant distress or impairment in social, occupational, or other important areas but who do not meet full criteria for gender dysphoria or (b) the individual meets the criteria for gender dysphoria, but duration of symptoms is less than 6 months.
■ Specified category is used in situations in which the reasons the individual does not meet the criteria for gender dysphoria are specified.

Unspecified Gender Dysphoria
■ Applies to individuals who present with symptoms characteristics of gender dysphoria that cause clinically significant distress or impairment in social, occupational or other important areas, but do not meet full criteria for gender dysphoria.
■ Unspecified category is used in situations in which the reasons the individual does not meet the criteria for gender dysphoria are unspecified and/or in which there is insufficient information available.

Etiology
■ Unknown etiology
■ One theory involves structure formation of the uncinate nucleus.
■ In gender dysphoria without a disorder of sex development, twin studies suggest an increased concordance for transsexualism among monozygotic twin pairs and some degree of heritability.
■ Possible androgen increase in some women
■ In gender dysphoria with a disorder of sex development, a prenatal androgen imbalance may increase vulnerability to gender dysphoria.
■ For individuals with gender dysphoria without a disorder of sex development, gender dysphoria may develop as early as preschool, with increased likelihood of persistence into adolescence and adulthood.
■ Males with gender dysphoria without a disorder of sex development are more likely to have older brothers.

Demographics
▦ Male-to-female (MtF) transsexualism is two to four times more prevalent than female-to-male (FtM) transsexualism (children).
▦ MtF transexualism has a 1% to 6% prevalence.
▦ Age of onset is often in early childhood with one report of onset in a child younger than 3 years old.
▦ FtM transsexuals and the homosexual MtF usually apply for gender reassignment surgery in their 20s.
▦ Heterosexual MtF patients usually apply for gender reassignment surgery much later.
▦ Heterosexual MtF patients usually have married and fathered children before applying.
▦ Those with this disorder will either continue to have unresolved issues with gender, will accept their birth gender, will have part-time cross-gender behavior, or will have gender reassignment surgery.
▦ For adult males, prevalence ranges from 0.005% to 0.014%. Adult females: 0.002% to 0.003%.
▦ Individuals with gender dysphoria have been reported across many countries and cultures.

Risk Factors
Age
▦ Age of development varies.
▦ Most common ages of onset of gender dysphoria reported are from younger than 3 years old to middle childhood.

Gender
▦ This disorder is found in both genders.
▦ Men are affected two to three times more often than women.

Stressful Events in Susceptible People
▦ Significant crisis or loss may worsen this disorder.

Having Another Mental Health Disorder
▦ Higher likelihood of having schizophrenia, affective psychosis, or adjustment disorder
▦ Patients with gender dysphoria are more likely to have substance abuse problems, although statistics vary on prevalence.
▦ Patients with gender dysphoria are more likely to have a personality disorder, have attempted suicide in the past, have engaged in self-harm behavior, have an increased risk for violence (assault, rape, attempted rape), HIV infection, and other sexually transmitted diseases (STDs).

DIAGNOSIS

Differential Diagnosis
▦ Nonconformity to gender roles
▦ Transvestic disorder
▦ Body dysmorphic disorder
▦ Schizophrenia and other psychotic conditions
▦ Other clinical presentations

ICD-10 Codes
Gender dysphoria in children (F64.2)
Gender dysphoria in adolescents and adults (F64.7)

Diagnostic Workup
- The diagnostic workup includes a comprehensive medical history, including a sexual history, a history of prior and current medications, a physical examination and pertinent laboratory work.
- Psychiatric assessment should account for family, school, and occupational settings and relationships with peers.

Initial Assessment
- Complete medical history
- Sexual history
- Psychiatric history
- Psychosexual development
- For how long have you felt you are of the opposite sex?
- What brought you to seek help now?
- What is your sexual orientation?
- How do you feel about your body?
- Are you currently in a relationship?
- Tell me your feelings related to your birth gender.
- How were you raised?
- Did your family raise you in your birth gender?
- Do you have a social support system?
- What is your occupation?
- What outcome are you looking for? (counseling, gender reassignment surgery, etc.).

Laboratory Tests
None is relevant to diagnosis of this disorder.

TREATMENT OVERVIEW

Acute Treatment
- Psychodynamic psychotherapy focused toward acceptance of birth gender has been the accepted therapy for years.
  - Multiple studies have been unable to determine exact efficacy of psychodynamic psychotherapy.
  - Patients with any of the following characteristics are most likely to respond to this therapy:
    - Patient treated and controlled for comorbid psychological problems
    - Religious beliefs inconsistent with gender reassignment surgery
    - Anatomic features prevent passing as the opposite gender despite sex reassignment surgery (extremely tall stature or very large size)
    - Fear of losing spouse, children, and alienating other family members
  - Individual psychotherapy can also help the patient
    - It provides a safe setting for the patient to discuss feelings and concerns.
    - This is recommended but not required during real-life experience.
  - Group psychotherapy is also helpful for patients.
    - It provides a supportive environment.

- Hormone therapy
  - This is used in those who decide not to undergo gender reassignment surgery but still want to be the opposite gender part time.
  - These patients will undergo either masculinizing or feminizing hormonal therapy.
  - Episodically they will live as the opposite sex.
  - This occurs more often in cross-dressing adult males and less often in adult females with this disorder.
- Real-life experience
  - Homosexual MtF transsexuals usually will undergo this "test."
  - Heterosexual MtF transsexuals are least likely to undergo this "test."
  - FtM transsexuals usually have an easier time with this "test" than the other two groups.
  - There are irreversible social consequences to living as the opposite sex without surgery.
  - This is usually done while taking hormone therapy.
- Gender reassignment surgery
  - This is a permanent solution.
  - The patient must have a thorough evaluation before being allowed to undergo surgery.
  - Patients must also have either completed at least 1 year of cross-sex hormone therapy or at least 1 year of real-life experience in their gender role.
  - The process to completely become the opposite sex takes years to decades.

Chronic Treatment

- Psychotherapy
  - About 50% of those undergoing evaluation or psychotherapy for this disorder will stop treatment.
  - Some, but not all, return to treatment at a later time.
  - Reasons for not continuing therapy include impatience, seeing the therapist as unempathetic, expensiveness of therapy, or decision not to resolve gender identity problem.
- Hormone therapy
- Gender reassignment surgery:
  - This is the most permanent solution.
  - The surgery takes place in stages.
  - The physical transition may take place over years but the complete emotional, psychological, and identity changes may take decades.

Recurrence Rate

- Rate depends on the patient, the outcome decided by the patient, and other factors.

Clinical Presentation

- No specific physical symptoms are related to this disorder.
- Patients may have symptoms related to hormonal therapy or surgical procedures.

PATIENT EDUCATION

■ Information on gender dysphoria disorder can be found at www.merck.com under the *Merck Manual of Diagnosis and Therapy* (psychiatric disorders, then sexuality and sexual disorders, then gender identity disorder).

■ E-medicine (emedicine.medscape.com) also has a good website with information under the topic of psychiatry and sexual and gender identity disorders.

MEDICAL/LEGAL PITFALLS

■ During acute psychotic episodes, those with bipolar disorder, schizophrenia, and other psychotic disorders may have delusions of becoming the opposite sex.

■ Care should be taken to diagnose and treat these conditions before jumping ahead toward treatment.

■ Treatment of the psychotic disorders will resolve the desire to become the opposite sex.

■ Those with antisocial or borderline personality disorders will also seek gender reassignment surgery for unrelated reasons.

■ Sex hormone therapy often leads to permanent sterilization, so patients should be counseled on sperm/egg preservation.

■ Estrogen therapy can cause thrombosis and pulmonary embolism; patients should also be monitored for insulin resistance.

■ Testosterone therapy may predispose the patient for cardiovascular disease; regular screening should be done, including lipid profiles and tests for insulin resistance.

■ Patients undergoing sex hormone therapy should be monitored for cancer.

■ Ovarian malignant changes and endometrial hyperplasia with testosterone therapy.

Voyeuristic Disorder

BACKGROUND INFORMATION

Definition of Disorder

■ Observation of an unsuspecting person who is naked, disrobing, or performing a sexual act

■ Most of the unsuspecting persons are strangers.

■ The act of "peeping" is intended for the observer to achieve sexual excitement.

■ Sexual activity with the unsuspecting person is not usually sought.

■ Orgasm may occur during the initial observation or later while reminiscing.

■ The voyeur may later have fantasies involving the person observed.

■ In reality, sexual acts with the observed person rarely occur.

■ The most severe form is the voyeur observing only sexual activity.

■ This behavior usually begins before 15 years of age and is a chronic condition.

■ In more severe forms, voyeurs will spend a very large amount of time seeking out observation opportunities.

■ Duration of at least 6 months

Specifications

■ In controlled environment (applies to individuals living in settings where opportunities to engage in voyeuristic activities are limited)

■ In remission—individual has not acted on urges with a nonconsensual person and there has been no distress in impairment in functioning for at least 5 years.

Etiology
▩ The exact etiology is unknown.
▩ May be due to an unfortunate learning history secondary to conditioning, modeling, and reinforcement
▩ From a psychoanalytical perspective, three key occurrences are present in voyeurs:
  ▩ Hypercathexis (preoccupation with visual function): this is often found in artists and mathematicians, but not solely in these two classes of people.
  ▩ Postnatal experience with the mother: this includes early visual exchanges and fear of loss of her and her breasts.
  ▩ Early trauma in the first or second year of life: this trauma must severely affect the mother-and-child relationship. This may lead to pregenital fixation and other problems with the ego and superego.
    ▩ From a biologic perspective, in the past, voyeurs have been thought to have high testosterone levels, although most current research shows that testosterone levels in voyeurs are in the normal range.
    ▩ It is currently thought that voyeurs have an abnormal androgen receptor, it is either enhanced or produces an abnormal response to androgens.
    ▩ Therapy causing hypoandrogenism has been highly effective in suppressing voyeuristic desires, behaviors, and the relapse of both.

Demographics
▩ The exact incidence and prevalence are unknown.
▩ Voyeurism is not included in national mental health questionnaires.
▩ Highest possible lifetime prevalence is thought to be 12% in males and 4% females.

Risk Factors
Voyeurism is a necessary precondition to voyeuristic disorder.

Age
▩ Begins to develop in adolescence and early adulthood
▩ Persists throughout life

Gender
▩ Men have this disorder at least twice as often as women.
▩ Men are more likely to have risk-taking behaviors associated with this disorder.

Family History
▩ There is no evidence that this disorder is directly related to family history.

Stressful Events in Susceptible People
Childhood sexual abuse, substance misuse, and sexual preoccupation/hypersexuality have been suggested though a causal relationship has not been established.

Having Another Mental Health Disorder
▩ Men with a hypersexual disorder are more likely to have voyeurism or another paraphilia or paraphilia-related disorder than the general population.
  ▩ Those diagnosed with voyeurism have a higher likelihood of having another mental health disorder than the general population.
  ▩ Voyeurs are also more likely to have another paraphilia than the general population.
  ▩ Those with voyeurism engage in more risk-taking behaviors (substance use and sexual behavior).

DIAGNOSIS

Differential Diagnosis
▦ Other paraphilia disorders
▦ Obsessive–compulsive disorder (OCD)
▦ Conduct disorder
▦ Antisocial personality disorder
▦ Substance use disorders
▦ Specified paraphilic disorder
▦ Unspecified paraphilic disorder

ICD-10 Code
Voyeuristic disorder (F65.3)

Diagnostic Workup
▦ The diagnosis is based on the patient's history and honesty.
▦ Legal records and other medical records can help identify voyeurs.
▦ Physical and mental evaluation.

Initial Assessment
▦ Medical history
▦ Family history
▦ Social history
▦ Sexual history
▦ Psychosexual history
▦ Psychiatric history
▦ Legal history
▦ For how long has the patient been having voyeuristic desires?
▦ For how long has the patient been acting out those desires?
▦ How is the behavior affecting personal relationships?
▦ Amount of time spent seeking out places to observe people?
▦ Amount of time spent seeking out people to observe?
▦ When and where do these experiences tend to occur?
▦ What effect do the experiences have on the patient's ability to function?

Laboratory Tests
▦ Physical examination
▦ Medical and psychiatric history
▦ Laboratory as needed to evaluate physical complaints:
    ▦ Thyroid function studies (triiodothyronine [T3], thyroxine [T4], thyroid-stimulating hormone [TSH])
    ▦ CMP, including glucose, calcium, albumin; total protein count; levels of sodium, potassium, CO_2 (carbon dioxide and bicarbonate), chloride, BUN, creatinine, ALP, ALT, AST), and bilirubin
    ▦ CBC with differentials: hemoglobin, hematocrit, RBC count, WBC count, WBC differential count, and platelet count
    ▦ Free and total serum testosterone levels
    ▦ The following should be done before medical treatment:
        ▪ Pregnancy test

TREATMENT OVERVIEW

Acute Treatment
▦ The goal of therapy is to decrease or completely extinguish voyeuristic desires and actions without a recurrence of these desires and behaviors.
▦ Treatment consists of psychotherapy and/or medication.
▦ Surgical castration has been used in the past but is not commonly used today due to ethical/legal concerns.
▦ Psychotherapy includes behavior, cognitive, and group therapy.
▦ Behavioral and cognitive strategies attempt to make the social context of voyeurism unfavorable.
  ▦ Use of aversion therapy:
    ● Pair the deviant but pleasurable stimulus with some painful stimulus.
  ▦ Classical conditioning:
    ● Patient masturbates to deviant but pleasurable stimulus (fantasy, etc.) and approaches orgasm, but, right before orgasm, changes the stimulus to a nondeviant and pleasurable stimulus.
    ● This links orgasm (pleasurable stimulus) with nondeviant and pleasurable stimuli.
▦ Group therapy works very well but, if used alone, may take 6 months to several years to extinguish behavior.
  ▦ Provides support from other voyeurs.
  ▦ Works well to reverse incorrect beliefs (all disrobing women like to be watched, even if they are unaware of it).
  ▦ Improves insight and knowledge base.
  ▦ Compared to group therapy for other topics, these groups take longer for members to become completely comfortable with each other.
▦ Medications commonly used in the United States are antiandrogenic (medroxyprogesterone acetate, nafarelin, leuprolide, flutamide, triptorelin) and psychotropic (fluoxetine, paroxetine, fluvoxamine).
▦ More double-blind controlled studies need to be done on medication use.
▦ Antiandrogens seem to produce better results than psychotropics.

Chronic Treatment
▦ Treatment consists of surgical castration or continuation of acute treatment (psychotherapy or medication).
▦ Surgical castration was used in the past but is now rarely used.
▦ It has the lowest relapse rate but is permanent as compared to other treatments.
▦ The effectiveness of chronic treatment with psychological and medical therapy depends on patient compliance.
▦ Group therapy is considered the best psychological therapy to use although behavioral and cognitive therapies are good as well.
▦ Patients with surgical castration or on antiandrogen therapy should be monitored for liver function changes and signs/symptoms related to hypogonadism and hypoandrogenism.
▦ Hypogonadism and hypoandrogenism caused by long-acting gonadotropin-releasing hormone (GNRH) analogues can be reversed with small doses of testosterone (25–50 mg) monthly.
▦ This regimen alleviates the side effects with no increase in voyeuristic desires or behaviors.

Recurrence Rate
▓ Recurrence rate depends on the method of treatment used.
▓ The highest recurrence rate found after surgical castration was 7.4%.
▓ Average recurrence rate for medical castration using antiandrogens reaches 6% to 7%.
▓ More research needs to be done on recurrence rate when using antidepressants.
▓ Those medically castrated with a long-acting GNRH inhibitor have the lowest rate of recurrence compared to the other antiandrogens.

Clinical Presentation
▓ No biologic symptoms or signs help diagnose this disorder.
▓ If following up for medication use, look for side effects (liver failure, etc.).
▓ Psychologic symptoms may include mental distress over the patients' behavior.
▓ May have stress-related symptoms if problem is interfering with important relationships.

PATIENT EDUCATION

▓ A good support system can help with rehabilitation and prevent relapse.
▓ Support systems can include spouse, partner, therapist, therapy group, counselor, and so forth.
▓ For patient education resources, visit MD Consult's patient education page on voyeurism.
▓ Contact a mental health specialist for information on treatment.

MEDICAL/LEGAL PITFALLS

▓ Voyeurs may be arrested and imprisoned; teens are less likely to be arrested than adults.
▓ Charges are more likely to be pressed if there are other concurrent legal problems or past legal issues.
▓ Those with this disorder are more likely to have psychological problems.
▓ Those with this disorder may have problems with interpersonal relationships, hypersexuality, or other paraphilias.
▓ Those with one paraphilia are more likely to have a second.
▓ Voyeurs also have a higher incidence of risk-taking behaviors, leading to STDs, substance-use-related issues, and other sequelae.

REFERENCE

American Psychiatric Association. (2013). *Diagnostic and statistical manual of mental disorders* (5th ed.). Washington, DC: American Psychiatric Press.

BIBLIOGRAPHY

Basson, R. (2002). A model of women's sexual arousal. *Journal of Sex and Marital Therapy, 28*, 1–10.

Basson, R., Leiblum, S., Brotto, L., Derogatis, L., Fourcroy, J., Fugl-Meyer, K., …Schultz, W. W. (2003). Definitions of women's sexual dysfunction reconsidered: Advocating expansion and revision. *Journal of Psychosomatic Obstetrics and Gynecology, 24*(4), 221–229.

Covington, S. (1991). *Awakening your sexuality*. San Francisco: Harper.

Dennerstein, L., & Lehert, P. (2004). Confronting the challenges: Epidemiological study of female sexual dysfunction and menopause. *Journal of Sexual Medicine, 2*(3), 118–132.

Graham, C. A., Sanders, S. A., Milhausen, R. R., & McBride, K. R. (2004). Turning on and turning off: A focus group study of the factors that affect women's sexual arousal. *Archives of Sexual Behavior, 33*(6), 527–538.

Masters, W. H., & Johnson, V. E. (1970). *Human sexual inadequacy*. London, England: Churchill.

Mathers, N., Bramley, M., Draper, K., Snead, S., & Tobert, A. (1994). Assessment of training in psychosexual medicine. *British Medical Journal, 308*, 969–972.

Nelson, S. (2005). Women's sexuality. In G. Andrews (Ed.), *Women's sexual health* (pp. 3–13). Edinburg, Scotland: Elsevier.

Pollack, M. H., Reiter, S., & Hammerness, P. (1992). Genitourinary and sexual adverse effects of psychotropic medication. *International Journal of Psychiatry in Medicine, 22*(4), 305–327.

Sobczak, J. A. (2009). Female sexual dysfunction: Knowledge development and practice implications. *Perspectives in Psychiatric Care, 45*(3), 161–173.

Chapter 16

Paraphilic Disorders

Paraphilic Disorders

DEFINITION OF TERMS

- Paraphilias are sexual acts or stimuli outside of what society considers normal.
- Paraphilias are not consciously chosen by the person experiencing them, but tend to be discovered during the maturation period (Halter & Carson, 2010).
- Paraphilic disorders are also known as sexual impulse disorders.
- Paraphilic disorders likely vary in severity throughout an affected individual's life (American Psychiatric Association [APA], 2013).

According to the *Diagnostic and Statistical Manual of Mental Disorders*, Fifth Edition (*DSM-5*; APA, 2013), paraphilic disorders are paraphilias, such as exhibitionism, voyeurism, fetishism, transvestic fetishism, pedophilia, sexual masochism, and sexual sadism,

- That cause distress or impairment to the individual experiencing them, or
- Whose satisfaction through a particular paraphilia has caused or risked personal harm to others.

DIAGNOSIS

Differential Diagnosis
- Dementia
- Personality changes due to general medical conditions
- Substance use disorder or intoxication
- Manic episodes
- Hypersexuality
- Conduct disorder
- Antisocial personality disorder
- Obsessive–compulsive disorder
- Gender dysphoria

Initial Assessment
- There is a problem in arousal in relation to a normal stimuli.
- Anxiety about normal sexual activity
- Anxiety about social interactions with adults

257

- Skills deficits in social interactions
- Skills deficits in normal sexual activity
- Whether the individual has an underlying gender role identity problem
- Nurse self-assessment is crucial in working with clients with paraphilic disorders, especially those considered heinous and criminal, such as pedophilic disorder.

Clinical Presentation
- Individuals present to the clinic due to referrals by law-enforcing agents.
- Individuals who are distressed by their paraphilias and/or experience impairment in functioning in expected social roles
- Individuals whose partners are distressed by their paraphilias
- Individuals who report erectile disorders or other dysfunctions, which are secondary to the person's paraphilia
- Individuals who report sexually transmitted diseases, unwanted pregnancy, or accidents/injuries sustained while being sexual

TREATMENT OVERVIEW

Clinical Management
- A general strategy is the combination of different types of treatments.

Behavioral/Psychotherapy
- Psychotherapy can be divided between group and individual therapy.
- With individual therapy, the focus is on insight-oriented, cognitive behavioral, and supportive psychotherapies.
- This is the most common form of treatment used.

Medical
- The majority of medical treatments are used for sexual offenders.
- Medroxyprogesterone acetate inhibits gonadotropin secretion, which inhibits sexual behavior.
  - Onset of action: 3 weeks, and the effects are reversible
  - Indicated to reduce recidivism in sexual offenders
- Antidepressants appear to reduce sexual behavior
  - These are usually prescribed at the depression-dose level.
- Long-acting gonadotropin-releasing hormone (GnRH) agonists are the most potent of the antiandrogen agents.
  - The use of GnRH agonists and psychotherapy is extremely effective in controlling selected paraphilias (pedophilia, exhibitionism, and voyeurism).
- Luteinizing hormone-releasing agents produce complete "chemical castration" with hypoandrogenism.
- Cyproterone acetate, a testosterone antagonist, is approved for reducing sex drive and hot flashes after orchiectomy.

Surgical
- Surgical castration (orchiectomy) involves removal of testes.
- Until the early decades of this century, surgical castration had been widely used in several countries, but it is practiced rarely these days because of ethical and legal issues.
- Surgical castration is still done in some countries, including some states in the United States.

Exhibitionistic Disorder

BACKGROUND

- Exhibitionistic urges tend to begin in adolescence.
- Urges and behaviors tend to decrease with age (APA, 2013).
- Occurs almost exclusively in men exposing genitalia to women
- Occurs nearly always in public places
- Rarely involves physical contact with victim (Halter & Carson, 2010)
- Desire is to shock or disgust victim (Frisch & Frisch, 2011).

DIAGNOSIS

ICD-10 Code
Exhibitionistic disorder (F65.2)

DSM-5 Diagnostic Guidelines
- For at least 6 months: recurrent and intense sexual arousal from the exposure of one's genitals to an unsuspecting person, whether through fantasies, urges, or behaviors
- Individual has acted on these urges with a nonconsenting person, or the urges are causing significant distress or impairment in functioning.

MEDICAL/LEGAL PITFALLS

- There are concerns that in an uninhibited individual, exhibitionism progresses to other, more serious types of sexual assault. In cases of individuals who expose a flaccid penis, the progression is less likely to occur than individuals who expose an erect penis.

Voyeuristic Disorder

BACKGROUND

- More common in males than females
- Entails sexual pleasure by observing unsuspecting people disrobing or engaging in sexual activity. Voyeurism not considered a disorder if it does not cause impairment of self or harm others.

DIAGNOSIS

ICD-10 Code
Voyeuristic disorder (F65.3)

DSM-5 Diagnostic Guidelines
- For at least 6 months: recurrent and intense sexual arousal from observing an unsuspecting person who is naked, disrobing, or engaging in sexual activity, whether through fantasies, urges, or behaviors
- Individual has acted on these urges with a nonconsenting person, or the urges are causing clinically significant distress or impairment in functioning.

- ▨ Must also cause distress or impairment in functioning in social roles or risk of harm to others.
- ▨ Individual is at least 18 years old.

MEDICAL/LEGAL PITFALLS

- ▨ Voyeuristic behaviors are most commonly potentially lawbreaking sexual behaviors (APA, 2013).
- ▨ Spying or "peeping tom" behavior may result in arrest.

Fetishistic Disorder

BACKGROUND

- ▨ Usuall onset is during puberty (APA, 2013).
- ▨ Common fetishes include shoes, gloves, pantyhose, leather, latex, women's clothing.
- ▨ Occur more often in men than women.

DIAGNOSIS

ICD-10 Code
Fetishistic disorder (F65.0)

DSM-5 Diagnostic Guidelines
- ▨ For at least 6 months: recurrent and intense sexual arousal from either nonliving objects or a nongenital body part, whether through fantasies, urges, or behaviors
- ▨ Causes clinically significant distress or impairment in functioning.
- ▨ Fetish objects are not limited to clothing used in cross-gender dressing or devices intended for stimulation, such as a vibrator.

MEDICAL/LEGAL PITFALLS

- ▨ About 25% of people with a fetish steal their objects (i.e., women's underwear).
- ▨ Majority of the individuals with fetishistic disorder try to avoid being caught by the law.

Transvestic Disorder

BACKGROUND

- ▨ May begin as early as childhood
- ▨ Most commonly occurs in heterosexual males (Frisch & Frisch, 2011)
- ▨ Does not necessarily indicate gender dysphoria (differential diagnosis)

DIAGNOSIS

ICD-10 Code
Transvestic disorder (F65.1)

DSM-5 Diagnostic Guidelines
▦ For at least 6 months: recurrent and intense sexual arousal from cross-dressing, whether through fantasies, urges, or behaviors
▦ Cause clinically significant distress or impairment in functioning.
▦ Fetishism within transvestic disorder is a specifier

MEDICAL/LEGAL PITFALLS

▦ Individuals rarely seek treatment for this paraphilia unless forced to by circumstances, such as stealing opposite-sex clothes to cross-dress or when their spouse seeks a divorce.

Frotteuristic Disorder

BACKGROUND

▦ While frotteuristic *acts* may be seen as fairly common, only 10% to 14% of adult males seeking outpatient treatment for paraphilias meet the criteria for frotteuristic *disorder* (APA, 2013).
▦ Often occurs in crowded public places where the offender can get away quickly.

DIAGNOSIS

ICD-10 Code
Frotteuristic disorder (F65.81)

DSM-5 Diagnostic Guidelines
▦ For at least 6 months: recurrent and intense sexual arousal through touching or rubbing up against a nonconsenting person, whether through fantasies, urges, or behaviors
▦ Individual has acted on these urges with a nonconsenting person *or* urges have caused clinically significant distress or impairment in functioning.

MEDICAL/LEGAL PITFALLS

▦ This individual may suffer legal consequences as a result of frotteuristic behavior, as contact is not usually with a consenting individual and often occurs in public places.

Pedophilic Disorder

BACKGROUND

▦ Highest possible prevalence among males is 3% to 5% (APA, 2013).
▦ Males with co-occurring antisocial personality traits are more likely to act on urges (APA, 2013).
▦ Most individuals with pedophilic disorder have at least one other co-occurring paraphilia (Frisch & Frisch, 2011).
▦ Considered to be the most common paraphilic disorder.

DIAGNOSIS

ICD-10 Code
Pedophilic disorder (F65.4)

DSM-5 Diagnostic Guidelines
▪ For at least 6 months: recurrent, intense fantasies, urges, or behaviors involving sexual activity with prepubescent child(ren)
▪ Individual has acted on these urges, or they cause significant distress or interpersonal difficulty.
▪ Individual is at least 16 years old and at least 5 years older than victim(s).
▪ Not intended to include an individual in late adolescence involved in a sexual relationship with a 12- or 13-year-old.

MEDICAL/LEGAL PITFALLS

▪ Note that terms that describe sex with a minor involve criminal actions, while pedophilia is a sexual attraction toward children. Without the actual act being done, this paraphilia would only be considered a psychiatric disorder. Hence an individual with pedophilia is not a sexual offender unless the person commits the act.
▪ This paraphilia, when enacted on a child, infringes on the child's right to physical and psychological integrity because children do not have the ability to give consent to a sexual relationship.
▪ Sex with a minor inhibits the child's sense of security and control of personal boundaries with daily relationships.
▪ Studies show that many pedophiles have themselves been victims of sexual abuse during childhood.
▪ Behavioral problems, suicidal ideation, and drug abuse appear to be the aftermath for people who have suffered childhood abuse.
▪ There is also an increased risk of childhood sexual-abuse victims being rape victims in their adolescence and adult life.

Sexual Masochism Disorder

BACKGROUND

▪ Mean age of onset is 19.3 years (APA, 2013).
▪ At risk for accidental death through asphyxiation or other injury while sexually active
▪ May tend to partner with an individual practicing sexual sadism

DIAGNOSIS

ICD-10 Code
Sexual masochism disorder (F65.51)

DSM-5 Diagnostic Guidelines
▪ For at least 6 months: recurrent and intense sexual arousal occurs from being humiliated, beaten, and other forms of suffering, whether through fantasies, urges, or behaviors

- Causes clinically significant distress or impairment in functioning.
- Asphyxiophilia is a specifier for individuals who engage in achieving sexual arousal related to a restricted airway.

MEDICAL/LEGAL PITFALLS

- This type of paraphilia can be dangerous because the individual is willfully submitting to harm, which may lead to injury or death.

Sexual Sadism Disorder

BACKGROUND

- Thought to be more common in men (APA, 2013)
- Rates and statistics related to this disorder are in large part measured in forensic settings (APA, 2013).
- Mean age of onset is thought to be 19.4 years for males (APA, 2013).

DIAGNOSIS

ICD-10 Code
Sexual sadism disorder (F65.52)

DSM-5 Diagnostic Guidelines
- For at least 6 months: recurrent and intense sexual arousal occurs as a result of another being physically or psychologically hurt, whether through fantasies, urges, or behaviors
- Individual has acted on these urges with a nonconsenting person *or* the urges have caused clinically significant distress, impairment in functioning, and/or risk of harm to another.

MEDICAL/LEGAL PITFALLS

- This type of paraphilia can be dangerous because the rights of others can be disregarded, which breeds criminal activity such as rape and death.

REFERENCES

American Psychiatric Association. (2013). *Diagnostic and statistical manual of mental disorders* (5th ed.). Arlington, VA: American Psychiatric Press.

Frisch, N., & Frisch, L. (2011). The client with disorders of self-regulation: Sleep disorders, eating disorders, and sexual disorders. In N. Frisch & L. Frisch (Eds.), *Psychiatric mental health nursing* (4thed.). Clifton Park, NY: Delmar Cengage Learning.

Halter, M., & Carson, V. (2010). Sexual dysfunction and sexual disorders. In E. Varcarolis & M. Halter (Eds.), *Foundations of psychiatric mental health nursing* (6th ed.). St. Louis, MO: Saunders Elsevier.

BIBLIOGRAPHY

Bossini, L., Fagiolini, A., Valdagno, M., Polizzotto, N. R., & Castrogiovanni, P. (2007). Sexual disorders in subjects treated for mood and anxiety diseases. *Journal of Clinical Psychopharmacology, 27*(3), 310–312.

Briken, P., & Kafka, M. (2007). Pharmacological treatments for paraphilic patients and sexual offenders. *Current Opinion in Psychiatry, 20,* 609–613.

Brown, G. R. (2006). Sexuality and sexual disorders. In M. H. Beers, R. S. Porter, T. V. Jones, J. V. Kaplan, & M. Berkwitz (Eds.),*The Merck manual of diagnosis and therapy* (18th ed.). Whitehouse Station, NJ: Merck Research Laboratories.

Faden, B. (2005). *Psychological therapies. BRS: Behavioral Science* (4th ed., pp. 163–164). Baltimore, MD: Lippincott, Williams & Wilkins.

Fedoroff, J. (2008). Sadism, sadomasochism, sex, and violence. *Canadian Journal of Psychiatry, 53*(10), 637–646.

Garcia-Falgueras, A., & Swaab, D. F. (2008). A sex difference in the hypothalamic uncinate nucleus: Relationship to gender identity. *Brain: A Journal of Neurology, 131*(12), 3132–3146.

Guay, D. (2008). Drug treatment of paraphilic and nonparaphilic sexual disorders. *Clinical Therapeutics, 31*(1), 1–31.

Hayes, R. D., Bennet, C. M., Fairley, C. K., & Dennerstein, L. (2006). What can prevalence studies tell us about female sexual difficulty and dysfunction? *Journal of Sexual Medicine, 3*(4), 589–595.

Hayes, R. D., Dennerstein, L., Bennet, C. M., & Fairley, C. K. (2008). What is the "true" prevalence of female sexual dysfunctions and does the way we assess these conditions have an impact? *Journal of Sexual Medicine, 5*(4), 777–787.

Kirsch, L., & Becker, J. (2007). Emotional deficits in psychopathy and sexual sadism: Implications for violent and sadistic behavior. *Clinical Psychology Review, 27,* 904–922.

Kreuger, R., & Kaplan, M. (1997). Voyeurism: Psychopathology and theory. In R. Laws & W. O'Donohue (Eds.), *Sexual deviance: Theory, assessment, and treatment* (pp. 305–319). New York, NY: Guilford Press.

Långström, N., & Hanson, R. K. (2006). High rates of sexual behavior in the general population: Correlates and predictors. *Archives of Sexual Behavior, 35,* 37–52.

Långström, N., & Seto, M. (2006).Exhibitionistic and voyeuristic behavior in a Swedish national population survey. *Archives of Sexual Behavior, 35,* 427–435.

Rowland, D. L., & Incrocci, L. (2008). *Handbook on sexual and gender identity disorders* (pp. 188–213). Hoboken, NJ: John Wiley & Sons.

Saleh, F. M., & Guidry, L. L. (2003). Psychosocial and biological treatment considerations for the paraphilic and nonparaphilic sex offender. *Journal of the American Academy of Psychiatry and the Law, 31,* 486–93.

Seagraves, R. (2007). Female sexual dysfunction. *Primary Psychiatry, 14*(2), 37–41.

Sharma, B. (2003). Disorders of sexual preference and medicolegal issues thereof. *American Journal of Forensic Medicine and Pathology, 24*(3), 277–282.

Thyer, B., & Wodarski, J. (2007).*Social work in mental health: An evidence-based approach.* Hoboken, NJ: John Wiley & Sons.

WEB RESOURCES

■ American Psychiatric Association: www.psych.org/
■ www.behavenet.com

Chapter 17
Feeding and Eating Disorders

Anorexia Nervosa

BACKGROUND INFORMATION

Definition of Disorder and Diagnostic Criteria

- Anorexia nervosa (AN), as defined in the *Diagnostic and Statistical Manual of Mental Disorders*, Fifth Edition, *(DSM-5; American Psychiatric Association, 2013)*, is the purposeful and persistent energy intake restriction, an intense fear of gaining weight or becoming fat or persistently engaging in behaviors that interfere with weight gain, and a disturbance in self-perceived weight or shape. The *DSM-5* criteria for the diagnosis of AN include:
  - A restriction of energy intake relative to energy requirements, leading to the patient being significantly below weight (weight that is less than minimally normal or minimally expected) in the context of patient norms.
  - An intense fear of gaining weight, becoming fat, and/or persistent behaviors that preclude normal weight gain, such as excessive exercise and/or purging.
  - A disturbance in the way the patient experiences his or her body weight, undue influence of body weight or shape on the evaluation of self or persistent nonrecognition of the graveness of his or her current low body weight.
  - In addition, specification in three areas is required. The areas are (a) subtype of AN, whether restricting or binge eating/purging; (b) remission status, partial or full: and (c) current level of severity, using body mass index (BMI) scoring. Severity levels are as follows: BMIs of 17 kg/m^2 or greater are mild, BMIs of 16 to 16.99 kg/m^2 are moderate, BMIs of 15 to 15.99 kg/m^2 are severe, and BMIs of 15 kg/m^2 or less are extreme.

Associated Features

- AN is not just a desire to be thin, but an overwhelming desire to be thin and to reduce weight to meet lower and lower weight targets. The individual, in lowering his or her weight, may thereby reduce stress and improve his or her sense of empowerment.
- Individuals are most often brought to medical attention by family members who are concerned with marked weight loss or failure to gain expected weight.

Individuals with AN lack insight into, or deny, a problem, making it important for the practitioner to obtain information from family members or other legitimate sources.

▓ Nutritional compromise seen in AN can affect most major organ systems and produce a wide range of disturbances. Depending on the specific behaviors the individual is engaging in, laboratory values may or may not reflect the disturbances.

▓ Depressive symptoms, such as a depressed mood, social withdrawal, irritability, insomnia, and diminished interest in sex, may be present. These features may be secondary to starvation or severe enough to warrant an additional diagnosis of clinical depression. Suicide risk is elevated in AN. A complete suicide assessment, including suicide-related ideation, behaviors, other risk factors, and history of attempts should be conducted.

▓ Obsessive–compulsive tendencies both related and unrelated to food are often present. As with depressive symptoms, food, body shape, and weight preoccupation are often secondary to starvation. Preoccupations commonly noted are rigid calorie counting, eating only low-calorie foods, cutting food into very small pieces, using only toothpicks to eat, recipe collecting, meal preparation without consumption, chewing food and spitting it out, repeated weighing of self, and frequent comments about feeling fat.

▓ When individuals with AN exhibit obsessions and compulsions not related to food, body shape, or weight, an additional diagnosis of obsessive–compulsive disorder may be warranted.

▓ Individuals with AN who use excessive exercise to control weight are at risk during treatment due to the difficulty in controlling physical activity.

▓ Medications may be misused by the individual with AN to avoid weight gain or achieve weight loss. Medications may include (a) diet pills containing caffeine, ephedrine, or phenylpropanolamine, and (b) medications that induce purging such as laxatives and emetics. Withholding or reducing insulin to minimize carbohydrate metabolism is seen in individuals with both AN and insulin-dependent diabetes mellitus (DM).

▓ Other features that may be associated with AN include feelings of ineffectiveness, a strong desire to control the environment, concerns about eating in public, inflexible thinking, limited social spontaneity, and overly restrained emotional expression.

▓ Individuals with binge-eating/purging type of AN have higher rates of impulsivity and are more likely to abuse alcohol and other drugs than those with the restricting type.

▓ The individual denies his or her weight problem and feels better as a result of continued weight loss.

▓ Younger individuals (preadolescent) may not lose weight but may fail to gain weight and to achieve their ideal weights. Younger children very often have a poor ability to express inner turmoil and may refuse to eat certain foods or to increase exercise activity.

▓ Approximately, half of the individuals with AN have experienced a phase of bingeing/purging. During bingeing, the amounts of food ingested may not be large, and the foods themselves are often "forbidden foods," high in calories or fat.

Prevalence and Etiology

▓ The average prevalence is 0.3% to 1% in women and 0.1% in men for the diagnosis in developed countries. The gender difference in the development of this disorder is a 10:1 female to male ratio. The disorder commonly begins during adolescence or young adulthood. Rarely does it begin before puberty or after the age of 40 years though both can occur. Hospitalization may be required to restore weight and stabilize medical complications. Most individuals with AN experience remission within 5 years of presentation. Mortality rate is approximately 5% per decade with the cause of death being medical complications associated with the disorder or suicide. The development of AN is associated with combinations of biological, psychological, and societal factors.

■ Any individual who participates in restrictive diets can trigger obsessive focus on food and feelings of loss of control, often seen with repeated weight loss and weight gains, "yo-yo dieting." Modern Western culture cultivates and reinforces a desire for thinness, compounded by the influence of the media of very thin models and actors and the emphasis on elite athletes. Individuals in this society may view thinness as "successful." AN, however, did exist prior to the sociocultural values of the modern Western culture.

■ Although social, economic, and cultural factors may be influencing factors, eating disorders have not been found among the majority of society.

■ Individuals with AN may have low self-worth and an obsessive–compulsive personality trait for perfectionism. In these cases, the individuals will never be the "perfect weight."

■ AN can be influenced by transitions in life experiences, requirements of sports, work, or artistic activity, and the media and society.

■ Studies have indicated the interplay of an imbalance of neurotransmitters, such as serotonin (5-HT) as a factor in AN. Whether changes in the brain are a causative factor or caused by the disorder is not yet clear.

Demographics

■ Eating disorders occur more in female patients, 90%; Whites, 95%; and first develops in adolescence in 75% of cases.

■ Although most patients are from middle or upper-socioeconomic status families, the disorders can be found among any gender, race, age, or socioeconomic group. In fact, recent studies suggested that the disorder among minority females and adolescents of color is higher than suspected.

Complications

■ Death: AN has the highest incidence of death related to starvation than any other mental illness.

■ Anemia

■ Cardiac problems, such as mitral valve prolapse, arrhythmias, and heart failure

■ Osteoporosis

■ Respiratory problems resembling emphysema

■ Renal insufficiency and/or renal failure

Risk Factors

Age

■ AN first occurs in middle school and then continues throughout adolescence.
  ■ Onset usually occurs in young girls of middle-school age. Dieting, either for legitimate reasons or as a result of a body image distortion, is in itself a risk factor for the development of AN.
  ■ Children who refuse to eat
  ■ Young children who do not gain weight as expected

Children who develop anxiety disorders or display obsessional traits are at risk for developing AN.

Gender
■ Young girls of the White race, most often adolescents.

Family History
■ In a study on risky eating disorders of mothers and sisters who had AN, the incidence of occurrence was eight times more often.
■ Genetic studies also have indicated an underlying biologic influence on eating disorders, especially in twins. AN and other anxiety disorders tend to run in families.
■ History of perfectionism coupled with compulsive behaviors

There is an increased risk for AN and bulimia nervosa (BN) among first-degree relatives of individuals with the disorder.

Stressful Events in Susceptible People
■ Females in late childhood and adolescence who feel a need to diet or lose weight are at risk of harmful weight-loss habits.
■ Transitioning events in childhood or adolescence, such as when entering high school or college.

Having Another Mental Health Disorder
■ Those with other mental health disorders, such as depression or substance abuse (alcoholism or drug abuse), have an increased risk for suicide or suicidal tendency. It is estimated that 30% of individuals seeking medical care are depressed or have depressive episodes, such as sadness or depressed mood, lack of interest or enjoyment, or reduced energy or fatigability.

DIAGNOSIS

Differential Diagnosis
■ Hyperthyroidism
■ Cardiac insufficiency or arrhythmias
■ Gastrointestinal disease
■ Malignancy, central nervous system (CNS) neoplasm
■ Pregnancy
■ AIDS/acute onset
■ Depression
■ Substance abuse
■ Schizophrenia
■ Social anxiety disorder
■ Obsessive–compulsive disorder
■ Body dysmorphic disorder
■ Avoidant/restrictive food intake disorder

ICD-10 Codes
Restricting type (F50.01 1)
Binge eating/purging type (F50.02)

Diagnostic Workup

- Low white blood cell count, increased margination of the leukocytes not related to an infection
- Blood plasma protein levels and prealbumin (determine malnourishment)
- Erythrocyte sedimentation rate is usually normal and may be elevated with organic illness, such as inflammatory bowel disease.
- Thyroid function studies—may be depressed
- CMP-14—biochemical profiles, especially for presence of electrolyte imbalance such as hypoglycemia, hypomagnesia, and hypokalemia
- Liver function studies—may be elevated with severe dehydration as much as two times the normal level.
- Cholesterol levels may be elevated, with starvation due to depressed triiodothyronine (T3); cholesterol binding with globulin is low and fatty infiltration and leakage of cholesterol into the hepatic system is possible.
- Complete blood count (CBC) with differential; elevated hemoglobulin levels may be related to dehydration.
- Electrocardiogram may reveal presence of bradycardia, prolonged QT interval.
- Transferritin and iron levels may be low.
- X-rays to rule out fracture, pneumonia, respiratory or infectious process

Initial Assessment

- Medical history
- Symptoms experienced
- Assess vital signs, especially for hypothermia and for presence of orthostatic hypotension
- Assess for hypovolemia
- Dental assessment for presence of dental enamel erosion
- Assess for Russell sign—abrasion or callus of metacarpophalangeal joint of the index of middle finger of dominant hand
- Assess for alopecia
- Assess for edema, especially peripheral, which is indicative of poor capillary integrity due to malnutrition.
- Assessment of weight and height is done by using standard growth charts for children or for those younger than 10 years of age; calculate BMI. Children, especially boys, have an increase of BMI with age. It is best to use standard growth charts
- BMI = (weight in kg)/(height in m^2).
- Physical, mental, and psychosocial evaluation; use of screening tools for depression, mood
- Nutritional intake history and assessments for weight loss or weight cycling
- Diet recall:
  - How does the patient feel about his or her weight?
  - Is the patient satisfied with eating his or her patterns?
  - Has the patient tried to control or lose weight by vomiting, diet pills, laxative, or starving?
  - Exercise practices of the patient
- Family history or sibling eating disorder patterns
- History of mental illness/affective disorders, inpatient, and/or of family members
- Physical symptoms:
  - Amenorrhea

- Cold hands and feet
- Constipation
- Dry skin and hair
- Headaches
- Fainting or dizziness
- Lethargy or lack of energy
- Anorexia
- Lanugo (body's attempt to maintain body heat)
- Low blood pressure for the age
■ Emotional and behavioral symptoms:
- Refusal to eat
- Denial of hunger
- Excessive exercise
- Flat mood, or lack of emotion
- Difficulty concentrating
- Preoccupation with food
- Black-and-white thinking (resistant to change)

DSM-5 Diagnostic Guidelines

■ Difficult disorder to diagnose because individuals with anorexia often attempt to hide the disorder.
■ Denial and secrecy
■ It is unusual for an individual with anorexia to seek professional help because the individual typically does not accept that he or she has a problem (denial).
■ In many cases, the actual diagnosis is not made until medical complications have developed.
■ The individual is often brought to the attention of a professional by family members only after marked weight loss has occurred.
■ Warning signs of developing anorexia or one of the other eating disorders include excessive interest in dieting or thinness
■ Restriction of energy intake relative to requirements, leading to a significantly low body weight
■ Weight in the context of age, sex, developmental trajectory, and physical health
■ Significantly low weight is defined as a weight that is less than minimally normal or, for children and adolescents, less than that minimally expected.
■ Intense fear of gaining weight or becoming fat, or persistent behavior that interferes with weight gain even though at a significantly low weight
■ Disturbance in the way body weight or shape is experienced, undue influence of body weight or shape on self-evaluation or persistent lack of recognition of the seriousness of the current low body weight

TREATMENT OVERVIEW

■ The psychiatrist may assume the leadership role within a program or team that includes other physicians, psychologists, registered dietitians, and social workers or may work collaboratively on a team led by others. Additionally, these same practice guidelines require that communication among all disciplines is essential (Recommendation I).
■ A team approach is recommended by the APA Practice Guidelines (Recommendation III) as well as using various resources for treatment: inpa-

tient, outpatient, psychological therapy, and pharmacotherapy, including patient education (Recommendation I).

▦ Obtain a history; schedule a physical that is comprehensive with a review of the patient's height and weight history, restrictive and binge eating and exercise patterns and their changes, purging and other compensatory behaviors, core attitudes regarding weight, shape, and eating, and associated psychiatric conditions (Recommendation I).

▦ Obtain a family history of eating disorders or other psychiatric disorders, including alcohol and other substance-use disorders; a family history of obesity; the family's reactions or interactions in relation to the eating disorder; and family attitudes toward eating, exercise, and appearance (Recommendation I).

▦ It is important to determine stressors that may trigger the eating disorders in order to facilitate amelioration of the eating disorder.

▦ When assessing children and adolescents, it is essential to involve parents, significant others, and, when appropriate, school personnel and health professionals who routinely work with the patient (Recommendation I).

▦ With older adults, although spouses and significant others should be part of the treatment program, the clinician should consider whether others should be involved (Recommendations II and III).

Acute Treatment

▦ Treatment is multifaceted and interprofessional.

▦ Goal is to stop weight loss and gain weight. The ultimate goal is to establish a structured pattern of three meals and one to three snacks daily.

▦ Breakfast is essential as this is the meal most often missed by dieters, anorexics, and adolescents. Patients who eat breakfast often have less chance of binge eating later in the day, are less hungry, and thus may avoid bingeing.

▦ In severe situations, acute treatment may be indicated for life-threatening conditions, such as cardiac arrhythmias, severe dehydration, or electrolyte imbalance. Intensive care has been instituted for life-threatening situations.

   ▦ Total parenteral nutrition may be indicated along with intravenous replacement of electrolytes.

   ▦ Albumin may be given to prevent sudden refeeding syndrome—a potentially fatal condition resulting from rapid changes in fluids and electrolytes in malnourished individuals given oral, enteral, or parenteral feeding. Monitor for hypophosphatemia occurring as a result of glycolysis.

   ▦ Hypophosphatemia can result in impairment of myocardial contractility.

   ▦ Heart failure can occur in the presence of fluid retention with an inadequate cardiac status.

   ▦ Hypokalemia may result as well from insulin secretion in response to an increase in calories, which shifts the potassium into the cells.

   ▦ A daily multivitamin with thiamine should be used to prevent Wernicke's encephalopathy.

   ▦ Nasogastric feeding may be necessary to replenish caloric requirements once the acute phase for refeeding occurs.

▦ Supervise and monitor weight daily; some patients with AN have learned how to increase weight by drinking fluids.

▦ Monitor vital signs for hypothermia and fluid and electrolytes, especially urine-specific gravity. Patients may try to falsify weight by wearing increased underclothing garments; however, urine-specific gravity can indicate dehydration or starvation.

■ A dietitian should be an integral part of the inpatient treatment to evaluate and treat specific deficiencies or excesses.

■ Food should be balanced with a flexible exchange system to allow for variety. All food consumption should be monitored. Diet must be balanced, and limit "fat-free foods" and emphasize healthy foods. Adolescents may perceive "fat-free foods" as "good" food, not realizing the increase in sugar and calories. Educate the patient on a balanced diet and nutritional concepts.

■ The patient can maintain a journal of eating patterns and identify dysfunctional eating patterns (purging) that occur during the inpatient episode. Provide feedback and encouragement for adherence to health; try not to stress the increase in food intake.

■ The individuals with AN may not think that they have a problem but rather that they have chosen a lifestyle.

■ Inpatient treatment in a mental health setting is necessary in patients with a suicidal ideation and plan, serious alcohol or sedative withdrawal symptoms, or when the differential includes other medical disorders that warrant admission (e.g., unstable angina, acute myocardial ischemia).

■ Cognitive behavioral therapy (CBT), including dialectical behavior therapy, allows patients to monitor progress and identify triggers for dieting, binge eating, and purging as well as refusal to eat. CBT focuses on restructuring thoughts that lead to distorted eating.

■ Psychotherapy that establishes trust is essential, as individuals with AN may not be willing to relinquish their coping mechanism or eating patterns. AN must be explained in terms of the patient's stage of psychosocial development. Reassure the patient that others need to be incorporated in care to assist with improving health and that the clinician is not abandoning the patient.

■ Family therapy can help resolve family conflicts or elicit support from concerned family members; this is especially important for children who live at home.

■ Group therapy can help persons with AN to connect with others facing similar complications, stressors, and coping behaviors. Group therapy must be carefully monitored as persons with AN may use it as a means to compete as to who is thinnest.

Chronic Treatment

■ A multidisciplinary approach with a psychologist, primary care provider, and a dietitian is essential. Any therapy can last for over 1 year while the individual attempts to gain insight into triggers that can induce the eating-disordered behavior.

■ Interpersonal therapy and family therapy have proven to be more effective than CBT, with or without pharmacotherapy, for AN.

■ A meta-analysis revealed that intervention was more successful if it was interactive and had multiple sessions.

■ Measurement of bone density should be evaluated initially and every 6 months. Findings demonstrate that depressive symptoms and anxiety are associated with low bone density.

■ Menses resumption occurs with return to at least 86% of ideal body weight; therefore, the goal should be to assist adolescents in acquiring a healthy habit of eating nourishing foods and exercising.

Pharmacotherapy Overview for AN

▒ Selective serotonin reuptake inhibitors (SSRIs) may be useful with AN to maintain weight gain and prevent relapse, such as fluoxetine (Prozac, Sarafem, with the initial dose of 20 mg once daily increased to 40 to 60 mg for maintenance).

▒ SSRIs are not useful in AN when patients are at low weights due to decreased protein levels, including tryptophan, which is needed for serotonin production.

▒ Although tricyclic antidepressants, such as clomipramine (Anafranil) and amitriptyline (Elavil), have been prescribed to individuals with AN, cardiac toxicity due to electrolyte abnormality, as seen in AN patients, can occur. This category of drugs can also cause sedation, tachycardia, constipation, dry mouth, and confusion.

▒ Cyproheptadine (Periactin), an antihistamine, and serotonin antagonists have proven beneficial in increasing food intake. Serotonin in the hypothalamus is responsible for decreased food consumption; therefore, it is hypothesized that a serotonin antagonist would have the opposite effects. Cyproheptadine has been successful in treatment of patients with inappropriate caloric intake, such as patients with HIV, cancer, and other chronic illnesses.

▒ Dronabinol (Marinol), a cannabinoid, has been used with patients to increase appetite (see Web Resources section).

▒ In some patients with AN, anxiolytic agents such as olanzapine (Zyprexa, Zyprexa Zydis), prior to eating, have been effective.

▒ Because gastric motility is impaired with AN, drugs such as metoclopramide (Reglan) and cisapride (Propulsid) help to accelerate gastric emptying and enhance gastric motor activity. Osmotic agents such as Gl-Lytely or Glycolax can help with constipation and bloating.

▒ Zinc supplementation, alone or along with a multivitamin, has been associated with weight gain.

▒ Rate, growth factors (insulin-like growth factor 1 [IGF-1]), and dehydroepiandrosterone (DHEA), a naturally occurring adrenal hormone, may be of some benefit in patients with severe bone loss.

▒ The Society for Adolescent Medicine has suggested 1,200 to 1,500 mg of elemental calcium, a multivitamin with 400 units of vitamin D, along with dual emission x-ray absorptiometry (DEXA) scans on baseline and to monitor bone regrowth.

▒ Natural herbs may improve appetite and have a placebo effect on weight gain; Kiddie Florish™ has been used by some parents with younger school-age children to improve appetite.

Note: The FDA has not approved natural remedies as pharmacological treatments for eating disorders.

▒ Appropriate pharmacological therapy and CBT, individually or in combination, are effective in more than 85% of cases.

▒ In general, pharmacotherapy has limited usefulness in the treatment of AN.

Recurrence Rate

▒ Rate of recurrence is approximately 15 to 25 percent. Individuals with AN who are hospitalized have a 75% to 85% chance of full recovery.

PATIENT EDUCATION

▒ Advise patients with AN to avoid nicotine, sympathomimetic or anticholinergic drugs, caffeine, and alcohol.

Drug Selection Table for Anorexia Nervosa

CLASS	DRUG
Tricyclic antidepressants	Drugs sometimes useful to treat symptomatology:
	Amitriptyline (*Apo-Amitriptyline, Elavil*)
	Clomipramine (*Anafranil*)
Selective serotonin reuptake inhibitors (SSRIs)	Drugs sometimes useful to treat symptomatology:
	Citalopram (*Celexa*)
	Fluoxetine (*Prozac*)
	Sertraline (*Zoloft*)
Antipsychotics, atypical (second-generation)	Drugs sometimes useful to treat symptomatology:
	Quetiapine (*Seroquel*)
	Olanzapine (*Zyprexa, Zyprexa Zydis*)

▪ Avoid weighing self, resist urge to isolate self from caring individuals.
▪ Provide information on healthy lifestyles, such as supplements and vitamins.
▪ Avoid proanorexia websites, chat rooms, or media that emphasize thinness.
▪ Avoid contact with friends who also have AN. Stick to your healthy lifestyle plan, use of cognitive behavioral interventions, such as participating in appropriate student organizations, journaling, identifying feelings and thoughts and linking to an Internet support program.
▪ Information regarding AN and support groups can be obtained from the National Institute of Mental Health (NIMH).

MEDICAL/LEGAL PITFALLS

▪ A common finding in those who commit suicide is the presence of more than one mental health disorder, such as mood disorder (i.e., depression), and personality disorder and other psychiatric disorders (WHO, 2000). Individuals with AN are at risk for depression due to their distorted body image and perfectionist psychological profile (Wattula, 2008).
▪ As of May 2, 2007, the National Clearing House has labeled all antidepressant drugs with a black box warning on the prescribing information to include warnings about the increased risks of suicidal thinking and behavior in young adults aged 18 to 24 years during the first months of treatment.
▪ In 2006, the antidepressant Paxil received the first warning—only to be followed by others in 2007; that is, a Clinical Worsening and Suicide Risk label in the prescribing information related to adult patients, especially younger adults.
▪ Individuals with an eating disorder display symptoms as a result of psychological problems; failure to recognize the relationship may result in inappropriate care.

Bulimia Nervosa and Binge-Eating Disorder

BACKGROUND INFORMATION

Definition of Disorder
- BN and binge-eating disorder (BED) occur when a large amount of food is eaten in a short time period. The essential features of BN include recurrent episodes of binge eating, recurrent inappropriate compensatory behaviors to prevent weight gain, and self-evaluation that is unduly influenced by body shape and weight. A diagnosis of BN can be made when the binge eating and inappropriate compensatory behaviors occur, on average, at least once per week for 3 months. With BN, weight is usually within or slightly above normal parameters.
- Individuals may not have a body image distortion or may actually see themselves as not as heavy as they actually are.
- Psychosocial factors may include family conflict or ineffective coping during stressful times, such as when entering high school or college. Conversely, an individual feels "power or control" while participating with weight-control behaviors, especially if there are secondary rewards, such as compliments or acceptance by peers. The studies suggest that females in late childhood and adolescence who feel a need to diet or lose weight are at a risk of adopting harmful eating disorders.

DSM-5 Diagnostic Criteria
- Recurrent episodes of binge eating, in a discrete period of time, an amount of food that is definitely larger than what most individuals would eat in a similar period of time under similar circumstances, and a sense of lack of control over eating during the episode.
- Recurrent inappropriate compensatory behaviors to prevent weight gain, such as self-induced vomiting; misuse of laxatives, diuretics, or other medications; fasting; or excessive exercise.
- The binge eating and compensatory behaviors both occur on average at least once a week for 3 months.
- Self-evaluation is unduly influenced by body weight and shape.
- The BN episodes do not occur exclusively during AN episodes.
- The diagnosis should include specifications of (a) remission status, partial or full, and (b) severity status, which is initially based on the frequency of inappropriate compensatory behaviors per week, with 1 to 3 episodes a week constituting mild severity; 4 to 7, moderate; 8 to 13, severe; and 14 or more considered extreme severity.
- The binge-eating episodes are associated with three or more of the following: (a) eating much more rapidly than normal; (b) eating until feeling uncomfortably full; (c) eating large amounts of food when not feeling physically hungry; (d) eating alone because of feeling embarrassed by how much one is eating; (e) feeling disgusted with oneself, depressed, or very guilty afterward.
- Marked distress regarding binge eating is present.
- The binge eating occurs on average at least once a week for 3 months.

Associated Features

■ BN may occur as part of experimentation with induced vomiting, use of laxatives, fasting, or rigorous exercise to prevent weight gain.

■ The patient's perceptions of body shape and body size have become distorted.

■ Purging is the compensatory behavior most often used to avoid weight gain. Binge eating, however, is the defining element of the diagnosis.

■ In adolescents, purging includes self-stimulation of the upper pharynx, pressure put on the abdomen, and the use of ipecac and laxatives.

■ Adolescents may also use rigorous exercise and fasting to prevent weight gain.

■ The individual with BN may exhibit attitudes of self-deprecation or have depressed mood after becoming aware of his or her anomalous eating patterns.

■ In contrast, those individuals with BED may use compensatory methods to avoid weight gain when other attempts to avoid weight gain have failed.

■ Individuals with BED often eat alone, as they are embarrassed about bingeing.

■ BED can be distinguished from BN in that, in BED, there is a recurring compensatory weight-control habit, such as dieting, when overeating occurs.

■ BED has been associated with male athletes' attempts to control weight during sports events.

Etiology

■ The pathogenesis believed to occur with an imbalance of serotonin is that at the hypothalamus, higher levels of 5-HT tend to decrease appetite and food intake, whereas lower levels are associated with decreased satiety. The CNS precursor to serotonin, 5-hyroxyindolacetic acid (5-HIAA), is lower in patients with AN when they are ill but returns to a higher level during recovery from AN. A similar process occurs with BN.

■ Two other factors associated with BN and BED are sexual trauma and depression. Patients with BN and BED have histories of depression. There is a higher incidence of sexual trauma among adolescents who have BN than in the general population. Depression is difficult to determine if it precedes BN or is associated with affective disorder.

■ BN has been associated with dissatisfaction with one's body after sexual abuse, poor attachment to others, and insecurity.

■ Athletes of any gender, especially gymnasts and runners who have low self-esteem, are predisposed to eating disorders.

■ Male patients with eating disorders, who constitute a much lower incidence than females, have either BN or BED. Male athletes with BED avoid weight gain or maintain a certain weight for sports activities. Male athletes will often engage in binge eating and vomiting.

■ Increased incidence or prevalence of BN may account for the increase in eating disorders.

■ Increased media attention, better screening of patients for eating disorders, and less stringent diagnostic criteria may also be responsible for the apparent increase in eating disorders.

■ Binge eating and purging allow patients to be in control when engaged in weight-control behaviors, especially if secondary gains occurs.

■ During binges, individuals tend to eat food high in calories or fat that they would otherwise avoid.

▦ Suicide risk is elevated in BN. A complete suicide assessment, including suicide-related ideation, behaviors, other risk factors, and history of attempts, should be conducted.

Demographics

▦ Of patients with BN 90% are female; 95% are White; and 75% first developed the disorder as adolescents. BED also occurs more in females but not to the same extent as BN does.

▦ BN and BED are more common in high school and college students, with a peak incidence occurring around 18 years of age.

▦ Many children do not meet stringent diagnostic criteria for BN but may exhibit partial symptoms.

▦ BN is found across racial and socioeconomic groups, with boys representing one fifth of adolescents and about one tenth of adult males. Recent data suggest that bingeing and/or purging may occur when the individual perceives an increase in food intake and not on a regular basis.

▦ Twenty-five percent of adolescents regularly engage in self-induced purging as a means to control weight.

▦ There is an increase in prevalence for eating disorders primarily due to media attention and improved detection.

▦ BN is thought to be a learned behavior, acquired from modeling of peer groups.

Risk Factors

Age
▦ Adolescents in high school and college, young adults
▦ Athletes who have specific weight requirements
▦ BN and BED patients often have episodes of dieting to lose weight rapidly.
▦ Patients who have BED often can be overweight and may have parents who are overweight, maternal control over feeding (restricting or urging) is seen.
▦ Patients may use the excuse of bingeing as an attempt to bulk up for sports repeatedly and then use purging or vomiting as an attempt to avoid weight gain.
▦ Children older than 2 years with a BMI of 85% are considered at risk of becoming overweight; children at the 95th percentile are overweight.

Gender
▦ Although both genders are at risk, female adolescents are more likely to participate in BN or BED.
▦ Postpubertal females constitute 5% to 10% of cases of mild variants of eating disorders.

Family History
▦ Genetic studies have indicated an underlying biologic influence on eating disorders, especially in twins. There is an association with BN and being a twin in up to 35% to 50% of cases.
▦ Overweight parents, especially fathers

Having Another Mental Health Disorder

- Those with other mental health disorders, such as depression or substance abuse (alcoholism or drug abuse), have an increased risk for suicide or suicidal tendency. It is estimated that 30% of individuals seeking medical care are depressed or have depressive episodes such as sadness, depressed mood, lack of interest or enjoyment, or reduced energy or fatigability.
- Individuals with a history of sexual abuse in childhood are at risk of developing BN.

DIAGNOSIS

Differential Diagnosis
- AN, binge-eating/purging type
- Major depressive disorder with atypical features
- Borderline personality disorder
- Kleine–Levin syndrome
- Bipolar disorder
- Insulin resistance
- Sleep apnea/daytime somnolence
- Pseudotumor cerebri
- Hyperthyroidism
- Inflammatory bowel disease
- Malignancy, CNS neoplasm
- Pregnancy
- AIDS/acute onset
- Systemic lupus erythematosum
- Substance abuse
- Obesity

ICD-10 Code
Bulimia Nervosa (F50.2)
Binge Eating Disorder (F50.8)

Diagnostic Workup
- Physical, mental, and psychosocial evaluation
- Nutritional intake history and assessments for weight loss or weight cycling
- Blood plasma protein levels and prealbumin (determine malnourishment)
- Erythrocyte sedimentation rate is usually normal and may be elevated with organic illness, such as inflammatory bowel disease.
- Thyroid function studies—may be depressed.
- Cholesterol levels may be elevated, with starvation due to depressed T3, cholesterol binding with globulin is low, and there is possible fatty infiltration and leakage of cholesterol into hepatic system.
- CBC with differential, elevated hemoglobulin levels may be related to dehydration and hemoconcentration.
- Transferrin and iron levels: levels may be normal.
- Electrolyte studies often indicate hypokalemia, hypochloremia, and/or metabolic alkalosis due to recurrent vomiting. The absence of abnormality in electrolytes does not exclude BN.

- Hypomagnesium may be present with excessive use of laxatives or water-diarrheal stools.
- CMP-14—biochemical profiles, especially for presence of electrolyte imbalance, such as hypoglycemia, hypomagnesia, and hypokalemia.
- Liver function studies may be elevated with severe dehydration, as much as two times the normal.
- EKG, presence of bradycardia, prolonged QT interval when BN occurs in low-weight individuals. U waves may be present secondary to hypokalemia and if cardiomyopathy has occurred due to alkaloid emetine contained in syrup of ipecac.
- Screening with appropriate instruments for depression

Clinical Presentation
- Binge eating
  - Weight gain or weight fluctuation
  - Bloating
  - Lethargy
  - Salivary gland enlargement (if vomiting)
  - Guilt
  - Depression
  - Anxiety
- Purging
  - Weight loss
  - Electrolyte imbalance: $\downarrow$ potassium, $\uparrow CO_2$
  - Hypovolemia
  - Guilt
  - Depression
  - Anxiety/guilt
  - Knuckle calluses (vomiting)
  - Dental enamel erosion (vomiting)
  - Any form of self-mutilation such as cutting
  - Frequent overeating used for coping
  - Self-induced vomiting, hematemesis
  - Excessive exercise

Diagnostic Guidelines
In BN, recurrent episodes of binge eating are characterized by:

- Eating amounts of food that are unquestionably larger than what most persons would consume in the same time period and under similar circumstances
- Absence of self-control during the episodes
- Presence of compensatory behaviors to prevent weight gain: induced vomiting, use of laxatives and diuretics, use of enemas, use of other medications, fasting, rigorous exercise
- Binge eating and the accompanying compensatory behaviors, both occurring at least twice a week for 3 months
- Self-evaluation is unduly influenced by body shape and weight.
- The episodes of BN do not occur exclusively during episodes of AN.

TREATMENT OVERVIEW

- Obtain a history and a physical that are comprehensive, with a review of the patient's height and weight history; restrictive and binge eating and exercise patterns and their changes; purging and other compensatory behaviors; core attitudes regarding weight, shape, and eating; and associated psychiatric conditions (Recommendation I).
- Obtain a family history of eating disorders or other psychiatric disorders, including alcohol and other substance-use disorders; a family history of obesity; the family's reactions or interactions in relation to the eating disorder; and family attitudes toward eating, exercise, and appearance (Recommendation I).
- It is important to determine stressors that may trigger the eating disorders in order to facilitate amelioration of the eating disorder.
- When assessing children and adolescents, it is essential to involve parents, significant others, and, when appropriate, school personnel and health professionals who routinely work with the patient (Recommendation I).
- With older adults, although spouses and significant others should be part of the treatment program, the clinician should consider whether others should be involved. Assess vital signs, especially for hypothermia and for presence of orthostatic hypotension.
- Assess for hypovolemia
- Dental assessment for presence of dental enamel erosion
- Assess for Russell sign—abrasion or callus of metacarpophalangeal joint of the index of middle finger of dominant hand
- Assessment for alopecia
- Assess for edema, especially peripheral, which is indicative of poor capillary integrity due to malnutrition.
- Assessment of weight and height is done by using standard growth charts for children or for those younger than 10 years old; calculate BMI. Children, especially boys, have an increase in BMI with age. It is best to use standard growth charts. BMI = (weight in kg)/(height in m^2).
- Assess for gastrointestinal irritability secondary to esophageal tears
- Auscultate for cardiac arrhythmias

Acute Treatment

- Treatment is multifaceted and interprofessional, including a mental health professional, a primary care provider or medical person, a dietitian, school personnel, and religious persons, if indicated.
- The medical personnel work to correct and manage medical issues, such as electrolyte imbalances and dental problems.
- The dietitian is essential in providing nutritional education and a rationale for selection of certain foods and a meal plan. In some organizations, a dietitian is supplemented by a sports physiologist or trainer to assist individuals with weight management.
- If exercise therapy is needed, proceed cautiously as, excessive exercising could occur along with binge–purge eating in susceptible individuals.
- The nutritional intake for those requiring a weight gain should consist of 2 to 3 lbs/wk (0.9–1.4 kg) of controlled weight gain; for outpatients, 0.5 to 1 lbs/wk. The intake should start at 3,040 kcal/kg (1,000–1,500 kcal/day) and advance progressively.

▪ In severe situations, acute inpatient treatment for BN may be indicated for of life-threatening conditions. Some of these conditions include cardiac arrhythmias, severe dehydration or electrolyte imbalance, arrested development, failure of out-patient treatment, acute food refusal, suicidal ideation, comorbid diagnosis such as depression, or severe family dysfunction.
▪ Intensive care has been instituted for life-threatening situations.
  ▫ Total parenteral nutrition may be indicated along with intravenous replacement of electrolytes.
  ▫ Albumin may be given to prevent sudden refeeding syndrome—a potentially fatal condition resulting from rapid changes in fluids and electrolytes in malnourished individuals given oral, enteral, or parenteral feeding. Monitor for hypophosphatemia occurring as a result of glycolysis.
  ▫ Hypophosphatemia can result in impairment of myocardial contractility.
  ▫ Heart failure can occur in the presence of fluid retention with an inadequate cardiac status.
  ▫ Hypokalemia may also result from insulin section in response to an increase in calories, which shifts the potassium into the cells.
  ▫ A daily multivitamin with thiamine should be used to prevent Wernicke's encephalopathy.
  ▫ Nasogastric feeding may be necessary to replenish caloric requirements once the acute phase for refeeding occurs.
▪ Caution should be provided that some patients may gain weight rapidly due to fluid retention, possibly due to low protein levels.
▪ Treat electrolyte or nutritional deficits first, inpatient treatment may be indicated.
  ▫ CBT emphasizes that thoughts and feelings may lead to distorted eating patterns. CBT has higher efficacy and lower cost, dropout rates, and relapse rates than pharmacological treatments.
  ▫ A combination of psychotherapy and antidepressant medications provide the best chance for remission.
  ▫ Appetite suppressants and psychological treatment have been effective in the treatment of individuals who are overweight or who have bulimia.
  ▫ Individuals with BED may need to be treated for other physical problems, such as sleep apnea, snoring, diabetes, hyperlipidemia, or cardiovascular disease.

Chronic Treatment
▪ Multidisciplinary approach with a psychologist, primary care provider, and a dietitian is essential. Any therapy can last for over 1 year while the individual attempts to gain insight into triggers that can induce the eating-disorder behavior.
  ▫ Use screening tools to determine the presence of depression, child abuse, or sexual abuse in older adolescents and use the SCOFF questionnaire:
    ◦ S—Do you make yourself Sick because you feel uncomfortably full?
    ◦ C—Do you worry you have lost Control over how much you eat?
    ◦ O—Have you recently lost more than One stone (14 lbs or 7.7 kg) in a 3-month period?
    ◦ F—Do you believe yourself to be Fat when others say you are too thin?
    ◦ F—Would you say that Food dominates your life?
  ▫ Use of cognitive behavioral interventions such as CBT, dialectical behavior therapy, participation in appropriate student organizations, journaling, identifying feelings, linking food and emotions to circumvent unwanted behavior, and an Internet support program have proven beneficial.

Pharmacotherapy Overview
▥ Antidepressants, with SSRIs as the first category of choice, may be useful with BN and BED to counteract the depressive symptoms associated with both disorders.
▥ The *DSM-5* identifies depressive disorders as the most common comorbid states associated with both BN and BED.
▥ Appropriate pharmacological therapy and CBT, individually or in combination, are effective in more than 85% of cases.
▥ Antiepileptic agents like topiramate (Topamax) have been useful in individuals with BN to improve binge–purge behaviors as well as improve depressive symptoms.
▥ Gastric motor activity. Osmotic agents such as Gl-Lytely or Glycolax can help with constipation and bloating.
▥ Zinc supplementation alone, or along with a multivitamin, has been associated with weight gain.

Recurrence Rate
▥ Poorer outcomes have been associated with later age of onset of eating disorders.
▥ Low self-esteem can impact the recurrence of binge–purge behaviors. Thirty percent of individuals may continue to engage in bingeing–purging up to 10 years after follow-up if substance abuse is coupled with the eating behavior.

PATIENT EDUCATION

These sites provide a description of outpatient and inpatient residential services available to individuals with eating disorders, dual diagnosis, and/or additive behaviors.

Drug Selection Table for Bulimia Nervosa

CLASS	DRUG
Selective serotonin reuptake inhibitors	First-line drug therapy:
	*Fluoxetine (Prozac)
	Citalopram (*Celexa*)
	Sertraline (*Zoloft*)
Benzodiazepines (BZDs)	Alprazolam (*Xanax IR* and *ER*) Clonazepam (*Klonopin*) Diazepam (*Valium*)
Mood-stabilizing anticonvulsants	Second-line drug therapy:
	Carbamazepine (*Tegretol*) Zonisamide (*Zonegran*)
Tricyclic antidepressants	Third-line drug therapy:
	Amitriptyline (*Elavil, Endep, Vanatrip*) Clomipramine (*Anafranil*)

*Food and Drug Administration (FDA)-approved for bulimia nervosa.

■ http://www.milestonesprogram.org/program.html
■ http://palmpartners3-px.rtrk.com
■ http://www.raderprograms.com

MEDICAL/LEGAL PITFALLS

■ A common finding in those who commit suicide is the presence of more than one mental health disorder.
■ Mood disorder (i.e., depression), personality disorder, and other psychiatric disorders may be overlooked. As of May 2, 2007, the National Clearing House has labeled antidepressant drugs with a black box warning on the prescribing information to include warnings about the increased risk of suicidal thinking and behavior in young adults aged 18 to 24 years during the first 1 to 2 months of treatment.
■ As of May 12, 2006, the National Clearing House has labeled paroxetine (Paxil) and Paxil CR with a Clinical Worsening and Suicide Risk advisory in the prescribing information related to adult patients, especially younger adults.

REFERENCES

American Psychiatric Association. (2013). *Diagnostic and statistical manual of mental disorders* (5th ed., pp. 329–354). Arlington VA: American Psychiatric Press.

Wattula, A. L. (2008). *Anorexia nervosa: Pharmacologic treatments.* Psychology Department, Vanderbilt University. Retrieved on December 26, 2008, from http://www.vanderbilt.edu/AnS/psychology/health psychology/anorexia drugs.htm

BIBLIOGRAPHY

American Psychiatric Association. (2006). *Practice guideline for the treatment of patients with eating disorders* (3rd ed.). Washington DC: American Psychiatric Press. Retrieved on January 5, 2009, from http://www.guideline.gov/summary/summary.aspx?doc id=9318&nbr=004987.

Berkman, N. D., Lohr, K. N., & Bulik, C. M. (2007). Outcomes of eating disorders: A systematic review of the literature. *International Journal of Eating Disorders, 40*(4), 293–309.

Boyd, M. A. (2012). *Psychiatric nursing: Contemporary practice* (5th ed.). Philadelphia, PA: Wolters Kluwer Health/Lippincott Williams & Wilkins.

Burns, C. E., Dunn, A. M., Brady, M. A., Starr, N. B., & Blosser, C. G. (2009). *Pediatric primary care* (4th ed.). St. Louis, MO: Saunders.

Dorn, L. D., Susman, E. J., Pabst, S., Huan, B., Kalkwarf, H., & Grimes, S. (2008). Association of depressive symptoms and anxiety with bone mass and density in ever-smoking and never smoking adolescent girls. *Archives of Pediatrics and Adolescent Medicine, 162*(12). Retrieved on January 12, 2009, from http://iiiprxy.library.miamie.edu

Forman, S. F. (2008). *Eating disorders: Treatment and outcome.* Up To Date. Retrieved on January 7, 2009, from www.uptodate.com/online/cotnent/topic.do?topicKeypsychiat//11503&view

Sanci, L., Coffey, C., Olsson, C., Reid, S., Carlin, J. B., & Patton, G. (2008). Childhood sexual abuse and eating disorders in females: Findings from the Victorian Adolescent Health Cohort Study. *Archives of Pediatrics and Adolescent Medicine, 162*(3). Retrieved on January 9, 2009, from http://iiiprxy.library.miami.edu

Stice, E., & Shaw, H. (2004). Eating disorder prevention programs: Ameta-analytic review. *Psychology Bulletin, 130*, 206.

Yager, J., Devlin, M. J., Halmi, K. A., Herzog, D. B., Mitchell, J. E., Powers, P., & Zerbe, K. J. (2012). *Guideline watch (August 2012): Practice guideline for the treatment of patients with eating disorders* (3rd ed.). Washington, DC: American Psychological Association. Retrieved on September 23, 2013 from http://psychiatryonline.org/pdfaccess.ashx?Re sourceID=5391825&PDFSource=6

WEB RESOURCES

- ▓ National Alliance of Mental Illness: http://www.nami.org/template.cfm? section=by illness& template=/contentmanagement/ This useful site provides information with discussions on diagnosis, treatment, and patient education for individuals with eating disorders.
- ▓ National Institute of Mental Health: http://www.nimh.nih.gov/ This site is a primary reference source for identification and classification of major mental health illnesses. Navigating through the site can lead to information on treatment and guidelines.

Chapter 18

Personality Disorders

Antisocial Personality Disorder

BACKGROUND INFORMATION

Definition of Disorder
- Persistent pattern of disregard for and defiance of the rights of others that begins in childhood or early adolescence and remains consistent into adulthood
- Deceit and manipulation are central features whereby the individual also lacks empathy as he or she has a tendency to disregard the feelings, rights, and suffering of others.
- History of pathological lying
- Inflated sense of self that appears confident and assured but is often to the determent of others as affected persons tend to be opinionated, coarse, and verbose, rambling about topics to impress others
- Cannot be diagnosed until the age of 18 years

Etiology
- Also known as sociopathy or psychopathy
- Previous research has debated whether the disorder is due to nature or nurture.
- Biological studies have identified that there are no known genetic risk factors for personality disorders in the cluster A, B, and C classifications.
- Psychosocial studies have identified that the lack of socialization; the increasing incidence of childhood traumas; as well as childhood maltreatment and neglect such as abuse, lack of empathy poverty, family instability, and community violence may be related to the development of this disorder.

Demographics
- Thirty to 70% of childhood psychiatric admissions are for disruptive behavior disorders. A small percentage of antisocial children (about 3% of males and 1% of females) grow up to become adults with antisocial personality disorder (ASPD), whereas the remainder of those individuals persist with severe problems with authority, maintaining gainful employment, and/or satisfying relationships.
- Research (meta-analysis) found irregularities in 5-HIAA metabolism, which is related to lower serotonin levels.
- Higher incidence in correctional and substance abuse facilities, forensic settings

Risk Factors

- Usually begins in childhood or adolescence
- Has been linked with head injuries in childhood
- Predominately affects males
- Low socioeconomic status and living in urban settings
- More common among first-degree biological relatives
- Familial linkage to female relatives is higher than to male relatives
- Children adopted into homes with parents who have ASPD increase the risk of developing this disorder.

DIAGNOSIS

Differential Diagnosis

- Pathological gambling
- Anxiety disorders
- Substance-related disorders
- Malingering
- Somatoform and factitious disorders
- Developmental and pervasive disorders
- Attention deficit hyperactivity disorder (ADHD)
- Schizophrenia and psychotic disorders
- Bipolar, mania

ICD-10 Code

Antisocial personality disorder (F60.2)

Diagnostic Workup

- Complete history and physical examination with consideration of previous neurological trauma
- No laboratory tests are indicated for this diagnosis.
- Psychiatric evaluation should specifically include a thorough focus on personal and social history as this area will highlight the individual's lack of empathy; his or her disregard of the feelings, rights, and suffering of others (i.e., multiple marriages, relationships, criminal history, lack of long-term plans or goals).
- Individuals will have underlying beliefs about the self and this will be manifested in their behaviors. The consideration of these beliefs or cognitive schemas can also be a useful way to validate the diagnosis. Therefore, here are a few examples of beliefs, thoughts, or sentiments that the individual may share with you as part of the diagnostic interview:
  - Force and cunning are the best ways to get things done.
  - People will get at me if I don't get them first.
  - It is not important for me to keep promises or honor debts.
  - What others think of me really does not matter.
  - I can get away with things, so I do not need to worry about bad consequences.
  - If it was not me, it would be someone else (on raping a woman).

Clinical Presentation

- Failure to conform to rules in society so that often behaviors are in direct violation with the law
- Deceitful, tells lies and distortions to the pleasure and advantage of the self

■ Lack of empathy and disregard for others
■ May be initially pleasant and cooperative but then becomes nasty and difficult
■ Impulsive, irritable, and aggressive physically as well as verbally
■ Lacks the ability to plan ahead; lacks goals
■ Consistently irresponsible and has lack of remorse for deviant activities and behaviors
■ Pathological lying

DSM-5 Diagnostic Guidelines
■ Since the age of 15 years, there has been a disregard for and violation of the rights of others as well as a disregard for those rights considered normal by the local culture.
■ At least three of the following must be present:
   ■ Failure to conform to the rules of society and disrespect for the law, leading to repeated acts that are the grounds for arrest
   ■ Deceitfulness (pathological lying, use of aliases, manipulation of others for personal profit or pleasure)
   ■ Inability to plan ahead or to set goals; engages in impulsive behaviors
   ■ History of assaults, aggressiveness, and irritability related to violent acts
   ■ Disregard for the safety of self and others; reckless
   ■ Irresponsible; unable to meet obligations, does not honor debts or meet financial obligations
   ■ Lack of regret or shame, indifferent regarding any hurt, damage, or theft
■ At least 18 years of age
   ■ Evidence of conduct disorder with onset before the age of 15 years
   ■ The incidence of the antisocial behaviors is not exclusively during the course of schizophrenia or a manic episode.

TREATMENT OVERVIEW

Acute Treatment
■ There is no acute treatment for this disorder as personality disorders such as ASPDs in part are persistent and pervasive patterns of maladaptive behaviors that require chronic treatment in the form of psychotherapy.
■ The individual with this personality disorder often ends up in the prison system or substance abuse treatment facility where the treatment focuses on detainment (due to their criminal activity) or withdrawal from substances (that he or she has become addicted to, not for the treatment of his or her antisocial behaviors).

Chronic Treatment
■ Previous studies have suggested that long-term intervention is the only form of treatment for this individual whether incarceration or long-term psychotherapy. There is no psychopharmacological treatment indicated specifically for ASPD.
■ Cognitive behavioral therapy (CBT) is one example of a modality of psychotherapy that has been suggested for individuals who present with antisocial behaviors and ASPD.

- Rather than attempt to change the *moral structure* of the individual as evidence in psychodynamic psychotherapy, CBT instead can be implemented to focus on improving moral and social *behaviors* through enhancement of cognitive functioning.
- Individuals with ASPD would need to (a) identify and address the possible negative outcomes for their behaviors and (b) have an increased awareness of their dysfunctional beliefs about themselves, the world, and the future before making cognitive changes. CBT would focus on assisting the individual with APD to make a transition from his or her concrete beliefs to a broader spectrum of possibilities and outcomes.
- A small percentage of children who have conduct disorder (about 3% of males and 1% of females) grow up to become adults with ASPD while the remainder of those individuals persist with severe problems with authority, maintaining gainful employment, and/or satisfying relationships.
- Individuals do not have episodes of a personality disorder; rather, they have these traits as lifelong behavioral patterns.

PATIENT EDUCATION

- Individuals would have to make personal life changes to correct their deviant behaviors through psychosocial education, CBT, ongoing long-term psychotherapy, and/or incarceration.
- In general, most individuals with this disorder have no interest in changing or understanding their behaviors. Education would most likely occur for family and friends who have been injured, deceived, or in some way manipulated by these individuals.
- Family therapy for those who have been affected by an individual with ASPD would include (a) understanding the diagnosis; (b) identifying the behaviors that are manipulative and deceitful; (c) being able to set limits with the individual with ASPD so as to not be hurt, abused, or deceived in the future.

MEDICAL/LEGAL PITFALLS

- These individuals are dangerous and often can fool even the most experienced clinician. It is best to consider a forensic evaluation or consultation with a forensic specialist (psychiatrist or psychologist) for further direction.
- Forensic psychiatry is a branch of medicine that focuses on the interface of law and mental health.
- Forensic psychiatrists have additional education, training, and/or experience related to the various interfaces of mental health (or mental illness) with the law and are able to distinguish between a personality disorder or a clinical syndrome (i.e., when violent and hostile/aggressive behaviors are criminal or immoral).
- Forensic psychiatrists often determine whether an individual is "clinically competent" to stand trial for his or her actions or provide expert evidence about his or her actions and behaviors.
- Clinicians can be at risk for violence directed at them by individuals through threats, physical or emotional abuse, or harm.
- Forensic research has identified three *key* principles when confronted with an individual with ASPD who is violent or has a history of violence: (a) in general, ASPDs

are rarely ego dystonic; (b) most patients and violent situations associated with clinical issues involve comorbid conditions; and (c) violence and violence risk are often associated with intoxication. In other words, most individuals with ASPD will not seek treatment for their symptoms of this PD, rather they will present to health care providers for other symptoms, illnesses, and/or treatment (i.e., related to their violent behaviors). In addition, treating or managing the coexisting conditions (which may include illness, substance abuse, or environmental factors such as being arrested and imprisoned) may alleviate some violence potential if they are incarcerated as they are out of the general public community. Finally, their outcome or prognosis for treatment of their substance abuse or dependence is poor.

■ Risk assessment includes being aware of a history of violence with the following antisocial behaviors: (a) *Purposeful, instrumental violence* (acts in which violence is a means to a conscious, gainful end such as a robbery as well as violence designed to manipulate or mislead another into some wanted behavior; (b) *purposeful, noninstrumental violence* is exemplified in seeking the pleasure of a stimulating or antisocial activity, but the actual injuring of others is not integral to the activity's purpose; and (c) *purposeful, targeted, defensive violence* is identified in an individual who fears abandonment or humiliation and strikes out in illogical ways, such as murder or injury. Examples are "paranoid stalkers" who follow their "victims" and are threatened by anything getting between their victims and themselves (i.e., police, children, spouse of victim).

■ Clinicians need to understand the importance of identifying these signs and symptoms in clinical practice, and how their relationship is defined in terms of the individual with ASPD.

■ The key is to recognize and assess risk in order to remain safe.

Borderline Personality Disorder (BPD)

BACKGROUND INFORMATION

Definition of Disorder
■ Persistent pattern of mood instability, intense interpersonal relationships, impulsivity, identity disturbance, recurrent suicidal acts and/or self-mutilating behaviors, intense anger and rage as well as the potential for dissociation and psychosis
■ Begins in adolescence and the behaviors vary throughout adulthood
■ Fear of abandonment
■ Idealizes and devalues people
■ Sees the world in black and white ("no gray areas")
■ Three specific components help to conceptualize the disorder: (a) an unstable sense of self, (b) impulsive thoughts, and (c) sudden shifts of mood.
■ Often confused with bipolar disorder due to impulsivity and mood instability.

Etiology
■ During the past 20 years, the literature has expanded with multiple reasons for the development of this personality disorder.
■ Includes a history of childhood abuse, unstable or otherwise detrimental family environment, and family history of psychopathology

■ Childhood sexual abuse (CSA) is the most significant correlation with severity; chronicity and age of onset of sexual abuse and co-occurrence (and severity) of other forms of abuse and neglect take a second place in the determination.

■ Psychoanalytic theories focus on poor parental/caretaker attachment and the individual's resulting difficulty with separation.

Demographics

■ BPD about 1% to 2% of the general population, 10% to 25% of patients presenting in clinical settings, and 20% of patients in hospital settings.

■ More common in females than males

■ No difference in ethnic origin or socioeconomic status

Risk Factors

■ Childhood physical, sexual, and emotional abuse

■ Children who experience childhood sexual abuse are four times more likely to BPD than those who do not.

■ Severity, chronicity, and age of onset of sexual abuse (the younger the abuse, the poorer the prognosis) as well as the co-occurrence of other forms of abuse and neglect place individual at greater risk.

■ Family factors such as difficult relationships, poor attachment, and poor parental care

■ Social factors such as low socioeconomic status of family, being raised in a single-parent family, welfare support of family, parental death, and social isolation

■ Temperament has been studied and findings suggest that children and adolescents who cope by "internalizing" symptoms such as anxiety and depression and "externalizing" symptoms such as impulsivity, defiance, and oppositional behavior are at greater risk for a poorer prognosis.

■ Genetic factors play a role in the potential for individual differences in BPD features in Western society. This finding surmised that the symptoms and presentation of this disorder were consistent across three countries studying twins.

■ Poor parenting and lack of attachment are frequently associated with the development of the symptoms of BPD in childhood, adolescence, and into adulthood.

DIAGNOSIS

Differential Diagnosis

■ Frequently comorbid with Axis I disorders, especially substance-use disorders in males, eating disorders in females, anxiety disorders, and mood disorders, so it is often missed or misdiagnosed

■ Due to the mood instability, impulsivity, and psychotic symptoms, bipolar disorder is often mistaken for personality disorder (although individuals can have both).

ICD-10 Code

Borderline personality disorder (F60.3)

Diagnostic Workup

■ Complete history and physical examination with consideration of previous neurological trauma and careful assessment of the potential for seizure disorder (i.e., temporal lobe epilepsy)

- Psychiatric evaluation with a focus on personal and social history, including history of abuse
- Physical and mental evaluation
- Thyroid function studies (thyroid-stimulating hormone [TSH], triiodothyronine [T3], thyroxine [T4])
- Complete metabolic panel (CMP) glucose, calcium, albumin; total protein; sodium; potassium; CO_2 (carbon dioxide, bicarbonate); chloride; blood urea nitrogen (BUN); creatinine
- Alkaline phosphatase (ALP); alanine aminotransferase (ALT, also called SGPT), aspartate amino transferase (AST, also called SGOT) bilirubin
- CBC with differential: hemoglobin, hematocrit, red blood cell (RBC) count, white blood cell (WBC) count; white blood cell differential count, platelet count
- Careful assessment for cuts, bruises, and scars where patient could have caused self-harm through cutting, burning, or self-injury

Clinical Presentation
- Three specific components help to conceptualize the disorder: (a) an unstable self of self; (b) impulsive thoughts; and (c) sudden shifts of mood.
- Reports mood instability, intense interpersonal relationships, impulsivity, identity disturbance, recurrent suicidal acts, and/or self-mutilating behaviors, intense anger, and rage as well as the potential for dissociation and psychosis
- Relates interpersonal issues in terms of extremes (black or white, good or bad, idealized or failed parenting or relationships)

DSM-5 Diagnostic Guidelines
A pervasive pattern of instability in interpersonal relationships, self-image, and affects; marked impulsivity beginning by early adulthood and present in a variety of contexts, as indicated by five (or more) of the following:

1. Frantic efforts to avoid real or imagined abandonment
2. A pattern of unstable and intense interpersonal relationships characterized by alternating between extremes of idealization and devaluation
3. Identity disturbance: markedly and persistently unstable self-image or sense of self
4. Impulsivity in at least two areas that are potentially self-damaging (e.g., spending, sex, substance abuse, reckless driving, binge eating)
5. Recurrent suicidal behavior, gestures, or threats, or self-mutilating behavior
6. Affective instability due to a marked reactivity of mood (e.g., intense episodic dysphoria, irritability, or anxiety usually lasting a few hours and only rarely more than a few days)
7. Chronic feelings of emptiness
8. Inappropriate, intense anger or difficulty controlling anger (e.g., frequent displays of temper, constant anger, recurrent physical fights)
9. Transient, stress-related paranoid ideation or severe dissociative symptoms

TREATMENT OVERVIEW

Acute Treatment
- Establish a trusting interpersonal professional relationship
- Stabilize symptoms that are the most distressing to the individual (mood instability, psychosis, suicidal thoughts and actions)

■ May consider atypical antipsychotics to assist with the transient psychosis and mood instability as well as selective serotonin reuptake inhibitors (SSRIs) for depression. Stay away from tricyclic and monoamine oxidase inhibitor (MAOI) antidepressants as they have a higher risk for overdose and lethality.

■ Crisis intervention is frequently the most common acute treatment along with brief hospitalizations for threats to self (i.e., suicidal ideation, plan, and intent), and others (homicidal ideation, plan, and intent); self-mutilating behaviors; brief psychosis

■ If individual is not in therapy, best to consider initiating this or referring to an experienced outpatient therapist as these individuals will present in crisis and need to know that there is a contact person.

■ Prescribe medications for short periods of time to avoid the potential for overdose of medications when individual is in crisis or impulsive

■ If not the therapist or prescriber, maintain an ongoing collaborative relationship with the therapist or prescriber as individuals with this disorder often split and play one against the other.

Chronic Treatment

■ Studies have shown that long-term psychodynamic psychotherapy is the most useful if not the most successful long-term form of treatment.

■ DBT is also very successful but often individuals need to repeat the group and individual sessions on a long-term basis to acquire the necessary skills to learn how to cope with their thoughts and feelings.

■ Medications for symptom relief are useful, such as SSRIs and/or mood stabilizers for management of mood instability. Cautious use of benzodiazepines or other addictive substances is needed.

■ This is a long-term pervasive personality disorder that does not "go away" and come back. It is frequently "crisis driven" and individuals with this disorder need to learn to live with the symptoms as well as learn to cope appropriately with their internalized emotions as well as the externalized behaviors.

■ Some individuals do mature and can move toward a healthier way of living and coping with stresses. This seems to be an outcome of long-term psychotherapy if the patient has insight and a willingness to change.

PATIENT EDUCATION

■ Multiple websites and "chat rooms" where individuals and families can learn about the disorder and also obtain support (see below)

■ Books that may help include:
1. *I Hate You, Don't Leave Me: Understanding the Borderline Personality* (1991; classic text; ISBN-10: 0380713055; ISBN-13: 978–0380713059)
2. *Stop Walking on Eggshells: Taking Your Life Back When Someone You Care About Has BPD* (1998; whole series of books for individuals, families and groups; ISBN-10: 157224108X; ISBN-13: 978–1572241084)
3. *Surviving a Borderline Parent: How to Heal Your Childhood Wounds & Build Trust, Boundaries, and Self-Esteem* (2003; ISBN-10: 1572243287; ISBN-13: 978–1572243286)
4. *Understanding the Borderline Mother: Helping Her Children Transcend the Intense, Unpredictable, and Volatile Relationship* (2002; ISBN-10: 0765703319; ISBN-13: 978–0765703316)

5. *Skills Training Manual for Treating BPD* (There is a whole series of books by Marsha Linehan, PhD, related to assessment and treatment using various psychotherapies, including DBT, starting in 1993; ISBN-10: 0898620341 ISBN-13: 978–0898620344)

MEDICAL/LEGAL PITFALLS

- It is extremely important to understand that patients who suffer from this disorder have difficulty with boundaries (personal, social, and professional) and will "test" the limits in their relationships.
- Hugging and/or touching the patient without some discussion of its meaning can be very dangerous for the clinician. It is best *not* to have physical contact with him or her and set this boundary early on in treatment.
- Individuals with BPD are, for the most part, likely to provoke various kinds of boundary violations, including sexual acting out and testing your "affection" for them (e.g., they may invite you to an event that they are attending or offer you tickets to a theater production).
- These individuals (sadly) also represent the majority of those patients who falsely accuse therapists of sexual involvement, touching, and inappropriate contact. Many clinicians choose not to work with these patients and also demoralize them because of their own lack of skill. Therefore, be aware of your own scope of practice and if you are not skilled, refer them to someone who is trained and/or skilled.
- In general, therapists can take advantage of developing an awareness of any repeating patterns of behaviors that occur with these individuals and in how they respond (both the patient and the clinician). With this knowledge, clinicians can then steer clear of the highly destructive litigation that can and will ensue.

Narcissistic Personality Disorder (NPD)

BACKGROUND INFORMATION

Definition of Disorder

- A persistent pattern of grandiosity (in fantasy or behavior), need for admiration, and lack of empathy, beginning by early adulthood and present in a variety of contexts
- Grandiose sense of self-importance (e.g., exaggerates achievements and talents, expects to be recognized as superior without commensurate achievements)
- Preoccupation with fantasies of unlimited success, power, brilliance, beauty, or ideal love
- Believes that he or she is "special" and unique and can only be understood by, or should associate with, other special or high-status people (or institutions)
- Requires excessive admiration
- Sense of entitlement, that is, unreasonable expectations of especially favorable treatment or automatic compliance with his or her expectations
- Interpersonally exploitative, that is, takes advantage of others to achieve his or her own ends
- Lacks empathy: is unwilling to recognize or identify with the feelings and needs of others

- Often envious of others or believes that others are envious of him or her
- Shows arrogant, haughty behaviors or attitudes

Etiology

- As with all personality disorders, early childhood development plays a role in the progression of the pathology that is inherent in each of the maladaptive behaviors listed in the definition of NPD.
- Some theories (i.e., psychoanalytic) focus on the lack of paternal availability and the strength (or lack) of the relationship between the mother and father as a determinant in the development of a narcissistic child, adolescent, and adult, as well as an outcome of the insufficient gratification of the normal narcissistic needs of infancy and childhood.
- Neoanalytical thinking takes an antithetical view that narcissism is the outcome of narcissistic overgratification during childhood. This view focuses on parents who overindulge their child, protect the child from disappointment and failure, and minimize the criticisms of others about their child. It also presents the child who displays difficulties in self-esteem regulation with a tendency toward massive externalization of emotions.

Demographics

- About 0.7% to 1% of the general population suffers from NPD.
- About 2% to 16% of the clinical population has NPD
- Between 50% and 75% has of those with NPD are males.

Risk Factors

- There have been no known genetic factors contributing to risk.
- An oversensitive temperament as a young child
- Children who are adopted and therefore struggle to cope with the loss and rejection of their biological parents, especially if there is dysfunction within the current family of origin
- Various developmental pathways may present a special risk for the formation of NPD: (a) having narcissistic parents, (b) being adopted, (c) being abused, (d) being overindulged, (e) having divorced parents, and/or (f) losing a parent through death.
- Some theorists believe that this is learned behavior and narcissistic children come from narcissistic parents or caretakers.

DIAGNOSIS

Differential Diagnosis

- Histrionic personality disorder (HPD)
- ASPD
- Obsessive–compulsive personality disorder (OCPD)

ICD-10 Code

Narcissistic personality disorder (F60.81)

Diagnostic Workup

- Complete history and physical examination with consideration of previous neurological trauma

■ No laboratory tests are indicated for this diagnosis.
■ Psychiatric evaluation, including a focus on personal and social history

Clinical Presentation
■ The essential features are grandiosity, lack of empathy, and need for admiration
■ A sense of superiority, a sense of uniqueness, exaggeration of talents, boastful and pretentious behavior, grandiose fantasies, self-centered and self-referential behavior, need for attention and admiration, arrogant and haughty behavior, and high achievement
■ Individuals with NPD can be at high risk for suicide during periods when they are not suffering from clinical depression periods.
■ The individual learns to use defenses, including projection and splitting into all good and all bad, and along with that, idealization.

DSM-5 Diagnostic Guidelines
NPD is defined as a pervasive pattern of grandiosity (in fantasy or behavior), need for admiration, and lack of empathy, beginning by early adulthood and present in a variety of contexts, as indicated by five (or more) of the following:

■ Has a grandiose sense of self-importance (e.g., exaggerates achievements and talents, expects to be recognized as superior without commensurate achievements)
■ Is preoccupied with fantasies of unlimited success, power, brilliance, beauty, or ideal love
■ Believes that he or she is "special" and unique and can only be understood by, or should associate with, other special or high-status people (or institutions)
■ Requires excessive admiration
■ Has a sense of entitlement, that is, unreasonable expectations of especially favorable treatment or automatic compliance with his or her expectations
■ Is interpersonally exploitative, that is, takes advantage of others to achieve his or her own ends
■ Lacks empathy: is unwilling to recognize or identify with the feelings and needs of others
■ Is often envious of others or believes that others are envious of him or her
■ Shows arrogant, haughty behaviors or attitudes

TREATMENT

Acute Treatment
■ Currently, there are no medications that have been developed specifically for the treatment of NPD.
■ Patients with NPD who are also depressed or anxious may be given medications for relief of those symptoms.
■ There are subjective reports in the literature that the SSRIs may reinforce narcissistic grandiosity and lack of empathy with others and thus worsen the disorder.

Chronic Treatment
■ Intensive psychoanalytic psychotherapy; requires referral to therapist with extensive training to implement this type of treatment

▓ The goals of treatment are to work on (a) the grandiose self, (b) the pathologic defense mechanisms that interfered with the patient's normal development, and (c) the patient's manipulative interactions with family and friends.

▓ CBT can be implemented in some cases to assist the individuals to identify their negative behaviors and replace them with more functional ways of interacting with others.

▓ Most individuals who suffer from NPD cannot form a sufficiently deep bond with a therapist to allow healing of early childhood injuries, so treatment is usually long term if the individual can tolerate it.

▓ This is a long-term pervasive personality disorder that originates in childhood and/or adolescence and is retained throughout adulthood.

PATIENT EDUCATION

Books

▓ Golomb, E. (1995). *Trapped in the mirror*. New York, NY: William Morrow & Company, Inc.

▓ Brown, N. (2001). *Children of the self absorbed: A grown-up's guide to getting over narcissistic parents*. Oakland, CA: New Harbinger Publications.

▓ Miller, A. (1996). *The drama of the gifted child: The search for the true self*. New York, NY: Basic Books.

MEDICAL/LEGAL PITFALLS

▓ Significant relationships were found between NPD and incarceration for violent crimes; therefore, obtain a thorough social and legal history.

BIBLIOGRAPHY

American Psychiatric Association. (2000). *Diagnostic and statistical manual of mental disorders* (4th ed., text rev.). Washington, DC: Author.

Beck, A., & Freeman, A. (2003). *Cognitive therapy of personality disorders* (2nd ed.). New York, NY: Guilford Press.

Bradley, R., Jenei, J., & Westen, D. (2005). Etiology of borderline personality disorder disentangling the contributions of intercorrelated antecedents. *Journal of Nervous & Mental Disorders, 193*, 24–31.

Cohen, P. (2008). Child development and personality disorder. *Psychiatric Clinics of North America, 31*(3), 477–93, vii.

Distel, M. A., Trull, T. J., Derom, C. A., Thiery, C. W., Grimmer, M. A., Martin, N. G.,...Boomsma, D. I. (2008). Heritability of borderline personality disorder features is similar across three countries. *Psychological Medicine, 38*(9), 1219–1229.

Fonagy, P., & Bateman, A. (2008). The development of borderline personality disorder—a mentalizing model. *Journal of Personality Disorders, 22*(1), 4–21.

Gutheil, T. A. (1989). Borderline personality disorder, boundary violations, and patient-therapist sex: medicolegal pitfalls. *American Journal of Psychiatry, 146*, 597–602.

Kendler, K. S., Aggen, S. H., Czajkowski, N., Røysamb, E., Tambs, K., Torgersen, S.,...Reichborn-Kjennerud, T. (2008). The structure of genetic and environmental risk factors for DSM-IV personality disorders: a multivariate twin study. *Archives General Psychiatry,* 65(12), 1438–1446.

Paris, J. (2009). The treatment of borderline personality disorder: Implications of research on diagnosis, etiology, and outcome. *Annual Review of Clinical Psychology, 5,* 277–290.

Reid, W. H., & Thorne, S. A. (2007). Personality disorders and violence potential. *Journal of Psychiatric Practice, 13*(4), 261–268.

Saddock, B. J., & Saddock, V. A. (2008). *Synposis of psychiatry* (10th ed.). Philadelphia, PA: Lippincott, Williams & Williams.

Smith, C. A., Ireland, T. O., Thornberry, T. P., & Elwyn, L. O. (2008). Childhood maltreatment and antisocial behavior: Comparison of self-reported and substantiated maltreatment. *American Journal of Orthopsychiatry, 78*(2), 173–186.

Torgersen, S., Kringlen, E., & Cramer, V. (2001). The prevalence of personality disorders in a community sample. *Archives of General Psychiatry, 58,* 590–596.

WEB RESOURCES

About Antisocial Personality Disorder:

▦ http://www.mentalhealth.com/dis/p20-pe04.html/
▦ http://www.ptypes.com/antisocialpd.html/

About Forensic Psychiatry:

▦ http://www.reidpsychiatry.com/index.html/
▦ http://www.umdnj.edu/psyevnts/forensic.html/

Chapter 19

Sleep Disorders

Insomnia Disorder

BACKGROUND INFORMATION

Definition of Disorder
- Insomnia disorder is associated with physical factors and physiological disorder, excluding anxiety or depression.
- Trouble falling asleep or maintaining sleep for 1 month
- Patient complains of not feeling rested.

Epidemiology
- Women are 1.5 times more likely to have insomnia-related office visits than men.
- Occurs predominantly between the ages of 18 and 64 years
- Ten to 14% of adults present with insomnia disorder in primary care

Risk Factors
- Acute stress
- Depression
- Anxiety
- Medications (nonprescription and prescription)
- Obesity
- Geriatric considerations:
  - Medications should be used only for short-term management.
  - Benzodiazepines (BZDs) or sedative-hypnotics increase risk of confusion, delirium, and/or falls.
- Pregnancy considerations:
  - Physiological changes associated with pregnancy may disrupt sleep.
  - Avoid medications.
  - Consider other comfort measures, such as a change to a softer bed or a change in sleeping position.

DIAGNOSIS

Differential Diagnosis
▧ Thyroid disorders
▧ Anxiety/stress
▧ Drug interactions
▧ Substance abuse
▧ Hypersomnia
▧ Parasomnia

Diagnostic Workup
▧ Subjective complaints of inability to fall asleep or maintain sleep
▧ Feeling of not being rested
▧ Impacts daytime functioning

Initial Assessment
▧ Sleep hygiene
▧ Related medical conditions
▧ Data on snoring, sleep movements, irregular breathing patterns, length of sleep, and changes in mood should be obtained from family.
▧ Length of time with sleep disturbance, difficulty falling asleep, thoughts racing, repeated awakenings, or early-morning awakening history should be obtained
▧ New stressors
▧ New medications, over-the-counter (OTC) medicines, or herbal supplements

Laboratory Tests
▧ Thyroid function studies (triiodothyronine [T3], thyroxine [T4], thyroid-stimulating hormone [TSH])
▧ Complete metabolic panel (CMP), including glucose, calcium, and albumin; total protein analysis; and levels of sodium, potassium, CO_2 (carbon dioxide, bicarbonate), chloride, blood urea nitrogen (BUN), creatinine, alkaline phosphatase (ALP), alanine amino transferase (ALT, also called SGPT), aspartate amino transferase (AST, also called SGOT), and bilirubin
▧ Complete blood count (CBC) with differentials: hemoglobin, hematocrit, red blood cell (RBC) count, white blood cell (WBC) count, WBC differential count, and platelet count

ICD-10 Code
Insomnia disorder (G47.0)

DSM-5 Diagnostic Guidelines
▧ Difficulty initiating and maintaining sleep
▧ Present for at least 3 months or early-morning awakening with inability to return to sleep
▧ Daily functioning is impaired.
▧ Occurs at least three nights per week despite the opportunity for sleep
▧ The insomnia is not caused by anxiety, depression, drug abuse, adverse effect of a medication, or other medical conditions related to sleep, such as obstructive sleep apnea.

TREATMENT OVERVIEW

Behavioral Modification
- Eliminate stressors or assist patient in developing coping strategies
- No caffeine after 3 p.m.
- No alcohol intake within 3 hours of bedtime
- Daily exercise (avoid 4 hours prior to sleep)
- Establish sleep routine

Pharmacotherapy for Sleep Disorders
Short-term use of non-BZD medications:

- Adult treatment only
  - Eszopiclone (Lunesta)
  - Zaleplon (Sonata)
  - Zolpidem (Ambien, Ambien CR, Edluar, Intermezzo, Zolpimist)
  - Ramelteon (Rozerem)

Short-term use of BZD medications:

- Flurazepam (Dalmane)
- Temazepam (Restoril)
- Triazolam (Halcion)

Follow-Up
- Consider psychiatric evaluation if mental, emotional, or behavioral disorder is suspected
- Consider sleep laboratory evaluation if symptoms persist

PATIENT EDUCATION

- Use bed for sleep or intimacy only.
- Encourage patient to establish a routine before sleep.

Drug Selection Table for Sleep Disorders

CLASS	DRUG
Non-benzodiazepine GABA receptor agonists	First-line drug therapy:
	Eszopiclone (*Lunesta*)
	Zaleplon (*Sonata*)
	Ramelteon (*Rozerem*)
	Zolpidem (*Ambien*)
Benzodiazepines (BZDs)	Second-line drug therapy:
	Flurazepam
	Temazepam (*Restoril*)
	Triazolam (*Halcion*)

GABA, gamma-aminobutyric acid.

- No caffeine 6 hours before sleep
- No exercise 4 hours before sleep
- Evaluate response to medication within 7 days
- Avoid diet high in protein or alcohol 3 to 6 hours before sleep.
- Exercise regularly at least 5 to 6 hours before bedtime.
- Avoid use of OTC antihistamines or alcohol to induce sleepiness.
- Create a calm, cool, quiet atmosphere for sleep.
- If unable to sleep for 30 minutes, leave bedroom and engage in a quiet activity, such as light reading.
- Pharmacologic agents are for short-term or intermittent use only.

Hypersomnolence Disorder

BACKGROUND INFORMATION

Definition of Disorder
- Self-reported excessive daytime sleepiness or prolonged nighttime sleep that impacts activities of daily living without central origin despite 7 hours of main sleep with at least one of the following:
  - Recurrent sleep period lapses within same day
  - Main sleep of more than 9 hr/day nonrefreshing
  - Difficulty being fully awake after abrupt wakening
    - Occurs a minimum of three times weekly for at least 3 months
    - Accompanied by significant distress or impairment with regard to social, cognitive, or occupational functioning
    - Not explained by other sleep disorders, substance abuse, adverse effects of medications, or other conditions

Etiology
- Idiopathic
- No genetic, environmental, or other relating factors are identified.

Demographics
- Most common onset is during adolescence.
- Rarely presents after age of 30 years
- Affects male and females equally
- Exact prevalence is unknown in the United States
- Five to ten percent of all patients referred to a sleep laboratory for evaluation are diagnosed with primary insomnia

Risk Factors
- Acute stress
- Depression
- Anxiety
- Medications (nonprescription and prescription)
- Physiological changes associated with pregnancy may disrupt sleep
- Poor sleep hygiene

DIAGNOSIS

Differential Diagnosis
- Sleep apnea
- Kleine–Levin syndrome
- Depression
- Head trauma
- Insomnia

ICD-10 Code
Hypersomnolence disorder (F51.11)

Diagnostic Workup
- Excessive daytime sleepiness requiring frequent naps
- Does not wake up feeling refreshed
- Night time sleep longer than 12 hours
- Difficult to awaken, once asleep
- Sleep hygiene
- Related medical conditions
- Data on snoring, sleep movements, irregular breathing patterns, length of sleep, and changes in mood should be obtained from family
- Length of time with sleep disturbance
- New medications, OTC medicines, or herbal supplements

Laboratory Tests
- Thyroid function studies (T3, T4, TSH)
- CMP, including glucose, calcium, albumin; total protein count; levels of sodium, potassium, CO_2 (carbon dioxide and bicarbonate), chloride, BUN, creatinine, ALP, ALT, AST, and bilirubin
- CBC with differentials: hemoglobin, hematocrit, RBC count, WBC count, WBC differential count, and platelet count
- Confirmed by multiple sleep latency test (MSLT)
- Mean initial sleep latency of less than 8 minutes without early onset of rapid eye movement (REM) sleep
- Polysomnography is used to exclude other sleep disorders
- Epworth Sleepiness Scale is used

Clinical Presentation
- Prolonged sleep patterns
- Sleep drunkenness
- Less common
  - Headache
  - Orthostatic hypotension
  - Syncope
  - Raynaud's phenomenon

DSM-5 Diagnostic Guidelines
Additional coding descriptors:

- Specify if (a) with mental disorder, (b) with medical condition, (c) with another sleep disorder

- Acute: Duration of less than 1 month
- Subacute: Duration of 1 to 3 months
- Persistent: More than 3 months
  - Mild: occurring 1 to 2 days weekly
  - Moderate: occurring 3 to 4 days weekly
  - Severe: occurring 5 to 7 days weekly

TREATMENT OVERVIEW

Behavioral
- Stimulants at the lowest dose produce optimal alertness and minimize side effects
- Avoidance of sleep deprivation
- Establish regular sleep and wake times
- Work in a stimulating environment
- Avoid shift work

Acute Treatment
- Trial stimulants at the lowest dose to produce optimal alertness and minimize side effects in combination with lifestyle modifications and regular work routine. Typically requires long-term treatment.

Chronic Treatment
- Stimulants (nonamphetamine or amphetamine) at the lowest dose to produce optimal alertness
- Reevaluate as indicated to ensure treatment compliance and relief of symptomatology
  - Methylphenidate
  - Amphetamine/dextroamphetamine (Adderall)
  - Dextroamphetamine (Dexedrine)
  - Modafinil (Provigil)

Follow-Up
- Consider psychiatric evaluation if mental, emotional, or behavioral disorder is suspected
- Consider sleep laboratory evaluation if symptoms persist

Drug Selection Table for Hypersomnolence Disorder

CLASS	DRUG
Stimulants, nonamphetamine	First-line drug therapy:
	Modafinil (*Provigil*)
	Armodafinil (*Nuvigil*)
Amphetamines	Second-line drug therapy:
	Amphetamine/dextroamphetamine (*Adderall*)
	Dextroamphetamine (*Dextrostat*)
	Methylphenidate (*Ritalin*)

Prognosis
- Responds poorly to treatment
- Disabling

PATIENT EDUCATION

- Eat three meals every day.
- Exercise regularly.
- Avoid use of OTC antihistamines or alcohol before bedtime.
- Use bedroom for sleep or intimacy only.

Narcolepsy

BACKGROUND INFORMATION

Definition of Disorder
- Chronic REM sleep disorder of central origin characterized by excessive daytime sleepiness
- Classic presenting symptoms include excessive daytime sleepiness, sleep paralysis, cataplexy, and hypnagogic hallucinations.
- Nocturnal sleep disturbances are common.

Etiology
- Associated with specific human leukocyte antigen (HLA) halotypes
- Possible autoimmune etiology resulting in the discrete loss of brain cells that produce hypocretin. Other factors include: infections, exposure to toxins, dietary factors, stress, hormonal changes, and alterations in a person's sleep schedule.

Demographics
- Male to female ratio is 1.64:1.
- First-degree relatives have a 10- to 40-fold higher risk than the general population.
- Age of peak presentation is 15 years.
- Narcolepsy is reported in children as young as 2 years.
- Affects 0.02% to 0.18% of the United States and Western population.
- Increases to 25 to 56 per 100,000 when cataplexy is not a required symptom for diagnosis.

Risk Factors
- Positive family history
- Age
- At risk for motor vehicle accidents and injuries
- Pregnancy considerations
- Pediatric consideration: children rarely present with all four symptoms.

DIAGNOSIS

Differential Diagnosis
- Absence seizures
- Benign childhood epilepsy

- Brainstem glioma
- Complex partial seizures
- Periodic limb movement disorder
- REM sleep behavior disorder
- Tonic–clonic seizures
- Transient global amnesia
- Syncope and related paroxysmal spells

ICD Code
Narcolepsy (G47.419)

Diagnostic Workup
- Symptoms
  - Nocturnal sleep disturbances
  - Short and frequent refreshing napping episodes
  - Excessive daytime sleepiness for 3 months or longer
  - Loss of muscle tone briefly
  - Extraocular movements (EOMs) and respiratory function remain intact with cataplexy
  - If cataplexy event is severe and generalized, patient may fall.
  - Cataplexy is often triggered by changes in emotions such as laughter or anger episodes.

Initial Assessment
- Sleep hygiene
- Related medical conditions
- Data on snoring, sleep movements, irregular breathing patterns, length of sleep, and changes in mood should be obtained from family.
- Length of time with sleep disturbance
- New medications, OTC medicines, or herbal supplements

Laboratory Tests
- Thyroid function studies (T3, T4, TSH)
- CMP, including glucose, calcium, albumin; total protein count; levels of sodium, potassium, CO_2 (carbon dioxide and bicarbonate), chloride, BUN, creatinine, ALP, ALT, AST, and bilirubin
- CBC with differentials: hemoglobin, hematocrit, RBC count, WBC count, WBC differential count, and platelet count
- Confirmed by MSLT as demonstrated by sleep latency of less than 8 minutes accompanied by REM sleep occurring within 15 minutes of sleep onset during at least two out of four nap opportunities
- Epworth Sleepiness Scale
- Polysomnography
- Actigraphy
- HLA typing
- Cerebrospinal fluid hypocretin-1 analysis

DSM-5 Diagnostic Guidelines
- The individual falls asleep irresistibly, occurring three times per week for at least 3 months.

■ The presence of one or both of the following:
1. Cataplexy (abrupt loss of muscle tone)
   ■ Patients with long-standing disease: cataplexy without loss of consciousness, precipitated by laughter or joking
   ■ Patients within 6 months of onset of symptoms: spontaneous facial grimacing and tongue movement without an emotional trigger
2. Hypocretin deficiency: confirmed with cerebrospinal fluid analysis without evidence of acute brain injury or meningitis
3. Confirmed REM sleep latency 15 minutes or less

   Specify:

   Mild: cataplexy occurring one episode per week or less, napping twice daily, less disturbed nocturnal sleep (vivid dreams, movement during sleep and insomnia)

   Moderate: cataplexy occurring daily or every few days, multiple napping episodes throughout the day, disturbed nocturnal sleep

   Severe: drug-resistant cataplexy, frequent daily episodes, nearly continual drowsiness with disturbed nocturnal sleep
   ■ Consistent incursions of elements of REM sleep into the transitions between sleep and wakefulness;
■ The disturbance is not the direct physiological effect of use of a substance or of other medical conditions.

TREATMENT OVERVIEW

Behavioral
■ Sleep hygiene
■ Scheduled naps
■ Reassurance for patient and family
■ Exercise programs
■ Avoidance of foods high in sugar

Psychopharmacotherapy Overview for Narcolepsy
Armodafinil Nuvigil, sodium oxybate (Xyrem 4.5–9 g/night) as well as:

■ Adjunct agents for cataplexy—fluoxetine (Prozac) 20 to 80 mg; imipramine (Tofranil) 50 to 250 mg; nortriptyline (Aventyl, Pamelor) 50 to 200 mg; protriptyline (Vivactil) 5 to 30 mg; venlafaxine (Effexor) 37.5 to 225 mg.

Acute Treatment
■ Trial stimulants at the lowest dose to produce optimal alertness and minimize side effects in combination with lifestyle modifications and regular work routine. Typically requires long-term treatment.

Chronic Treatment
■ Stimulants (nonamphetamine or amphetamine) at the lowest dose to produce optimal alertness
■ Reevaluate as indicated to ensure treatment compliance and relief of symptomatology.

Follow-Up
■ Pediatric patients should be followed by a pediatrician and pediatric neurologist.

Drug Selection Table for Narcolepsy

CLASS	DRUG
Stimulants, nonamphetamine	First-line drug therapy:
	Modafinil (*Provigil*)
	Armodafinil (*Nuvigil*)
Amphetamines	Second-line drug therapy:
	Amphetamine/dextroamphetamine (*Adderall*)
	Dextroamphetamine (*Dextrostat*)
	Methylphenidate (*Ritalin*)

Prognosis
▨ With medications and treatment, the patient may lead a productive life.

Complications
▨ Adverse effects of medications
▨ Injury

Patient Monitoring
▨ Monthly follow-up is recommended to monitor response to medications.

PATIENT EDUCATION

▨ Advise adult patients regarding driving responsibilities.
▨ Educate patient regarding long-term effects of medications and need for safety precautions.

Nightmare Disorder

BACKGROUND INFORMATION

Definition of Disorder
▨ Is associated with REM sleep
▨ Occurs at any age
▨ Patient describes bizarre dream plot.
▨ Patient is arousable from sleep.
▨ Remembers event
▨ Nightmare disorder is exacerbated by stress

Etiology
▨ Occurs equally in males and females
▨ Twenty to 39% of children between ages 5 and 12 years are affected.
▨ Five to 8% of adults are affected.

Risk Factors
▨ Stress
▨ Sleep deprivation

NIGHTMARE DISORDER ■ 309

■ Psychiatric and neurological disorders in adults
■ Medications affecting neurotransmitter levels, such as antidepressants, narcotics, or barbiturates

DIAGNOSIS

Differential Diagnosis
■ Sleep terrors
■ Sleep-disordered breathing
■ Restless leg syndrome

ICD-10 Code
Nightmare disorder (F51.5)

Initial Assessment
■ Sleep hygiene
■ Related medical conditions
■ Data on snoring, sleep movements, irregular breathing patterns, length of sleep, and changes in mood should be obtained from family.
■ Length of time with sleep disturbance, difficulty falling asleep, repeated awakenings, or early-morning awakening history should be obtained.
■ New stressors
■ New medications, OTC medicines, or herbal supplements

Clinical Presentation
■ Abrupt awakening
■ Frightened and able to describe fears

DSM-5 Diagnostic Guidelines
■ Frequent awakenings from major sleep or naps, with detailed recall of extended and ominous dreams (usually involving threats to survival, personal security, or self-esteem).
■ The awakenings generally occur during the latter part of the sleep period.
■ On waking, the person rapidly becomes oriented and alert.
■ The disturbance that is experienced on waking causes notable distress for the individual or impairment of social functioning.
■ The nightmares do not occur concurrently with and exclusively during the course of another mental health disorder (e.g., delirium, posttraumatic stress disorder) and are not the direct physiological effect of substance use or another medical condition.
■ Coexisting mental and medical disorders do not explain dysphoric dreams.
■ Specify if:
  ▫ During sleep onset
  ▫ With associated nonsleep disorder
  ▫ Associated with other medical condition
  ▫ Associated with other sleep disorder
■ Specify if:
  ▫ Acute—frequency of nightmares is 1 month
  ▫ Subacute—frequency of nightmares greater than 1 month and less than 6 months
  ▫ Persistent—frequency of nightmares greater than 6 months

■ Specify if:
  ■ Mild: less than one episode weekly
  ■ Moderate: one or more episodes per week, not occurring nightly
  ■ Severe: occurring nightly

TREATMENT OVERVIEW

Behavioral
■ Comfort and reassurance are given.
■ Behavioral strategies or counseling, if episodes are frequent and severe.

Pharmacotherapy
■ None indicated

Follow-Up
■ Referral to psychiatrist may be indicated if a psychiatric disturbance is suspected.
■ Referral to sleep laboratory, if history does not correlate with clinical findings to rule out sleep-disordered breathing, parasomnia, or restless legs syndrome
■ Nightmares should resolve with time.
■ Insomnia from fear of sleeping may occur.
■ Daytime sleepiness may occur.
■ Cognitive dysfunction with protracted sleep disruption

PATIENT EDUCATION

■ Reassure parents that the disorder should resolve with maturity.
■ Reinforce the need for security to parents.
■ Adult patients should decrease stressors.

Nonrapid Eye Movement Sleep Arousal Disorders

BACKGROUND INFORMATION

Definition of Disorder
Reoccurring episodes of incomplete awakening from sleep occurring within the first 2 to 3 hours of major sleep, accompanied by (a) sleepwalking and/or (b) sleep terrors

■ Sleep disturbance arising from slow-wave sleep, nonrapid eye movement (NREM) sleep, stage III or IV
■ Occurs 60 to 90 minutes after onset of sleep in children
■ Patient does not remember the event and is often confused and disoriented afterward.

Behaviors
■ Screaming, sitting upright in bed, or sleepwalking
■ May involve complex motor activity, such as eating or driving
■ May be precipitated by fever, stress, sleep deprivation, and medications
■ Occurs most often in school-age children
■ Frequently, will have pallor, pupil dilation, tachycardia, and sweating

▪ Occurs most often in children age 4 to 12 years
▪ Typically, a strong family history of parasomnias

Etiology
▪ Occurs in 3% of children ages 18 months to adolescence
▪ Prevalence 1% to 4% of population
  ▪ Genetic component is linked with *HLA* gene.
▪ Occurs typically between ages 3 and 10 years
▪ Occurs in 10% to 20% of all children
▪ Occurs in 1% to 4% of adults who had somnambulism as a child

Risk Factors
▪ Adults are likely to have psychopathology, such as substance abuse and affective disorders.
  ▪ Sleep deprivation
▪ Psychotropic medications may raise risk of somnambulism.
▪ Changes in routine
▪ Fatigue
▪ Daily stress

DIAGNOSIS

Differential Diagnosis
▪ Nocturnal panic attacks occur.
▪ Nocturnal dissociative episodes
▪ Frontal lobe seizures
▪ Delirium is associated with medical or neurologic disorder
▪ Sleep-disordered breathing occurs.
▪ Restless leg syndrome

ICD-10 Code
Sleepwalking (F51.3)

Initial Assessment
▪ Sleep hygiene should be examined.
▪ Related medical conditions should be determined.
▪ Data on snoring, sleep movements, irregular breathing patterns, length of sleep, and changes in mood should be obtained from family.
▪ Length of time with sleep disturbance, difficulty falling asleep, repeated awakenings, or early-morning awakening history should be obtained.
▪ New stressors should be recorded.
▪ New medications, OTC meds, or herbal supplements should be considered.

Clinical Presentation
▪ Patient abruptly awakens from sleep with screaming during the first one third of major sleep or has frequent episodes of rising from bed during sleep and walking about.
▪ Tachycardia, rapid breathing, pupil dilation, and sweating may occur with sleep terrors.

■ Patient is unresponsive to family; with sleepwalking may have a blank face and
  stare straight ahead.
■ Does not recall event
■ Frequent episodes of rising from bed during sleep and walking about
■ Usually occurs in first third of major sleep episode
■ Is unresponsive to verbal or tactile stimuli
■ May have short period of confusion, once awakened

Laboratory Tests
■ Polysomnography
■ Electroencephalogram (EEG) with time-synchronized video monitoring

DSM-5 Diagnostic Criteria
■ Abrupt awakenings from sleep, usually occurring during the first third of the sleep
  episode
■ A frightened scream often accompanies the awakening.
■ Intense fear occurs on waking.
■ Signs of autonomic stimulation: tachycardia, rapid breathing, and sweating.
■ Relative unresponsiveness of the individual to the efforts of others to comfort him
  or her.
■ The episodes result in notable distress for the individual or impairment of social
  functioning.
■ The disturbance is not the direct physiologic effect of substance use or another
  medical condition.
■ Additional coding descriptors:
■ Specify if:
   ▪ Sleepwalking type
   ▪ Involves sleep-related eating
   ▪ Involves sleep-related sexual behaviors
   ▪ Sleep terror type

TREATMENT OVERVIEW

Behavioral
■ Rule out sleep-disordered breathing.
■ Parent reassurance should be given.
■ Ensure safe environment; sleepwalkers should be directed back to bed quietly.
■ Timed awakening
■ Suggest afternoon nap for children
■ Self-hypnosis
■ Short course of therapy of BZD or tricyclic in adults
■ Do follow-up.
■ Referral to psychiatrist may be indicated if psychiatric disturbance is suspected.
■ Referral to sleep laboratory if history does not correlate with clinical findings to
  rule out sleep-disordered breathing, parasomnia, or restless leg syndrome.
■ Avoid precipitating factors.
■ No medications are indicated for children.

Acute Treatment

■ No Food and Drug Administration (FDA)-approved medications for non-REM sleep arousal disorders

Chronic Treatment

■ For persistent symptoms, tricyclic antidepressants (TCAs) or BZDs may improve symptoms.
■ Use lowest dose possible to control symptoms.

Prognosis

■ Sleep terrors should resolve with maturity.
■ Complications may occur.
■ Daytime sleepiness may occur.
■ Cognitive dysfunction with protracted sleep disruption.

Patient Monitoring

■ Reassess for protracted symptomatology.

PATIENT EDUCATION

■ Family, partner reassurance should be given.
■ Adult patients must avoid substances that trigger events.

Part IV

Syndromes and Treatments in Child and Adolescent Psychiatry

Chapter 20

Disorders Presenting in Infancy or Early Childhood (0–5 Years of Age)

Attention Deficit Hyperactivity Disorder (ADHD)

BACKGROUND INFORMATION

Definition of Disorder
A biochemically based disorder of behavior and attention that results in a persistent pattern of difficulty affecting a child's functioning at home, school, and socially. Symptoms must be outside of the range of normal behavior for developmental level.

- An inability to pay attention or to sustain attention
- Always on the move, as if driven by a motor
- Impulsivity—verbally and physically
- Symptoms interfere with multiple life domains:
  - School, social, home, or work
  - Symptoms must be present before the age of 7 years.

Etiology
- ADHD is not fully understood.
- It is hypothesized that inefficient neurochemical processing in the following areas account for the complex symptoms of ADHD
  - Dorsal anterior cingulate cortex—selective attention
  - Dorsal lateral prefrontal cortex—sustained attention and problem solving
  - Prefrontal motor cortex—hyperactivity
  - Orbital frontal cortex—impulsivity

Demographics
- About 4.7% of school-age children have ADHD.
- Rates are higher among boys than girls.
  - This may be secondary to boys having higher rates of disruptive behavior due to hyperactivity and impulsivity.

■ Girls are less likely to be hyperactive and if they have good social skills, they often do not come to the attention of parents, teachers, or health care providers.

Risk Factors

Gender
■ Male

Family History
■ Family members with ADHD
■ Heritability is estimated at greater than or equal to 75%.

Precipitating Factors
■ Infections
■ Head injury
■ Hypoxia
■ Exposure to drugs or alcohol in utero
■ Low birth weight

Comorbidity Factors
■ Higher incidence of chronic health conditions than in nonaffected children
■ High incidence of substance use and abuse
■ Six times more likely to have psychiatric comorbidities
  ■ ODD and conduct disorder (CD)
  ■ Developmental disorders
  ■ Learning disorders
  ■ Anxiety disorders
  ■ Mood disorders
  ■ Sleep problems
  ■ Difficulty winding down and falling asleep

Socioeconomic Factors
■ Children from single-mother families are more likely to have an ADHD diagnosis.
■ Children with Medicaid are more likely to have an ADHD diagnosis than privately insured children.
■ Adolescents with ADHD are more likely to drop out of school.
■ Higher rates of pregnancy among high school girls
■ Higher incidence of legal involvement
■ Higher incidence of auto accidents

DIAGNOSIS

ICD-10 Codes
ADHD, Predominantly Inattentive Type (F90.0)
ADHD, Predominantly Hyperactive Type (F90.1)
ADHD, Combined Type (F90.2)
ADHD, Unspecified Type (F90.9)

Diagnostic Workup
■ Vision and hearing screen may be indicated.

- Complete blood count (CBC), complete metabolic panel (CMP), thyroid-stimulating hormone (TSH), free thyroxine (T4), liver function test (LFT) are all recommended.
- Complete physical may be indicated.
- Consider an EKG if contemplating using a stimulant (this is not standardized practice).
- A complete psychiatric assessment is recommended.
  - Overall behavior, mood, sleep, drug, and alcohol use/abuse
- Rating scales for ADHD
  - Parents and teachers to complete rating scale
    - ADHD rating scale (ages 6–12 years)
    - Connor's Parent and Teacher Rating Scale (reliable with criterion validity)
    - Strengths and Weaknesses of ADHD Symptoms and Normal Behavior (SWAN) Rating Scale (helps differentiate type of ADHD)
    - Vanderbilt (ages 6–12 years with parent and teacher scales)
- School records

Initial Assessment
- Prenatal and postnatal care
- Growth and development
- Medical history
- Onset of symptoms
- Establish baseline symptoms
- Severity of symptoms
  - At home, school, work, and socially

Clinical Presentation
Symptom clusters: inattention, impulsive, and hyperactive

- Combined type has features of inattention, impulsivity, and hyperactivity.
- Children often do not grasp how their behavior impacts others.
  - Kids can feel demoralized by how their symptoms affect their ability to function at home, school, and at play.

DSM-5 Diagnostic Guidelines
Inattention Symptoms
- Six or more of the following symptoms of inattention are present for at least 6 months, to a degree that is maladaptive:
  - The individual fails to give attention to details, in schoolwork, or other activities.
  - Has difficulty in sustaining attention in performance of tasks
  - Does not seem to be listening when spoken to directly
  - Fails to follow through on instructions, fails to complete school work or other duties (with failures not attributable to confrontational behavior or failure to understand instructions)
  - Has difficulty in organizing tasks and other activities
  - Seeks ways to circumvent tasks that require mental effort
  - Often loses things
  - Individual is easily distracted by stimuli of many kinds.
  - Individual is, more often than not, forgetful in daily activities.

The *DSM-5* lists these symptoms as being diagnostic of ADHD:

- Has difficulty finishing any activity that requires concentration

- Does not seem to listen to anything said to him or her
- Is excessively active—running or climbing at inappropriate times, squirming in or jumping out of his or her seats
- Is very easily distracted
- Talks incessantly, often blurting out responses before questions are finished
- Has serious difficulty waiting his or her turn in games or groups
- May have specific learning disabilities

Hyperactivity–Impulsivity Symptoms

- Six or more of the following symptoms have persisted for at least 6 months, to a degree that is maladaptive:
  - The individual fidgets or squirms when seated.
  - Leaves seat in classroom or in other situations in which remaining seated is required
  - Runs about in environments in which it is inappropriate to do so
  - Has difficulty in engaging in leisure activities quietly
  - Is always on the go
  - Talks excessively
  - Gives answers to questions before questions have been fully verbalized
  - Has difficulty in waiting for his or her turn
  - Interrupts the speech of others or intrudes in the activities of others
  - In adolescents and adults: the presence of feelings of extreme restlessness
- Symptoms are present before the age of 7 years.
- Social deficits are present in two or more settings.
- Clear evidence of impairment in social functioning
- The symptoms do not occur concurrently with and exclusively during the course of a PDD, schizophrenia, or other psychotic disorder, and are not more readily ascribed to another psychiatric condition.

TREATMENT OVERVIEW

Acute Care

- Health care providers should be familiar with the multiple medications available to treat ADHD. Stimulant medications are first-line agents. Atomoxetine (Strattera) is a second-line agent and has been shown to be effective in placebo-controlled trials. Other medications with less extensive evidence to support their use include alpha-2-agonists (Intuniv).

Chronic Care

- Behavior modification, also called behavior therapy, is recommended as part of a total treatment.
- Plan for ADHD
- It is based on rewarding an individual for desired behaviors and having consequences for undesired behaviors. Rewards and point systems are effective when used consistently at school and home.
- It can help build self-esteem and guide the patient toward good behavior patterns.
- Create schedules and follow routines daily
- Keep tasks simple

- Help the child become organized
- Use brief and clear instructions
- Limit distractions (e.g., TV, radio, games) when the child is doing homework.
- Set SMART goals to track the child's progress:
  S = Specific: Develop specific goals that are clearly stated.
  M = Measurable: A goal is measurable if progress is made toward reaching it.
  A = Agreed upon: Talk about the goal with the child and agree on actions.
  R = Realistic: The goals should be within reach.
  T = Timely: A timely goal is one that can be achieved within a time frame that is meaningful.
- Stimulants
  - Immediate release
  - Extended release
    - Medications to treat ADHD can create sleep disturbance.
    - Rebound appetite
  - Twenty percent of patients do not respond to stimulants.
  - For patients with substance abuse issues choose stimulants with nonabuse formulations.
    - Lisdexamfetamine (Vyvanse)
    - dexamphetamine (Focalin)

Drug Selection Table for ADHD

CLASS	DRUG
Amphetamines	Short-acting stimulants: Dextroamphetamine/amphetamine (*Adderall*) Dextroamphetamine (*Dexedrine* and *Dextrostat*) Long-acting stimulants Dextroamphetamine (*Spansule*) Dextroamphetamine/amphetamine (*Adderall XR*) Lisdexamfetamine (*Vyvanse*)
Methylphenidates (amphetamine derivatives)	Short-acting stimulants: Dexmethylphenidate (*Focalin*) Methylphenidate (*Methylin*) Methylphenidate (*Ritalin SR* and *LA*) Intermediate-acting stimulants Methylphenidate (*Metadate ER* and *CD*) Methylphenidate (*Methylin ER*) Methylphenidate (*Ritalin SR* and *LA*) Long-acting stimulants Methylphenidate (*Concerta*) Methylphenidate transdermal (*Daytrana Patch*) Dexmethylphenidate (*Foaclin XR*)
Selective norepinephrine reuptake inhibitors (SNRIs)	Nonstimulant: Atomoxetine (*Strattera*)
Selective alpha-2a-adrenergic receptor agonist (SARIs)	Nonstimulant: Guanfacine (*Intuniv*)

■ Nonstimulants
  ■ Atomoxetine (Strattera)
    ● Black box warning
    ● Analysis of 12 studies revealed that 4 out of 1,000 children experienced sui-
      cidal thoughts. There were no actual suicides in the studies.
    ● Bupropion (Wellbutrin)
      – Contraindicated in patients with anorexia nervosa and bulimia nervosa
      – Can exacerbate tics
      – *Caution*—lowers seizure threshold
    ● Guanfacine
      – Longer duration of action than with clonidine (Catapres)
      – Immediate and extended release formulation
    ● Clonidine (Catapres)

Recurrence Rate

■ ADHD is a lifelong condition.
  ■ Hyperactive symptoms often dissipate with age as the brain matures and
    patients develop coping skills.
    ● Symptoms of inattention persist into adulthood.
  ■ For algorithm for treating ADHD by American Academy of Pediatrics, go to
    ● http://aappolicy.aappublications.org/cgi/reprint/pediatrics;108/4/ 1033.pdf

PATIENT EDUCATION

■ Nonpharmacological intervention
  ■ Psychoeducation
    ● Understanding of ADHD
    ● Coping skills
      – Preplanning
      – Organize study time
      – Break up big tasks into smaller parts
    ● Parenting strategies
      – Give one direction at a time
      – A light touch can help refocus attention
      – Provide a predictable and consistent schedule
      – Get kids ready for school the night before
      – Keep in close contact with teachers to proactively solve problems
  ■ Psychosocial support for child and parent
    ● Higher rates of divorce are found among parents of children with ADHD.
■ Urge structure, structure, structure.

MEDICAL/LEGAL PITFALLS

■ Comorbid illness: medical and psychiatric
■ Treating ADHD with stimulants can exacerbate other conditions, such as bipolar
  mood disorder, thought disorders, and chemical dependency issues.
■ Off-label prescribing
  ■ Medication education includes indications, dose, route, schedule, potential side
    effects, class effects, off-label use, black box warnings, and alternatives.

▩ Diversion of stimulants for abuse
  ▨ A new fad among adolescent babysitters is to go through medicine cabinets and steal prescription medications.
▩ Persons diagnosed with ADHD are protected under the Americans with Disabilities Act of 1990 and have recourse, should they experience discrimination at school or work.

Autism Spectrum Disorders

BACKGROUND INFORMATION

Definition of Disorder
Spectrum disorders now include autistic disorders, Asperger's syndrom, childhood disintegrative disorder, and pervasive development disorder (PDD). Autism is a PDD, is usually evident in the initial years of life (by age 3 years), and is often observed with other medical abnormalities, such as chromosomal abnormalities, congenital infections, and central nervous system (CNS) abnormalities. According to the *DSM-5*, symptoms of Autism include

▩ Markedly abnormal or impaired development of social interaction, including at least two of the following:
  ▨ Impaired nonverbal behaviors (e.g., eye contact, facial expression, body postures, and gestures)
  ▨ Failure to develop age-appropriate peer relationships
  ▨ Lack of spontaneous activity to share enjoyment, interests, or achievements with others (e.g., play)
▩ Marked impairment in communication as indicated by at least one of the following:
  ▨ Delay or lack of development of spoken language
  ▨ In individuals with adequate speech, the lack of ability to initiate or sustain conversations
  ▨ Stereotyped or repetitive use of language, or idiosyncratic language
  ▨ Lack of spontaneous play
▩ Restricted repetitive or stereotyped patterns of behavior, as indicated by at least one of the following:
  ▨ Narrowed range of interests
  ▨ Inflexible adherence to specific, nonfunctional routines or rituals
  ▨ Stereotyped and repetitive motor mannerisms
  ▨ Persistent preoccupation with parts of objects

Etiology
There is no one known single cause of autism, but it is generally accepted that it is caused by abnormalities in the brain structure or functioning.

▩ A number of theories are being investigated, including the links among heredity, genetics, and medical problems. In many families, there appears to be a pattern of autism or related disabilities, further supporting a genetic basis for the disorder, but no one gene has been identified as causing autism.
▩ It also appears that some children are born with a susceptibility to autism, but researchers have not yet identified a single "trigger" that causes autism to develop.

It is possible that under certain conditions a cluster of unstable genes may interfere with brain development.

■ Other research focuses on pregnancy or delivery problems as well as environmental problems, including viral infections, metabolic imbalances, and exposure to environmental chemicals.

Demographics
■ A total of 1 case in 150 births, with a median rate of 5 cases per 10,000
■ Affect 1 to 1.5 million Americans; it is the fastest growing developmental disability.
■ Lifelong cost of care can be reduced by two thirds with early diagnosis and intervention.

Note: It is unclear whether the higher reported rates reflect differences in methodology, increased awareness, or an increase in the frequency of autism.

Risk Factors
■ Gender: rates are four to five times higher in males. Females with the disorder are more likely to exhibit more severe mental retardation (MR).
■ Familial pattern: increased risk of autism among siblings (approximately 5%) and some risk for various developmental difficulties in affected siblings.
■ Stressors
  ■ Having another mental disorder
  ■ In most cases, there is an associated diagnosis of MR, ranging from mild to profound.
  ■ Having a child with autism can be a significant stressor for families.
  ■ Change in routine can be a major stressor for the autistic child.

DIAGNOSIS

Differential Diagnosis
■ Rett's disorder
■ Childhood disintegrative disorder
■ AS
■ Selective mutism (SM)
■ Language disorders
■ MR
■ Stereotypic movement disorder
■ Attention deficit hyperactivity disorder
■ Schizophrenia

ICD-10 Code
Childhood Autism (F84.0)

Diagnostic Workup
■ Autism tends to occur more frequently than expected among children with certain medical conditions, including Fragile X syndrome, tuberous sclerosis, congenital rubella syndrome, and untreated phenylketonuria (PKU).
■ Some harmful substances ingested during pregnancy also have been associated with increased risk of autism.
■ Seizures may develop, especially in adolescence, in up to 25% of cases.
■ Microcephaly and macrocephaly may be observed.

Initial Assessment

▩ Medical history, including assessing for
  ▢ Maternal infections, bleeding, or other problems during gestation
  ▢ Experiences in pre-, peri-, and neonatal periods
  ▢ Potentially brain-damaging events in the postnatal period
  ▢ Medical illnesses of infancy
  ▢ Growth patterns normal
▩ Physical examination, including head circumference, weight, and height measurements for growth patterns, and neurological examination

Considerations include posture, gait, and what the child is grasping in his or her hand. Is child rocking or whirling? Or catatonic? Observe for movements, such as self-biting, hands over ears, hand flapping, clasping, wringing, and clapping. Fingers or other objects in the mouth? Is there facial grimacing? Is child performing visual self-stimulation on a pattern in your office? Note and record any myoclonic jerks. If possible, observe spontaneous handedness. Record spoken language by child, if any. Observe information processing, overstimulation, or distraction by visual/auditory information, tactile defensiveness, or delay in response.

▩ Hearing tests can determine whether hearing problems may be causing developmental delays, especially those related to social skills and language use.
▩ Behavioral questionnaires are commonly used, and use varies according to age and informant, and presenting symptoms. Commonly used tests are as follows:
  ▢ Modified Checklist for Autism in Toddlers: evaluates infants who are at least 24 months old, and is used to identify milder autistic symptoms.
  ▢ Pervasive Development Disorders Screening Test: this questionnaire is completed by parents to evaluate early signs of autism.
  ▢ Autism Screening Questionnaire: used for children 4 years and older.
  ▢ Autism Behavior Checklist: a screening tool that is completed by the teacher.
  ▢ Childhood Autism Rating Scale: rates how much a child's behavior differs from that of other children the same age (older than 24 months).
  ▢ Autism diagnostic interview: parents provide information about their child's behaviors during this wide-ranging, structured interview.
  ▢ Autism observation schedule: observation of the child performing activities, including communication, interaction, play, and other behaviors.
▩ If a metabolic disorder is suspected, the DAN (Defeat Autism Now!) protocol may be used to pinpoint it; see http://www.healing-arts.org/children/assessment.htm#Metabolic for more information/

Clinical Presentation

▩ Symptoms of autism vary, but contain core deficiencies in social and communication skills and behaviors, as previously described. CNS abnormalities will typically be present.
▩ Assess for known medical conditions, refer for specialty assessment.
▩ When other medical conditions are present, note on Axis III.
▩ Assess for sleep problems, as fatigue and attention deficits are often the result of sleep problems or exacerbated behavioral problems.
▩ There is an increased frequency of gastroesophageal reflux disease (GERD), food allergies, and vitamin deficiencies in children with ASD.
▩ Assess for pain related to a wide range of physical and physiological risk factors, as pain can be a contributor to an increase in emotional and behavioral problems.

Laboratory Tests

When autism is associated with a general medical condition, laboratory findings consistent with the general medical condition will be tested.

■ There are no medical tests for autism, but it should be diagnosed with a team of professionals.
■ There are some differences with measures of serotonergic activity, but no specific pattern is clearly identified.
■ Imaging studies may be abnormal.
■ EEG abnormalities are common, even in the absence of a seizure disorder.
■ A laboratory and clinical assessment of malabsorption problems and nutritional deficiencies is prudent, especially if nutrition supplements are being considered.
■ Test for lead poisoning, especially if a condition called pica (a craving for substances that are not food, such as dirt or flecks of paint) is present. Children with developmental delays usually continue putting items in their mouths after this stage has passed. This practice can result in lead poisoning, which should be identified and treated as soon as possible.

TREATMENT OVERVIEW

Autism follows a continuous course. Language skills and intelligence are the strongest factors related to progress. In the school-age years, gains in some areas are common, however, some adolescents deteriorate and some improve. In general, autistic children respond best to highly structured and specialized treatment. A program that addresses helping parents and caregivers in improving communication, social, behavioral, adaptive, and learning aspects of a child's life will be most successful. Treatments can be broken down into the following five categories.

Behavioral and Communication Approaches

■ Use positive reinforcement, self-help, and social skills training to improve behavior and communication
■ Many types of treatments have been developed, including applied behavioral analysis (ABA), treatment and education of autistic and related communication-handicapped children (TEACCH), and sensory integration.

Biomedical and Dietary Approaches

■ Medicines are most commonly used to treat related conditions and problem behaviors, including depression, anxiety, hyperactivity, and obsessive–compulsive behaviors.
■ Some studies (most unreplicated) have found the following supplements to improve functioning: cod liver oil (with vitamins A and D), vitamins C and B, biotin, selenium, zinc, and magnesium.
■ Other studies suggest avoiding copper and taking extra zinc to boost the immune system, and a need for more calcium.

Community Support and Parent Training

■ Educating family members about autism and how to effectively manage the symptoms has been shown to reduce family stress and improve the functioning of the child with autism.

▦ Some families will need more outside assistance than others, depending on their internal functioning, established support systems, and financial situation.

Specialized Therapies

▦ Speech, occupational, and physical therapies are important for managing autism and should all be included in various aspects of the child's treatment program.
▦ Speech therapy improves language and social skills.
▦ Occupational and physical therapy can help improve coordination and motor skills, and help in learning to process information from the senses (sight, sound, hearing, touch, and smell) in more manageable ways.

Complementary Approaches

▦ Music, play, art, and animal therapy may be used.
▦ All can help to increase communication, develop social interaction, and provide a sense of accomplishment; these therapies can provide a nonthreatening way to develop a positive relationship with a therapist in a safe environment. Art and music are useful in sensory integration, providing tactile, visual, and auditory stimulation. Music therapy enhances speech development and language comprehension. Songs can teach language and increase the ability to put words together.
▦ Art therapy can provide a nonverbal, symbolic way for expression.
▦ Animal therapy, including horseback riding, provides improved coordination and motor development while creating a sense of well-being and self-confidence.

Note: With most complementary approaches, there may be little scientific research that has been conducted to support the particular therapy.

Chronic Treatment

▦ There is no known cure, and chronic treatment is necessary and depends on associated symptoms. There are no approved medications for autism. Targeted therapies for specific symptoms have included serotonin-specific reuptake inhibitors (SSRIs) for rituals and compulsive behaviors, stimulants for attentive problems, neuroleptics for agitation and aggression, and benzodiazepines for anxiety.
▦ Be aware of interactions among multiple medications and assess for interactions.
▦ Treatment needs often change over time, as growth and development occur, and include the above-mentioned treatment approaches as well as vocational training and independent living skills, when appropriate, for older youth.

Recurrence Rate

▦ Follow-up studies indicate that only a small percentage of individuals with autism live and work independently as adults.
▦ In about one third of cases, partial independence is possible, and in the highest functioning adults some degree of social, and communication problems exists, along with markedly restricted interests and activities.

Drug Selection Table for Autism Spectrum Disorder

CLASS	DRUG
Amphetamines	Short-acting stimulants: Dextroamphetamine/amphetamine (*Adderall*) Dextroamphetamine (*Dexedrine* and *Dextrostat*) Long-acting stimulants Dextroamphetamine (*Spansule*) Dextroamphetamine/amphetamine (*Adderall XR*) Lisdexamfetamine (*Vyvanse*)
Methylphenidates (amphetamine derivatives)	Short-acting stimulants: Dexmethylphenidate (*Focalin*) Methylphenidate (*Methylin*) Methylphenidate (*Ritalin SR* and *LA*) Intermediate-acting stimulants Methylphenidate (*Metadate ER* and *CD*) Methylphenidate (*Methylin ER*) Methylphenidate (*Ritalin SR* and *LA*) Long-acting stimulants Methylphenidate (*Concerta*) Methylphenidate transdermal (*Daytrana Patch*) Dexmethylphenidate (*Foaclin XR*)
Selective norepinephrine reuptake inhibitors (SNRIs)	Nonstimulant: Atomoxetine (*Strattera*)
Selective alpha-2a-adrenergic receptor agonist (SARIs)	Nonstimulant: Guanfacine (*Intuniv*)

PATIENT EDUCATION

It is important for families to actively seek assistance from whatever sources are available. The following measures are helpful for all families who have a member with autism:

- Schedule breaks for caregivers. Daily demands of caring for an autistic child can be overwhelming. Trained personnel can relieve family members from these duties as needed. Breaks can help families communicate in a less stressful context and allow parents to focus on their relationships with other children and significant others. Regular breaks may also help a family continue to care for a child at home, rather than considering out-of-home care. Government programs exist to help families with limited resources.

- Seek assistance for a child with autism who is entering adolescence. Community services and public programs can help families during what can be an especially difficult time for their child. An adolescent child may benefit from group home situations, special employment, and other programs designed to help the transition into adulthood.

- Make contact with other families who have a child with autism. Local and national groups can help connect families and provide much-needed sources of information. The Internet and targeted web sites (e.g., www.autism-society.org) can be an important tool, that helps individuals with limited community resources (e.g., in rural areas) connect with others.

MEDICAL/LEGAL PITFALLS

- Given the complexity of medications, drug interactions, and the unpredictability of how each patient may react to a particular drug, parents should seek out and work with a provider with expertise in the area of medication management and experience with individuals with ASD.
- The FDA has advised that antidepressants may increase the risk of suicidal thinking in some patients, especially children and adolescents, and all young people being treated with them should be monitored closely for unusual changes in behavior.
- Individuals with ASD may be eligible for specialized education services under the Individuals with Disabilities Education Act (IDEA), which mandates the creation of an individualized education program (IEP). The IEP sets goals and objectives and describes what services a child will receive as part of his or her special education program. There is a process to determine eligibility, requiring an evaluation by the child's school district. See http://www.nichcy.org/InformationResources/Documents/ for more information.

Asperger's Syndrome

BACKGROUND INFORMATION

Definition of Disorder
- Neurodevelopmental disorder
- Characterized by significant social impairment
- Restricted interests and stereotyped movements
- Similar to autism but no significant delay in language or cognitive abilities
- Similar characteristics to nonverbal learning disability

Etiology
- Most studies are of autism in general; Asperger's syndrome (AS) is included in these studies.
- Not caused by immunizations, as previously speculated
- Compelling genetic evidence
- Neuroimaging shows abnormalities in frontal and temporal lobes and amygdala.
- Megalencephaly is a consistent finding.
- Not fully understood

Demographics
- A total of 3 cases per 10,000 births
- Nine times more frequent in males
- Five times less common than autism

Risk Factors
- Gender: males
- No apparent socioeconomic factors
- Family history
  - Parental psychiatric history (not specifically of autism)
  - Family history of an autoimmune disease
  - Advanced paternal age, older than 40 years
  - Risk increases with every 10 years of maternal/paternal age

DIAGNOSIS

Comorbidities
■ Attention deficit hyperactivity disorder (ADHD)
■ Anxiety disorders
■ Depression
■ Obsessive–compulsive disorder (OCD)
■ Oppositional-defiance disorder (ODD)
■ Schizophrenia

ICD-10 Code
Asperger's Disorder (F84.5)

Initial Assessment
■ Developmental history
■ Milestones met or delayed
■ How significant is the delay?
■ Onset age/symptoms
■ Symptoms/severity
■ Medical history

Diagnostic Evaluation
■ Interview is based on *DSM-5:* talking to the child and asking questions about the parents and other caregivers
■ Most interviews, testing, and scales require specialized training.
■ Autism Diagnostic Interview—Revised—semistructure interview is based on the *DSM.*
■ Neuropsychological testing
■ Cognitive/IQ testing
■ Childhood AS test (CAST)—available online through Autistic Research Centre (ARC)
■ Autism Spectrum Screening Questionnaire (ASSQ); 27-question screen must be purchased.
■ Gilliam Autism Rating Scale available through PRO-ED
■ Modified Checklist for Autism in Toddlers (M-CHAT) can be given at well-child preventive visits before age 3 years.

Clinical Presentation
■ Poor eye contact
■ Poor social skills
■ Interest in specific area that is restrictive
■ Difficulty with transitions
■ Sensory sensitivity
■ Routine and rule driven
■ Cognitively/academically on track
■ Early motor clumsiness
■ *DSM-5* lists the following as symptoms:
　　■ Communication problems: difficulty using or understanding language; children focus attention and conversation on a few topic areas, some frequently repeat phrases, and some have very limited speech

- Difficulty relating to people, things, and events: They have trouble making friends and interacting with people, difficulty reading facial expressions, and may not make eye contact
- Repetitive body movements or behaviors: Children with Asperger's engage in hand flapping or repeating sounds or phrases.

DSM-5 Diagnostic Guidelines

- Notable difficulty in social interaction, as manifested by two of the following:
  - Presence of a range of restrictions in nonverbal expression/behaviors, including eye contact, facial expression, body posture, and gestures
  - Failure to develop peer relationships commensurate with age and developmental level
  - Absence of spontaneous activity
  - Limited social or emotional reciprocity; limited empathy
- Restricted and repetitive activities and interests, as manifested by at least one of the following:
  - A very narrowed range of interests, patterns of interest that are aberrant in intensity
  - Rigid adherences to routines or rituals
  - Persistent preoccupation with parts of objects (versus objects in their entirety)
- The overall disturbance engenders a notable impairment in social functioning.
- Linguistic development and cognitive development are relatively unaffected.
- Criteria for another pervasive developmental disorder (PDD) or schizophrenia are not met.

TREATMENT OVERVIEW

Behavioral Therapy

- Individual, family, and group therapies—developmentally appropriate
- Behavioral therapy
- Social skills training
- Monitor for sedation, hypotension, dystonia, akathisia, oculogyric crisis, neuroleptic malignant syndrome, elevated prolactin, galactorrhea, amenorrhea, hyperglycemia, insulin resistance, and weight gain.
- Monthly, administer an abnormal involuntary movement scale (AIMS) or a Dyskinesia Identification System: Condensed User Scale (DISCUS) rating scale to monitor side effects
- Educate parents about the risk/benefit profile of atypical antipsychotic.
- Educate parents on how to recognize extrapyramidal side effects and neuroleptic malignant syndrome.

Chronic Treatment of ASD

Behavior Modification

There are several methods of behavior modification that are used to treat inappropriate, repetitive, and aggressive behavior and to provide autistic patients with skills necessary to function in their environment. Most types of behavior modification are based on the theory that rewarded behavior is more likely to be repeated than behavior that is ignored. This theory is called applied behavior analysis (ABA).

Successful behavior modification must involve the following:

▪ Highly structured, skill-oriented activities that are based on the patient's needs and interests
▪ Intense, one-on-one training with a therapist
▪ Extensive caregiver involvement
▪ *Sensory integration therapy* is a type of behavior modification that focuses on helping autistic patients cope with sensory stimulation. Treatment may include having the patient handle materials with different textures or listen to different sounds.
▪ *Play therapy* is a type of behavior modification that is used to improve emotional development. This type of therapy improves social skills and learning. Play therapy involves adult–child interaction that is controlled by the child.
▪ *Social stories* can also be used to improve undeveloped social skills. Stories are designed to help autistic patients understand the feelings, ideas, points of view of others, or to suggest an *alternate* response to a particular situation. They also may be used to help patients understand and cope with their own feelings.

Psychopharmacotherapy Overview
▪ Fluoxetine (Prozac) and fluvoxamine (Luvox) are helpful for rigid/obsessive thinking/irritability
▪ Fluvoxamine (Luvox) had significant side effects
▪ Fluoxetine (Prozac) is Food and Drug Administration (FDA) approved for depression and OCD in children younger than 7 years.
▪ Fluoxetine (Prozac)—initiate at 10 mg, children up to 30 mg, adolescents up to 60 mg
▪ Risperidone (Risperdal) is FDA approved for use in children aged 5 to 16 years for irritability, aggression, deliberate self-harm, temper tantrums, and mood fluctuations in autistic disorders
  ▪ Less than 20 kg (44 lb), 0.25 to 0.5 mg
  ▪ Greater than 20 kg (44–99 lb) 0.5 to 1.0 mg
▪ An increase of risperidone (Risperdal) of 0.25 to 0.5 mg can be considered at 2-week intervals. Maximum daily dose is 3 mg.
▪ Initiate risperidone (Risperdal) at 0.5 mg once daily, titrate up to 3 mg/day, divided dose.
▪ Treat comorbid disorders as appropriate.

PATIENT EDUCATION

▪ Explain diagnosis and prognosis
▪ Community resources
▪ Social skills education for patient
▪ Academic education with accommodations for developmental needs

MEDICAL/LEGAL PITFALLS

▪ Depending on severity of illness, may require guardian as patient approaches adulthood.
▪ Informed consent for medications, most are not FDA approved for use in children; this should be part of consent.

Disruptive Behavior Disorders (Not Otherwise Specified)

BACKGROUND INFORMATION

Definition of Disorders

Disruptive behavior disorders comprise three disorders:

- Conduct disorder (CD)
- Oppositional defiant disorder (ODD)
- Attention deficit disorder (ADD)

Research indicates that CD is a more severe form of ODD. Severe ODD can lead to CD. Milder ODD usually does not. The common thread that separates CD and ODD is safety. If a child has CD, there are safety concerns, either the personal safety of others in the school, family, or community, or the safety of the child with CD. These three disorders will be presented as a group to help compare and contrast the similarities and differences among the three.

Conduct Disorder

CD is a repetitive and persistent pattern of behavior in which the basic rights of others or major rules are of society violated. At least three of the following criteria must be present in the last 12 months, and at least one criterion must have been present in the last 6 months:

- Aggression to people and animals
- Often bullies, threatens, or intimidates others
- Often initiates physical fights
- Has used a weapon that can cause serious physical harm to others (a bat, brick, broken bottle, knife, gun)
- Is physically cruel to animals or people
- Has stolen while confronting a victim (mugging, purse snatching, extortion, armed robbery)
- Destruction of property
- Deliberate fire setting with the intention of causing serious damage
- Deceitfulness or theft
- Has broken into someone else's house, building, or car
- Often lies to obtain goods or favors or to avoid work
- Theft is committed without confronting a victim (shoplifting, forgery)
- Seriously violates rules
- Often stays out at night despite parental prohibitions, beginning before the age of 13 years
- Running away from home overnight at least twice for a lengthy period
- Often skips school before the age of 13 years

Note: The above problems cause significant impairment in social, academic, and occupational functioning.

Oppositional Defiant Disorder

ODD is a psychiatric disorder that is less severe than CD and is beyond the range of simple stubbornness. The criteria for ODD are as follows. A pattern of negativistic, hostile, and defiant behavior lasting at least 6 months, during which four or more of the following are present:

- Often loses temper
- Often argues with adults

▪ Often actively defies or refuses to comply with adults' requests or rules
▪ Often deliberately annoys people
▪ Often blames others for his or her mistakes or misbehavior
▪ Is often touchy or easily annoyed by others
▪ Is often angry and resentful
▪ Is often spiteful and vindictive

Note: The disturbance in behavior causes clinically significant impairment in social, academic, family, or occupational functioning.

All of the criteria above include the word "often." Although research indicates that these behaviors occur to a varying degree in all children, for the behavior to be considered "often," apply the following criteria:

1. Has occurred during the last 3 months:
   ▪ Is spiteful and vindictive
   ▪ Blames others for his or her mistakes or misbehavior
2. Occurs at least twice a week:
   ▪ Is overly touchy or easily annoyed by others
   ▪ Loses temper
   ▪ Argues with significant others
   ▪ Actively defies or refuses to comply with adults' requests or rules
3. Occurs at least four times per week
   ▪ Is angry and resentful
   ▪ Deliberately annoys people

ADD/ADHD

ADHD is one of the most common disorders diagnosed in youth. The essential feature is a persistent pattern of inattention and/or hyperactivity and impulsivity that is more frequent and severe than typically observed in individuals at a comparable level of development. ADHD has been associated with impaired academic achievement, rejection, and family resentment and antagonism.

The most common symptoms of ADHD are as follows:

▪ Impulsiveness: acting before thinking of consequences, jumping from one activity to another, disorganization, tendency to interrupt other people's conversations
▪ Hyperactivity: restlessness, often characterized by an inability to sit still, fidgeting, squirminess, climbing on things, restless sleep
▪ Inattention: distracted, daydreaming, not finishing work, difficulty listening

Etiology

▪ Problematic behaviors are the result of both difficult temperament qualities (e.g., low frustration tolerance, demanding, inflexibility, low psychophysiological arousal) of the child and environmental influences, including poor parenting, family stress, and adversity, association with deviant peers, and trauma.
▪ Some theorists believe ODD is the result of disruption of normal behavioral development, and that children may get stuck in the 2- to 4-year-old stage of development.
▪ Cognitions may also influence the development of CD, as these youth have been found to misinterpret or distort social cues during interactions and have deficits in social problem solving. Thus, they generate fewer alternate solutions to social problems, seek less information, see problems as having a hostile basis, and anticipate fewer consequences than children without CD.

▪ A specific cause of ADHD and other behavior disorders is not known. There are, however, a number of factors that may contribute to ADHD, including genetics, diet, and social and physical environments.

▪ Genetic factors: Twin studies indicate that the disorder is highly heritable and that genetics are a factor in about 75% of ADHD cases. It is believed that a large majority of ADHD cases arise from a combination of various genes, many of which affect dopamine transporters. The broad selection of targets indicates that ADHD does not follow the traditional model of a "genetic disease" and should therefore be viewed as a complex interaction between genetic and environmental factors. Twin studies suggest 9% to 20% of the variance in ADHD symptoms can be attributed to nonshared environmental or nongenetic factors.

▪ Environmental factors: ingestion of alcohol and tobacco smoke by the mother during pregnancy as well as environmental exposure. Premature birth may play a role. A meta-analysis found that elimination of artificial food coloring and preservatives may provide a benefit to children with ADHD. Also, children who grow up in an environment where there is poverty, alcohol or drug use, or violence are more likely to develop ODD.

Demographics

▪ Six percent of children in the United States may have CD. The incidence varies. For example, in a New York sample, 12% had a moderate level of CD and 4% had severe CD. Prevalence is based primarily on referral rates and because many youth are never referred for mental health services, the actual incidence may be higher.

▪ Prevalence of ODD ranges from 2% to 16% and is strongly associated with later development of CD, if untreated; about 52% continue to exhibit problems.

▪ For youth with CD, the co-occurrence with ADHD is at least 50%.

▪ High comorbidity (32% to 37%) exists between behavior disorders and anxiety and depression, and learning disorders and academic failure.

▪ Prevalence estimates of ADHD vary according to methods of assessment, diagnostic criteria, informants, and population sampled, and prevalence in school-age children is 3% to 16%.

Risk Factors

▪ Gender: ADHD occurs twice as commonly in boys as in girls. However, there is some evidence that it is underdiagnosed in girls because they may be less likely to exhibit aggressive behaviors and so go unnoticed.

▪ Family history: the majority of studies performed to assess genetics in ADHD have supported a strong familial nature of this disorder. Family studies have identified a two- to eightfold increase in the risk for ADHD in parents and siblings of children with ADHD.

▪ Maternal smoking during pregnancy

▪ Some theorists have proposed that a lack of empathic concern, or callous disregard for the welfare of other people, is a risk factor for CD.

▪ Stressors, including increased violence in media, social status competition, and decreased parental involvement, increase risk for disruptive behavior disorders.

▪ Having another mental disorder

▪ Increased risk for CD exists in children with an adoptive or biological parent with antisocial personality, alcohol dependence, mood disorder, schizophrenia, ADD, or CD or a sibling with CD.

▪ Increased risk for CD when there is marital conflict and child abuse/neglect, and inconsistent or harsh parenting style.

DIAGNOSIS

Differential Diagnosis
Conduct Disorder
- Childhood mood disorder or bipolar disorder
- ADHD
- ODD

Oppositional Defiant Disorder
- CD
- Mood disorder
- Psychotic disorder
- ADD
- MR
- Impaired language comprehension

ADD/ADHD
Problems with the diagnosis and treatment of ADD/ADHD can arise because approximately 65% of ADHD patients may have at least one of the following comorbid disorders:

- Anxiety, communication, mood, and learning disorders
- Tourette's syndrome
- Subnormal intelligence
- ODD (35%) and CD (26%)
- Primary disorder of vigilance: Characterized by poor attention and concentration, as well as difficulties staying awake. These children tend to fidget, yawn, and stretch, and appear to be hyperactive in order to remain alert and active.
- Bipolar disorder: As many as 25% of children with ADHD have bipolar disorder. Children with this combination may demonstrate more aggression and behavioral problems than those with ADHD alone.
- Posttraumatic stress disorder (PTSD)
- Medical conditions:
  - Medical conditions that must be excluded include hypothyroidism, anemia, lead poisoning, chronic illness, hearing or vision impairment, substance abuse, medication side effects, sleep impairment, and child abuse.
- Sleep conditions:
  - The relationship between ADHD and sleep is complex and includes an overlap in the central nervous system centers that regulate sleep and those that regulate attention and arousal. Sleep disorders play a role in the clinical presentation of symptoms of inattention and behavioral dysregulation. Mechanisms that account for excessive daytime sleepiness include chronic sleep deprivation, fragmented or disrupted sleep, sleep apnea, and circadian rhythm disorders.

ICD-10 Codes
CD (F91.8), Specify Type: childhood or adolescent onset; mild, moderate, or severe

ODD (F91.3) ADD: NOS (F90.9), Combined Type (F90.9), Predominantly Inattentive Type (F98.8), Predominantly Hyperactive/Impulsive Type (F90.0)

Diagnostic Workup
■ Assessing a child for disruptive behavior disorders begins with complete school and family histories and a medical examination to exclude other causes. A number of medical conditions may cause signs and symptoms similar to those of ADHD, including learning disabilities, mood disturbances, hyperthyroidism, seizure disorders, fetal alcohol syndrome, vision or hearing problems, and Tourette's syndrome.
■ Psychiatric interview, including substance use
■ Sleep patterns
■ Nutritional assessment
■ Check for heart conditions before treatment with stimulant medications.
■ An evaluation for ADHD should also include checking for learning or language problems, depression, anxiety, and sleep disorders. These and other coexisting conditions are found in as many as one in three children with ADHD.
■ Symptoms may not be obvious in an office setting, so questionnaires and interviews will be needed; including the parent, teachers, and other people who know the child well, such as babysitters and coaches, may be interviewed.
■ Rating scales, such as the Vanderbilt Questionnaire, the Conners Rating Scales or the Achenbach Child Behavior Checklist (CBCL), are helpful in diagnosing behavior disorders.
■ It is important to determine not just behavior but also whether the behavior is long-standing or temporary, and when it occurs. Children with behavior disorders exhibit these behaviors over a long period of time and have particular trouble in stressful, demanding situations or in activities that require sustained attention, such as reading, doing math problems, or playing board games.
■ Brain scans are not a reliable way to diagnose the disorder, nor are a child's responses to a psychostimulant medication.
■ The behaviors do not occur simultaneously with a psychotic disorder.

Clinical Presentation
■ Symptoms can vary greatly and are related to cognitive, emotional, and behavioral signs previously described.
■ Sleep problems may be reported.
■ Culture may influence how children and families communicate symptoms.

Laboratory Tests
■ There are currently no laboratory tests assessing chemical status of the living brain.
■ CBC with differential and platelet counts are needed periodically when using stimulants to assess for side effects such as leucopenia.
■ EKG prior to, and then periodically, when stimulants are prescribed.
■ Use of clonidine (Catapres) requires monitoring of blood pressure and cardiovascular parameters.
■ Depending on age and assessment, test for substance use.

TREATMENT OVERVIEW

Conduct Disorder
■ Bupropion (Wellbutrin) has been shown to improve symptoms in ADHD and CD, and SSRIs have been shown to be effective in youth with disruptive disorders and associated major depression.

■ Stimulants, antidepressants, lithium, anticonvulsants, risperidone (Risperdal), and clonidine (Catapres) have all been used in the treatment of CD.

■ No medications have been found consistently effective in the treatment of CD alone without other disorders such as ADHD or mood disorders.

■ Initial intervention is to teach all family members clear, direct, and specific communication techniques, and how to consistently set rules, limits, and expectations. A home rules contract, set up with the help of a therapist, can provide the high level of structure that is needed.

■ It is helpful to set aside time each day for interacting with children or teens with CD (e.g., play, sports, shopping).

■ In extreme cases, intensive behavior modification in a residential setting may be needed. The World Wide Association of Programs' six-level behavior modification programs can offer hope to parents who are dealing with teens diagnosed with either CD or ODD.

■ Teens with CD are poorly bonded to people and institutions, including broader social rules; they may come into contact with the juvenile justice system. Unfortunately, experiences with other deviant peers often worsen the behavior, as do group therapy programs.

■ Residential programs such as military-style camps (e.g., boot camps) are popular but studies of their effectiveness indicate poorer outcomes in the young-adult years, with lower employment rates and higher rates of felony arrests.

Oppositional Defiant Disorder

■ Treatments for ODD and other behavior disorders are tailored specifically to the individual child and different treatments are used for preschoolers, school-age children, and adolescents.

■ Parent-training programs, individual and family therapy, social skills training, cognitive behavioral therapy (CBT), and social skills training are useful in combination.

■ An approach developed by Russell Barkley (Barkley & Benton, 1998) uses a parent-training model that focuses on positive approaches to increase compliance, only later introducing methods to extinguish negative or noncompliant behaviors.

■ One study examined the use of Ritalin to treat children with both ADHD and ODD. This study found that 90% of the children treated with methylphenidate (Ritalin) no longer had the ODD by the end of the study. The study had a significant amount of dropouts, but even if these children are included as treatment failures, the study still showed a 75% success rate.

■ One study showed that 80% of children with explosive behavior improved when given the mood stabilizer divalproex (Depakote).

ADD/ADHD

■ Methods of treatment often involve some combination of behavior modifications, lifestyle changes, counseling, and medication.

■ Stimulant medications (e.g., methylphenidate and amphetamine) are the most clinically and cost-effective methods of treating ADHD but are not recommended for preschool children. Stimulants improved teachers' and parents' ratings of disruptive behavior, but did not improve academic achievement. Stimulants neither increased nor decreased rates of delinquency. No significant differences among the various drugs in terms of efficacy or side effects have been found. About 70% of children improve after being treated with stimulants. Stimulants, in the short term, have been found to be safe in the appropriately selected patient and appear well tolerated over 5 years of treatment. Long-term safety has not been determined. Amphetamines such as Adderall have warnings about potential for abuse, drug dependence, and sudden death.

- It may take some time to find the best medication, dosage, and schedule. Some children respond to one type of stimulant but not another. The amount of medication needed may be adjusted over time, and scheduled on the target outcome (e.g., performance at school given on school days).
- Side effects occur sometimes with stimulant medication. These tend to happen early in treatment and are usually mild and short-lived. The most common side effects include the following: decreased appetite/weight loss, sleep problems, headaches, jitteriness, social withdrawal, and stomachaches.
- Comorbid disorders or substance abuse can make the diagnosis and treatment of ADHD more difficult. Psychosocial therapy is useful in treating some comorbid conditions.
- Behavioral interventions:
  - Psychological therapies used to treat ADHD include psychoeducational input, behavior therapy, cognitive behavioral therapy, interpersonal psychotherapy, family therapy, school-based interventions, social skills training, and parent management training.
- Parent training and education have been found to have short-term benefits. Family therapy has shown to be of little use in the treatment of ADHD.
- Support groups

Chronic Treatment

Behavior therapy, in addition to medication management, enables parents, teachers, and other caregivers to learn better ways to work with and relate to the child with ADHD. There are three basic principles to any behavior therapy approach:

- Set specific goals. Set clear goals such as staying focused on homework for a certain time or sharing toys with friends.
- Provide rewards and consequences. Give a specified reward (positive reinforcement) when the child shows the desired behavior. Give a consequence (unwanted result or punishment) when the child fails to meet a goal.
- Keep using the rewards and consequences. Using the rewards and consequences consistently for a long time will impact behavior in a positive way.

Recurrence Rate

- Treatment of disruptive behavior disorders is important because persistent symptoms are linked to difficulty in school, social development, and adult health.
- Children with disruptive behavior disorders who respond to initial risperidone (Risperdal) treatment continue to have decreased symptoms when continued on long-term treatment.
- ADHD diagnosed in childhood resolves in 40% to 90% of individuals by the time they reach adulthood. Those affected are likely to develop coping mechanisms as they mature, thus compensating for their previous ADHD. Thirty-seven percent of those with ADHD do not get a high school diploma even though many will receive special-education services. The combined outcomes of the expulsion and dropout rates indicate that almost half of all ADHD students never finish high school, and

less than 5% of individuals with ADHD get a college degree as compared to 28% of the general population.
■ People with ADHD tend to work better in less structured environments with fewer rules. Self-employment or jobs with greater autonomy are generally well suited for them. Hyperactive types are likely to change jobs often due to their constant need for new interests and stimulations to keep motivated.

PATIENT EDUCATION

Conduct Disorder
■ Emphasize the seriousness of CD and the possibility of a poor prognosis if there is not significant family intervention.
■ Any comorbid substance abuse should be treated first.
■ Multisystemic treatment addresses serious antisocial behavior, is targeted to the home, school, and community environment; is carried out in the child's natural settings; and has been shown to reduce juvenile incarcerations and out-of-home placements.

Oppositional Defiant Disorder
■ All children with disruptive behavior disorders may be eligible for special-education services.
■ The most effective way to address ODD is through parent management training and programs specific to the child's age. These programs can be quite expensive. They often cost $100/week or more and last from several months up to half a year. Insurance may not pay for such programs. However, some online and home-based programs exist that have been shown to be effective.
■ Generally, the younger the child is when enrolled in such a program, the better the outcome will be.

Attention Deficit Disorder/Attention Deficit Hyperactivity Disorder
■ Maintain a daily schedule. Try to keep the time that the child wakes up, eats, bathes, leaves for school, and goes to sleep the same each day.
■ Cut down on distractions. Loud music, computer games, and television can be overstimulating. Make it a rule to keep the TV or music off during mealtime and while doing homework.
■ Organize the house. If there are specific and logical places to keep schoolwork, toys, and clothes, they are less likely to be lost.
■ Reward positive behavior. Offer kind words, hugs, or small prizes for reaching goals in a timely manner or for good behavior.
■ Set small, reachable goals. Aim for slow progress rather than instant results. Use charts and checklists to track progress with homework or chores. Keep instructions brief. Offer frequent, friendly reminders.
■ Limit choices to two or three options at a time.
■ Find activities at which the young person can succeed. All children need to experience success to feel good about themselves.
■ Use calm discipline. Use consequences such as time-out, removing the child from the situation, or distraction. Sometimes, it is best to simply ignore the behavior. Physical punishment, such as spanking or slapping, is not helpful. Discuss the behavior when all parties are calm.

MEDICAL/LEGAL PITFALLS

▦ There is a significantly higher risk for injury-producing automobile accidents in older adolescents and adult drivers. The major factors contributing to this higher risk were higher rates of drunken driving, street racing, and traffic violations. Those with more severe ADHD symptoms are more likely to be in danger.

▦ Regular checkups are needed to evaluate medication and assess for side effects.

▦ Due to the potential for abuse with some medications (e.g., stimulants), it is important to address this issue with the patient and family. Drug dependence with stimulants can occur and drug holidays should be considered.

▦ Children with disruptive behaviors are often qualified to receive specialized education services through the local school system.

▦ Early sexual activity is associated with emotional and physical health risks. Sexual activity increases risk of contracting sexually transmitted infections and pregnancy. In 2005, 18% of students in grades 9 to 12 who had sexual intercourse in the past 3 months reported that they used birth control pills before their prior sexual intercourse and 63% reported condom use.

▦ It is important to note that the FDA has advised that antidepressants may increase the risk of suicidal thinking in some patients, especially children and adolescents, and all people being treated with them should be monitored closely for unusual changes in behavior.

▦ Risperidone (Risperdal) treatment of children with disruptive behavior disorders can lead to initial weight gain, elevated prolactin levels, and somnolence.

▦ Youth with behavioral problems often become involved in the juvenile court system.

▦ Nurses are mandated reporters of suspected child abuse or neglect.

Dyslexia

BACKGROUND INFORMATION

Definition of Disorder
▦ Language-based reading disorder
▦ Dys = difficulty, lexia = language
▦ Difficulty with written language: writing, spelling, and reading
▦ Combination of phonological and letter-processing errors
▦ Persons with reading disorders have normal intellect.

Etiology
▦ Neurobiological disorders
▦ Inherited genetic connections

Demographics
▦ Evenly distributed among sexes, cultures, and social groups
▦ All languages are affected
▦ Twenty percent of any given population is likely to have some degree of reading difficulty.

Risk Factors

■ Boys are affected twice as likely as girls.
■ Family history of reading and learning disabilities
■ Families with histories of autoimmune disease (asthma and diabetes)

DIAGNOSIS

ICD-10 Code
Specific Reading Disorder (F81.0)

Diagnostic Workup
■ Functional hearing examination
■ Functional eye examination

Testing is standardized: refer to psychologist, education specialist, or specialist dyslexia teacher.

Initial Assessment
■ Was there any birth trauma?
■ Growth and development: Were milestones met on time for speaking?
■ Is there a family history of learning disabilities?
■ History of chronic ear infections
■ Has the child attended school regularly?
■ Specialist

Clinical Presentation
■ Delay in language acquisition—late to speak
■ Does not hear sound patterns
■ Difficulty with learning the names and sounds of letters
■ Can read a word on one page, but not recognize it on another
■ Reading comprehension is well below expected grade level; inaccurate, slow, and effortful reading
■ Classic warning signs of dyslexia before the age of 5 years:
  ■ Speech delay
  ■ Slow to get words out
■ Warning signs in school-age children:
  ■ Stuttering and articulation issues
  ■ Mixes up letters
  ■ Produces sounds out of sequence (animal = aMinal)
  ■ Difficulty with letters R, L, M, and N
  ■ Adds or eliminates words while reading
  ■ Difficulty with learning how to write
  ■ Difficulty with memorizing sequences
  ■ Poor written expression that lacks clarity
  ■ Difficulties remembering number facts
  ■ Inaccurate mathematical reasoning

DSM-5 Diagnostic Guidelines

▩ An individual's ability to read is impaired.
▩ Reading achievement, as measured by standardized tests of reading accuracy and comprehension, is substantially below age-appropriate reading achievement levels.
▩ The deficit in reading achievement interferes with academic achievement and activities of daily living that require reading skills.
▩ If a sensory deficit is also present, the impaired reading ability is in excess of impairments associated with the sensory deficit.
▩ Note: If a general medical condition (e.g., a neurological condition) or sensory deficit is present, the disorder should be classified as such.
▩ *DSM-5* says an individual's specific learning disorder is diagnosed by:
  ▩ Clinical review of the individual's developmental, medical, educational, and family history
  ▩ Reports of test scores and teacher observations
  ▩ Response to academic interventions
  ▩ The diagnosis requires persistent difficulties in reading, writing, and arithmetic or mathematical reasoning skills during formal years of schooling.

TREATMENT OVERVIEW

▩ Individual education should plan for accommodations at school.
▩ Small-group education
▩ Focus on repetition
▩ Therapies that integrate auditory, visual, and motor inputs

PATIENT EDUCATION

▩ Dyslexia is a lifelong condition.
▩ Severity of disability is variable.
▩ Treatment is important as children who have difficulty learning often believe they are incapable of learning, give up, and risk failure.
▩ Foster the child's strengths and creativity.

MEDICAL/LEGAL PITFALLS

▩ Higher incidence of autoimmune disease in families with a history of language disorders
▩ Protected under the IDEA http://idea.ed.gov/

Mental Retardation

BACKGROUND INFORMATION

Definition of Disorder

▩ Disorder of intellectual functioning
▩ Limitations in adaptive skills, such as communication, self-care, and social skills

▩ Mild MR is IQ 50–55 to 70.
▩ Moderate MR is IQ 35–40 to 50–55.
▩ Severe MR is IQ 20–25 to 35–40.
▩ Profound MR is IQ below 20–25.

Etiology

▩ Thirty-five percent of cases have a genetic cause.
▩ Ten percent are caused by malformation syndrome.
▩ Thirty-three percent are external or trauma related (prenatal, perinatal, or postnatal factors).
▩ Causes of 20% of cases are unknown.

Demographics

▩ One percent of total population is affected.
▩ Eighty-five percent have mild MR.
▩ Two times more likely to have medical conditions than other populations with mental issues

Risk Factors

▩ Parental age at birth
▩ Congenital heart disease
▩ Parental education/occupation/income
▩ Trauma
▩ PKU
▩ Hydrocephalus
▩ Infection
▩ Increased lead levels
▩ Pre- or postcerebral hemorrhage

DIAGNOSIS

Comorbidities

▩ Increased level of MR severity—increased medical comorbidity
▩ Hypothyroidism, congenital cataracts, or cardiac defects
▩ Fifteen to thirty percent have seizures.
▩ Twenty to thirty percent have a motor handicap such as cerebral palsy.
▩ Ten to twenty percent have a sensory impairment such as a vision handicap.
▩ Five times more likely to have a diagnosable psychiatric illness
▩ Anxiety disorder, CD, depression, eating disorder (pica and ruminations)
▩ Seventy-five percent of autistic children have comorbid MR.
▩ Seventy-five percent of people with Down syndrome may have Alzheimer's by the age of 60 years.
▩ ADHD rates are similar to the general population.

ICD-10 Codes

Mild MR (F70)
Moderate MR (F71)
Severe MR (F72)
Profound MR (F73)

Diagnostic Workup
- IQ testing
- Physical examination
- Chromosomal analysis
- Brain imaging (MRI or computed tomography [CT])
- EEG
- Urinary amino acids, blood organic acids, lead levels
- Biochemical tests for inborn errors of metabolism

Initial Assessment
- Parent/child early development
- Including prenatal or perinatal development, postnatal development
- Physical assessment
- Milestones
- Motor/coordination
- Medical history
- Onset of symptoms
- Severity of symptoms (communication, social, behavioral)

Assessment Tools
- The Aberrant Behavior Checklist—moderate to severe MR
- The Reiss Scales—eight psychopathology scales and six maladaptive behaviors

Clinical Presentation
- Decreased cognitive functioning
- Concrete thinking
- May have stereotypical movements
- Difficulty with change/transitions

DSM-5 Diagnostic Guidelines
- Notably substandard intellectual functioning: IQ of approximately 70 or below (for infants, a judgment of substandard intellectual functioning must be based on a clinical evaluation).
- The individual cannot fulfill standards of adaptive functioning for his or her age group. Presence of deficits in adaptive functioning in at least two of the following areas: communication, care of self, home living, social and interpersonal skills, self-direction, use of community resources, academic skills, work, leisure, health, and safety.
- The onset is prior to 18 years.

ICD-10 Code: Based on Degree of Severity Reflecting Level of Intellectual Impairment
- Mild MR: IQ level, 50–55 to approximately 70 (F70)
- Moderate MR: IQ level, 35–40 to 50–55 (F71)
- Severe MR: IQ level, 20–25 to 35–40 (F72)
- Profound MR: IQ level below 20 or 25 (F73)
- MR, Severity Unspecified: when there is strong presumption of MR but the person's intelligence cannot be tested using standard IQ tests (F79)

TREATMENT OVERVIEW

- ▥ Parent education programs
- ▥ Habilitation focusing on attempts to care for individuals in the community
- ▥ Behavior therapy
- ▥ Social skills training
- ▥ Special education
- ▥ Ancillary therapies—occupational therapy and physical therapy
- ▥ There are no specific medicines used for MR but treat coexisting medical and psychological conditions. There are no FDA-approved medications for use in children with MR.
- ▥ Neuroleptic/antipsychotics such as risperidone (Risperdal) have been used as first-line treatment for behavior problems associated with MR but due to the patients' limited verbal skills, monitoring side effects is difficult. Strongly weigh the risk/benefit of these medicines.
- ▥ People with Down syndrome are particularly sensitive to anticholinergics.
- ▥ People with MR may be disinhibited by sedative-hypnotics and benzodiazepines, which is aparadoxical reaction.
- ▥ Benzodiazepines are not used as first-line treatment.

PATIENT EDUCATION

- ▥ Educate about diagnosis, including prognosis
- ▥ Treatment options
- ▥ Available community resources
- ▥ Importance of support systems for the family

MEDICAL/LEGAL PITFALLS

- ▥ Most people with MR will require guardianship as they enter adulthood.
- ▥ IDEA guarantees children with disabilities diagnostic, educational, and support service until the age of 21 years.
- ▥ Public Law 94–142 mandates provision of free appropriate education up to the age of 21 years.
- ▥ Informed consent required for medications, most are not FDA approved for use in children; this should be part of consent.

Reactive Attachment Disorder

BACKGROUND INFORMATION

Definition of Disorder

Reactive attachment disorder (RAD) is a developmental disorder that is a direct response to abuse, neglect, and disruptions in early caretaking. Attachment and social interaction are rooted in infancy and early childhood. Failures of attachment occur when a child's basic needs for emotional and physical safety, security, and predictability are not met. This failure to attach results in children being incapable of developing normal loving relationships and they exhibit maladaptive and disruptive behaviors. This disorder can be diagnosed as early as 1 month of age.

Etiology
▦ Maternal deprivation
▦ Birth to 36 months is a hallmark period for attachment

Demographics
Estimate of prevalence is 1% of the general population. This is hard to estimate as abuse and neglect are seriously underreported in the United States.

Risk Factors
▦ Birth to the age of 5 years
▦ Emotional, physical, sexual abuse, and inconsistent care providers
▦ Genetic vulnerability is unclear
▦ Being removed from neglectful or abusive homes
▦ Children do attach to abusive care givers
▦ Postpartum depression in a mother
▦ Unwanted pregnancy
▦ Living in an orphanage or institution
▦ Parents with abuse histories, mental illness, MR, substance abuse, and behavioral disturbance
▦ Long medical hospitalizations with separation from parent
▦ Failure to thrive
▦ Poverty

DIAGNOSIS

Differential Diagnosis
▦ ADHD
▦ Autistic disorder
▦ CD
▦ MR
▦ ODD
▦ PDD

ICD-10 Code
RAD of Infancy or Early Childhood (F94.1)

Diagnostic Workup
▦ Full psychological evaluation with a multidisciplinary approach
  ▦ Psychosocial history
  ▦ Intellectual functioning
  ▦ Psychometric assessment

Initial Assessment
▦ Destruction of property
▦ Hoarding food
▦ Highly controlling of others and situations
▦ Lying about things or issues that the child does not need to lie about or when it would be easier to tell the truth
▦ Refusal to make eye contact

- Does not seek comfort from caregiver
- Failure to initiate or respond to social interactions
- Being demonstrative with strangers and refusing to be separated from new acquaintances
- Dangerous behavior with a lack of remorse
  - Assaulting others
  - Fire setting
  - Injury to self
    - Head banging
    - Hitting and biting oneself
  - Stealing
  - Sexual acting out
  - Learning problems
  - Stereotyped behaviors
    - Nose picking
    - Nail biting
    - Rocking
- The child's negative behaviors are much easier to assess than their attachment.
- Ask parents whether they are afraid of their child.
- Randolph Attachment Disorder Questionnaire (RADQ) is standard.

Clinical Presentation
- Inhibited: inability to initiate or respond to social interactions
  - Emotionally withdrawn
  - Guarded
  - Disinterested in others
  - Does not seek comfort
  - Minimal eye contact
  - Avoidance of physical touch
- Disinherited: inability to identify an appropriate attachment figure
  - Indiscreet and superficial attachments to others
  - Knows no stranger
  - Exaggerates need for help
  - Anxious—seeks reassurance
  - Excessive childlike behaviors

DSM-5 Diagnostic Guidelines
- Two types
  - Inhibited type: if inhibitions predominate in the clinical presentation
  - Disinhibited type: if indiscriminate sociability predominates in the clinical presentation
- Disturbed and developmentally inappropriate ways of relating to others, beginning before the age of 5 years, as evidenced by either of the following:
  - Failure to initiate social interaction or failure to respond in a developmentally appropriate fashion to many social stimuli, as manifested by excessively inhibited or ambivalent/contradictory responses
  - Indiscriminate sociability, with the individual showing a marked inability to form appropriate selective attachments (e.g., excessive familiarity with strangers).

▪ The social deficits cannot be ascribed to developmental delay (as in MR) and do not meet criteria for a PDD.
▪ Care of the child or infant is very likely to have included at least one of the following:
  ▪ Persistent disregard of the child's basic emotional needs, disregard of the child's need for affection
  ▪ Persistent disregard of the child's physical needs
  ▪ Repeated changes of primary caregiver (e.g., frequent changes in foster care setting)
▪ There is a presumption that the unmet needs are responsible for the failures of social interaction.

TREATMENT OVERVIEW

Behavioral
▪ There is no "gold standard" treatment for RAD.
▪ Focus treatment effort on parents or primary caregiver.
▪ Play therapy for patient
▪ Residential treatment
▪ Behavior management therapy
  ▪ Provides psychoeducation and parenting strategies
▪ Holding therapy
  ▪ This is not well researched and is highly controversial
▪ It is not mandatory that children be removed from their previously neglectful parents if those parents have changed their behavior and are now capable of providing a loving, stable relationship, and environment.

Psychopharmacotherapy Overview
▪ Mood stabilizer/antiseizure medications—off label
  ▪ Aggression
  ▪ Mood instability
▪ Atypical antipsychotics—off label
  ▪ Mood stabilization
  ▪ Disorganized behavior
  ▪ Behavior disturbance
  ▪ Comorbid diagnosis
  ▪ See specific diagnosis

Recurrence Rates
▪ Lifelong condition

PATIENT EDUCATION

▪ RAD children need consistent, predictable relationships and a stable environment.
▪ Parents must be flexible.
▪ Coach parents on how the child's behavior is not personal and rather a response to failures of empathy and protection.

- Older RAD kids often have behavioral disturbances resulting in legal difficulties.
- Parents are encouraged to spend time and money resources on themselves as children will get the benefit of parents who feel capable and supported.
- Work closely with school and incorporate interventions into the child's individual education plan

MEDICAL/LEGAL PITFALLS

- It is not unusual that adopted children with RAD will be "un-adopted" by their families.
- Follow mandatory reporting guidelines for abuse and neglect

Rett Disorder/Rett Syndrome

BACKGROUND INFORMATION

Definition of Disorder
- Neurodevelopmental disorder
- Onset is after a period of seemingly normal development at the age of 6 to 8 months
  - Loss of previously acquired motor and social skills
  - Severe impairment in language development
  - Poor coordination
- First stage: precocious stagnation
  - Age: 6 to 18 months
  - Developmental stagnation
  - Lasting a few months
- Second stage: rapidly destructive
  - Age: 1 to 3 years
  - Regression, irritability, and crying
  - Autistic behaviors and stereotyped hand movements
  - Breathing irregularities and epilepsy may be present.
- Third stage: pseudostationary
  - Ages 2 to 10 years
  - Some improvement in socialization
  - Medical difficulties present—ataxia and apraxia, spasticity, scoliosis, and tooth grinding
  - Aerophagia, forced air and saliva expulsions
- Fourth stage: later motor deterioration
  - Age: 10 years
  - Significant motor impairments: scoliosis, dystonia, and choreoathetosis
  - Will usually need a wheelchair

Etiology
- Degenerative disease of the white matter
- Reductions in the frontal lobe, caudate nucleus, and mesencephalus
- Seventy-five to eighty percent have mutation of the X-linked *MECP2* gene

Demographics
▥ About 6 to 7 cases per 100,000 females
▥ Almost exclusively seen in females
▥ Males with Rett syndrome (RS) usually die
▥ Equal among race and ethnic groups

Risk Factors
▥ Gender: female
▥ Family history
　▥ No specific precipitating factors

DIAGNOSIS

Comorbidities
▥ Epilepsy
▥ Scoliosis
▥ Cardiac-prolonged QT and bradycardia
▥ Breathing difficulties, that is, apnea
▥ Motor difficulties, that is, dystonia, spasticity
▥ Premature death may come from scoliosis, respiratory infection, or sudden death.

ICD-10 Code
Rett Disorder (F84.2)

Diagnostic Workup
▥ Interview based on *DSM-5* criteria
▥ EKG—normal initially but becomes slower as illness progresses
▥ Molecular genetic testing—CDKL5 mutation testing is not routinely available through most diagnostic laboratories; go to International Rett Syndrome Foundation (IRSF) web site (see below) for laboratories.
▥ Physical-assessing motor, seizure, cardiac respiratory, scoliosis
▥ Assessment of language delays
▥ Consult neurologist to address seizures and for help with differential diagnosis.
▥ Type 1 excludes AS and other childhood disintegrative disorders.

Initial Assessment
▥ Growth and development including socialization
▥ Medical history
▥ Onset of symptoms
▥ Severity of symptoms
▥ Timeline of development/regression
▥ Compare head circumference (head circumference at birth is normal)

Clinical Presentation
▥ In younger children, may look like autism—often misdiagnosed early
▥ Significant deterioration in motor, abilities, speech, and socialization
▥ Few are able to speak

■ Frequently present with epilepsy
■ Patients often have stereotypic hand movement, that is, hand-washing movements.
■ Breathing difficulties, that is, hyperventilation, air swallowing, breath holding
■ Wide gait if able to walk (50% gain independent mobility)
■ Scoliosis
■ Small hands and feet, may be discolored due to poor circulation

DSM-5 Diagnostic Guidelines

■ A neurodevelopmental syndrome characterized by all of the following:
  ▪ Apparently normal prenatal and perinatal development
  ▪ Apparently normal psychomotor development for the first 5 months
  ▪ Normal head circumference at birth
■ The onset of all of the following after a period of normal development:
  ▪ Deceleration of head growth between the ages of 5 months and 48 months
  ▪ Loss of previously acquired focused hand skills, between the ages of 5 months and 30 months, with the subsequent development of stereotyped hand movements (e.g., hand wringing)
  ▪ Loss of social engagement early in the course of the disorder
  ▪ Poor gait and poorly coordinated trunk movements
  ▪ Markedly impaired language development and markedly poor muscle function

TREATMENT OVERVIEW

■ Symptom relief
■ Physical therapy for muscular difficulties
■ Medications for comorbidities/complications, that is, epilepsy
■ No effective medical treatment for RS exists

PATIENT EDUCATION

■ Educate about diagnosis
■ Available community resources
■ Prognosis
■ Prenatal screening is available for subsequent pregnancies.

MEDICAL/LEGAL PITFALLS

■ Most people with Rett's syndrome will require guardianship as they enter adulthood.
■ Public Law 94–142 mandates the provision of free appropriate education up to the age of 21 years.
■ Informed consent needed for medications, most of which are not FDA approved for use in children; this should be part of consent.

Selective Mutism

BACKGROUND INFORMATION

Definition of Disorder
Selective mutism (SM) is a condition in which children are unable to speak in situations where talking is an expected behavior. These children are able to talk freely at home and in situations where they are comfortable. They may have articulation problems or a medical condition that affects speech, but overall, SM is an anxiety-based disorder.

Etiology
- The exact etiology is unknown.
- Children with SM are likely to have issues related to shyness, avoidance, and anxiety.

Demographics
- About 0.2% to 2% of population

Risk Factors
- Age: onset between the ages of 3 and 6 years
- Gender: boys and girls
- Family history
  - Parent with history of SM
  - Parents with anxiety disorders
- Precipitating factors
  - Traumatic events during the time of language development
  - Multiple moves in homes or school
  - Being threatened or bullied at school

DIAGNOSIS

Comorbidities
- Developmental disorders
- Elimination disorders
- Learning disabilities
- ODD
- Separation anxiety disorder
- Social phobia

ICD-10 Code
Selective Mutism (F94.0)

Diagnostic Workup
- Dental examination
- Hearing evaluation
- Rule out language disorders:
  - Consultation with a speech language pathologist
- Rule out medical causes:
  - Asthma—being short of breath makes it difficult to speak

▩ Rating scales
  ▩ Anxiety Disorder Interview Schedule for Children
  ▩ Social Anxiety Scale for Children–R

Initial Assessment
▩ Baseline level of functioning
▩ Onset of symptoms
  ▩ Difficulties may not come into focus until the child enters school.
▩ Environments and situations where the child is mute
▩ How does the child communicate at home, school, and in social situations?
  ▩ Gestures, writing, whispering
  ▩ Will child talk on the phone?
  ▩ Will child talk to people in one situation, but not in another?
    ● Talks to a friend in the child's home, but not at school.

Clinical Presentation
Refuses to speak in situations where talking is appropriate and expected.

DSM-5 Diagnostic Criteria
▩ Consistent inability to speak in specific social situations in persons who are capable of speech in other situations
▩ The disturbance interferes with educational/occupational/social functioning.
▩ A duration of at least 1 month (excluding the first month of school attendance)
▩ The failure cannot be ascribed to a lack of familiarity or comfort with the spoken language.
▩ The disturbance is not more easily ascribed to a communication disorder (e.g., stuttering) and does not occur concurrently with and exclusively during the course of a PDD, schizophrenia, or other psychotic disorder.

TREATMENT OVERVIEW

▩ Individual and family therapy
▩ Behavioral therapy
▩ Cognitive therapy
▩ Exposure therapy
▩ Skills training
  ▩ Communication skills
  ▩ Anxiety management
▩ Speech language pathologist
▩ SSRIs may be appropriate to treat anxiety symptoms
  ▩ Case studies report benefit
    ● Fluoxetine is most studied
  ▩ Coordinate services with school

PATIENT EDUCATION

▩ SM can remit on its own without treatment
▩ Treatment may take several months before benefit is noted.

■ Reinforce positive accomplishment.
■ Educational pitfalls
■ Hinders social development
■ Interferes with reading language developmental tasks
■ Hinders a child's ability to engage in regular and extracurricular activities

Separation Anxiety Disorder

BACKGROUND INFORMATION

Definition of Disorder
■ Anxiety disorder of childhood and early adolescence
■ Characterized by unrealistic fear of separation from attachment figures
■ Interferes significantly with daily life and development
■ Begins before the age of 18 years

Etiology
■ Genetic link but only in girls
■ Temperamental traits
■ Parental rearing styles
■ Caregiver stress/support
■ Life events

Demographics
■ Most common anxiety disorder in childhood
■ Prevalence is 2.4%
■ Peak onset is 7 to 9 years of age

Risk Factors
■ Female
■ Family history of anxiety disorder or depression
■ African American
■ Lower-socioeconomic-status homes
■ Child temperament
■ Parenting styles
■ Life events such as death or threat of separation

DIAGNOSIS

Comorbidities
■ Another anxiety disorder such as OCD, overanxious disorder
■ Depression

ICD-10 Code
Separation Anxiety Disorder (F93.0)

Diagnostic Workup
■ Clinical interview using *DSM-5* criteria

▦ Anxiety disorder interview schedule for *DSM-5*—child/parent (ADIS-C/P)
▦ Screen for child anxiety-related emotional disorders (SCARED)—parent and child

Initial Assessment

▦ Growth and development
▦ Current or recent life stressors for child and caregivers
▦ Significant losses
▦ Onset of symptoms
▦ Severity of symptoms
▦ Medical history
▦ School reports

Clinical Presentation

▦ Physical complaints, that is, stomach or head, particularly on schooldays
▦ Distress upon separation
▦ Fears that something bad will happen to parent(s) or attachment figure
▦ School refusal
▦ Severe anxiety/worry
▦ Difficulty with sleep

DSM-5 Diagnostic Guidelines

▦ Disproportionate or extreme anxiety related to separation from the home or from persons to whom the individual is attached, as manifested by three or more of the following:
  ▦ Distress for the individual, when separation from the home or "attachment figures" occurs or is anticipated
  ▦ Frequent worry about losing attachment figures; worry about harm coming to attachment figures
  ▦ Frequent worry that an untoward event will lead to separation from attachment figures (e.g., getting lost)
  ▦ Reluctance or refusal to go to school or elsewhere because of fear of separation
  ▦ Reluctance or refusal to be alone or without attachment figures, at home or in other settings
  ▦ Reluctance or refusal to go to sleep in the absence of proximity to an attachment figure, or to sleep away from home
  ▦ Repeated nightmares that include the element of separation
  ▦ Physical symptoms (such as headache, nausea, vomiting) when separation from attachment figures occurs or is anticipated
▦ A duration of 4 weeks or more
▦ Onset before age of 18 years
▦ The disturbance causes significant distress for the individual, or impairment in social functioning.
▦ The disturbance does not occur exclusively during the course of a PDD, schizophrenia, or other psychotic disorder.
▦ In adults and adolescents, the disturbance is not more easily ascribed to panic disorder with agoraphobia.

TREATMENT OVERVIEW

- Consensus exists that CBT is treatment of choice
- Exposure-based CBT is preferable—refer out
- Psychopharmacology is recommended treatment for resistant separation anxiety disorder (SAD).
- SSRI antidepressants are effective.
- Sertraline (Zoloft) and fluoxetine (Prozac) are shown to be effective in randomized controlled trials (RCTs).
- Fluoxetine (Prozac; if older than 7 years), initiate 10 mg/day; adolescents, initiate 20 mg/day, FDA approved for use in depression and OCD
- Sertraline (Zoloft; if older than 6 years), initiate 25 mg/day, FDA approved for use in OCD
- Monitor antidepressants for side effects such as nausea, agitation, sleep disturbance, suicidal thoughts, changes in appetite, and drowsiness.
- SSRIs carry black box warning for increased suicidal ideation.
- Results on tricyclic antidepressants (TCA) are mixed—increased risks for cardiac problems.
- Benzodiazepines are effective but, due to risk/benefit considerations, are not often used in pediatric population.

PATIENT EDUCATION

- About diagnosis
- Treatment options
- Strategies for management of symptoms such as school refusal; accommodation of symptoms makes problem worse
- Community/national resources and supports

MEDICAL/LEGAL PITFALLS

- School refusal may lead to problems with truancy.

Drug Selection Table Separation Anxiety Disorder

CLASS	DRUG
Selective serotonin reuptake inhibitors (SSRIs)	First-line drug therapy: Sertraline (*Zoloft*) Fluoxetine (*Prozac*) Paroxetine (*Paxil*) Paroxetine mesylate (*Pexeva*) Fluvoxamine (*Luvox*) Citalopram (*Celexa*) Escitalopram (*Lexapro*)
Tricyclic antidepressants (TCAs)	Drugs for treatment-resistant cases: Imipramine (*Tofranil*) Desipramine (*Norpramin*) Clomipramine (*Anafranil*)
Benzodiazepines (BZDs)	Drugs used for short-term treatments: Alprazolam (*Xanax/Xanax XR/Niravam*) Lorazepam (*Ativan*) Diazepam (*Valium*) Chlordiazepoxide (*Librium*)

REFERENCE

Barkley, R., & Benton, C. (1998). *Your defiant child.* New York, NY: Guilford Press.

BIBLIOGRAPHY

American Academy of Child and Adolescent Psychiatry. (2007). Practice parameters for the assessment and treatment of children and adolescents with anxiety disorders. *Journal of American Academy of Child and Adolescent Psychiatry, 46*(2), 267–283.

American Psychiatric Association. (2000). *Diagnostic and statistical manual of mental disorders* (4th ed., text revision). Washington, DC: American Psychiatric Press.

Barkley, R., & Benton, C. (1998). *Your defiant child.* New York, NY: Guilford Press.

Biederman, J. (2005). Attention-deficit/hyperactivity disorder: A selective overview. *Biological Psychiatry, 57*, 1215–1220.

Buckner, J. D., Lopez, C., Dunkle, S., & Joiner, T. E., Jr. (2008). Behavior management training for the treatment of reactive attachment disorder. *Child Maltreatment, 13*(3), 289–297. Retrieved September 1, 2009, from http://www.pubmedcentral.nih.gov/articlerender.fcgi?tool=pubmedandpubmedid=18490700

Carr, E. G., & Herbert, M. R. Integrating behavioral and biomedical approaches: A marriage made in heaven. *Autism Advocate, 50*(1), 46–52.

DuCharme, R. W., & McGrady, R. W. (2003). What is Asperger syndrome? In R. W. DuCharme & T. P. Gullotta (Eds.), *Asperger syndrome: A guide for professionals and families* (pp. 1–20). New York, NY: Plenum Publishers.

Farone, S. V., Perlis, R. H., Doyle, A. E., Smoller, J. W., Goralnick, J. J.,…Sklar, P. (2005). Molecular genetics of attention-deficit/hyperactivity disorder. *Biological Psychiatry, 57*, 1313–1323.

Ferguson-Noyes, N., &Wilkinson, A. M. (2008). *Caring for individuals with ADHD throughout the lifespan: An introduction to ADHD.* Ridgewood, NJ: Delaware Media Group.

Filipek, P. (2005) Medical aspects of autism. In F. Volkmar, R. Paul, A. Klin, & C. Donald (Eds.), *Handbook of autism and pervasive developmental disorders* (pp. 534–578). Hoboken, NJ: Wiley.

Fombonne, E. (2002). Prevalence of childhood disintegrative disorder. *Autism, 6*(2), 149–157.

Fombonne, E. (2005). Epidemiological studies of pervasive developmental disorders. In F. Volkmar, R. Paul, A. Klin, & C. Donald (Eds.), *Handbook of autism and pervasive developmental disorders* (pp. 42–69). Hoboken, NJ: Wiley.

Ghaziuddin, M. (2005). A family history study of Asperger syndrome. *Journal of Autism and Developmental Disorders, 35*, 177–182.

Gillberg, C., Gillberg, C., Rastam, M., & Wentz, E. (2001). The Asperger syndrome (and high-functioning autism) diagnostic interview (ASDI): A preliminary study of a new structured clinical interview. *Autism, 5*, 57–66.

Hall, S. E. K., & Geher, G. (2003). Behavioral and personality characteristics of children with reactive attachment disorder. *Journal of Psychology, 137*(2), 145–163.

Kearny, C. A., & Vecchio, J. L. (2007). When a child won't speak. *Journal of Family Practice, 56*(11), 917–921.

Kessler, R. C., Adler, L., Barkley, R., Biederman, J., Connors, C. K., Demler, O., . . . Zaslavsky, A. M. (2006). The prevalence and correlates of adult ADHD in the United States: Results from the National Comorbidity Survey Replication. *American Journal of Psychiatry, 163*(4), 716–723.

Kristensen, H. (2000). Selective mutism and comorbidity with developmental disorder/delay, anxiety disorder, and elimination disorder. *Journal of the American Academy of Child and Adolescent Psychiatry, 39*(2), 249–256.

MacDonald, H. Z., Beeghly, M., Grant-Knight, W., Augustyn, M., Woods, R. W., Cabral, H . . . Frank, D. A. (2008). Longitudinal association between infant disorganized attachment and childhood posttraumatic stress symptoms. *Developmental Psychopathology, 20*(2), 493–508.

Muter, V., & Snowling, M. J. (2009). Children at familial risk of dyslexia: Practical implications for an at-risk study. *Children and Adolescent Mental Health, 14*(1), 37–41.

Sakolsky, D., & Birmaher, B. (2008). Pediatric anxiety disorders: Management in primary care. *Current Opinion in Pediatrics, 20*(5), 538–543.

Silverman, W. K., & Dick-Niederhauser, A. (2004). Separation anxiety disorder. In T. L. Morris & J. S. March (Eds.), *Anxiety disorders in children and adolescents* (2nd ed., pp. 212–240). New York, NY: Guilford Press.

Silverman, W. K., & Ollendick, T. H. (2005). Evidence-based assessment of anxiety and its disorders in childhood. *Journal of Clinical Child and Adolescent Psychology, 34*(3), 380–411.

Scahill, L., & Martin, A. (2005). Psychopharmacology. In F. Volkmar, R. Paul, A. Klin, & C. Donald (Eds.), *Handbook of autism and pervasive developmental disorders* (pp. 1102–1120). Hoboken, NJ: Wiley.

Schum, R. L. (n.d.). Selective mutism: An integrated treatment approach. *The ASHS Leader Online.* Retrieved December 22, 2008, from http://www.asha.org/about/publications/leader-archives/2002/q3/020924ftr.htm.

Seida, J. K., Ospina, M. B., Karkhaneh, M., Hartling, L., Smith, V., & Clark, B. (2009). Systematic reviews of psychosocial interventions for autism: an umbrella review. *Developmental Medicine and Child Neurology, 51*(2), 95–104.

Swiezy, N., & Korzekwa, P. (2008). Bridging for success in autism: Training and collaboration across medical, educational, and community systems. *Child and Adolescent Psychiatric Clinics of North America, 17*(4), 907–922, xi, Review.

Woodbury-Smith, M. R., & Volkmar, F. R. (2008). Asperger's syndrome. *European Child and Adolescent Psychiatry, 18*(1), 1–11.

U.S. Department of Health and Human Services. (2008). *Vital and health statistics. Diagnosed attention deficit hyperactivity disorder and learning disability: United States, 2004–2006.* Series 10(237). Atlanta, GA: Centers for Disease Control and Prevention. Retrieved from http://www.cdc.gov/nchs/data/series/sr 10/Sr10 237 .pdf.

Volkmar, F., Koenig, K., & State, M. (2005). Childhood disintegrative disorder. In F. R. Volkmar, R. Paul, A. Klin, & D. J. Cohen (Eds.), *Handbook of autism and pervasive developmental disorders* (pp. 70–87). Hoboken, NJ: Wiley.

Ziegler, J. C., Castel, D., Georget-Pech, C., George, F., Alario, F. X., & Perry C. (2008). Developmental dyslexia and the dual role model of reading: Simulating individual differences and subtypes. *Cognition, 107,* 151–178.

WEB RESOURCES

- http://www.autismcenter.org/treatmentinterventions.aspx/
- http://www.asatonline.org/resources/articles/evidencebasedpractice.htm/
- http://www.csha.org/protecteddirectories/magazinearticles/EvidenceBasedPracticeAutism.pdf/
- http://www.ahrq.gov/clinic/epcsums/adhdsum.htm/
- American Academy of Child and Adolescent Psychiatry: http://www.aacap.org/
- American Association on Intellectual and Developmental Disabilities (AAIDD) for professionals: http://www.aaidd.org/
- American Association on Mental Retardation: http://www.aamr.org/
- American Psychiatric Association: http://www.psych.org/
- American Speech-Language-Hearing Association: http://www.asha.org/default.htm/
- Anxiety Disorders Association of America (ADAA): http://www.adaa.org/
- ARC of the United States: http://www.thearc.org/
- Association for the Treatment and Training in the Attachment of children: http://www.ATTACh.org/
- Autism Society of America: www.autism-society.org/
- CHADD (Children and Adults with Attention Deficit/Hyperactivity Disorder): http://www.chadd.org/
- Dyslexia Institutes of America: http://www.diaread.com/dyslexiafacts.htm/
- International Dyslexia Association: http://www.interdys.org/
- International Rett Syndrome Foundation (IRSF): http://www.rettsyndrome.org/
- MAAP Services for Autism and Asperger Syndrome: http://www.asperger.org/
- National Alliance on Mental Illness: http://www.nami.org/
- National Autism Association: http://www.nationalautismassociation.org/
- National Center for Health Statistics: http://www.cdc.gov/nchs/fastats/adhd.htm/
- National Guideline Clearinghouse: http://www.guideline.gov/summary/summary.aspx?doc id=11375andnbr=005912andstring=adhd/
- National Institute of Neurological Disorders and Stroke: http://www.ninds.nih.gov/disorders/
- U.S. Autism and Asperger Association: http://www.usautism.org/
- RAdKid.org: http://radkids.org/
- Selective Mutism Foundation Inc.: http://www.selectivemutismfoundation.org/about.shtml/
- Selective Mutism Group: http://www.selectivemutism.org/faq/faqs?full=1/
- Southeastern Rett Syndrome Alliance (SRSA): http://www.serett.org/

Chapter 21

Disorders Presenting in Middle Childhood (6–11 Years of Age) or Adolescence (12–18 Years of Age)

Childhood-Onset Fluency Disorder

BACKGROUND INFORMATION

Definition of Disorder
- Speech disorder characterized by disruptions in speech
- Syllable repetition
- Syllable prolongation
- Halted or interrupted flow of speech

Etiology
- Disorder is not fully understood.
- Research suggests heritability: Chromosome 12q
- Pathology is the lack of integration between language development and the motor ability needed for a forward flow in speech production
- Auditory processing has also been implicated as a potential factor in stuttering.
- Dysfluency can be normal in children just learning to talk and stuttering can abate on its own.
- Stuttering is not caused by an emotional disturbance.

Demographics
- Occurs in 1% of the general population
- About 2.5% of preschoolers are afflicted
- Male-to-female ratio is 3:1
- Some research supports higher prevalence in African American children

Risk Factors
- Age of onset is prior to ages 3 to 3.5 years
- Male

■ Brain damage
■ Twice as likely in families with a history of stuttering

DIAGNOSIS

Differential Diagnosis
■ Normal stuttering: dysfluency beginning before 3 years of age is likely to abate on its own.

ICD-10 Code
Childhood Onset Fluency Disorder (F80.81)

Diagnostic Workup
■ Functional hearing evaluation
■ Oral examination

Initial Assessment
■ Prenatal care
■ Labor and delivery
■ Growth and development
■ Age of onset of dysfluency
■ Has stuttering lasted longer than 6 to 12 months?
■ Symptoms of anxiety relating to speaking situations
■ Does the child stutter while singing, whispering, or talking to a pet?
■ Previous treatment for stuttering

Degrees of Dysfluency
Below is a guideline; the actual degree of impairment is to be determined by a speech pathologist.

■ Normal stuttering (onset prior to the age of 3 years):
  ■ Occasional repetition of sounds, syllables, or short words
  ■ Periodic hesitation or insertion of fillers ("uh, um")
  ■ Increases when the child is tired
  ■ No distress to the child

■ Mild stuttering:
  ■ Frequent repetition of sound, long syllables, or short words
  ■ Physical manifestations: closing eyes, muscle strain in lips
  ■ Occurs more of the time than not
  ■ No distress to mild frustration noted in the child

■ Severe stuttering:
  ■ Recurring long, repeated sounds: prolongations and blockages
  ■ Pitch of utterances may increase
  ■ Difficulty in most speaking circumstances
  ■ Anxious, fearful, or embarrassed when speaking

Clinical Presentation
▦ Onset between the ages of 2 and 7 years with a peak occurrence at 5 years
▦ Difficulty starting a word
▦ Repeating the sound of a letter or word (usually vowels)
▦ Repeating sounds more than once every 8 to 10 sentences
▦ Use of filler words or utterances ("um, uh")
▦ Change in pitch
▦ Rapid blinking
▦ Facial grimacing
▦ Lip pressing
▦ Hands about the face
▦ Use of physical gestures to get words out
▦ Looking to the side when speaking
▦ Emotional distress or embarrassment when speaking

DSM-5 Diagnostic Guidelines
▦ Abnormalities in the fluency, rhythms, and intonations of speech, characterized by frequent occurrences of one or more of the following:
  ▦ Sound and/or syllable repetitions
  ▦ Sound prolongations
  ▦ Interjections, outbursts
  ▦ Pauses within a word
  ▦ Blocking (filled or unfilled pauses in speech)
  ▦ Circumlocutions (word substitutions as a way of avoiding problematic words)
  ▦ The individual exhibits a notable stress in the utterances of words.
▦ The deficits in language fluency impede academic and occupational achievement.
▦ If a motor deficit related to speech or sensory deficit is present, the difficulties with language fluency are in excess of those usually associated with these deficits.
Note: If a motor deficit related to speech, sensory deficit, or neurological condition is present, the condition should be diagnosed as such.

TREATMENT OVERVIEW

▦ Refer to a speech/language pathologist (SLP)—first-line treatment
▦ SLPs evaluate speech and language issues and establish a hierarchy of speaking challenges.
▦ SLPs may recommend mechanical devices such as delayed or altered auditory feedback: patients with dysfluency can often speak fluently when talking in unison with someone else. These devices resemble a hearing aid with a pocket converter. The converter feeds back the patient's voice on a slight delay or an altered pitch and replicates the experience of speaking in unison.
▦ There is no gold-standard pharmacological intervention for stuttering.
▦ Assess for comorbid psychiatric disorders and implement appropriate pharmacological treatments (i.e., anxiety).
▦ Medication studies for stuttering are for adults.
▦ No medication has been shown to consistently improve, decrease, or mediate social, emotion, or cognitive symptoms of stuttering.

▧ All medications prescribed for stuttering are "off label" and not Food and Drug Administration (FDA) approved for the treatment of dysfluency—especially in children.
▧ Dopamine antagonist
   ▧ Risperidone (Risperdal): 0.25 to 1.0 mg daily
   ▧ Monitor for sedation, hypotension, dystonia, akathesia, oculogyric crisis, elevated prolactin, galactorrhea, amenorrhea, insulin resistance, and weight gain.
   ▧ Monthly, administer an abnormal involuntary movement scale (AIMS) or a Dyskinesia Identification System: Condensed User Scale (DISCUS) rating scale to monitor for side effects.
   ▧ Educate parents about the risk/benefit profile of an atypical antipsychotic.
   ▧ Educate parents on how to recognize extrapyramidal side effects.

PATIENT EDUCATION

▧ Help the child to feel less anxious or self-conscious.
▧ Wait while the child finishes a sentence.
▧ Speak slowly to the child.
▧ Limit questions to the child.
▧ Practice taking and listening sessions with the child.
▧ Foster acceptance.
▧ Collaborate with school teachers and counselors—kids who stutter are often teased.
▧ Support the child in practicing fluency skills.
▧ Clarify that the word "therapy" in speech therapy does not relate to counseling.
▧ Adolescents may benefit from group speech interventions as peers are a major influence in this developmental stage.
▧ The child's course of dysfluency often follows a family pattern in terms of whether stuttering abates on its own or requires treatment.

MEDICAL/LEGAL PITFALLS

▧ Child is protected under the Individuals with Disabilities Act and antidiscrimination laws. Go to: http://www.stutterlaw.com/index.htm/

Pervasive Developmental Disorder— Unspecified

BACKGROUND INFORMATION

Definition of Disorder
▧ Disorder is characterized by delayed social development, verbal, and nonverbal language delays, repetitive nonpurposeful behaviors, restricted range of interest, and unusual sensory responses.
▧ Clinical presentation is atypical in that there may be a later age of onset after the age of 3 years.
▧ Child has some but not all of the features of autism or his or her symptoms are a subsyndrome.

Etiology
- Not fully understood
- Multiple potential factors: genetic, neurologic, immunologic, environmental, and obstetrical
- Possible abnormal brain development in first months of life
- Serotonin, norepinephrine, and dopamine may play a role

Demographics
- Three to four times more males are affected than females.
- Occurs in all racial and ethnic groups

Risk Factors
- Low-birth weight
- Gestational age is less than 35 weeks
- Lower socioeconomic status
- Older parents (moms older than 30 years and dads older than 35 years)
- Parents with psychiatric disorders
- Parents with schizoid personality traits
- Ten to fifteen percent of children with fragile X have autistic traits.

DIAGNOSIS

Differential Diagnosis
- Childhood disintegrative disorder: rare, two cases in 100,000
- Rett syndrome: rare, one case in 10,000 to 15,000, and almost exclusively affecting girls
- Autism disorder
- Asperger's syndrome
- Fragile X: most common form of inherited mental retardation
- Attention deficit hyperactivity disorder
- Obsessive–compulsive disorder (OCD)
- Oppositional deviant disorder

ICD-10 Codes
Pervasive developmental disorder, unspecified (F84.9)
Pervasive developmental disorder (F84.8).

Diagnostic Workup
- Well-child screening hearing examination
- Laboratory: heavy metal—lead
- Laboratory: fragile X mental retardation 1 (FMR-1) DNA gene test for fragile X
- Childhood Autism Rating Scale (ages 2 years and above)
- Autism Diagnosis Interview–Revised
- Autism Diagnostic Observation Schedule
- Aberrant Behavior Checklist

Initial Assessment
- Prenatal care
- Labor and delivery

■ Growth and development
■ Age at onset or when parent first thought that something was not "quite right"
■ History of self-harm behaviors during fits/tantrums
■ History of seizure activity: one in four children has co-occurring seizures that begin in childhood or adolescence
■ Did child seem to develop normally, but has tapered off in further language and social skill acquisition?

Clinical Presentation
■ Minimal eye contact
■ Limited interest in others
■ Delay in language acquisition (speaking first word after 2 years of age and no phrases until after 3 years)
■ Does not pick up on social cues
■ Sensitive to sounds, lights, touch, taste, smell, and textures
■ Does child know how to play with toys or use toys for intended purpose?
■ The child lines up toys or objects.
■ Overly attached to a specific toy or item
■ When overstimulated, can lose control of behavior.
■ Difficulty in making transitions
■ Forced transitions can result in agitation or out-of-control behavior.

DSM-5 Diagnostic Guidelines
■ A conspicuous and pervasive impairment in the development of reciprocal social skills, associated with impairment of verbal or nonverbal communication skills and/or the presence of a narrowed range of interests and behaviors.
■ The criteria for a specific developmental disorder, schizophrenia, schizotypal personality disorder, or avoidant personality disorder are not met.
Note: This category includes "atypical autism"—in which patient histories do not meet the criteria for autistic disorder because of late age at onset, atypical symptomatology, partial symptomatology, or all of these.

■ Disorder characterized by severe and profound impairment in social interaction, communication, and the presence of stereotyped behaviors, interests, and activities

TREATMENT OVERVIEW

■ No cure
■ Younger than 3 years: early intervention (EI) programs
■ Greater than or equal to 3 years: school-based EI (individual education plan [IEP])
■ Specialized according to impairment and need
■ Speech therapy
■ Occupational therapy
  ■ Risperidone (Risperdal)
  ■ FDA approval for ages 5 to 16 years
  ■ For irritability, aggression, deliberate self-harm, temper tantrums, and mood fluctuations
  ■ An increase of risperidone (Risperdal) can be considered at 2-week intervals. Monitor for sedation, hypotension, dystonia, akathesia, oculogyric crisis,

Drug Selection Table for Pervasive Developmental Disorder

CLASS	DRUG
Selective serotonin reuptake inhibitors (SSRIs)	First-line drug therapy: Sertraline (*Zoloft*) Fluoxetine (*Prozac*) Paroxetine (*Paxil*) Paroxetine mesylate (*Pexeva*) Fluvoxamine (*Luvox*) Citalopram (*Celexa*) Escitalopram (*Lexapro*)

      neuroleptic malignant syndrome, elevated prolactin, galactorrhea, amenorrhea, hyperglycemia, insulin resistance, and weight gain.
- Monthly, administer an AIMS or a DISCUS rating scale to monitor for side effects.
- Educate parents about the risk/benefit profile of an atypical antipsychotic.
- Educate parents on how to recognize extrapyramidal side effects and neuroleptic malignant syndrome.
- SSRIs may decrease repetitive and ritualistic behavior and may improve social reciprocity, off-label use, black box warning.
  - FDA approval for treating depression and OCD
  - Monitor for nausea, agitation, sleep disturbance, suicidal thoughts, changes in appetite, and drowsiness.
- Assess for other comorbid Axis I diagnosis.
- Consider referral to community mental health center for case management as child will need a multidisciplinary treatment approach.

PATIENT EDUCATION

- Parents with a child who has autism and fragile X may want to consider genetic testing as there is a 50% likelihood that other boys will have the same constellation of autism and mental retardation.
- EI programs are mandated through the Individuals with Disabilities Education Act (IDEA), Part C (Program for Infants and Toddlers with Disabilities).
- EI programs vary from state to state.

MEDICAL/LEGAL PITFALLS

- Protected under the Individuals with Disabilities Act and antidiscrimination laws.

Conduct Disorder

BACKGROUND INFORMATION

Definition of Disorder
Conduct disorder (CD) is a severe form of oppositional defiant disorder (ODD). CD is characterized by a persistent pattern of behavior that ignores the rights of others with consistent violations of rules and age-appropriate behavior. A hallmark feature of CD is antisocial behavior without court involvement.

Etiology

▨ It is speculated that children with CDs have elevated sensory thresholds and engage in high-stimulus risk-taking behavior for optimal excitement.

▨ Serotonin may play a role in this excitatory process. Additionally, there is decreased communication between the amygdale and the ventromedial prefrontal context (VMPF).

▨ The amygdala is responsible for interpreting distress, whereas the VMPF processes emotion and cognitions.

▨ Cultural factors may influence behavior where urban decay and violence shape the beliefs and behaviors of children in those communities.

Demographics

▨ One to four percent of children, aged 9 to 17 years

Risk Factors

▨ Male:female (boys:girls), 5:1
▨ Low birth weight
▨ History of abuse and neglect
▨ Poverty
▨ Urban environments
▨ Decreased parental involvement
▨ Comorbidity:
  ▨ Attention deficit hyperactivity disorder (ADHD)
  ▨ ODD as a previous diagnosis
  ▨ Substance abuse

DIAGNOSIS

Differential Diagnosis

▨ ODD
▨ ADHD
▨ Substance use/abuse
▨ Depression
▨ Bipolar mood disorder
▨ Intermittent explosive disorder

ICD-10 Codes

Conduct disorder, childhood-onset type (F91.1)
Conduct disorder, adolescent-onset type (F91.2)
Conduct disorder, unspecified onset (F91.8)

Diagnostic Workup

▨ Physical
▨ Prenatal care
▨ Growth and development
▨ School history
▨ Family history
▨ Previous psychiatric history
▨ Legal history

Initial Assessment
▦ Establish baseline behavior.
    ▧ History of ODD
▦ Lack of empathy and guilt

Clinical Presentation
▦ Consistent disregard for social norms and behavioral expectation
▦ Onset of symptoms in childhood and early adolescence
▦ Patients typically have a previous diagnosis of ODD.
▦ Often have legal charges by adolescents

DSM-5 Diagnostic Guidelines
▦ Patterns of behavior in which the fundamental (human) rights of others are violated or in which established codes of conduct are violated, as evidenced by the presence of three or more of the following within the most recent 12-month period and one of the following in the most recent 6 months:
▦ Behavior that violates either the rights of others or major societal norms m ust be present for at least 3 months with one symptom present for the past 6 months:
    ▧ Bullies or threatens others
    ▧ Initiates physical fights
    ▧ Has used a weapon that can bring serious physical harm to others (e.g., a broken bottle)
    ▧ Has been physically cruel to people
    ▧ Has been physically cruel to animals
    ▧ Has stolen (e.g., has mugged someone)
    ▧ Has forced someone into sexual activity
    ▧ Has deliberately engaged in fire setting
    ▧ Has deliberately destroyed property (other than by fire setting)
    ▧ Has broken into a house, business, building, or car
    ▧ Has lied to obtain goods or favors, or to avoid obligations
    ▧ Has stolen items of some value without confronting a victim (e.g., shoplifting)
    ▧ Stays out late, despite parental or other prohibitions (starting before the age of 13 years)
    ▧ Has "run away from home," overnight, at least twice (or once without returning for a lengthy period)
    ▧ Is often truant from school (starting before the age of 13 years)
▦ The disturbances in behavior engender impaired social/academic/occupational functioning.
▦ In individuals 18 years or older, the criteria for antisocial personality disorder are not met.
▦ Type, based on age of onset:
    ▧ Childhood onset: onset of at least one criterion characteristic of CD prior to the age of 10 years
    ▧ Adolescent onset: absence of any criteria characteristic of CD prior to the age of 10 years
    ▧ CD—unspecified onset: when the age of onset is unknown
▦ Severity:
    ▧ Mild: Fewer conduct problems than are needed to make the diagnosis, and conduct problems bring only minor harm to others

Drug Selection Table for Conduct Disorder

Stimulants	Dextroamphetamine *(Dexedrine)*
	Methylphenidate *(Ritalin)*
Antidepressants	Bupropion *(Wellbutrin)*
	Fluoxetine *(Prozac)*
Alpha-adrenergicdrenergic receptor agonist	Clonidine

  ■ Moderate: Number of conduct problems and effects on others are intermediate between "mild" and "severe."
  ■ Severe: A greater number of conduct problems than is needed to make the diagnosis, or conduct problems bring considerable harm to others.

TREATMENT OVERVIEW

  ■ Medications to address aggression, inattention, hyperactivity, and impulsivity:
    ■ Caution: avoid formulations that have abuse potential or street value.

Behavior Therapy
  ■ Parent training courses
    ■ Intensive individual, family, and in-home therapy
  ■ Treatment is often difficult because kids typically first interface with the juvenile justice system.

PATIENT EDUCATION

  ■ Several studies have found that families that participate in therapy and training courses significantly reduce the amount of time their child spends in psychiatric and legal institutions.
  ■ Lower rates of sibling offenders in families that seek mental health services
  ■ Patients need education on the importance of following through with community services to reduce the risk of detention or incarceration.

MEDICAL/LEGAL PITFALLS

  ■ Patients are more likely to engage in risk-taking and potentially lethal behavior than in any other psychiatric diagnosis.
  ■ Chemical use, abuse, and dependence are rampant.
    ■ Often being under the influence of a substance is a compounding factor in illegal activity.

Oppositional Defiant Disorder

BACKGROUND INFORMATION

Definition of Disorder
  ■ Disorder presents with a consistent pattern of negative, hostile, and disobedient behavior.
  ■ Children with ODD are described as being "stubborn to a fault" and their disruptive behavior is exhibited at home and school.

▦ These children have difficulty in complying with the most simple requests or directives from adults or persons in authority.

Etiology
▦ Unknown

Demographics
▦ Five to fifteen percent in the general population
▦ Eight percent lifetime prevalence
▦ Up to half of all referrals for outpatient mental health services are related to ODD and conduct-related issues.

Risk Factors
▦ Age: prior to the age of 8 years
▦ Gender:
  ▦ Boys more than girls
    ● ODD criteria may not fully capture symptoms in girls.
▦ Family history:
  ▦ Exposure to alcohol or in utero toxins may contribute, but this is unclear
  ▦ Maternal depression may be a contributing factor in the development of ODD
  ▦ Parenting style of being harsh, punitive, and inconsistent
  ▦ Parents with alcohol abuse and legal issues
    ● These children are 18% more likely to have ODD.

DIAGNOSIS

Differential Diagnosis
▦ ADHD
  ▦ Fifty percent comorbidity
▦ Mood disorders
▦ Substance abuse

ICD-10 Code
Oppositional Defiant Disorder (F91.3)

Diagnostic Workup
▦ Physical
▦ Establish baseline level of functioning.
  ▦ Understand that stubborn and uncooperative behavior can be normal behaviors, depending on the child's developmental stage when compared with peers.
▦ Instruments as reported in American Academy of Child and Adolescent Psychiatry (AACAP) practice parameter
  ▦ http://www.aacap.org/galleries/PracticeParameters/JAACAP ODD 2007 .pdf/
    ● Conners' Parent Rating Scale (CPRS)
    ● Vanderbilt ADHD Diagnostic Parent Rating Scale
    ● Eyberg Child Behavior Inventory

Initial Assessment
■ Prenatal care
■ Growth and development
■ Medical history
■ Psychiatric history
■ Family history
■ School history

Clinical Presentation
■ Difficult temperament
■ Argumentative
■ Stubborn
■ Refuses even the simplest request
■ Explosive when told "no"
■ Blames others for difficulty, failures, or negative behavior
　■ "You made me do that."
■ Behavioral difficulties are consistent and not within the context of mood symptoms.

DSM-5 Diagnostic Guidelines
■ A pattern of antagonism toward others lasting at least 6 months, during which four or more of the following are present:
　■ Loses temper easily.
　■ Is likely to be argumentative
　■ Refuses to comply with, or actively defies, adults' requests
　■ Goads others
　■ Is likely to blame others for his or her mistakes or misdeeds
　■ Is easily annoyed by others
　■ Is often angry or resentful
　■ Is often spiteful or vindictive

Note: A criterion is met if the behavior occurs more frequently than is typically observed in individuals of comparable age and emotional development.

■ The disturbance in behavior engenders notable impairment of social, academic, or occupational functioning.
■ The antagonistic behavior does not occur concurrently with and exclusively during the course of a psychotic disorder or mood disorder.
■ The criteria for CD are not met, and if the individual is 18 years or older, the criteria for antisocial personality disorder are not met.

TREATMENT OVERVIEW

Behavioral Therapy
■ ODD is not an acute presentation.
■ Individual therapy:
　■ Skills training
　　● Coping skills for anger management, conflict resolution, and peer issues
■ Family therapy:
　■ Parent skills training
　　● Teaching flexibility

Psychopharmacotherapy
▓ Medications
  ▓ Irritability
  ▓ Comorbid diagnosis

PATIENT EDUCATION

▓ Start parent skills training as soon as possible.
▓ Target and reward good behavior.
▓ Reasonable behavioral expectations
▓ Logical consequences
  ▓ Time-out
    ● Use a kitchen timer
    ● Time starts when the children are in their room or on chairs.
▓ Be consistent
  ▓ The rules are the rules
▓ Be flexible
  ▓ Offer a choice
    ● "I need you to take out the trash. Do you want to do it now or in 15 minutes?"
▓ Be very clear.
  ▓ General statements like "straighten up" are too imprecise
    ● "I need you to stop hitting your sister."
▓ Make sure that the child is getting adequate sleep.
▓ Monitor the content of video games and television programs.
  ▓ Aggressive content can normalize violent behavior.

MEDICAL/LEGAL PITFALLS

▓ Children may need an IEP with a behavioral component to address issues at school.
▓ Children are more likely to interface with school and legal authorities.

Learning Disorders

BACKGROUND INFORMATION

Definition of Disorder
▓ Learning disorders (LDs) are diagnosed when achievements on standardized tests are substantially below (at least two standard deviations) what is expected for age, schooling, and level of intelligence, and learning problems significantly interfere with academic achievement and activities of daily living.
▓ These can be categorized as reading disorder, mathematics disorder, and disorder of written expression and LDs (not otherwise specified [NOS]).
▓ Children with LDs have specific impairments in acquiring, retaining, and processing information. Standardized tests place them well below their IQ range in their area of difficulty.
▓ If a sensory deficit is present, the difficulties are in excess of those usually associated with it.
▓ Problematic areas may include the following:

■ Language development and language skills (listening, speaking, reading, writing, and spelling)
■ Social studies
■ Mathematics
■ Social skills
■ Motor skills (fine motor skills, as well as coordination)
■ Cognitive development and memory
■ Attention and organization
■ Test taking

Etiology

■ There may be abnormalities in cognitive processing, including deficits in visual perception, linguistic processes, attention, or memory that precede or are associated with LD.
■ Central nervous system (CNS) damage (prenatal or postnatal)
■ LD may also be caused by such medical conditions as a traumatic brain injury or brain infections, such as encephalitis or meningitis.
■ LD is frequently found in association with a variety of general medical conditions (e.g., lead poisoning, fetal alcohol syndrome, or fragile X syndrome).
■ Prenatal factors that may play a role in LDs include eclampsia, placental insufficiency, cord compression, malnutrition, and bleeding during pregnancy.
■ School dropout rates for children with LDs are 40% (or 1.5 times the average).
■ Prevalence of specific disorders is difficult to determine because many studies focus on the prevalence of LDs in general.
■ Reading disorders are the most common form of LD.
■ Gender: from 60% to 80% of children with reading disorders are males, but when stringent criteria are used, the disorder has been found to occur at more equal rates in males and females. Males more often display disruptive behaviors in association with LDs.
■ Family history: LD aggregates among family members and 40% of first-degree biological relatives of LD children have LDs themselves.
■ Demoralization, low self-esteem, and social skill deficits are associated with LD.
■ Inadequate teaching
■ Learning problems are often stressful for family members and can strain relationships.
■ Children with LDs are more likely to have disruptive behavior disorders.

DIAGNOSIS

Differential Diagnosis

■ Differentiate from normal variations in academic achievement, lack of opportunity, poor teaching, and cultural factors.
■ Impaired vision or hearing may affect learning, and the learning disability cannot be due to sensory impairment.
■ Mental retardation
■ Pervasive developmental disorder
■ Math and written-expression disorders most commonly occur in combination with reading disorders.

▦ ADHD
▦ Ruling out substance use as the most common feature of substance abuse is an impairment in psychosocial and academic functioning.

ICD-10 Codes

Reading disorder specific reading disorder (F81.0)
Mathematics disorder (F81.2)
Disorder of written expression (F81.81)
Developmental disorder of scholastic skills, unspecified (F81.9)

Diagnostic Workup

▦ Individualized testing reflecting attention to ethnic or cultural background
▦ Rule out inadequate teaching and cultural barriers to learning
▦ Because standardized group testing is not accurate enough, it is important that special, psychoeducational tests be individually administered to the child to determine whether he or she has an LD. In administering the test, give special attention to the child's ethnic and cultural background
▦ Commonly used tests include the Wechsler Intelligence Scale for Children (WISC-III), the Woodcock-Johnson Psychoeducational Battery, the Peabody Individual Achievement Test–Revised (PIAT-R), and the California Verbal Learning Test (CVLT).
▦ For substance use as indicated by assessment
▦ To rule out acute infection when problems occur abruptly

Initial Assessments

▦ Medical history and physical examination, including hearing and vision tests
▦ Psychological assessment to include self-esteem and self-confidence
▦ Youth with LDs may also have CD, ADD, or depression
▦ A complete medical examination is needed to rule out an organic cause of the problem. This may include an eye examination by an ophthalmologist, a psychological examination by a psychologist, and an otolaryngology examination

TREATMENT OVERVIEW

Behavioral

▦ Because youth with LDs have higher rates of depression and anxiety and behavior disorders, concurrent treatment for these symptoms must be considered.
▦ Skill development specific to the child's limitations (e.g., social skills, problem solving, study skills, anger control, and leisure skills)
▦ LDs are treated with special educational methods and students with LDs frequently benefit from individualized tutoring focusing on their specific learning problem.
▦ Initial strategies focus on improving a child's recognition of the sounds of letters and language through phonics training. Later strategies focus on comprehension, retention, and study skills. Students with disorders of written expression are often encouraged to keep journals and to write with a computer keyboard instead of a pencil. Instruction for students with mathematical disorders

emphasizes real-world uses of arithmetic, such as balancing a checkbook or comparing prices.
- In the academic setting, short, brief assignments with time for feedback, preferential seating, reduced written tasks, support in organization and study skills, untimed tests and assignments, and colored cued materials and techniques
- Symptoms may occur as early as kindergarten.
- Up to 40% of LD youth drop out of school, so chronic counseling, special education services, and other support are often needed.

Recurrence Rate
- LDs can continue into adulthood, but with treatment and special accommodations, symptoms can be decreased.
- Children with undiagnosed LDs or who are improperly treated/educated may never achieve functional literacy. They often develop serious behavior problems as a result of their frustration with school.

PATIENT EDUCATION

- Parents of children with LDs should stay in close contact with educators and school administrators to ensure that their child's IEP undergoes a regular review and continues to provide the maximum educational benefit.
- School evaluations that include observations of the child in class can offer crucial information about coexisting issues.
- Mental health services may be required in addition to special academic services. Issues addressed in counseling children with LDs can include frustration, anxiety related to school performance, poor peer relationships, and depression.

MEDICAL/LEGAL ISSUES

- Federal legislation mandates that testing be free of charge within the public school system. The IDEA guides the actions of school committees on special education in determining the eligibility for special services of students through the age of 21 years.
- Parents may need legal assistance to ensure their child's needs are met by the school system.

Disorder of Written Expression

BACKGROUND INFORMATION

Definition of Disorder
- Writing abilities that fall below the expected level of performance based on the child's age, education, and intellectual ability
- Difficulty with putting thoughts on paper
- Difficulty with organizing grammatically correct sentences, paragraphs, or narratives
- Poor spelling and poor handwriting

Etiology
- Genetic influences
- Deficits in writing are attributed to faulty interactions between sensory inputs and motor outputs.

Demographics
- Estimated at 4% of schoolchildren
- Equal among boys and girls

Risk Factors
- Family history of LDs: reading, writing, mathematics
- Family history of developmental disorders

DIAGNOSIS

ICD-10 Codes
Disorder of written expression (F81.81)
Developmental disorder of scholastic skills, unspecified (F81.9)

Diagnostic Workup
- Performed by an education or language specialist
- Evaluation of affective states (anxiety and worry) that impact writing ability
- Takes into consideration the following:
  - Legibility
  - Speed of writing
  - Spelling
  - Vocabulary
  - Punctuation and usage
  - Sentence construction
  - Organization and planning
  - Attention and concentration
- Evaluates writing ability in context of different writing components: copying, dictating, spontaneity
- Standardized testing:
  - Test of written language
  - Test of early written language
  - Standardized intelligence testing

Initial Assessment
- Initial referral often made by a teacher
- Has the child attended school regularly?
- Review of child's academic record: Is the child's level of performance below the expected level when compared with the peers?

Clinical Presentation
- Frequent spelling errors
- Punctuation errors
- Grammatical errors
- Poor handwriting

■ Letters may be reversed, backward, or undistinguishable
■ Does not like school because child feels inadequate
■ Reluctant to participate in activities that require writing
■ May have social problems

DSM-5 **Diagnostic Guidelines**
Disorder of Written Expression

■ Writing skills as measured by standardized tests (or functional assessments of writing skills) are notably inferior to what would be expected on the basis of the individual's chronological age, intelligence (as measured by intelligence tests), and age-appropriate educational level.
■ This disorder is applicable to specific spelling disorder.
■ The presence of weak writing skills significantly interferes with academic performance and academic achievement, as well as activities of daily living that require the composition of written sentences.
■ If a sensory deficit is present, the reduction in writing ability is in excess of that usually associated with that deficit.

Note: If a sensory deficit or another medical condition (such as a neurological condition) is present, the condition should be diagnosed as such.

Learning Disorder—NOS

■ To be used for disorders in learning that do not meet the criteria for a specific learning disorder.
■ Very likely to include impairment in three areas (reading, written expression, mathematics), which, together, significantly hinder academic achievement even though performances on tests that measure the three skills individually are not substantially below what is expected on the basis of the individual's chronological age, intelligence (as measured by intelligence tests), and age-appropriate educational level.

TREATMENT OVERVIEW

■ No medical interventions
■ Writing plan is developed by an education and writing specialist in collaboration with teachers and parents.
■ Family support addresses anxiety or worry related to writing performance.
■ IEP, which sets goals and identifies interventions for improving performance
■ School accommodations: scribes, keyboards, computers, help with class notes, longer test-taking times

PATIENT EDUCATION

■ EI is paramount in preventing the potential long-term consequences of LDs, such as poor self-esteem, decreased learning, and academic failure.
■ Incorporate the child's interest into writing.

MEDICAL/LEGAL PITFALLS

■ Protected under the IDEA, http://idea.ed.gov/

Mathematics Disorder

BACKGROUND INFORMATION

Definition of Disorder
▦ Difficulty with mathematics in a manner that is not consistent with a child's age, intellect, education, and motivation to learn

Etiology
▦ Heritability: genetic connection
▦ Cognitive deficits in visual spatial ability

Demographics
▦ Six to seven percent of school-age children are estimated to have mathematics disorder (MD).
▦ Impacts boys and girls equally
▦ Two thirds of all children with MD have a comorbid diagnosis of language delay, dyslexia, or ADHD.

Risk Factors
▦ Lower social economic status
▦ Poor learning environment
▦ Family history of math disorders
▦ Preexisting reading disorders: children with reading problems often have difficulty with comprehension problems, which impacts mathematics.

DIAGNOSIS

ICD-10 Code
Mathematics disorder (F81.2)

Diagnostic Workup
▦ Functional eye examination
▦ Can the child name the number (flash cards with numbers on them)?
▦ Does the child understand numbering, counting?
▦ Does the child understand math concepts (base 10)?
▦ Does the child understand math procedures (−, +, ×, ÷) or borrowing and carrying numbers?
▦ Does the child transpose numbers?
▦ Can the child retrieve math facts from memory (times tables)?
▦ Testing is standardized: refer to psychologist or education specialist.

Initial Assessment
▦ Is there a family history of learning disability?
▦ Has the child regularly attended school?
▦ Is there a consistent pattern of decreased performance in math as compared to other subjects?

Clinical Presentation

- Difficulty with reading and writing numbers
- Difficulty with retaining and retrieving math facts
- Math grades are consistently lower than expected.
- Child may be feel demoralized by inability to achieve in mathematics.
- Difficulty may not become evident until third grade, when math reasoning is required.

DSM-5 Diagnostic Guidelines

- Mathematical ability, as measured by standardized tests, is notably inferior to what would be expected on the basis of the individual's chronological age, intelligence (as measured by intelligence tests), and age-appropriate educational level.
- The reduced mathematical ability hinders academic performance, academic achievement, and activities of daily living that require mathematical ability.
- If a sensory deficit is present, the reduction in mathematical ability is in excess of the losses that are usually associated with the deficit.

Note: If a general medical condition (such as a neurological condition) or a sensory deficit is present, the disturbance should be diagnosed as such.

- This disorder is applicable to developmental acalculia, developmental arithmetical disorder, and developmental Gerstmann's syndrome.
- This disorder excludes arithmetical difficulties associated with a reading disorder, a spelling disorder, and arithmetical disorders due to inadequate teaching.

TREATMENT OVERVIEW

- IEP with accommodations as needed
- Teaching strategies as identified by an education specialist
- Address all areas of weakness to foster success (language processing and working memory).
- Develop the child's strengths and abilities to promote resilience.
- Screen for comorbid diagnosis.

PATIENT/FAMILY EDUCATION

- Organize homework space at home to be free of distractions.
- Allow the child to use the fingers or other items to count.
- Break down assignments into manageable parts.
- Check his or her work at each step.
- Incorporate the child's interest into examples (sports statistics).
- Some children may benefit from talking math problems out or having visual learning aids.
- Computer programs can be a fun, creative, and effective way of learning and practicing math skills.

MEDICAL/LEGAL PITFALLS

- Protected under the IDEA, http://idea.ed.gov/

Mixed Receptive–Expressive Language Disorder

BACKGROUND INFORMATION

Definition of Disorder
■ A mixed receptive–expressive language disorder is a language disability that causes impairment of both the understanding and the expression of language.

Etiology
■ Communication disorders may be developmental or acquired.
■ The cause is believed to be based on biological problems, such as abnormalities of brain development, or possibly by exposure to toxins during pregnancy, such as abused substances or environmental toxins such as lead.
■ A genetic factor is sometimes considered a contributing cause in some cases.
■ Some causes of speech and language disorders include hearing loss; neurological disorders; brain injury; mental retardation; drug abuse; physical impairments, such as a cleft lip or palate; and vocal abuse or misuse.
■ Frequently, however, the cause is unknown.
■ For unknown reasons, boys are diagnosed with communication disorders more often than girls.
■ Children with communication disorders frequently have other developmental disorders as well.
■ Most children with communication disorders are able to speak by the time they enter school; however, they continue to have problems with communication. School-age children often have problems understanding and formulating words.
■ Teens may have more difficulty with understanding or expressing abstract ideas.
■ Diagnosis for receptive–expressive language disorder:
  ■ Most children with communication disorders are first referred for speech and language evaluations when their delays in communicating are noted.
  ■ A child psychiatrist is usually consulted, especially when emotional or behavioral problems are also present.
  ■ A comprehensive evaluation also involves psychometric testing (testing designed to assess logical reasoning abilities, reactions to different situations, and thinking performance, not tests of general knowledge) and psychological testing of cognitive abilities.
  ■ There are varied language disorders—for example, receptive language may be mildly delayed and expressive language may be severely delayed.
  ■ Knowing the type of mixed receptive–expressive language delay is important because the split may impact academics.
  ■ For once, the child may exhibit severely delayed receptive language skills and only mildly delayed expressive language.
  ■ The receptive language difficulties will most likely have a significant impact on being able to follow directions and understand classroom instruction.
  ■ This child will need extra help (written directions, one-on-one time) in order to be successful.
  ■ Many speech problems are developmental rather than physiological, and as such they respond to remedial instruction.
  ■ Language experiences are vital to a young child's development. In the past, children with communication disorders were routinely removed from the regular class for individual speech and language therapy.

■ This is still the case in severe instances, but the trend is toward keeping the child in the mainstream as much as possible.

■ In order to accomplish this goal, teamwork among the teacher, the speech and language therapist, the audiologist, and parents is essential.

■ Speech improvement and correction are blended into the regular classroom curriculum and the child's natural environment.

■ It is a communication disorder in which both the receptive and expressive areas of communication may be affected in any degree, from mild to severe.

■ If someone is being assessed on the Wechsler Adult Intelligence Scale, for instance, this may show up in relatively low scores for information, vocabulary, and comprehension (perhaps below the 25th percentile). If the person has difficulty with spatial concepts, such as "over," "under," "here," and "there," he or she may have arithmetic difficulties, difficulty in understanding word problems and instructions, or have difficulties using words.

■ He or she may also have a more general problem with words or sentences, both understanding and speaking them.

■ If someone is suspected to have a mixed receptive–expressive language disorder, then that person can go to a speech therapist or pathologist, and receive treatment. Most treatments are short term and rely on accommodations made in the person's environment, so as to interfere minimally with work and school functioning.

■ Three to five percent of all children have either a receptive or an expressive language disorder, or both.

■ These children have difficulty understanding speech (language receptivity) and using language (language expression).

■ The cause is unknown, but there may be genetic factors and malnutrition may play a role.

■ Problems with receptive language skills usually begin before the age of 4 years.

■ Some mixed-language disorders are caused by brain injury, and these are sometimes misdiagnosed as developmental disorders.

DIAGNOSIS

Differential Diagnosis
■ Dyslexia
■ Autism
■ LDs
■ Mental retardation

ICD-10 Code
Mixed receptive–Expressive language disorder (F80.2)

Clinical Presentation
The following are the most common symptoms of communication disorders. However, each child may experience symptoms differently.

■ May not speak at all, or may have a limited vocabulary for his or her age
■ Has difficulty in understanding simple directions or is unable to name objects
■ Shows problems with socialization

▦ Inability to follow directions but shows comprehension with routine, repetitive directions
▦ Echolalia (repeating back words or phrases either immediately or at a later time)
▦ Inappropriate responses to "why" questions
▦ Difficulty in responding appropriately to "yes/no" questions, "either/or" questions, "who/what/where" questions, or "when/why/how" questions
▦ Repeats back a question first and then responds to it
▦ High activity level and not attending to spoken language
▦ Jargon (e.g., unintelligible speech) is used.
▦ Uses "memorized" phrases and sentences
▦ The child may have a problem with words or sentences, in both understanding and speaking them.
▦ Learning problems and academic difficulties occur.
▦ Although many speech and language patterns can be called "baby talk" and are part of a young child's normal development, they can become problems if they are not outgrown as expected.
▦ In this way, an initial delay in speech and language or an initial speech pattern can become a disorder, which can cause difficulties in learning. Because of the way the brain develops, it is easier to learn language and communication skills before the age of 5 years.
▦ The symptoms of communication disorders may resemble other problems or medical conditions.
▦ Always consult your child's physician for diagnosis of the following:
  ▦ Problems with language comprehension
  ▦ Problems with language expression
  ▦ Speech containing many articulation errors
  ▦ Difficulty recalling early sight or sound memories

DSM-5 Diagnostic Guidelines
▦ Impairment in both receptive and expressive language development, as demonstrated by lowered scoring on standardized tests (e.g., IQ tests)
▦ Characterized by reductions in receptive language skills whereby a child has difficulty in extracting usable information from spoken language
▦ Characterized by reductions in expressive language skills whereby a child has a diminished vocabulary, has difficulty in producing words and sentences, and uses verb tenses incorrectly
Note: Measures/tests of language development must be appropriate to and relevant to language use in the specific cultural group.

▦ Onset is generally before the age of 4 years. However, this disorder can also occur if there is physical trauma later in childhood, for example, head injury.
▦ With positive input, some affected children may develop normal language.
▦ Associated features and disorders are as follows:
  ▦ Conversational skills (e.g., waiting one's turn to speak, staying with a topic of conversation) are lacking.
  ▦ A deficit in some aspect of sensory information processing is common (especially in auditory information processing).
  ▦ Difficulties with the language's sound system are often present.
  ▦ LDs are often present.
  ▦ Memory impairments

■ May occur concurrently with attention deficit hyperactivity disorder, developmental coordination disorder, or enuresis
■ The ability to process verbal output is reduced. The individual may find it difficult to absorb and recall a simple list of instructions.
■ There may be high levels of competence in non-language-based problem solving.
■ Note: A school psychologist, clinical psychologist, psychiatrist, or other qualified specialist should make this diagnosis. If there is a head injury or another medical problem (e.g., encephalitis), a physician should be on the diagnostic team.
■ This is applicable to developmental dysphasia or aphasia, receptive type, and developmental Wernicke's aphasia.
■ Type 1 excludes central auditory processing disorder, dysphasia or aphasia NOS, expressive language disorder, expressive type dysphasia or aphasia, and word deafness.
■ Type 2 excludes acquired aphasia with epilepsy, pervasive developmental disorders, selective mutism, and intellectual disabilities.

Laboratory Tests
■ Standardized receptive and expressive language tests can be given to any child suspected of having this disorder.
■ An audiogram should also be given to rule out the possibility of deafness as it is one of the most common causes of language problems.
■ All children diagnosed with this condition should be seen by a neurologist or a developmental pediatric specialist to determine whether the cause can be reversed.
■ If someone is being assessed on the Wechsler Adult Intelligence Scale, for instance, this may show up in relatively low scores for information, vocabulary, and comprehension (perhaps below the 25th percentile). If the person has difficulty with spatial concepts, such as "over," "under," "here," and "there," he or she may have arithmetic difficulties, have difficulty understanding word problems and instructions, or have difficulties using words.

TREATMENT OVERVIEW

■ Speech and language therapy are the best approach to this type of language disorder.
■ A coordinated effort among parents, teachers, and speech/language and mental health professionals provides the basis for individualized treatment strategies that may include individual or group remediation, special classes, or special resources.
■ Special-education techniques are used to increase communication skills in the areas of the deficit.
■ A second approach helps the child build on his or her strengths to overcome his or her communication deficit.
■ Specific treatment for communication disorders will be determined by your child's physician, special-education teachers, and speech/language and mental health professionals on the basis of the following:
    ▪ Your child's age, overall health, and medical history
    ▪ Extent of the disorder
■ Psychotherapy is also recommended because of the possibility of associated emotional or behavioral problems.

- Type of disorder
- Your child's tolerance for specific medications or therapies
- Expectations for the course of the disorder
- Your opinion or preference
■ SLPs assist children who have communication disorders in various ways.
  - They provide individual therapy for the child, consult with the child's teacher about the most effective ways to facilitate the child's communication in the class setting, and work closely with the family to develop goals and techniques for effective therapy in class and at home.
  - Early detection and intervention can address the developmental needs and academic difficulties to improve the quality of life experienced by children with communication disorders.
  - The SLP may assist vocational teachers and counselors in establishing communication goals related to the work experiences of students and suggest strategies that are effective for the important transition from school to employment and adult life.

PATIENT EDUCATION

- The outcome varies based on the underlying cause.
- Brain injury or other structural pathology is generally associated with a poor outcome with chronic deficiencies in language, whereas other, more reversible causes can be treated effectively.
- Difficulty in understanding and using language can cause problems with social interaction and inability to function independently as an adult.
- The outcome varies based on the underlying cause.
- Brain injury or other structural pathology is generally associated with a poor outcome with chronic deficiencies in language, whereas other, more reversible causes can be treated effectively.
- Difficulty understanding and using language can cause problems with social interaction and ability to function independently as an adult.

BIBLIOGRAPHY

American Academy of Child and Adolescent Psychiatry. (1997). *Practice parameter for the assessment and treatment of children and adolescents with conduct disorder*. Retrieved on January 2, 2009, from http://www.aacap.org/galleries/PracticeParameters/Conduct.pdf/

American Academy of Family Physicians. (2008). Oppositional defiant disorder. *American Family Physician, 78*(7), 861–868.

American Psychiatric Association. (2000). *Diagnostic and statistical manual of mental disorders* (4th ed., text revision). Washington, DC: American Psychiatric Press.

Berninger, V. W., Abbott, R. D., Abbott, S. P., Graham, S., & Richards, T. (2002). Writing and reading: Connections between language by hand and language by eye. *Journal of Learning Disabilities, 35*(1), 39–56.

Bernstein, B. E. (2008). *Learning disorder: Written expression*. Retrieved on February 15, 2009, from http://emedicine.medscape.com/article/918389-overview/

Bothe, A. K., Davidow, J. H., Bramlett, R. E., Franic, D. M., & Ingham, R. J. (2006). Stuttering treatment research 1970–2005: II. Systemic review incorporating trial quality assessment of pharmacological approaches. *American Journal of Speech-Language Pathology, 15*(4), 342–352.

Chandler, J. (n.d.). *Oppositional defiant disorder (ODD) and conduct disorder (CD) in children and adolescents: diagnosis and treatment.* Retrieved on January 2, 2009, from http://www.klis.com/chandler/pamphlet/oddcd/oddcdpamphlet.htm# Toc121406159/

Department of Health and Human Services. (1999). *Mental health: A report of the Surgeon General.* Retrieved on December 27, 2008, from http://www.surgeongeneral.gov/library/mentalhealth/chapter3/sec7.html/

Department of Health and Human Services. (2008). *Autism spectrum disorders: Pervasive developmental disorders.* NIH Publication No. 08–5511. Bethesda, MD: Department of Health and Human Services.

Feifer, S. G. (2007). *The neuropsychology of math disorders: Diagnosis and intervention.* Retrieved on February 12, 2009, from http://www.ahi-online.com/schoolpsychhandouts2008/lasvegas/feiffer-mathematics.pdf/

Fitz, K. (2003). Review of theoretical and applied issues in written language expression. *Canadian Journal of School Psychology, 18*(12), 203–222.

Grigorenko, E. L. (2006). Learning disabilities in juvenile offenders. *Child and Adolescent Psychiatric Clinics of North America, 15*(2), 353–71, viii.

Hadley, P. A. (2006). Assessing the emergence of grammar in toddlers at risk for specific language impairment. *Seminars in Speech and Language, 27*(3), 173–186, Review.

Hamilton, S. S., & Glascoe, F. P. (2006). Evaluation of children with reading difficulties. *American Family Physician, 74*(12), 2079–2084.

Hearne, A., Packman, A., Onslow, M., & Quine, S. (2008). Stuttering and its treatment in adolescence: The perceptions of people who stutter. *Journal of Fluency Disorders, 33*, 81–98.

Howell, P., Davis, S., & Williams, S. M. (2006). Auditory abilities of speakers who persisted, or recovered, from stuttering. *Journal of Fluency Disorders, 31*, 257–270.

Jones, A. P., Laurens, K. R., Herba, C. M., Barker, G. J., & Viding, E. (2009). Amygdala hypoactivity to fearful faces in boys with conduct problems and callous-unemotional traits. *American Journal of Psychiatry, 166*(1), 95–102.

Koenig, K., & Scahill, L. (2001). Assessment of children with pervasive developmental disorders. *Journal of Child and Adolescent Psychiatric Nursing, 14*(4), 159–166.

Lavigne, J. V., LeBailly, S. A., Gouze, K. R., Cicchetti, C., Jessup, B. W., Arend, R., ... Binns, H. J. (2008). Predictor and moderator effects in the treatment of oppositional defiant disorder in pediatric primary care. *Journal of Pediatric Psychology, 33*(5), 462–472.

McGlaughlin, S. M., Knoop, A. J., & Holliday, G. A. (2005). Differentiating students with mathematics difficulty in college: Mathematics disabilities vs. no diagnosis. *Learning Disability Quarterly, 28*(3), 223–232.

Miller, J. L. (2000). *Written expression disorder.* Retrieved on February 3, 2009, from http://www.athealth.com/consumer/disorders/writtenexp.html/

Rubia, K., Rozmin, H., Smith, A. B., Mohammed, M., Scott, S., Giampietro, V., ... Brammer, M. J. (2008). Dissociated functional brain abnormalities of inhibition in boys with pure conduct disorder and in boys with pure attention deficit hyperactivity disorder. *American Journal of Psychiatry, 165*(7), 889–897.

Rubia, K., Smith, A. B., Halari, R., Matsukura, F., Mahammad, M., Taylor, E., . . . Brammer, M. J. (2009). Disorder-specific dissociation of orbitofrontal dysfunction in boys with pure conduct disorder during reward and ventrolateral prefrontal dysfunction in boys with pure ADHD during sustained attention. *American Journal of Psychiatry, 166*(1), 83–94.

Searright, H. R., Rottnek, F., & Abby, S. L. (2001). Conduct disorder: Diagnosis and treatment in primary care. *American Family Physician, 63*(8), 1579–1588.

Stigler, K. A., & McDougle, D. J. (2008). Pharmacotherapy of irritability in pervasive developmental disorders. *Child and Adolescent Psychiatric Clinics of North America, 17*(4), 739–752.

Tynan, W. D. (2008). *Oppositional defiant disorder.* eMedicine. Retrieved on January 2, 2009, from http://emedicine.medscape.com/article/918095-overview/

Van Loosbroek, E., Dirkz, G., Hulstijn, W., & Janssen, F. (2009). When the mental number line involves a delay: The writing of numbers by children of different arithmetical abilities. *Journal of Experimental Child Psychology, 102,* 26–39.

Von Aster, M. G., & Shalev, R. S. (2007). Number development and developmental dyscalculia. *Developmental Medicine &Child Neurology, 49*(11), 868–873.

Woolfenden, S. R., Williams, K., & Peat, J. K. (2002). Family and parenting interventions for conduct disorder and delinquency: A meta-analysis of randomized controlled trials. *Archives of Disease in Childhood, 86*(4), 251–256.

WEB RESOURCES

- Athealth.com: http://www.athealth.com/consumer/disorders/writtenexp.html/
- Early Intervention Programs for Infants and Toddlers with Disabilities (Part C of IDEA): http://www.nectac.org/partc/partc.asp#overview/
- eMedicine, Learning Disabilities: http://emedicine.medscape.com/
- Family Self-Help Groups: http://www.nami.org/
- Family Village: http://www.familyvillage.wisc.edu/lib stut.htm/
- The Interactive Guide to Learning Disabilities for Parents, Teachers, and Children: http://www.ldonline.org/
- Learning Disability Association of America: http://www.ldanatl.org/
- Learning Disability Forum: Learning Disability Information and Rights: http:// learningdisabilityforum.com/
- Learning Disabilities Online Page: http://www.ldonline.org/
- National Center for Learning Disabilities (NCLD): http://www.ncld.org/
- National Education Association, IDEA/Special Education: http://www.nea.org/ specialed/
- National Institute of Neurological Disorders and Stroke: http://www.ninds. nih.gov/disorders/pdd/pdd.htm/
- National Stuttering Association: http://www.nsastutter.org/content/ index.php?catid = 1/
- National Youth Violence Prevention Resource Center: http://www.safeyouth.org/ scripts/topics/conduct.aspnternet Support/
- Oppositional Defiant Disorder (ODD) and Conduct Disorder (CD) in Children and Adolescents: Diagnosis and Treatment: http://www.klis.com/chandler/ pamphlet/oddcd/oddcdpamphlet.htm# Toc121406159/
- Our Defiant Kids: http://ourdefiantkids.com/
- The Stuttering Foundation: http://www.stutteringhelp.org/

Drug Monographs

ALPRAZOLAM (*XANAX/XANAX XR/NIRAVAM*; ALSO *APO-ALPRAZ, APO-ALPRAZ TS, NOVO-ALPRAZOL, NU-ALPRAZ*)

Classification
Benzodiazepine (BZD), anxiolytic

Indications
Short-acting BZD is used to treat generalized anxiety disorder and panic disorder. It may be used as a short-term adjunct to a selective serotonin reuptake inhibitor (SSRI) while waiting for the therapeutic effects of the SSRI to develop.

Available Forms
Tablet, 0.25, 0.5, 1, and 2 mg; orally disintegrating tablets (ODTs)—0.25, 0.5, 1, 2, and 3 mg; oral solution, extended-release capsule, 0.5, 1, and 2 mg; melt, 0.25, 0.5, 1, 2, and 3 mg. oral solution 1 mg/mL.

Dosage
▦ *Xanax*: Starting dose, 0.25 to 0.5 mg up to two to three times daily; maximum, 4 mg daily. It can be increased every 3 to 4 days. Treatment should be limited to as short a period as possible (less than 4 months) and/or reevaluated for continued use.
▦ *Xanax XR*: Starting dose, 0.5 to 1 mg PO, daily. It can increase up to 1 mg/day every 3 to 4 days.
▦ *Niravam (melt)*: Starting dose, 0.25 to 0.5 mg up to two to three times daily; maximum, 4 mg daily. It can be increased every 3 to 4 days.

Administration
▦ PO with a glass of water.
▦ Do not crush, cut, or chew extended-release tablets.
▦ Orally disintegrating form *(Niravam)* has special instructions.
▦ Concentrated liquid must be measured with a special dose-measuring spoon or cup. It comes with a calibrated dropper. Measured portion should be squeezed into liquid or semi-solid food. Do not store for future use.

Side Effects
▦ Drowsiness, lightheadedness, dry mouth, headache, changes in bowel habits, diarrhea, amnesia, changes in appetite, changes in sexual desire, constipation, increased saliva production, tiredness, trouble concentrating, unsteadiness, and weight changes.
▦ Some other side effects are syncope, tachycardia, seizures, respiratory depression, dependency, withdrawal syndrome, and suicidal ideation, and hypomania/mania.

Drug Interactions
▦ Contraindicated in patients with known sensitivity to this drug or other BZPs.
▦ Avoid grapefruit juice when using this drug.
▦ It may be used in patients with open-angle glaucoma who are receiving appropriate therapy but is contraindicated in patients with acute narrow-angle glaucoma.

NOTE: For some drugs, off-label use is reported. It is the responsibility of the practitioner to evaluate the efficacy of such use.

◼ This is contraindicated with ketoconazole and itraconazole, as these medications significantly impair the oxidative metabolism mediated by cytochrome P450 3A (CYP3A).

Pharmacokinetics

The drug metabolizes in the liver (CYP450) and is excreted in the urine. It binds to BZP receptors and enhances gamma-aminobutyric acid (GABA) effects.

BZDs enhance the activity of GABA, a major central nervous system (CNS) neurotransmitter, known to open CNS Cl-channels, leading to an inhibition of subsequent CNS neuronal signaling. BZDs with similar action can differ in their potency and rate of absorption.

◼ *Metabolism:* by the liver in the CYP450 3A4
◼ *Excretion:* urine
◼ *Peak:* 1 to 2 hours
◼ *Half-life:* Xanax half-life-immediate release: 11.2 hours; extended-release: 10.7 to 15.8 hours; 13 hours for oral disintegrating tablets

Precautions

◼ Do not abruptly stop taking the medication.
◼ It is not prescribed for children.
◼ Use lowest effective dose for shortest duration.
◼ It can be habit forming; do not increase dosage without checking patient compliance and review of chief complaints.
◼ Keep out of light in a tightly closed container.
◼ Store securely at room temperature.
◼ See patients as often as necessary to ensure that the drug is working on the panic attacks, determine compliance, and review side effects.
◼ Instruct patients and their families to watch for worsening depression or thoughts of suicide. Also, watch out for sudden or severe changes in feelings, such as feeling anxious, agitated, panicky, irritated, hostile, aggressive, impulsive, severely restless, overly excited, hyperactive, or not being able to sleep. If this happens, especially at the beginning of antidepressant treatment or after a change in dose, patient should call the health care provider.
◼ *Drowsiness or dizziness:* Patients should not drive or use machinery or do anything that needs mental alertness until the effects of this medicine are known.
◼ Caution patients not to stand or sit up quickly, especially if older. This reduces the risk of dizziness or fainting spells. Alcohol may interfere with the effect of this medicine. Avoid alcoholic drinks.
◼ Do not abruptly withdraw this drug as it may cause seizures.
◼ Caution should be exercised in the following:
  ◼ Major depressive disorder, psychosis, or bipolar affective disorder
  ◼ Respiratory disease
  ◼ Sleep apnea
  ◼ Heart disease
  ◼ Liver disease
  ◼ Seizures (convulsions)
  ◼ Suicidal thoughts, plans, or attempts by patients or a family member

---

NOTE: For some drugs, off-label use is reported. It is the responsibility of the practitioner to evaluate the efficacy of such use.

■ An unusual or allergic reaction to alprazolam, other medicines, foods, dyes, or preservatives

Patient and Family Education

■ Tell the health care provider of glaucoma, hepatic or renal impairment, drug-abuse history, salivary flow decrease (interferes with ODT absorption), or pregnancy.

■ Missed doses should be taken as soon as possible; however, if it is too close to next dose, then it should be skipped.

■ Take the medicine as prescribed and do not stop it abruptly, without first discussing with health care provider.

■ Store alprazolam at room temperature away from moisture, heat, and light. Remove any cotton from the bottle of disintegrating tablets, and keep the bottle tightly closed. Discard liquid 90 days after first opening.

■ Before taking this medicine, tell the health care provider of medical history of liver disease, kidney disease, lung/breathing problems, drug or alcohol abuse, or any allergies.

■ Do not drive, operate heavy machinery, or perform dangerous activities until it is known how this medicine will exert its effects.

■ This drug may be habit forming and should be used only by the person for whom it was prescribed. Alprazolam should never be shared with another person, especially someone who has a history of drug abuse or addiction. Keep the medication in a secure place where others cannot get to it.

Special Populations

■ *Elderly:* Older patients may be more sensitive to the effects of BZDs. Give 0.25 mg PO BID or TID. Use lowest, most effective dose. Dose adjustment is necessary for patients with liver impairment and/or renal disease due to excessive metabolites excreted by the kidney. Due to increased risk of sedation leading to falls and fractures, all BZDs are included on the Beers List of Potentially Inappropriate Medications for Geriatrics.

■ *Renal impairment:* No adjustment needed.

■ *Hepatic impairment:* With advanced hepatic disease, start at 0.25 mg PO BID or TID and titrate gradually.

■ *Pregnancy:* Category D; can cause teratogenic fetal effects. Infants born to mothers taking BZDs may be at risk for withdrawal symptoms contraindicated in the postnatal period.

■ *Lactation:* Excreted in human breast milk; infants can become lethargic and lose weight.

■ *Children:* Not indicated for use in children younger than 18 years of age.

AMITRIPTYLINE HYDROCHLORIDE (*ELAVIL*)

Classification
Tricyclic antidepressant (TCA)

Indications
The drug is used to treat adults with depression. It has been used off label for anxiety disorders, post herpetic neuralgia, prevention of chronic headache, prevention of migraine, and fibromyalgia.

Available Forms
Tablet, 10, 25, 50, 75, 100, and 150 mg

Dosage
▦ *Adults and adolescents:* Between 25 to 75 mg PO at bedtime. Dosage can be increased by 25 to 50 mg/day every week up to 200 mg until desired effect occurs. Maximum daily dose for hospitalized patients is 300 mg.
▦ *Elderly:* Starting dose, 10 to 25 mg PO at night in elderly patients; dosage can be increased by 10 to 25 mg/day every week. Maximum daily dose is 150 mg/day.
▦ *Children (9–12 years old):* 1 to 3 mg/kg/day PO divided TID with gradual increase by 0.5 mg/kg/day every 2 to 3 days. The dosage must be tapered gradually to discontinue. There is a black box warning. Not for use in children younger than 12 years of age.

Administration
▦ PO with a glass of water
▦ Do not abruptly stop taking the medication.
▦ Use lowest effective dose for shortest duration.

Side Effects
▦ *Most common:* Drowsiness, dry mouth, dizziness, constipation, blurred vision, palpitations, tachycardia, lack of coordination, appetite increase, nausea/vomiting, sweating, weakness, disorientation, confusion, restlessness, insomnia, anxiety/agitation, urinary retention/urinary frequency, rash/urticaria, pruritus, weight gain, libido changes, impotence, gynecomastia, galactorrhea, tremor, hypo/hyperglycemia, paresthesias, and photosensitivity
▦ *Less common:* Hypertension or orthostatic hypotension, ventricular arrhythmias, extrapyramidal symptoms, thrombocytopenia

Drug Interactions
▦ There are many drugs that may interact with amytriptiline.
▦ Some of the most common drugs that react with amytriptitline are arbutamine, disulfiram, levodopa, thyroid supplements, and other drugs that can cause bleeding/bruising (including antiplatelet drugs such as clopidogrel, nonsteroidal anti-inflammatory drugs such as ibuprofen, "blood thinners" such as warfarin),

---

NOTE: For some drugs, off-label use is reported. It is the responsibility of the practitioner to evaluate the efficacy of such use.

anticholinergic drugs (such as benztropine, belladonna alkaloids), some antihypertensive drugs such as clonidine, guanabenz, reserpine.

■ Avoid taking monoamine oxidase inhibitors (isocarboxazid, linezolid, methylene blue, moclobemide, phenelzine, procarbazine, rasagiline, selegiline, tranylcypromine) within 2 weeks before, during, and after treatment with this medication.

■ Avoid cimetidine, fluconazole, terbinafine, drugs to treat irregular heart rate (such as quinidine/propafenone/flecainide), and antidepressants (such as SSRIs, including paroxetine/fluoxetine/fluvoxamine). These drugs can affect the removal of amitriptyline from the body, thereby affecting how amitriptyline works.

■ Many drugs besides amitriptyline may affect the heart rhythm (QT prolongation in the EKG), including amiodarone, cisapride, dofetilide, pimozide, procainamide, quinidine, sotalol, macrolide antibiotics (such as erythromycin), among others.

■ Avoid drugs that may cause drowsiness, such as alcohol, antihistamines (such as cetirizine, diphenhydramine), drugs for sleep or anxiety (such as alprazolam, diazepam, zolpidem), muscle relaxants, and narcotic pain relievers (such as codeine).

■ Seizure risk may increase when amitriptyline is combined with isoniazid (INH), phenothiazines (such as thioridazine), theophylline, or TCAs (such as nortriptyline), among others.

Pharmacokinetics

■ TCAs are thought to work by inhibiting reuptake of norepinephrine and serotonin in the central nervous system, which potentiates the neurotransmitters. They also have significant anticholinergics, antihistaminic, and alpha-adrenergic activity on the cardiac system. These classes of antidepressants also possess Class 1A antiarrhythmic activity, which can lead to depression of cardiac conduction, potentially resulting in heart block or ventricular arrhythmias.

■ *Metabolism:* Extensively by the liver within the CYP450: 1A2, 2D6 (primary), 3A4 substrate; active metabolites include nortriptyline

■ *Peak*: 2 to 12 hours

■ *Excretion:* Primarily in urine (18% unchanged), feces

■ *Half-life:* 10 to 50 hours (amitriptyline)

Precautions

■ See patients as often as necessary to ensure that the drug is working on the panic attacks, determine compliance, and review side effects.

■ Instruct patients and families to watch for worsening depression or thoughts of suicide. Also, watch out for sudden or severe changes in feelings, such as feeling anxious, agitated, panicky, irritated, hostile, aggressive, impulsive, severely restless, overly excited, hyperactive, or not being able to sleep. If this happens, especially at the beginning of antidepressant treatment or after a change in dose, patient should call the health care provider.

■ *Drowsiness or dizziness*: Patients should not drive, use machinery, or do anything that needs mental alertness until the effects of this medicine are known. Caution patients not to stand or sit up quickly, especially if older. This reduces the risk of dizziness or fainting spells. Alcohol may interfere with the effect of this medicine. Avoid alcoholic drinks.

NOTE: For some drugs, off-label use is reported. It is the responsibility of the practitioner to evaluate the efficacy of such use.

- Do not abruptly withdraw this drug, as it may cause headache, nausea, and malaise.
- Advise to protect skin from ultraviolet light due to increased skin sensitivity.
- Grapefruit and grapefruit juice may interact with drug. Caution should be exercised in the following:
    - Major depressive disorder, psychosis, or bipolar affective disorder
    - Contraindicated in patients with a recent myocardial infarction
    - Blood dyscrasias
    - Respiratory disease
    - Heart disease
    - Liver disease, diabetes mellitus, asthma, and increased intracranial pressure
    - Seizures (convulsions)
    - Suicidal thoughts, plans, or attempts by patients or a family member

Patient and Family Education

- Do not stop taking this medicine without notifying the health care provider.
- Notify doctor or pharmacist promptly if any of these effects persist or worsen.
- To relieve dry mouth, suck on (sugarless) hard candy or ice chips, chew (sugarless) gum, drink water, or use a saliva substitute.
- To prevent constipation, maintain a diet adequate in fiber, drink plenty of water, and exercise. In case of constipation, consult pharmacist for help in selecting a laxative (e.g., stimulant type with stool softener).
- Inform clinician immediately if any of these unlikely but serious side effects occur: mental/mood changes (e.g., confusion, depression, hallucinations, memory problems), enlarged/painful breasts, unwanted breast milk production, irregular/ painful menstrual periods, muscle stiffness/twitching, feelings of restlessness, ringing in the ears, sexual problems (e.g., decreased sexual ability, changes in desire), shakiness (tremors), numbness/tingling of the hands/feet, trouble urinating, and severe vomiting.
- Inform clinician immediately if any of these rare but very serious side effects occur: easy bruising/bleeding, signs of infection (e.g., fever, persistent sore throat), unusual/uncontrolled movements (especially of the tongue/face/lips), severe stomach/abdominal pain, dark urine, and yellowing of eyes/skin.
- Seek immediate medical attention if any of these rare but very serious side effects occur: black stools, chest pain, fainting, high fever, slow/fast/irregular heartbeat, seizures, vomit that looks like coffee grounds.
- Store amitriptyline at room temperature away from moisture and heat.
- Stopping this medication suddenly could result in unpleasant side effects.
- Take the missed dose as soon as remembered. If it is almost time for the next dose, skip the missed dose and take the medicine at the next regularly scheduled time. *Do not* take extra medicine to make up the missed dose.

Special Populations

- *Elderly:* Elderly patients may need a reduced dose for they may be more sensitive to usual dosages. For elderly patients, 10 to 25 mg each day with increases of 10 to 25 mg at bedtime every 2 to 3 days may be sufficient. Amitriptyline is included in the Beers List of Potentially Inappropriate Medications for Geriatrics.

▪ *Renal impairment:* Use with caution when renal impairment is suspected. Confer with renal specialist.
▪ *Hepatic impairment:* Dosing in the presence of hepatic dysfunction is not given; caution is advised; strong anticholinergic properties; lower dosage initially and cautious titration recommended.
▪ *Pregnancy:* Safety has not been established. Use with Category C caution.
▪ *Lactation:* Excreted in human breast milk
▪ *Children:* Monitor closely for suicidal ideation with children, adolescents, and young adults with major depressive or other psychiatric conditions. Safety not established for children under 12 years.

NOTE: For some drugs, off-label use is reported. It is the responsibility of the practitioner to evaluate the efficacy of such use.

ARIPIPRAZOLE (*ABILIFY, ABILIFY DISCMELT, ABILIFY MAINTENA*)

Classification
Second-generation (atypical) antipsychotic, quinolone derivative

Indications
Schizophrenia (13 years and older), manic and mixed episodes associated with bipolar I disorder, adjunctive treatment to antidepressants for major depressive disorder, agitation associated with schizophrenia or bipolar disorder, manic or mixed

Available Forms
Tablet, 2, 5, 10, 15, 20, and 30 mg; tablet, orally disintegrating, 10 and 15 mg; solution, oral, 1 mg/mL; IM injection, solution, 9.75 mg/1.3 mL; long-acting injectable new on market, Abilify Maintena

Dosage
▦ 15 to 30 mg/day; 10 to 15 mg/day initially; maximum 30 mg/day
▦ IM 9.75 mg as a single dose (range: 5.25–15 mg). Repeated doses may be given with or without food.
▦ Parenteral administration is intended for IM use only at greater than 2-hour intervals to max of 30 mg/day.
▦ Maintena IM once monthly at 300 or 400 mg. This preparation needs a 14-day overlapping oral antipsychotic treatment for first dose.
▦ Not indicated for children under age 10 years, except for autistic disorder, which can be medicated at the age of 6 years.

Administration
▦ IM or PO; do not administer IV or SC; inject slowly, deep into muscle mass.
▦ *IM injection has not been evaluated in children.*
▦ Oral solution may be substituted for tablets on a mg-per-mg basis up to a 25-mg dose. Patients receiving 30-mg tablets should receive 25 mg of solution.
▦ Dosing for the orally disintegrating tablet is the same as the oral tablet.
▦ Do not open the ODTs until ready to administer. The ODT should be taken without liquid. Do not split the ODT.
▦ Use oral aripiprazole 10 to 30 mg/day instead of IM aripiprazole as soon as possible if ongoing therapy is indicated.

Side Effects
Nausea, vomiting, dizziness, insomnia, akathisia, activation, headache, asthenia, sedation, constipation, orthostatic hypotension (occasionally during initial phase), increased risk of death and cerebrovascular events in elderly with dementia-related psychosis, tardive dyskinesia, neuroleptic malignant syndrome (rare), seizures (rare), metabolic syndrome, QTc prolongation, suicide risk increase, bradycardia.

Drug Interactions
Major substrate of CYP450 3A4, CYP2D6, and CYP3A4. Caution with other CYP2D6 inhibitors (e.g., nefazodone, fluvoxamine, fluoxetine), CYP450 2D6 or CYP3A4 inhibitors. Avoid with metoclopramide (e.g., paroxetine, fluoxetine, duloxetine) and quinidine. It may increase plasma levels of aripiprazole.

NOTE: For some drugs, off-label use is reported. It is the responsibility of the practitioner to evaluate the efficacy of such use.

- Carbamazepine and other CYP450 3A4 inducers may decrease plasma levels of aripiprazole.
- Aripiprazole may enhance effects of antihypertensive medications by causing orthostatic hypotension.
- Aripiprazole may antagonize levodopa and dopamine agonists.
- *Alert:* This list may not describe all possible interactions. Instruct clients to provide a list of all medicines, herbs, nonprescription drugs, or dietary supplements they use.

Pharmacokinetics

- *Excretion:* About 25% of a single oral dose is excreted in urine (less than 1% unchanged) and 55% is excreted in feces (18% as unchanged drug).
- *Metabolism:* It is primarily metabolized by CYP450 2D6 and CYP450 3A4. Hepatic 50% to 60% glucuronidation.
- *Absorption:* IM, 100%; PO, 87%
- *Onset:* IM, 1 hour; PO, 1 to 3 weeks
- *Peak*: IM, 1 to 3 hours; PO, 3 to 5 hours
- *Duration:* 2 hours for injectable
- *Half-life:* 75 hours (aripiprazole) and 94 hours (active aripiprazole metabolite)

Precautions

- Cardiovascular disease; dementia
- Dysphagia is associated with use of aripiprazole. Use with caution in patients who are at risk for aspiration pneumonia.
- Use with caution in patients with conditions that may develop hypotension (dehydration, overheating, etc.).
- Do not use in patients who are allergic to aripiprazole, seizures; Parkinson's disease; sedation.

Patient and Family Education

- Store aripiprazole at 59°F to 86°F. It can be used for up to 6 months after opening. Protect injection from light by storing in carton until use.
- Same precautions are to be taken for neonates as with other antipsychotics.
- If client becomes pregnant, contact provider. Discuss with provider if you have any of these conditions. A dose adjustment or special tests to safely take aripiprazole may be needed:
  - Liver or kidney disease
  - Heart disease, high blood pressure (BP), heart rhythm problems
  - History of heart attack or stroke
  - History of low white blood cell counts
  - History of breast cancer
  - Seizures or epilepsy
  - A personal or family history of diabetes
  - Trouble swallowing
- Client should be encouraged to talk to provider if he or she has signs of hyperglycemia, such as increased thirst or urination, excessive hunger, or weakness. If he or she has diabetes, check blood sugar levels on a regular basis while taking aripiprazole.
- Avoid alcohol. Maintain adequate hydration; caution when changing position from lying to sitting.

NOTE: For some drugs, off-label use is reported. It is the responsibility of the practitioner to evaluate the efficacy of such use.

Special Populations

There is a black box warning for use with the elderly with dementia with psychosis

- ■ *Elderly:* Dosage adjustment is generally not required. Elderly with dementia-related psychosis treated with atypical antipsychotics are at higher risk of death and cerebrovascular events.
- ■ *Renal impairment:* No dosage adjustment is needed.
- ■ *Hepatic impairment:* No dosage adjustment is required.
- ■ *Cardiac impairment:* Use with caution because of the risk of orthostatic hypotension.
- ■ *Lactation:* Although there are no data on the excretion of aripiprazole into human milk, it is suggested that women receiving aripiprazole should not breastfeed.
- ■ *Children and adolescents:* Approved for schizophrenia (age 13 years and older) and manic/mixed episodes (age 10 years and older). It should be monitored more frequently than adults. Children may tolerate lower doses better.
- ■ *Pregnancy:* Category C

ARMODAFINIL (*NUVIGIL*)

Classification
Central nervous system stimulant

Indications
It is used primarily to treat sleep disorders that result in excessive sleepiness, such as narcolepsy, obstructive sleep apnea, hypopnea syndrome, and shift work sleep disorder.

Available Forms
Tablet, 50, 150, and 250 mg

Dosage
▨ *Narcolepsy/Obstructive Sleep Apnea (Adults and children 17 years and older):* PO: 150 or 250 mg as a single dose in the morning.
▨ *Shift Work Sleep Disorder (Adults and children 17 years and older):* PO:150 mg daily approximately 1 hour prior to the start of work shift.
▨ *Elderly:* PO: Consider using lower doses.
▨ *Hepatic function impairment:* PO: Reduce dose in severe hepatic impairment.

Administration
▨ PO with a glass of water. Take in morning to get maximum effects during waking hours and to avoid sleep later in the evening.
▨ Take without food.

Side Effects
Palpitations, increased heart rate, headache, insomnia, dizziness, anxiety, depression, fatigue, agitation, attention disturbance, depressed mood, migraine, nervousness, paresthesia, tremor, rash, contact dermatitis, hyperhidrosis nausea, dry mouth, diarrhea, dyspepsia, upper abdominal pain, anorexia, constipation, decreased appetite, loose stools, vomiting, increased Gamma-glutamyl transferase (GGT), increased alkaline phosphatase, dyspnea, influenza-like illness, pain, polyuria, pyrexia, seasonal allergy, and thirst.

Drug Interactions
▨ Avoid concomitant use with alcohol.
▨ When used with dextroamphetamine/methylphenidate, absorption may be delayed approximately 1 hour; the same effect may be applicable to armodafinil.
▨ Drugs metabolized by CYP2C19 (e.g., clomipramine, diazepam, midazolam, omeprazole, phenytoin, propranolol, triazolam) for plasma concentration may be elevated by armodafinil, increasing the risk of adverse reactions.

NOTE: For some drugs, off-label use is reported. It is the responsibility of the practitioner to evaluate the efficacy of such use.

▦ Drugs metabolized by CYP3A4/5 (e.g., cyclosporine, ethinyl estradiol, midazolam, triazolam) for plasma concentrations may be reduced by armodafinil, decreasing efficacy.

▦ Food may delay the armodafinil T_{max} by approximately 2 to 4 hours. Because the delay in T_{max} is associated with elevated plasma concentrations later in time, food can potentially affect the onset and time course of the pharmacologic action of armodafinil.

▦ The efficacy of hormonal contraceptives may be reduced during and for 1 month after armodafinil coadministration. Use of alternative or concomitant methods of contraception are recommended during and for 1 month after coadministration with armodafinil.

▦ Use caution when administering monoamine oxidase inhibitors (MAOIs) and armodafinil.

▦ Potent inducers of CYP3A4/5 (e.g., carbamazepine, phenobarbital, rifampin) may reduce drug efficacy

▦ Potent inhibitors of CYP3A4/5 (e.g., erythromycin, ketoconazole) may increase drug concentration increasing the risk of adverse reactions.

▦ Possible decrease in armodafinil levels due to prazosin; larger doses of armodafinil may be needed.

▦ A pharmacodynamic interaction cannot be ruled out. Monitor prothrombin time (PT) and international normalized ratio (INR) more frequently when armodafinil is administered with warfarin.

Pharmacokinetics

▦ This medicine is a stimulant; the exact mechanism of action is unknown. It is believed to have similar wake-promoting actions as sympathomimetic agents.

▦ There is rapid absorption in absence of food.

▦ Peak plasma levels are reached in 2 hours in the fasted state: food delays peak plasma concentrations by 2 to 4 hours.

▦ Steady state reached within 7 days of dosing.

▦ *Excretion*: Urine 80%

▦ *Half-life:* Average is 15 hours once steady state is reached.

Precautions

▦ See client as often as necessary to ensure drug is promoting wakefulness, determine compliance, and review side effects.

▦ Advise patient to report any new rashes immediately.

▦ Discontinue drug immediately if any rash is reported.

▦ Advise patient of risk for transient psychosis-like symptoms (ideas of reference, paranoid delusions, and auditory hallucinations).

▦ May experience transient palpitations and EKG changes.

▦ Avoid using in clients with left ventricular hypertrophy or mitral valve prolapsed.

Patient and Family Education

▦ Do not operate heavy machinery or equipment until reasonably certain that drug will not affect ability to engage in such activities.

▦ Discontinue medication immediately if a rash is noted and follow up with provider.

▦ Patients may experience palpitations.

NOTE: For some drugs, off-label use is reported. It is the responsibility of the practitioner to evaluate the efficacy of such use.

▨ Have patient monitor blood pressure (BP) at home and notify provider of persistent BP elevations.

▨ Store securely at room temperature between 20°C and 25°C (68°F–77°F).

Special Populations

▨ *Elderly*: Clearance has been reduced in older adults. Use lowest effective dose. Safety in those above the age of 65 years has not studied.

▨ *Hepatic impairment*: Modify dosage by one-half accordingly.

▨ *Pregnancy*: Category C

▨ *Lactation*: No human studies have been performed. The medicine is not recommended in breastfeeding mothers.

▨ *Children*: This medicine is not for use in pediatric patients.

NOTE: For some drugs, off-label use is reported. It is the responsibility of the practitioner to evaluate the efficacy of such use.

ASENAPINE (*SAPHRIS*)

Classification
Dopamine and serotonin antagonist; antipsychotic drug, atypical (second generation)

Indications
Schizophrenia, manic or mixed episodes associated with bipolar I disorder as mono-therapy or as adjunctive therapy with either lithium or valproate.

Available Forms
Sublingual tablets, 5 and 10 mg

Dosage
Initial dose, 5 mg BID; after 1 week may increase to 10 mg BID. Can decrease back to 5 mg BID based on tolerability.

Administration
■ The drug comes in tablet form. Place the tablet under the tongue and allow to dissolve completely.
■ The tablet dissolves within seconds.
■ Do not eat or drink anything for 10 to 30 minutes after administration.
■ Tablets should not be crushed, chewed, or swallowed.

Side Effects
Akathisia, oral hypoesthesia (numbness), somnolence, dizziness, other extrapyramidal symptoms excluding akathisia, weight gain, insomnia, headache, may induce ortho-static hypotension and syncope in some patients, especially early in treatment, rare neuroleptic malignant syndrome (rare), TD (rare) and metabolic changes.

Drug Interactions
■ The drug may enhance effects of certain antihypertensive drugs because of its alpha-1-adrenergic antagonism with potential for inducing hypotension.
■ Inhibitor of P450 CYP2D6: subject also to induction/inhibition of 1A2. Manufacturer recommends caution with other QTc drugs and may contribute to increased levels of other drugs acting as substrates of 2D6. Dextromethorphan, paroxetine may increase both these drug levels.
■ It appears to decrease prolactin from baseline.

Pharmacokinetics
■ Rapidly absorbed within 0.5 to 1.5 hours.
■ *Half-life:* Approximately 24 hours

Precautions
■ Caution should be used when the drug is taken in combination with other centrally acting drugs or alcohol. EKG should be taken prior to starting this medication.
■ Caution should be used with other drugs that are both substrates and inhibitors for CYP 2D6. For example, CYP2D6 may double the level of paroxetine.

NOTE: For some drugs, off-label use is reported. It is the responsibility of the practitioner to evaluate the efficacy of such use.

- The drug may cause transient increases in serum transaminase; therefore, it needs to be monitored during the initial months.
- Elderly patients with dementia-related psychosis treated with antipsychotic drugs are at an increased risk of death. Asenapine is not approved for the treatment of patients with dementia-related psychosis. Note: Black box warning.
- Patients with a preexisting low white blood cell (WBC) or a history of drug-induced leukopenia/neutropenia should have their complete blood count monitored frequently during the first few months of therapy, and asenapine should be discontinued at the first sign of decline in WBC in the absence of other causative factors.
- The use of asenapine should be avoided in combination with other drugs known to prolong the QTc interval, including Class 1A antiarrhythmics (e.g., quinidine, procainamide) or Class 3 antiarrhythmics (e.g., amiodarone, sotalol), antipsychotic medications (e.g., ziprasidone, chlorpromazine, thioridazine), and antibiotics (e.g., gatifloxacin, moxifloxacin).
- Like other drugs that antagonize dopamine D2 receptors, asenapine can elevate prolactin levels, and the elevation can persist during chronic administration. As with other antipsychotic drugs, asenapine should be used with caution in patients with a history of seizures or with conditions that potentially lower the seizure threshold; for example, Alzheimer's dementia. Conditions that lower the seizure threshold may be more prevalent in patients 65 years or older.

Patient and Family Education

- Take exactly as prescribed by the provider. Do not take in larger or smaller amounts or for longer than recommended.
- Asenapine tablets must be placed under the tongue and be allowed to dissolve. Do not crush, chew, or swallow.
- No eating or drinking for at least 10 to 30 minutes after the drug is absorbed.
- *Avoid drinking alcohol.*
- *Stop using this medication and call provider immediately* if you have very stiff (rigid) muscles, high fever, sweating, confusion, fast or uneven heartbeats, tremors; feel like you might pass out, have jerky muscle movements you cannot control, trouble swallowing, problems with speech, have blurred vision, eye pain, or see halos around lights; have increased thirst and urination, excessive hunger, fruity breath odor, weakness, nausea and vomiting; have fever, chills, body aches, flu symptoms; or have white patches or sores inside your mouth or on your lips.
- Do not stop taking this drug suddenly without first talking to your provider, even if you feel fine. You may have serious side effects if you stop taking the drug suddenly.
- Call provider if symptoms do not improve or get worse.
- Store at room temperature away from moisture and heat.

Special Populations

- *Elderly:* The elderly may tolerate lower doses better and are more sensitive to adverse effects. It is not approved for treatment of elderly patients with dementia-related psychosis, and such patients are at increased risk of cardiovascular events and death.
- *Renal impairment*: No adjustment is needed.
- *Hepatic impairment*: Lower dose for mild-to-moderate impairment is to be administered. It is not recommended with severe liver impairment.

NOTE: For some drugs, off-label use is reported. It is the responsibility of the practitioner to evaluate the efficacy of such use.

- *Cardiac impairment:* Use with caution due to risk of orthostatic hypotension and QTc potential prolongation.
- *Pregnancy:* Category C. There are no adequate and well-controlled studies of asenapine in pregnant women. It is not recommended for this population.
- *Lactation:* Asenapine is excreted in the milk of rats during lactation. It is not known whether asenapine or its metabolites are excreted in human milk. As many drugs are excreted in human milk, caution should be exercised when asenapine is administered to a nursing woman. It is recommended that women receiving asenapine should not breastfeed.
- *Children and adolescents:* This medicine is not indicated for use in children.

NOTE: For some drugs, off-label use is reported. It is the responsibility of the practitioner to evaluate the efficacy of such use.

ATOMOXETINE HYDROCHLORIDE (*STRATTERA*)

Classification
Serotonin–norepinephrine reuptake inhibitor (SNRI), attention deficit hyperactivity disorder (ADHD) drug

Indications
This is the first nonstimulant drug approved for the treatment of ADHD of children aged 6 years and above and adults. Although nonstimulants are considered second-line therapy, they may be a safer alternative than stimulants for patients with a history of substance abuse.

Available Forms
Capsule, 10, 18, 25, 40, 60, 80, and 100 mg

Dosage
▦ Dosage should be individualized according to the therapeutic needs and response of the patient.
▦ *Children older than 6 years:* less than 70 kg; start, 0.5 mg/kg PO QAM × 3 days, then increase to 1.2 mg/kg PO QAM; maximum, 1.4 mg/kg/day, doses greater than 0.5 mg/kg/day may be divided bid. *Greater than 70 kg:* Start, 40 mg PO QAM × 3 days, then increase to 80 mg PO QAM, may increase to 100 mg/day after 2 to 4 weeks if needed; maximum, 100 mg/day.
▦ *Adults:* 80 mg QAM; start, 40 mg PO QAM × 3 days, then increase to 80 mg PO QAM, may increase to 100 mg/day after 2 to 4 weeks if needed. Maximum: 100 mg/day.

Administration
Taking the drug with food may alleviate gastrointestinal side effects, requires slower titration if patient is poor CYP2D6 metabolizer or on strong CYP2D6 inhibitor. For poor CYP2D6 metabolizers, initiate at 40 mg/day but not exceed 80 mg/day. Periodically reassess need for treatment during maintenance.

Side Effects
Nausea and/or vomiting, fatigue, decreased appetite, abdominal pain, somnolence, constipation, dry mouth, insomnia, priapism, urinary hesitancy or retention or dysuria, dysmenorrheal, hot flashes, severe liver injury, serious cardiovascular events (myocardial infarction, stroke, sudden death), rapid heart rate and increased blood pressure (BP), suicidal ideation, allergic reactions, and decreased growth.

Drug Interactions
The drug may interact with monoamine oxidase inhibitors (MAOIs), CYP2D6 inhibitors, SSRIs, quinidine BP agents, albuterol, and other beta-2 agonists. The action of albuterol on cardiovascular system can be potentiated.

Pharmacokinetics
▦ The precise mechanism by which atomoxetine produces its therapeutic effect is unknown.

NOTE: For some drugs, off-label use is reported. It is the responsibility of the practitioner to evaluate the efficacy of such use.

■ Its therapeutic effect may be related to selective inhibition of the presynaptic nor-epinephrine transporter.
■ Minimally affected by food intake.
■ Maximal plasma concentration is reached within 1 to 2 hours after dosing.
■ Mainly excreted in the urine (80%); feces (17%)
■ *Half-life:* Approximately 21 hours
■ Bioavailability: 63% to 94%

Precautions
■ Do not prescribe to patients with cardiomyopathy and pheochromocytoma.
■ Hypersensitivity to atomoxetine or other constituents of the product.
■ Use within 2 weeks of taking or discontinuing MAOIs.
■ Narrow-angle glaucoma.

Patient and Family Education
■ Do not crush, open, or chew capsules.
■ Avoid touching a broken capsule: Powder is a known ocular irritant and if gets into eyes needs to be flushed out immediately.
■ It can be taken with or without food.
■ Do not double the dose if a day is missed.
■ Call poison control/seek medical attention for overdose.
■ Seek medical attention for chest pain, shortness of breath, elevated BP, erections that last more than 4 hours, or any other concerning symptoms.
■ Children, adolescents, or adults who are being considered for treatment with atom-oxetine should have a careful history (including assessment for a family history of sudden death or ventricular arrhythmia) and physical exam to assess for the presence of cardiac disease, and should receive further cardiac evaluation if findings suggest such disease (e.g., electrocardiogram and echocardiogram). Patients who develop symptoms such as exertional chest pain, unexplained syncope, or other symptoms suggestive of cardiac disease during atomoxetine treatment should undergo a prompt cardiac evaluation.
■ Store at room temperature.
■ Routinely assess weight and BP.

Special Populations
■ *Elderly:* Safety has not been studied in geriatric patients.
■ *Pregnancy:* Category C
■ *Lactation:* Safety is unknown in lactating mothers.
■ *Children: Not recommended for use in children.* It has not been studied in children younger than 6 years.

NOTE: For some drugs, off-label use is reported. It is the responsibility of the practitioner to evaluate the efficacy of such use.

B COMPLEX (*VITAMIN B₁/THIAMINE HYDROCHLORIDE*)

Classification
Vitamin

Indications
Treat and prevent thiamine deficiency, including thiamine-specific deficiency, Wernicke–Korsakoff syndrome (common in patients diagnosed with alcoholism)

Available Forms
Tablets, 50, 100, 250, 500 mg; injection: 100 mg/mL; enteric coated tablets, 20 mg

Dosage
1 to 2 mg of thiamine per day is commonly used. The daily recommended daily allowances (RDAs):

- *Infants:* 0 to 6 months: 0.2 mg; 7 to 12 months: 0.3 mg
- *Children:* 1 to 3 year: 0.5 mg; 4 to 8 years: 0.6 mg
- *Males:* 9 to 13 years: 0.9 mg; 14 years and older: 1.2 mg
- *Females:* 9 to 13 years: 0.9 mg; 14 to 18 years: 1 mg; over 18 years: 1.1 mg; pregnat women: 1.4 mg; lactating breastfeeding women: 1.5 mg

Administration
- PO with a glass of water.
- It may be taken with or without food.

Side Effects
Feelings of warmth, restlessness, nausea, and pruritus.

Drug Interactions
None indicated.

Pharmacokinetics
The drug is widely distributed. It is eliminated in urine.

Precautions
- Watch for anaphylaxis reaction.

Patient and Family Education
- Take medication at same time every day.

Special Populations
- *Elderly:* No contraindications.
- *Renal impairment:* Use with caution.
- *Hepatic impairment:* Use with caution.
- *Pregnancy:* Category A.
- *Lactation:* American Academy of Pediatrics classifies Thiamine as compatible with breastfeeding
- *Children and adolescents:* Multivitamin use in children determined by nutritional deficiency noted. Dose contingent is based on weight.

NOTE: For some drugs, off-label use is reported. It is the responsibility of the practitioner to evaluate the efficacy of such use.

BISMUTH SUBSALICYLATE

Classification
Antidiarrheal

Indications
▪ Used for mild, nonspecific diarrhea

Available Forms
▪ Caplets, 262 mg
▪ Liquid, 87 mg/5 mL, 87.3 mg/5 mL, 130 mg/15 mL, 175 mg/5 mL, 262 mg/15 mL, 524 mg/15 mL
▪ Oral suspension, 525 mg/15 mL
▪ Tablets (chewable), 262 mg

Dosages
For patients with mild, nonspecific diarrhea

▪ Adults and children age 12 years and older: 30 mL or 2 tablets every 30 minutes to 1 hour, up to maximum of 8 doses for no longer than 2 days
▪ Children aged 9 to 11 years: 15 mL or 1 chewable tablet every 30 minutes to an hour, up to maximum of 8 doses and for no longer than 2 days
▪ Children aged 6 to 8 years: 10 mL or two thirds chewable tablet PO every half hour to an hour up to maximum of 8 doses and no longer than 2 days
▪ Children aged 3 to 5 years: 5 mL or one third chewable tablet PO every half hour to an hour, up to 8 doses and no longer than 2 days

For traveler's diarrhea:

▪ Adults: 30 mL PO every half hour for 8 doses/day; 4 doses maximum strength

Administration
▪ Shake liquid well before administration. Have patient chew or dissolve tablets in the mouth.
▪ Liquid formulation works more effectively for relief of severe symptoms.
▪ Avoid use prior to radiologic procedures because drug is radioopaque and may interfere with x-rays.
▪ Liquid form is preferred for children to give more accurate dosing.

Side Effects
▪ Gastrointestinal: temporary darkening of tongue and stools, salicylic with high doses
▪ Effects on lab test results: none reported

Drug Interactions
▪ Aspirin/other salicylates: may cause salicylate toxicity. Monitor patient.
▪ Oral anticoagulants, oral antidiabetics: may increase effects of these drugs after high doses of bismuth. Monitor patient closely.
▪ Tetracycline: may decrease tetracycline absorption. Separate doses by at least 2 hours.

NOTE: For some drugs, off-label use is reported. It is the responsibility of the practitioner to evaluate the efficacy of such use.

Pharmacokinetics
- Drug may have antisecretory, antimicrobial, and anti-inflammatory effects against bacterial and viral enteropathogens.
- Onset of action: 1 hour, peak unknown, duration and half-life unknown.

Precautions
- It is contraindicated in patients hypersensitive to salicylates.
- Use the drug cautiously in patients taking aspirin.
- Stop therapy if tinnitus occurs.
- Use cautiously in children and in patients with bleeding disorders or salicylate sensitivity.

Patient and Family Education
- Advise patient that drug contains salicylate.
- Instruct patient to shake liquid before measuring dose and to chew tablets well before swallowing.
- Tell patient to call prescriber if diarrhea lasts longer than 2 days, accompanied by high fever.
- Advise patient to drink plenty of clear fluids to avoid dehydration, which may accompany diarrhea.
- Avoid red-colored hydration fluids as this may be misinterpreted as bleeding from rectum.
- Inform the patient that tongue and stools may temporarily turn gray-black.
- Urge patient to consult with prescriber prior to giving the drug to children or teenagers during or after recovery from flu or chicken pox.
- Tell the patient to watch for hives, ringing in the ears, or rectal bleeding.

Special Populations
- *Elderly:*
  - Caution is recommended for the elderly because of the risk of fluid and electrolyte loss; also, elderly are more likely to have age-related renal function impairment, which may increase the risk of salicylate toxicity.
  - Bismuth is more likely to cause impaction in elderly patients.
- *Pediatric:*
  - Avoid use in children or teenagers who have or are recovering from influenza or varicella.
  - *Use cautiously in infants and debilitated patients due to increased risk of constipation with impaction.*
  - Use cautiously in children and in patients with bleeding disorders or salicylate sensitivity.
- *Pregnancy:*
  - Drug has not been officially assigned to a pregnancy category.
  - The effects of the drug are unknown.

NOTE: For some drugs, off-label use is reported. It is the responsibility of the practitioner to evaluate the efficacy of such use.

BROMOCRIPTINE MESYLATE (*PARLODEL, CYCLOSET*)

Classification
Ergot derivative with potent dopamine receptor agonist activity; antiparkinsonian

Indication
Hyperprolactinemia-Associated Dysfunctions
▦ Indicated in disorders associated with hyperprolactinemia, including amenorrhea with or without galactorrhea, infertility or hypogonadism, with prolactin-secreting adenomas.

Acromegaly
▦ It is indicated in the treatment of acromegaly.
▦ The drug is used alone or as adjunctive therapy with pituitary irradiation or surgery.

Parkinson's Disease
▦ The drug is used for the treatment of the signs and symptoms of idiopathic or post-encephalitic Parkinson's disease.
▦ It is used as adjunctive treatment to levodopa (alone or with a peripheral decarboxylase inhibitor).
▦ It is also used for traumatic brain injury.

Available Forms
Tablet, 0.8 and 2.5 mg; capsule, 5 mg

Dosage
Hyperprolactinemia
Initial: 1.25 to 2.5 mg orally daily
Titration: Add 2.5 mg orally, as tolerated, to the treatment dosage every 2 to 7 days.
Maintenance: 2.5 to 15 mg orally daily

Acromegaly
Initial: 1.25 to 2.5 mg orally once daily, with food, at bedtime for 3 days
Titration: Add 1.25 to 2.5 mg orally, as tolerated, to the treatment dosage every 3 to 7 days.
Maintenance: 20 to 30 mg orally daily
The maximum dosage should not exceed 100 mg/day.

Parkinson's Disease
Initial: 1.25 mg twice daily with meals.
Titration: Add 2.5 mg/day, with meals, to dosage regimen every 14 to 28 days.
Maximum dosage: 100 mg/day

Hyperprolactinemia
For 11- to 15-years-olds:
Initial: 1.25 to 2.5 mg orally daily
Maintenance: 2.5 to 10 mg orally daily

NOTE: For some drugs, off-label use is reported. It is the responsibility of the practitioner to evaluate the efficacy of such use.

Administration
PO: Take the drug with food to avoid gastrointestinal (GI) distress; take in evening with food to minimize adverse reactions.

Drug Interactions
▨ Metoclopramide will antagonize the effects of this drug and should be avoided.
▨ Use with caution ergot alkaloids (e.g., ergonovine); "triptans" (e.g., sumatriptan, frovatriptan); medications for high blood pressure (e.g., methyldopa, reserpine, beta-blockers such as metoprolol/propranolol); antipsychotic medication (e.g., haloperidol, pimozide); metoclopramide; nitrates (e.g., nitroglycerin); octreotide; cimetidine; delavirdine; efavirenz; telithromycin; azole antifungals, including keto-conazole; macrolide antibiotics, including erythromycin; HIV protease inhibitors, such as ritonavir; rifamycins, including rifabutin, can affect concentrations of the drug. Salicylates may increase adverse reactions.
▨ St. John's wort; certain antiseizure medicines, including carbamazepine; drugs that cause drowsiness, such as certain antihistamines (e.g., diphenhydramine), anti-seizure drugs (e.g., phenytoin), medicine for sleep or anxiety (e.g., alprazolam, diazepam, zolpidem), and muscle relaxants; narcotic pain relievers (e.g., codeine); psychiatric medicines (e.g., chlorpromazine, risperidone, nortriptyline, trazodone) will also affect efficacy.
▨ Patients need to check the labels on all their medicines (e.g., cough-and-cold products) because they may contain drowsiness-causing ingredients.

Pharmacokinetics
▨ *Absorption:* 28% bioavailable
▨ *Onset:* 1 to 3 hours
▨ *Peak*: 8 hours
▨ *Metabolism:* Via CYP3A4 (major)
▨ *Excretion:* 85% feces; urine 2.5% to 5%
▨ *Half-life:* 15 hours

Precautions
▨ Bromocriptine is contraindicated for use in patients with uncontrolled hypertension due to risk of acute myocardial infarction. It is also contraindicated for use in the prevention of physiological lactation.
▨ Bromocriptine should be used with caution in patients with a history of psychosis or cardiovascular disease.
▨ Patients should be evaluated frequently during dose titration to determine the low-est dosage possible to achieve the desired therapeutic effects.
▨ Patients treated with pituitary irradiation should be withdrawn from bromocrip-tine therapy on a yearly basis to assess both the clinical effects of radiation on the disease process, as well as the effects of bromocriptine. Usually a 4- to 8-week withdrawal period is adequate for this purpose.
▨ With elderly patients, starting at the lower end of the dose range, reflecting the greater frequency of decreased hepatic, renal, or cardiac function, and of concomi-tant disease, or other drug therapy in this population.
▨ Patients with cardiac valvular fibrosis and other cardiovascular diseases need to be carefully assessed to determine risk/benefit.
▨ This drug may cause impulse control disorders.
▨ It may increase the risk of melanoma

NOTE: For some drugs, off-label use is reported. It is the responsibility of the practitioner to evaluate the efficacy of such use.

Patient and Family Education
- ■ The patient needs to know that he or she should not discontinue this medicine without consulting the prescriber.
- ■ Take with meals to avoid gastrointestinal (GI) distress.
- ■ Urine or perspiration may appear darker.

Special Populations
- ■ *Elderly*: Clinical studies for Parlodel did not include sufficient numbers of subjects aged 65 years and older to determine whether the elderly respond differently from younger subjects.
- ■ *Pregnancy*: Category B. Withdraw unless medically impossible—such as rapidly expanding macroadenoma that necessitates continued use.
- ■ *Lactation*: Breastfeeding is not recommended.
- ■ *Children:* The safety and effectiveness of bromocriptine for the treatment of prolactin-secreting pituitary adenomas have been established in patients aged 16 years to adult. There are available data on bromocriptine use in pediatric patients under the age of 8 years. This medicine is not indicated for children under the age of 11 years.

NOTE: For some drugs, off-label use is reported. It is the responsibility of the practitioner to evaluate the efficacy of such use.

BUPRENORPHINE, BUPRENORPHINE HCl, BUPRENEX, BUTRANS, AND NALOXONE HCl DIHYDRATE (*SUBUTEX, SUBOXONE*)

Classification
Opiate partial agonists, opioid analgesic

Indications
- The drug is used sublingually for treatment of opiate dependence.
- It is preferred for the initial (i.e., induction) phase of opiate-dependence treatment.
- It is also used for controling pain (acute and chronic).

Available Forms
Sublingual tablets, *Subutex:* 2 and 8 mg; *Suboxone*: 2 mg/0.5 mg, 4/1 mg, 8 mg/2 mg, 12/3 mg; injectable, *Subutex:* 0.3 mg/mL; transdermal patch, 5 mcg/hr, 10 mcg/hr, 20 mcg/hr.

Dosage
Pediatric
Intravascular or Intramuscular
- *Children 2 to 12 years of age:* 2 to 6 mcg/kg every 4 to 6 hours; monitor effects of the drug before establishing fixed doses
- *Children 13 years of age or older:* 0.3 mg given at intervals of up to every 6 hours prn. Can repeat initial dose (up to 0.3 mg) once in 30 to 60 minutes, if control is not achieved.
- Exercise particular caution with IV administration, especially with initial doses.

Adults
Intravascular or Intramuscular
- Administer 0.3 mg every 6 hours prn. Repeat initial dose (up to 0.3 mg) once in 30 to 60 minutes, if needed.
- A regimen, including an initial dose of 0.3 mg followed by another 0.3-mg dose repeated in 3 hours, is as effective as a single 0.6-mg dose in relieving postoperative pain.
- Decrease dosage by approximately 50% in patients who are at increased risk of respiratory depression.

Opiate Dependence
Induction
Sublingual

- Begin with 8 mg on day 1 and 16 mg on day 2. From day 3 onward, administer buprenorphine in fixed combination with naloxone at the same buprenorphine dose as on day 2.
- To avoid precipitating withdrawal, give the first dose when the patient is objective and clear signs of opiate withdrawal are evident.
- Manufacturer recommends that an adequate maintenance dosage, titrated to clinical effectiveness, be achieved as rapidly as possible to prevent undue opiate withdrawal symptoms.

NOTE: For some drugs, off-label use is reported. It is the responsibility of the practitioner to evaluate the efficacy of such use.

Maintenance
Sublingual

▓ Target dosage of buprenorphine in fixed combination with naloxone is 16 mg daily; however, dosages as low as 12 mg daily may be effective in some patient. Adjust dosage in increments/decrements of 2 or 4 mg daily to a dosage that suppresses opiate withdrawal symptoms and ensures that the patient continues treatment.

▓ Usual dosage: 4 to 24 mg daily depending on the individual patient.

▓ If switching between buprenorphine/naloxone sublingual tablets and sublingually dissolving strips, continue same dosage/However, not all doses and dose combinations are bioequivalent; monitor for efficacy and tolerability and adjust dosage if needed.

Administration

▓ Administer sublingually as a single agent or in fixed combination with naloxone for management of opiate dependence.

▓ Also administered by continuous IV infusion by IM or IV injection using a patient-controlled infusion device, and by epidural injection† for pain relief. Incompatibilities: diazepam, furosemide, lorazepam

Sublingual Tablets

▓ Place tablets under the tongue and allow to dissolve; swallowing the tablets reduces bioavailability. Drinking warm fluids prior to administration may aid dissolution.

▓ For doses requiring more than two tablets, all the tablets may be placed under the tongue at once.

▓ Alternatively, patients may place two tablets under the tongue at a time if unable to place more than two tablets comfortably.

▓ To ensure consistent bioavailability, patients should adhere to the same dosing schedule with continued use.

IV Injection
Rate of Administration
Administer over greater than or equal to 2 minutes.

Transdermal

▓ Apply the transdermal system to a dry, intact, nonirritated, hairless or nearly hairless surface on the upper chest, upper back, side of chest, or upper outer arm.

▓ Firmly press the system by hand for 15 seconds with the adhesive side touching the skin and ensuring that contact is complete, particularly around the edges.

▓ Clip, do not shave hair at the application site prior to application, if indicated.

▓ Only water should be used if the site must be cleaned before transdermal application; do *not* use soaps, oils, lotions, alcohol, or abrasive devices that could alter absorption of the drug.

▓ System is intended to be worn continuously for 7 days.

▓ Apply subsequent systems to a different site each time administered.

▓ At least 21 days should elapse before reusing any single application site.

Note: Restricted Distribution Program
The Drug Addiction Treatment Act (DATA) of 2000 allows qualifying physicians to prescribe and dispense opiates in Schedules III, IV, and V of the Federal Controlled Substances Act, which have been approved by the FDA for detoxification or maintenance treatment of opiate dependence.

Side Effects
- Somnolence, dizziness, alterations in judgment, or alteration in level of consciousness, including coma
- Use with caution in comatose patients or in patients with central nervous system (CNS) depression.
- It may impair mental alertness and/or physical coordination needed to perform potentially hazardous activities, such as driving or operating machinery.
- Concurrent use of other CNS depressants may potentiate CNS depression, increased intracranial pressure, and bradycardia.

Drug Interactions
- CNS depression
- Respiratory depression
- Diazepam may cause respiratory distress or cardiac arrest
- Macrolide antibiotics may increase drug levels

Pharmacokinetics
- *Metabolism:* Liver by CYP 3A4
- *Peak:* IV, 2 minutes; IM, 1 hour; sublingual, unknown; transdermal, 3 to 6 days
- *Half-life:* 37 hours; 1 to 7 hours, transdermal, 26 hours

Precautions
- Watch for respiratory depression.
- Supervise ambulation due to sedative effects.

Patient and Family Education
- Do not drive or engage in other hazardous activities until response to drug is known.
- Avoid alcohol or other CNS depressants.
- It may cause constipation.

Special Populations
- *Elderly:* Use with caution due to sedative effects.
- *Renal impairment:* Use with caution.
- *Hepatic impairment:* Use with caution; patients may require lower dosage.
- *Pregnancy:* Category C
- *Lactation:* Safety has not been established.
- *Children and adolescents:* Safety has not been established.

NOTE: For some drugs, off-label use is reported. It is the responsibility of the practitioner to evaluate the efficacy of such use.

BUPRENORPHINE/NALOXONE (*SUBOXONE*)

Classification
Opioid (narcotic) partial agonist–antagonist

Indications
It is indicated for maintenance treatment of opioid dependence

Available Forms
Sublingual film, 2 mg/0.5 mg; 4 mg/1 mg; 8 mg/2 mg; 12 mg/3 mg

Dosage
■ Recommended dosage is 16 mg/4 mg a day as a single daily dose.
■ Dosage adjusted in increments/decrements of 2 mg/0.5 mg or 4 mg/1 mg to a level that obtains optimum results and avoids withdrawal.
■ Maintenance dose is 4 mg/1 mg to 24 mg/6 mg per day.

Administration
■ It cannot be cut, chewed, or swallowed.
■ It should be placed under the tongue until the film is completely dissolved.
■ Rotate places where film is placed.
■ Do not move film once it is placed under tongue.

Side Effects
■ Most common side effects are headache, stomach pain, constipation, vomiting, difficulty falling asleep or staying asleep, and sweating.
■ Some side effects can be serious. The following symptoms are uncommon but serious possible effects:
  ▪ Hives, skin rash, itching, difficulty breathing or swallowing, slowed breathing, upset stomach extreme tiredness, unusual bleeding or bruising, lack of energy, loss of appetite, pain in the upper right part of the stomach, yellowing of the skin or eyes, and flu-like symptoms

Drug Interactions
■ Monoamine oxidase inhibitors
■ Itraconazole, ketoconazole, erythromycin, clarithromycin, ritonavir, indinavir
■ Saquinavir
■ Local anesthetics
■ Avoid use with benzodiazepines
■ Alcohol
■ Medicine for sleep
■ Antianxiety drugs
■ Narcotic pain relievers
■ Phenothiazines
■ Tricyclics
■ Antiseizure drugs
■ Muscle relaxants
■ Antihistamines

NOTE: For some drugs, off-label use is reported. It is the responsibility of the practitioner to evaluate the efficacy of such use.

Note: Interactions are extensive and providers need to educate patients on not taking over-the counter (OTC) medications without informing their providers.

Pharmacokinetics
- Mean elimination half-life from plasma ranging from 24 to 42 hours
- Naloxone has a mean elimination half-life from plasma ranging from 2 to 12 hours.

Precautions
- Check all known allergies
- Use with extreme caution in patients with histories of lung disease, liver disease, serious head injury or CNS diseases, hypothyroidism, Addison's disease, psychosis, benign prostatic hypertrophy (BPH), acute alcoholism, kyphoscoliosis, and biliary tract disease.
- Check for a history of vertigo and syncope.
- Avoid alcoholic beverages.
- Respiratory depression
- Lethargy
- New studies show difficulty in weaning patients off Suboxone.
- For patients with hepatic impairment: higher plasma levels in patients with moderate and severe hepatic impairment
- Dosage should be adjusted and patients should be watched for signs and symptoms of opioid withdrawal.
- Fot with renal impairment: effects are unknown.

Patient Education
- Instruct patient that if he or she misses a dose to take it as soon as possible unless it is almost time for next dose; if so, then patient needs to be instructed to wait until then to use the medicine and skip the missed dose. Do not use extra medicine to make up for a missed dose.
- Medication should be stored in a closed container at room temperature, away from heat, moisture, and direct light.
- *OTC medications should not be used without conferring with provider. This includes vitamins and herbal products.*
- Do not drink alcohol while you are using this medicine.
- Be aware that there are numerous drug–drug interactions with this drug.
- Explore with patient history of any mental or emotional problems.
- This medication cannot be abruptly stopped. Provider will slowly decrease dose before stopping it completely.
- All dentists and providers need to be aware that patient is on this drug.
- Necessary to draw blood levels at specific intervals, therefore all appointments need to be kept.

Special Populations
- *Elderly*
  - There is little clinical data on safety and efficacy in the elderly.
  - If used in the elderly do so with caution. Start at the low end of the dosing range and monitor carefully.

NOTE: For some drugs, off-label use is reported. It is the responsibility of the practitioner to evaluate the efficacy of such use.

- There are higher plasma levels in patients with moderate and severe hepatic impairment.
- Dosage should be adjusted and patients should be watched for signs and symptoms of opioid withdrawal. For those with renal impairment, providers need to use caution for its unknown effects.
- *Pregnancy: Category C*
  - There is no adequate information regarding efficacy and safety in pregnant women.
  - This drug should be used during pregnancy only if the potential benefit justifies the potential risk to the fetus.
- *Nursing Mothers*
  - Drug passes into breast milk.
  - Breastfeeding is not recommended.
- *Pediatric*
  - It is not recommended for pediatric patients. Safety and effectiveness have not been established in pediatric patients.

NOTE: For some drugs, off-label use is reported. It is the responsibility of the practitioner to evaluate the efficacy of such use.

BUPROPION (*WELLBUTRIN*) BUPROPION HYDROBROMIDE (*APLENZIN*) AND BUPROPION HYDROCHLORIDE (*WELLBUTRIN, WELLBUTRIN SR, WELLBUTRIN XL, ZYBAN*)

Classification
Norepinephrine/dopamine reuptake inhibitor (NDRI); antidepressant, aminoketone

Indications
Used for the treatment of major depression of adults; used for smoking cessation, seasonal affective disorder (SAD)

Available Forms
Tablet, 75 and 100 mg; sustained-release (SR) tablet, 100 and 150 mg; extended-release tablet, 100, 150, 200, and 300 mg; 450 mg XL newly available. Plain bupropion is still available.

Dosage
Adults: 100 mg PO TID; start, 100 mg PO BID, dose increase after 3 days; maximum, 150 to 450 mg/dose , 450 mg/day

Administration
Depending on formulation prescribed, taken TID (rapid release), BID; second dose not to be given within 5 to 6 hours of bedtime to avoid insomnia (SR) and to prevent seizures. SR without food and XL formulations are most commonly used, and XL formulation is recommended if available. Extended-release formulations to be taken once daily.

Side Effects
- Dry mouth, headache, agitation
- Seizure threshold significantly decreased particularly at greater than 300 to 450 mg/day dosage. Use of SR or XL formulation is also helpful in reducing risk of seizure, suicidal behavior, and arrythmias
- Headache, anxiety, tremor, tachycardia, and insomnia; cognitive impairment and mental clouding; delayed hypersensitivity reactions; tachycardia; nausea; increased sweating; blurred vision; dry mouth; weight loss are the other side effects

Drug Interactions
It can be fatal when combined with monoamine oxidase inhibitors (MAOIs). Caution: Use with *Phenergan* with codeine, Linezolid, and ethanol. Avoid other medications that lower seizure threshold, including benzodiazepine withdrawal.

- The drug can elevate tricyclic antidepressant activity; use with caution.
- It potentially increases plasma levels of other 2D6 metabolites.
- Risk of seizure may be increased by concomitant use of inhibitors of CYP2D6 (e.g., desipramine, sertraline, paroxetine, fluoxetine), due to increased bupropion blood levels. Nausea; dizziness; constipation; tremor; sweating; abnormal dreams; insomnia; tinnitus; pharyngitis; anorexia; weight loss; infection; abdominal pain; diarrhea; anxiety; flatulence; rash; palpitations; myalgia/arthralgia; chest pain; blurred vision; urinary frequency; suicidality; depression, worsening; psychiatric

NOTE: For some drugs, off-label use is reported. It is the responsibility of the practitioner to evaluate the efficacy of such use.

disorder exacerbation; behavioral disturbances; agitation; psychosis; hallucinations; paranoia; mania; seizures; hepatotoxicity; arrhythmias; tachycardia; hypertension (HTN), severe; elevated intraocular pressure; migraine; Stevens–Johnson syndrome; erythema multiforme; anaphylactic/anaphylactoid reactions

Pharmacokinetics
- It inhibits activity of CYP450 2D6, potentially increasing plasma levels of other 2D6 metabolites.
- It has been converted to an active metabolite.
- Mechanism for smoking cessation is unknown.
- The exact mechanism of action for depression is unknown.
- The drug inhibits neuronal uptake of norepinephrine and dopamine.
- *Metabolism:* Liver, excreted mainly in the urine
- *Half-life:* Parent compound, 10 to 24 hours; active metabolite, 20 to 24 hours
- 8 to 24 hours, *peak:* 3 to 5 hours

Precautions
- Use with caution in patients with cardiovascular disease, hepatic impairment, or renal impairment.
- Do not use in patients with seizure disorders, alcoholism, or hypersensitivity to drug/class.
- Do not use with MAOI until off the drug for 14 days.
- Seizure disorder
- Bulimia
- Anorexia nervosa
- Sexual dysfunction: less sexual dysfunction with bupropion
- Black box warning: Drug may cause hostility, agitation, and depressed mood. It may increase risk of suicidal thinking and behavior in children, adolescents, and young adults with major depressive disorder or other psychiatric disorder. It is not for use in children. Bupropion hydrobromide (Aplenzin is not approved for smoking cessation).
- *Patients at risk for seizure disorders: The drug may* lower seizure threshold.
- Avoid combinations with other central nervous system stimulants, injury/intracranial lesion, alcohol or drug abuse, psychiatric disorder, bipolar disorder, suicidality history, suicidal ideation.
- Use with caution in case of diabetes mellitus, cirrhosis, severe hepatic impairment, renal impairment, recent myocardial infarction, and HTN.

Patient and Family Education
- The medicine should be taken about the same time every day, preferably in the morning (for XL formulation) with or without food.
- If taking rapid-release or SR formulation, take last dose more than 5 to 6 hours from bedtime, as late dosing can precipitate insomnia.
- The drug may take up to 4 to 8 weeks to show its maximum effect, but some may see symptoms of dysthymia improving in as little as 2 weeks.
- If patient plans on becoming pregnant, discuss the benefits versus the risks of using this medicine while pregnant.
- This medicine is excreted in the breast milk, and hence, nursing mothers should not breastfeed while taking this medicine without prior consultation with a psychiatric

---

NOTE: For some drugs, off-label use is reported. It is the responsibility of the practitioner to evaluate the efficacy of such use.

nurse practitioner or psychiatrist. Newborns may develop symptoms, including feeding or breathing difficulties, seizures, muscle stiffness, jitteriness, or constant crying.

▪ Do not stop taking this medication unless your health care provider directs you to do so. Report side effects or worsening dysthymia symptoms to your health care provider promptly.

▪ Treatment should continue for 6 to 12 months following last reported dysthymic experience.

▪ Keep these medications out of the reach of children and pets.

▪ Store at room temperature.

▪ Monitor the patient for worsening psychiatric complaints.

Special Populations

▪ *Elderly:* Older individuals tend to be more sensitive to medication side effects, such as hypotension and anticholinergic effects. They often require adjustment of medication doses for hepatic or renal dysfunction. Begin at a lower dosage; XL formulation is recommended. Caution with use due to polypharmacy and comorbid conditions.

▪ *Pregnancy:* Psychotherapy is the initial choice for most pregnant patients with depression disorder (DD). Category C; not recommended during pregnancy, especially first trimester, as there are no adequate studies during pregnancy.

▪ *Lactation:* Unsafe

▪ *Children:* It is recommended that the dose begin in the lower range. Monitor the patient closely for suicidal ideation. Psychiatric consultation is recommended due to black box warning of increased suicidal ideation using selective serotonin reuptake inhibitor (SSRI) therapy in children. It may be useful in treating children with comorbid attention deficit hyperactivity disorder; ages 6 to 17 years.

NOTE: For some drugs, off-label use is reported. It is the responsibility of the practitioner to evaluate the efficacy of such use.

CARBAMAZEPINE (*TEGRETOL, CARBATROL, TERIL, TEGRETOL XR, EQUETRO*)

Classification
Mood-stabilizing anticonvulsant, iminostilbene derivative

Indications
Used alone or in combination with other medications for seizures and neuropathic pain. Additional uses include the treatment of trigeminal neuralgia. It can be used as extended-release capsules to treat episodes of mania or mixed episodes in patients with bipolar I disorder. It can be also used for tonic–clonic seizures, complex partial seizures, mixed seizure patterns (except Carbatrol and Equetro), borderline personality disorder, and alcohol withdrawal.

Available Forms
Tablet: 100 mg, 200 mg; extended-release (XR) capsule: 100, 200, 300, and 400 mg; oral suspension: 100 mg/5 mL; XR tablet: 200 mg, no 400 mg capsule; XR tablets: 100, 200, and 400 mg

Dosage
Trigeminal Neuralgia
- *Adults:* Begin with either 100 mg BID for tablets or XR tablets, or ½ teaspoon QID for suspension, for a total daily dose of 200 mg. This daily dose may be increased by up to 200 mg/day using increments of 100 mg every 12 hours for tablets or XR tablets, or 50 mg (½ teaspoon) QID for suspension, only as needed to achieve freedom from pain.
- Do not exceed 1,200 mg daily.
- *Maintenance:* Control of pain can be maintained in most patients with 400 to 800 mg daily. However, some patients may be maintained on as little as 200 mg daily, whereas others may require as much as 1,200 mg daily. At least once every 3 months throughout the treatment period, attempts should be made to reduce the dose to the minimum effective level or even to discontinue the drug.

Epilepsy
Adults and Children Above 12 Years of Age
- *Initial*: Either 200 mg BID for tablets and XR tablets, or 1 teaspoon QID for suspension (400 mg/day).
- Increase at weekly intervals by adding up to 200 mg/day using a BID regimen of Tegretol-XR or a TID or QID until the optimal response is obtained.
- It should not exceed 1,000 mg daily in children 12 to 15 years of age, and 1,200 mg daily in patients above 15 years of age.
- *Maintenance:* Usually 800 to 1,200 mg daily.

Children 6 to 12 Years of Age
- *Initial*: Either 100 mg BID for tablets or XR tablets, or ½ teaspoon QID for suspension (200 mg/day).
- Increase at weekly intervals by adding up to 100 mg/day BID of Tegretol-XR or a TID or QID of other formulations until the optimal response is obtained.
- Dosage generally should not exceed 1,000 mg daily.
- *Maintenance:* Usually 400 to 800 mg daily. Maximum dose can be 1,000 mg/day.

NOTE: For some drugs, off-label use is reported. It is the responsibility of the practitioner to evaluate the efficacy of such use.

Children Below 6 Years of Age
- *Initial:* 10 to 20 mg/kg/day BID or TID as tablets, or QID as suspension.
- Increase weekly to achieve optimal clinical response administered TID or QID.
- *Maintenance:* Optimal clinical response is achieved at daily doses below 35 mg/kg. If satisfactory clinical response has not been achieved, plasma levels should be measured to determine whether or not they are in the therapeutic range.

Administration
- Store at room temperature.
- Give with meals to reduce the risk of gastrointestinal (GI) distress.
- Shake oral suspension well.
- Do not administer with grapefruit juice.
- Do not crush capsules or tablets. If switching from tablets to capsules, maintain the same dose.
- Contents of extended-release capsules may be sprinkled over applesauce if the patient faces difficulty in swallowing.

Side Effects
- *Central nervous system (CNS):* Fatigue, lethargy, coma, epileptiform seizures, tremors, drowsiness, headache, confusion, restlessness, dizziness, psychomotor retardation, blackouts, electroencephalogram changes, worsened mental syndrome, impaired speech, ataxia, and incoordination
- *Cardiovascular:* Arrhythmias, bradycardia, reversible ECG changes, and hypotension.
- *EENT:* Tinnitus and blurred vision
- *GI:* Vomiting, anorexia, diarrhea, thirst, nausea, metallic taste, dry mouth, abdominal pain, flatulence, and indigestion
- *Genitourinary:* Polyuria, renal toxicity with long-term use, glycosuria, decreased creatinine clearance, and albuminuria
- *Hematologic:* Anemia, agranulocytosis, and leukocytosis with leukocyte count of 14,000 to 18,000/mm
- *Metabolic:* Transient hyperglycemia, goiter, hypothyroidism, and hyponatremia.
- *Musculoskeletal:* Muscle weakness
- Serious and sometimes fatal dermatologic reactions, including toxic epidermal necrolysis (TEN) and Stevens–Johnson syndrome (SJS), have been reported with Tegretol treatment.
- *Psychiatric:* Increase the risk of suicidal thoughts or behavior, possibility of activation of a latent psychosis and, in elderly patients, of confusion or agitation should be borne in mind.
- *Other:* Mild anticholinergic activity and use with caution in patients with increased intraocular pressure.
- The use of Tegretol should be avoided in patients with a history of hepatic porphyria (e.g., acute intermittent porphyria, variegate porphyria, and porphyria cutanea tarda).

Drug Interactions
- CYP 3A4 inhibitors inhibit Tegretol metabolism, which can increase plasma carbamazepine levels.
- Drugs that increase plasma carbamazepine levels include: cimetidine, danazol, diltiazem, macrolides, erythromycin, troleandomycin, clarithromycin, fluoxetine,

fluvoxamine, nefazodone, trazodone, loxapine, olanzapine, quetiapine, lorata-dine, terfenadine, omeprazole, oxybutynin, dantrolene, isoniazid, niacinamide, nicotinamide, ibuprofen, propoxyphene, azoles (e.g., ketaconazole, itraconazole, fluconazole, voriconazole), acetazolamide, verapamil, ticlopidine, grapefruit juice, protease inhibitors, valproate.

■ CYP 3A4 inducers can increase the rate of Tegretol metabolism.

▦ Drugs that decrease plasma carbamazepine levels include cisplatin, doxorubicin HCl, felbamate, fosphenytoin, rifampin, phenobarbital, phenytoin, primidone, methsuximide, theophylline, aminophylline.

■ Tegretol is a potent inducer of hepatic CYP 3A4 and may therefore reduce plasma concentrations of other drugs mainly metabolized by 3A4 through induction of their metabolism resulting in decreased levels of the following: acetaminophen, alprazolam, bupropion, dihydropyridine calcium channel blockers (e.g., felo-dipine), citalopram, cyclosporine, corticosteroids (e.g., prednisolone, dexametha-sone), clonazepam, clozapine, dicumarol, doxycycline, ethosuximide, everolimus, haloperidol, imatinib, itraconazole, lamotrigine, levothyroxine, methadone, meth-suximide, midazolam, olanzapine, oral and other hormonal contraceptives, oxcar-bazepine, phensuximide, phenytoin, praziquantel, protease inhibitors, risperidone, theophylline, tiagabine, topiramate, tramadol, trazodone, tricyclic antidepressants (e.g., imipramine, amitriptyline, nortriptyline), valproate, warfarin, ziprasidone, zonisamide.

■ Coadministration of carbamazepine with nefazodone results in insufficient plasma concentrations of nefazodone and its active metabolite to achieve a therapeutic effect. Coadministration of carbamazepine with nefazodone is contraindicated.

■ Concomitant administration of carbamazepine and lithium may increase the risk of neurotoxic side effects.

■ Concomitant use of carbamazepine and isoniazid has been reported to increase isoniazid-induced hepatotoxicity.

■ Concomitant medication with Tegretol and some diuretics (hydrochlorothiazide, furosemide) may lead to symptomatic hyponatremia.

■ Carbamazepine may antagonize the effects of nondepolarizing muscle relaxants.

■ Alterations of thyroid function have been reported in combination therapy with other anticonvulsant medications.

■ Concomitant use of Tegretol with hormonal contraceptive products (e.g., oral, and levonorgestrel subdermal implant contraceptives) may render the contraceptives less effective because the plasma concentrations of the hormones may be decreased.

■ Breakthrough bleeding and unintended pregnancies have been reported. Alternative or back-up methods of contraception should be considered.

■ Lamotrogine (may lower lamotrigine level and increase carbamezapine level)

■ *Peak action:* 30 minutes to 1 hour; PO: 1.5 to 12 hours, PO extended release: 4 to 8 hours

■ *Half-life:* 18 hours (adolescents); 36 hours (elderly). Twenty-five to 65 hours with single dose, 8 to 29 hours with long-term use

■ *Excretion:* Urine

Precautions

■ Before initiating therapy, perform a detailed history and physical examination.

■ Use with caution in patients with a mixed seizure disorder that includes atypical absence seizures due to increased frequency of seizures.

NOTE: For some drugs, off-label use is reported. It is the responsibility of the practitioner to evaluate the efficacy of such use.

- Use with caution in patients with a history of cardiac conduction disturbance, including second- and third-degree AV heart block; cardiac, hepatic, or renal damage; adverse hematologic or hypersensitivity reaction to other drugs, including reactions to other anticonvulsants.
- There are possible elevations of liver enzymes.
- Before initiating the drug, obtain a history of hypersensitivity reactions to other drugs for there is a high probability of sensitivity to this drug.
- Patients of Asian background should be screened for serious skin reactions before starting carbamazepine.
- Black box warning: Aplastic anemia and agranulocytosis have been reported. Obtain complete pretreatment hematologic testing as baseline. If patient in course of treatment exhibits low or decreased white blood cell or platelet counts, monitor closely. The drug may have to be discontinued if there is significant bone marrow depression.

Patient and Family Education

- Patients should be made aware of the early toxic signs and symptoms of a potential hematologic problem, as well as dermatologic, hypersensitivity or hepatic reactions.
- The patient should be advised that he or she must report any occurrence of side effects immediately to a provider.
- In addition, the patient should be advised that any side effects should be reported, even if mild or when occurring after extended use.
- Patients, their caregivers, and families should be counseled on increased risk of suicidal thoughts and behavior or worsening of symptoms of depression; any unusual changes in mood or behavior; or the emergence of suicidal thoughts, behavior, or thoughts about self-harm.
- Patients should be advised that serious skin reactions have been reported in association with Tegretol. In the event a skin reaction should occur while taking Tegretol, patients should consult with their physician immediately.
- Tegretol may interact with some drugs. Therefore, patients should be advised to report to their doctors the use of any other prescription or nonprescription medications or herbal products.
- Caution should be exercised if alcohol is taken in combination with Tegretol therapy, due to a possible additive sedative effect.

Special Populations

- *Elderly:* Use with caution in men with benign prostatic hyperplasia (BPH) due to increased urinary retention; monitor for dizziness and falls secondary to sedation.
- *Pregnancy/lactation:* Do not use if breastfeeding.
- *Children:* Approved for use in epilepsy, therefore safety profile exists. Used off label for aggression.

NOTE: For some drugs, off-label use is reported. It is the responsibility of the practitioner to evaluate the efficacy of such use.

CHLORDIAZEPOXIDE HYDROCHLORIDE (*LIBRIUM*)

Classification
Benzodiazepine (BZD), anxiolytic

Indications
Used to achieve sedation during hypnosis, relieve anxiety, and prevent withdrawal from alcohol; used on a temporary (tapering) basis.

Available Forms
Capsule, 5, 10, and 25 mg

Dosage
Adults: 5 to 10 mg PO TID to QID. *Children aged 6 years or older:* 5 mg BID or QID; may be increased/day in 3 to 10 mg BID or TID.
For withdrawal symptoms of acute alcoholism: 50 to 100 mg PO, up to 300 mg/day

Administration
▥ Administered PO
▥ Use exactly as prescribed.
▥ Do not increase the dose, take it more frequently, or use it for a longer period of time
▥ Take with full glass of water.
▥ The drug should not be stopped abruptly, but tapered off slowly.
▥ When used for an extended period of time this medicine may not work as well and may require different dosing.
▥ Write prescription for the shortest duration possible to prevent potential dependence.
▥ *Missed dose:* Take as soon as remembered. Skip the missed dose if it is almost time for the next scheduled dose. Do not take extra medicine.

Side Effects
Drowsiness, ataxia, confusion, skin eruptions, edema, menstrual irregularities, nausea, constipation, extrapyramidal effects, libido changes, or paradoxical stimulation, depression, fatigue, sedation, dizziness, slurred speech, weakness, confusion, nervousness, hyperexcitability, hypersalivation, dry mouth; hallucinations (rare), and agranulocytosis.

Drug Interactions
▥ Avoid sodium oxybate as it can increase CNS and respiratory rate.
▥ There are increased CNS depressive effects when taken with other CNS depressants.
▥ Fluconazole and similar drugs can increase and prolong chlordiazepoxide levels. Avoid its use altogether.
  ▥ Cimetidine: This medicine may decrease chlordiazepoxide clearance and increase risk of adverse reactions.
  ▥ Digoxin: It may increase digoxin level and risk of toxicity.
  ▥ Disulfiram: It may decrease clearance and increase half-life of chlordiazepoxide.
  ▥ Herbs: Kava may increase sedation.

NOTE: For some drugs, off-label use is reported. It is the responsibility of the practitioner to evaluate the efficacy of such use.

Pharmacokinetics

- *Half-life:* 5 to 30 hours. Metabolites can range from 14 to 100 hours. It can last for weeks in the blood after the initial dosing interval.
- *Peak:* 0.5 to 4 hours
- Metabolized in the liver (CYP450) and excreted in the urine.
- Binds to BZD receptors and enhances gamma-aminobutyric acid effects.

Precautions

In general, concomitant administration of chlordiazepoxide and other psychotropic drugs is not recommended. Caution should be exercised in administering chlordiazepoxide to patients with a history of psychosis, depression, suicidal ideation, porphyria, or alcohol/drug substance abuse.

- Use with caution in patients with pulmonary impairment/disease.
- History of substance abuse increases risk of dependency.
- Some patients present with disinhibiting behaviors after administration.
- Since dependence may develop, use with caution in patients with history of depression. The action of BZDs may be potentiated by barbiturates, narcotics, phenothiazines, monoamine oxidase inhibitors, or other antidepressants, and can be used if depression, porphyria, suicidal ideation, alcohol/drug-abuse, or psychosis is present.

Patient and Family Education

- Inform the health care provider of glaucoma, hepatic or renal impairment, drug-abuse history, salivary flow decrease, or pregnancy.
- Take medicine as prescribed and do not abruptly stop without first consulting with provider.
- Before taking this medicine, tell provider of medical history of liver disease, kidney disease, lung/breathing problems, drug or alcohol abuse, or any allergies.
- Do not drive, operate heavy machinery, or perform dangerous activities until it is known how this medicine will exert its effects.
- This drug may be habit forming and should be used only by the person for whom it was prescribed.
- It can be taken with or without food.
- Do not drink alcohol.
- Smoking may decrease drug's effectiveness.

Special Populations

- *Elderly:* Start with 5 mg every day BID and then gradually increase to 5 mg PO BID or QID. Due to the sedative effects and increased risk of falls, all BZDs are included on Beers List of Potentially Inappropriate Medications for Geriatrics.
- Use with caution; it may require smaller dosage due to comorbid modalities.
- *Renal impairment:* CrCl greater than or equal to 10, no dose adjustment needed—for less than 10, decrease by 50%
- *Hepatic impairment:* Use with caution with hepatic impairment.
- *Pregnancy:* Category D; positive evidence of human fetal risk.
- *Lactation:* It is contraindicated for breastfeeding mothers.
- *Children and adolescents:* This drug is not recommended for children below 6 years of age. In children above 6 years, initial 10 to 20 mg/day in two to four doses: may increase to 20 to 30 mg/day in two to three divided doses if needed.

NOTE: For some drugs, off-label use is reported. It is the responsibility of the practitioner to evaluate the efficacy of such use.

CITALOPRAM HYDROCHLORIDE (*CELEXA*)

Classification
Selective serotonin reuptake inhibitor (SSRI), antidepressant

Indications
This medicine is used for major depressive disorder, premenstrual disorders, and obsessive compulsive disorder.

Available Forms
Oral tablet, 10, 20, and 40 mg; oral solution, 10 mg/5 mL

Dosage
- *Children:* The safety and effectiveness of using this drug to treat depression have not been established in children under 18 years of age. Black box warning: Not for use in children.
- *Adults:* Starting dose, 20 mg initially once daily in the morning or evening; then increase in 20-mg increments at intervals of no less than 1 week.
- *Elderly:* 20 mg/day initially; then slowly increase to 40 mg/day for nonresponding patients only. Increase dose incrementally 20 mg only once per week. Most patients reach efficacy at 40 mg daily.

Administration
- Give PO with a glass of water.
- Take the medicine with or without food.
- Scored tablets may be crushed.
- Take at regular intervals.
- Caution patients not to stop taking drug except on provider's advice.
- This drug is not prescribed for children.
- Instruct patients to take missed dose as soon as possible. If it is almost time for the next dose, advise to take only that dose.

Side Effects
Most common: The most common side effects are somnolence, headache, asthenia, dizziness, sweating, dry mouth, drowsiness, tremor, diarrhea, abnormal ejaculation, decreased libido, nausea, agitation, and suicide attempt.

Drug Interactions
Linezolid or MAOIs may cause anorexia, nervousness, anxiety, abnormal vision change in appetite, change in sex drive or performance, diarrhea, constipation, indigestion, and nausea.

- *Less common*: The less common side effects are suicidality, worsening depression, serotonin syndrome, seizures, hyponatremia, extrapyramidal symptoms, priapism, and acute-angle glaucoma.
- Most of the interactions occur with over-the-counter cough and cold preparations. This medicine may also interact with the following medications:
  - Absolute contraindications include concurrent use with MAOIs such as phenelzine (*Nardil*), tranylcypromine (*Parnate*), isocarboxazid (*Marplan*, and selegiline (*Eldepryl*).

NOTE: For some drugs, off-label use is reported. It is the responsibility of the practitioner to evaluate the efficacy of such use.

▦ Avoid using with other SSRIs due to serotonin effect; SNRI drugs such as desvenlafaxine (*Pristiq*) and venlafaxine (*Effexor*); drugs with sympathomimetic properties, such as phenylpropanolamine, pseudoephedrine, St. John's wort, diazepam (*Valium*), any other antidepressants; and clopidogrel (*Plavix*), amoxicillin, erythromycins, and lansoprazole (*Prevacid*).

▦ Exercise caution with cold medications, nonsteroid anti-inflammatory drugs (NSAIDs), and drugs used for analgesia with opioid properties, diabetes (DM), and serotonin syndrome.

▦ Use with caution due to increased risk of bleeding with NSAIDs, aspirin (ASA).

▦ *Alert:* This list may not describe all possible interactions. Instruct patients to provide a list of all medicines, herbs, nonprescription drugs, or dietary supplements used, and whether they smoke, drink alcohol, or use illegal drugs.

Pharmacokinetics

▦ *Onset:* 1 to 2 weeks

▦ *Peak:* 4 hours

▦ *Metabolism:* Citalopram is extensively metabolized in the liver into DCT, DDCT, and citalopram-N-oxide. The CYP enzymes that are responsible for the metabolism of citalopram are CYP2C19 and CYP3A4.

▦ *Excretion:* Primarily excreted in the urine (10% unchanged), feces Liver in CYP450 2C19, 3A4 substrate; 2D6 (weak) inhibitor.

▦ *Half-life:* 35 hours

Precautions

Contraindications

Sensitivity to citalopram; MAOI use within 14 days.

Cautions

While prescribing this drug be cautious of hepatic/renal impairment, history of seizures, mania, and hypomania.

▦ See patients as often as necessary to ensure that the drug is working on the panic attacks, determine compliance, and review side effects.

▦ Make sure patients realize that they need to take prescribed doses even if they do not feel better right away. It can take several weeks before they feel the full effect of the drug.

▦ Instruct patients and their families to watch for worsening depression or thoughts of suicide. Also, watch out for sudden or severe changes in feelings, such as feeling anxious, agitated, panicky, irritated, hostile, aggressive, impulsive, severely restless, overly excited, hyperactive, or not being able to sleep. If this happens, especially at the beginning of antidepressant treatment or after a change in dose, patient should call the health care provider.

▦ Drowsiness or dizziness: Patients should not drive or use machinery or do anything that needs mental alertness until the effects of this medicine are known.

▦ Caution patients not to stand or sit up quickly, especially if older. This reduces the risk of dizzy or fainting spells. Alcohol may interfere with the effect of this medicine. Avoid alcoholic drinks.

▦ Caution patients not to treat themselves for coughs, colds, or allergies without asking a health care professional for advice. Some ingredients, such as dextromethorphan, can increase possible side effects.

NOTE: For some drugs, off-label use is reported. It is the responsibility of the practitioner to evaluate the efficacy of such use.

- Dry mouth: Chewing sugarless gum, sucking hard candy, and drinking plenty of water may help. Contact health care provider if the problem persists or is severe.
- Caution should be exercised in the following:
  - Bipolar disorder or a family history of bipolar disorder
  - Diabetes
  - Heart disease
  - Liver disease
  - Electroconvulsive therapy
  - Seizures (convulsions)
  - Suicidal thoughts, plans, or attempts by patients or a family member
  - An unusual or allergic reaction to citalopram, other medicines, foods, dyes, or preservatives
  - Pregnancy or trying to get pregnant
  - Breastfeeding

Patient and Family Education
- Do not stop taking medication abruptly or increase dosage without notifying health care provider.
- Store at room temperature. Avoid alcohol use.
- Avoid tasks that require alertness and motor skills until response to drug is established.
- Try to take the medicine at the same time each day. Follow the directions on the prescription label. To get the correct dose of liquid citalopram, measure the liquid with a marked measuring spoon or medicine cup, not with a regular tablespoon. If there is no dose-measuring device available, ask the pharmacist for one.

Special Populations
- *Elderly*: The elderly are more sensitive to anticholinergic effects. They are more likely to experience dizziness, sedation, confusion, hypotension, and hyperexcitability. They are generally able to tolerate citalopram better than other SSRIs.
- *Children*: Citalopram may cause increased anticholinergic effects and hyperexcitability. It is not indicated for children.
- *Renal and hepatic impairment:* The initial dose should be reduced in patients with severe renal and/or hepatic impairment. Half-life is doubled in patients with hepatic impairment. Titration upward should be slow and at intervals.
- *Pregnancy:* Category C; potential for persistent pulmonary hypertension if the patient is at more than 20 weeks' gestation.
- *Lactation:* Drug is excreted in human breast milk, some reports of infant somulence. Lactation is not recommended.

NOTE: For some drugs, off-label use is reported. It is the responsibility of the practitioner to evaluate the efficacy of such use.

CLOMIPRAMINE (*ANAFRANIL*)

Classification
Tricyclic antidepressant (TCA)

Indications
■ This drug is not used much anymore; it is off many formularies due to high risk of suicidality and completion.
■ It is indicated for obsessive compulsive disorder (OCD) B.

Available Forms
Capsule, 25, 50, and 75 mg

Dosage
The dose ranges from 75 to 300 mg. Generally, 150 to 250 mg is the most effective dosage for OCD. A dosage of 75 to 100 mg is usually only used in women weighing in the 100-pound range. Starting dose of 25 to 50 mg, which can then be increased by 25 to 50 mg every 1 to 3 days. It takes 6 to 10 weeks for the full effect to be realized. A dose close to 250 mg taken over 10 weeks, on average, produces the best results.

Administration
Take this medicine PO with or without food. Do not abruptly discontinue medication.

Side Effects
Dry mouth, nausea, vomiting, diarrhea, constipation, nervousness, decreased sexual ability, decreased memory or concentration, headache, stuffy nose, and change in appetite or weight. *The following side effects should be immediately reported to the clinician:* Extrapyramidal syndrome/dystonia seizures; fast, irregular, or pounding heartbeat; difficulty urinating or loss of bladder control; believing things that are not true, hallucinations (seeing things or hearing voices that do not exist), eye pain; shakiness; difficulty breathing or fast breathing; severe muscle stiffness, unusual tiredness or weakness; and sore throat, fever, and other signs of infection.

Drug Interactions
■ The following drugs are contraindicated: antiarrhythmics Class IA such as procainamide, quinidine gluconate, quinidine sulfate, disopyramide (*Norpace*) as these may increase risk of side effects or increase the risk of a QT prolongation.
■ Specific medications that may interact with the agent include cimetidine (*Tagamet*); guanethidine monosulfate (*Ismelin*; methylphenidate [Concerta, Ritalin, Daytrana]); phenytoin (*Dilantin*); warfarin (*Coumadin*); heart or blood pressure medication, such as clonidine (*Catapres*) or digoxin (*Lanoxin*); heart rhythm medications, such as flecainide (*Tambocor*), quinidine (*Cardioquin, Quinidex, Quinaglute*); or antipsychotic medications, such as chlorpromazine (*Thorazine*), haloperidol (*Haldol*), thioridazine (*Mellaril*), clozapine (*Clozaril*), olanzapine (*Zyprexa, Zydis*), quetiapine (*Seroquel*), risperidone (*Risperdal*), or ziprasidone (*Geodon*). Cisapride (*Propulsid*) may increase risk of QT prolongation, cardiac arrhythmias; dronedarone (*Multaq*) may increase TCA levels and risk of adverse effects, increase risk of QT prolongation, cardiac arrhythmias; may increase risk of cardiac arrhythmias, seizures.

NOTE: For some drugs, off-label use is reported. It is the responsibility of the practitioner to evaluate the efficacy of such use.

▧ Monoamine oxidase inhibitors (MAOIs) such as selegiline (*Eldepryl/Zelapar*), pro-carbazine (*Matulane*), phenelzine (*Nardil*), tranylcypromine (*Parnate*), isocarboxazid (*Marplan*), selegiline transdermal (*Eldepryl/Zelapar*), and rasagiline (*Azilect*) may result in central nervous system (CNS) overstimulation, hyperpyrexia, seizures, or death.

▧ Pimozide (*Orap*) may increase risk of CNS depression and psychomotor impair-ment, QT prolongation, arrhythmias, anticholinergic effects, hyperpyrexia; potassium salts such as potassium acid phosphate, potassium citrate, potassium chloride, potassium iodide, potassium phosphate/sodium phosphate, potassium acid, phosphate/sodium acid phosphate, and potassium phosphate are contraindi-cated for solid potassium dose forms.

▧ Weigh risk/benefit of thyroid protection with solid iodide salt forms, may delay solid potassium passage through gastrointestinal (GI) tract, increase risk of ulcer-ative/stenotic lesions.

▧ Use with caution in patients with altered GI motility.

▧ Monitor the patient for anticholinergic symptoms.

Pharmacokinetics

This drug is presumed to influence obsessive and compulsive behaviors through its effects on serotonergic neuronal transmission.

▧ It is metabolized in the liver extensively (CYP450, 1A2, 2C19, 2D6) and is excreted in the urine (66%) and in the feces (32%).

▧ *Half-life:* 32 hours

▧ *Peak:* 2 to 6 hours

▧ The exact neurochemical mechanism of action is unknown, but its capacity to inhibit the reuptake of serotonin (5-HT) is thought to be important.

Precautions

▧ It is contraindicated with recent myocardial infarction.

▧ Do not use the drug if MAOI used within past 14 days.

▧ Do not use the drug if patient is allergic to similar drugs (TCAs).

▧ Monitor the patient for suicidal thoughts.

▧ Report new or worsening symptoms of mood or behavior changes, anxiety, panic attacks, insomnia, or feelings of impulsivity, irritability, agitation, hostility aggres-siveness, restlessness, hyperactivity, increased depression, or suicidal thoughts. It inhibits norepinephrine and serotonin reuptake.

Patient and Family Education

▧ Anxiety symptoms may temporarily worsen when you first start taking clomipramine.

▧ Do not stop taking this medicine without notifying the health care provider.

▧ Anxiety symptoms may temporarily worsen when first starting.

▧ Notify doctor or pharmacist promptly if any of these effects persist or worsen.

▧ To relieve dry mouth, suck on (sugarless) hard candy or ice chips, chew (sugarless) gum, drink water, or use a saliva substitute.

▧ To prevent constipation, maintain a diet adequate in fiber, drink plenty of water, and exercise. In case of constipation, consult your pharmacist for help in selecting a laxative (e.g., stimulant-type with stool softener).

NOTE: For some drugs, off-label use is reported. It is the responsibility of the practitioner to evaluate the efficacy of such use.

- Notify your clinician immediately if any of these unlikely but serious side effects occur: mental/mood changes (e.g., confusion, depression, hallucinations, memory problems), enlarged/painful breasts, unwanted breast milk production, irregular/painful menstrual periods, muscle stiffness/twitching, feelings of restlessness, ringing in the ears, sexual problems (e.g., decreased sexual ability, changes in desire), shakiness (tremors), numbness/tingling of the hands/feet, trouble urinating, and severe vomiting.
- Notify your clinician immediately if any of these rare but very serious side effects occur: easy bruising/bleeding, signs of infection (e.g., fever, persistent sore throat), unusual/uncontrolled movements (especially of the tongue/ face/lips), severe stomach/abdominal pain, dark urine, and yellowing of eyes/skin.
- Seek immediate medical attention if any of these rare but very serious side effects occur: black stools, chest pain, fainting, high fever, slow/fast/irregular heartbeat, seizures, vomit that looks like coffee grounds.

Special Populations
- *Elderly:* Lower doses are recommended.
- *Renal impairment:* Significant caution is warranted with renal impairment.
- *Hepatic impairment:* Caution is advised in children with hepatic impairment.
- *Pregnancy/Lactation*: This is a category C drug; animal studies have shown adverse fetal effects.
- *Children and adolescents 12 to 17 years*: There is an increased risk of suicidality in children, adolescents, and young adults. Gradual increase in dose is recommended.

NOTE: For some drugs, off-label use is reported. It is the responsibility of the practitioner to evaluate the efficacy of such use.

CLONAZEPAM (*KLONOPIN*)

Classification
Benzodiazepine (BZD)

Indications
■ This is an antianxiety medication.
■ It is also used to prevent seizures.

Available Forms
Tablets, 0.5, 1, and 2 mg; disintegrating tablets, 0.125, 0.25, 0.5, 1, and 2 mg

Dosage
■ For seizures in adults the initial dose is 1.5 mg daily in three divided doses.
■ Dosage may be increased by 0.5 to 1 mg daily every 3 days until seizures are controlled or side effects preclude further increases in dose.
■ The maximum dose is 20 mg daily.
■ The initial dose for panic disorders is 0.25 mg twice daily.
■ The dose may be increased to the target dose of 1 mg daily after 3 days.

Administration
■ The dose is tailored to the patient's needs.
■ It can be taken with or without food.

Side Effects
■ Sedation, dizziness weakness, and unsteadiness
■ Depression, loss of orientation, headache, and sleep disturbance

Drug Interactions
■ Other BZDs can accentuate the effects of other drugs that slow the brain's processes, such as alcohol, barbiturates, and narcotics, and leads to increased sedation.

Pharmacokinetics
■ Act by enhancing the effects of GABA in the brain. GABA inhibits brain activity.
■ Excessive activity in the brain can cause anxiety or mood disorders.

Precautions
■ Sudden cessation of the drug can cause seizures, tremors, muscle cramping, vomiting, and/or sweating, severe depression, agitation, and insomnia.
■ The dose should be reduced slowly.
■ It can cause increased risk of suicidal thinking and behavior.
■ Observe patient for clinical worsening, suicidal thoughts, or unusual changes in behavior.

Patient Education
■ This drug can cause physical dependence.
■ Never stop taking the drug, as sudden cessation of the drug can cause serious side effects.
■ Report all side effects to provider.

NOTE: For some drugs, off-label use is reported. It is the responsibility of the practitioner to evaluate the efficacy of such use.

Special Populations

▨ *Elderly:* Elderly patients are more sensitive to this drug's CNS effects.

▨ *Pregnancy:* Category D

▢ There is documented evidence of fetal damage, including congenital malformations, when taken by pregnant women in their first trimester.

▢ It is not recommended throughout pregnancy.

▨ *Lactation:*

▢ BZDs are secreted in breast milk.

▢ It is not recommended for mothers who are breastfeeding.

▨ *Children:* The drug is not indicated for treatment of panic disorder or restless legs syndrome.

CLONIDINE HYDROCHLORIDE (*CATAPRES, DIXARIT, DURACLON, JENLOGA, KAPVAY, CATAPRES-TTS*)

Classification
Alpha-agonist, antihypertensive

Indications
- ▦ Essential and renal hypertension, severe cancer pain new indication* attention deficit hyperactivity disorder (ADHD) as monotherapy or adjunct to stimulant medications.
- ▦ It is used for ADHD, control of pain, and has been used off label for control of withdrawal symptoms for opiates and ETOH.

Available Forms
- ▦ Tablet, 0.1, 0.2, and 0.3 mg; 0.025 mg, 0.1 mg, 0.2 mg, 0.3 mg; extended-release tablets, 0.1 mg, 0.17 mg, 0.2 mg, and 0.26 mg.
- ▦ Topical patch (7-day administration): 0.1 mg/24 hr, 0.2 mg/24 hr, and 0.3 mg/24 hr; extended-release tablets and injection and as Nexiclon oral suspension: 0.09 mg/mL.

Dosage
Oral: 0.1 to 0.3 mg given in two to three divided doses prn (as needed). Maximum dose is dependent on clinical response but should not exceed 0.6 mg.
Topical: Apply once every 7 days and based on indications for use.

Administration
Oral: Take the medicine with a full glass of water; it may be taken with or without food.
Topical: Apply patch on skin without hair. Leave it in place for 7 days. It may require special covering. Take last dose immediately before bedtime.

Side Effects
Dry mouth, sedation, dizziness, constipation, weakness, fatigue, insomnia, headache, impotence, loss of libido, major depression, hypotension, nervousness, agitation, nausea, vomiting, rashes with patches, bradycardia, and severe rebound hypertension are the side effects of the drug.

Drug Interactions
- ▦ Do not administer the medicine with a beta-blocker due to cardiovascular symptoms. It may cause the paradoxical hypertensive effect.
- ▦ It causes increased sedative and depressive symptoms when given with another CNS depressant.
- ▦ Administration with drugs that affect sinus node or AV function may result in bradycardia or AV block. Herbs such as capsicum and ma huang may reduce antihypertensive effectiveness; digoxin, verapamil, and diuretics may increase hypotensive effect; levodopa may reduce effectiveness of levodopa; monoamine oxidase inhibitors: may decrease antihypertensive effect.

NOTE: For some drugs, off-label use is reported. It is the responsibility of the practitioner to evaluate the efficacy of such use.

Pharmacokinetics
- Inhibit central vasomotor centers, lowering peripheral vascular resistance, blood pressure, and heart rate
- *Metabolism:* Liver, excreted by kidney (urine 72%)
- *Peak:* PO = 2 to 4 hours; transdermal = 2 to 3 days
- *Half-life:* 6 to 20 hours

Precautions
- There have been rare cases of hypertensive crisis and stroke after abrupt discontinuation.
- If used with a beta-blocker, the beta-blocker should be stopped several days before tapering drug.

Patient and Family Education
- Make position changes slowly and in stages. Dangle feet over bed prior to standing.
- Lie down immediately if feeling faint or dizzy.
- Avoid potentially hazardous activities until effect of medication has been determined.
- *Missed dose:* Take the dose as soon as remembered. If it is almost time for next dose, wait until next regularly scheduled dose. Do not take extra medicine to make up the missed dose.

Special Populations
- *Elderly:* Use with caution due to sedative effects.
- *Renal impairment:* Use with caution. It may require smaller dosage.
- *Hepatic impairment*: Use with caution.
- *Pregnancy:* Category C
- *Lactation:* Some drug is found in mother's breast milk; discontinue drug or bottle-feed.
- *Children and adolescents*: Safety and efficacy not established for children under 12 years; children are more likely to experience CNS depression with overdose.

NOTE: For some drugs, off-label use is reported. It is the responsibility of the practitioner to evaluate the efficacy of such use.

CLORAZEPATE (*TRANXENE*)

Classification
Benzodiazepine (BZD)

Indications
Clorazepate is used to achieve sedation during hypnosis and to relieve anxiety.

Available Forms
Tablet, 3.75, 7.5, and 15 mg

Dosage
Adults: 15-to 60-mg dose PO every day divided into BID or TID, or 15 to 30 mg at bedtime.

Children (9 to 12 years): Start 7.5 mg PO BID. Maximum, 60 mg/day. Alternatively, dose can begin at 0.3 mg/kg/day PO divided into BID or QID.

Administration
The drug is taken as per PO. It should not abruptly stop taking this drug. To discontinue this drug, client must consult with health care provider.

Side Effects
Drowsiness, dizziness, various GI complaints, nervousness, blurred vision, dry mouth, headache, and confusion.

Drug Interactions
- Avoid antacids.
- Avoid sodium oxybate as it can increase CNS and respiratory depression.
- Chloramphenicol, cimetidine (*Tagamet*), clarithromycin (*Biaxin*), conivaptan (*Vaprisol*), cyclosporine (*Gengraf/Neoral*), delavirdine (*Rescriptor*), imatinib (*Gleevec*), isoniazid, itraconazole (*Sporanox*), ketoconazole, nefazodone (*Serzone*), posaconazole (*Noxafil*), protease inhibitors, telithromycin (*Ketek*), voriconazole (*Vfend*), and use of antacids for they may increase BZD levels, risk of CNS depression, and psychomotor impairment.
- The action of BZDs may be potentiated by barbiturates, narcotics, phenothiazines, monoamine oxidase inhibitors, or other antidepressants. The concomitant use of other CNS depressant drugs is contraindicated.

Pharmacokinetics
- Drug is metabolized in the liver (CYP 450) and excreted primarily through the urine and feces.
- This drug has depressant effects on the CNS by binding to BZD receptors and enhancing GABA effects.
- *Half-life:* 40 to 50 hours
- *Onset:* 1 to 2 hours
- *Duration:* Variable 8 to 24 hours

NOTE: For some drugs, off-label use is reported. It is the responsibility of the practitioner to evaluate the efficacy of such use.

Precautions

Serious reactions to the drug include hepatotoxicity, respiratory depression, seizure exacerbation, suicidality, dependency, and abuse.

Patient and Family Education

- Do not abruptly stop taking the drug without consulting the prescriber; the dose must be carefully tapered.
- It may increase the risk of suicidal thoughts and behavior; be alert for the emergence of or worsening of signs and symptoms of depression, unusual changes in mood or behavior, or emergence of suicidal thoughts.
- Avoid taking this drug if there is a known hypersensitivity to the drug or if there is acute narrow-angle glaucoma.
- Do not drive, operate heavy machinery, or do other dangerous activities until it is known how clorazepate exerts its effects.
- Do not drink alcohol or take other drugs that may cause sleepiness or dizziness while taking clorazepate without first talking to the provider.
- Avoid becoming pregnant while on this drug; if pregnancy occurs, alert health care provider immediately.

Special Populations

- *Elderly*: The elderly or debilitated patients need to start at 7.5 to 15 mg/day. Due to its sedative effect and increased risk of falls, all BZDs are included on Beers List of Potentially Inappropriate Medications for Geriatrics.
- *Renal impairment:* No adjustment needed.
- *Hepatic impairment:* Not defined at this time.
- *Pregnancy*: Category D; trimester specific. There is an increased risk of congenital malformations associated with the use of this drug during the first trimester of pregnancy.
- *Lactation:* It is probably safe during lactation but caution is advised.
- *Children*: Pediatric dosing is currently unavailable or not applicable. It is not recommended for children under 9 years of age.

NOTE: For some drugs, off-label use is reported. It is the responsibility of the practitioner to evaluate the efficacy of such use.

CLOZAPINE (*CLOZARIL, FAZACLO*)

Classification
Antipsychotic drug, atypical (second generation); dibenzapine derivative

Indications
It is used for treatment-resistant schizophrenia, reduction in risk of recurrent suicidal behavior in patients with schizophrenia, or schizoaffective disorder.

Available Forms
Orally disintegrating tablet, 12.5, 25, 100, 150, and 200 mg

Dosage
Taper to goal dose.

Children: This is a drug not for pediatric use.

Adults: 150 to 300 mg BID; start, 12.5 mg PO daily, BID, increase 25 to 450 mg/day every 3 to 7 days; maximum, 900 mg/day; taper dose gradually over 1 to 2 weeks to discontinue.

Administration
▦ The drug is subject to restricted distribution in the United States; permission for its use should be granted through the FDA. It requires registration. White blood cell (WBC) levels should be drawn weekly and reported to the dispensing pharmacy prior to drug being dispensed. After 6 months of normal WBC counts, blood draws reduced to every 2 weeks, monitor complete blood count, glucose, and cholesterol throughout treatment course—WBC/absolute neutrophil count (ANC) at baseline, then every week × 6 months, then every 2 weeks × 6 months, then every 4 weeks for treatment duration and every week × 4 weeks after discontinuing drug; fasting glucose at baseline if diabetes risk factors, then periodically; see package insert for additional recommendations based on results of WBC/ANC monitoring.

Side Effects
Hypotension, severe; syncope; extrapyramidal symptoms, severe; tardive dyskinesia; neuroleptic malignant syndrome; hyperglycemia, severe; diabetes mellitus; seizures; priapism; stroke; transient ischemic attacks (TIA); QT prolongation; hypersensitivity reaction; anaphylactic reaction; angioedema; erythema multiforme; leukopenia; neutropenia; agranulocytosis; suicidality; somnolence; increased appetite; fatigue; rhinitis; upper respiratory infections; nausea/vomiting; cough; urinary incontinence; salivation; constipation; fever; dystonia; abdominal pain; anxiety; dizziness; dry mouth; tremor; rash; akathisia; dyspepsia; tachycardia; hyperprolactinemia/gynecomastia; weight gain; dysphagia.

Drug Interactions
▦ The drug interacts with Haldol, sodium oxybate, and ziprasidone. Caution is required with diabetes and HTN.

▦ Tablets may be given with or without food. Take the regular oral tablet with a full glass of water.

NOTE: For some drugs, off-label use is reported. It is the responsibility of the practitioner to evaluate the efficacy of such use.

▓ The orally disintegrating tablet (*Fazaclo*) can be taken without water. Advise patients to keep the tablet in its blister pack until ready to take. The patient should gently peel back the foil from the blister pack and drop the tablet onto dry hand; place the tablet in mouth; it will begin to dissolve right away; allow it to dissolve in the mouth without chewing; swallow several times as the tablet dissolves. If desired, advise patients to drink liquid to help swallow the dissolved tablet.

▓ If one half of an orally disintegrating tablet is prescribed, advise patients to break the tablet in half and throw the other half away. DO NOT save the other half for later use.

▓ If patients stop taking clozapine for more than 2 days in a row, caution patients to call providers before starting to take it again.

▓ Store clozapine at room temperature away from moisture and heat.

▓ Risk or severity of bone marrow suppression may be increased if the drug is given in conjunction with medications that suppress bone marrow.

▓ Use with caution if given in conjunction with alcohol, central nervous system (CNS) depressants, or general anesthesia.

▓ It may enhance effects of antihypertensive drugs.

▓ It may need to reduce clozapine dose if given in conjunction with CYP450 1A2 inhibitors (e.g., fluvoxamine) or with smoking cessation.

▓ There may be a need to increase clozapine dose if given in conjunction with CYP450 1A2 inducers (e.g., cigarette smoke).

▓ CYP450 2D6 inhibitors (e.g., paroxetine, fluoxetine, and duloxetine) and CYP450 3A4 inhibitors (e.g., nefazodone, fluvoxamine, and fluoxetine) can raise clozapine levels, but usually dosage adjustment is not required.

▓ *Alert:* This list may not describe all possible interactions. Instruct clients to provide a list of all the medicines, herbs, nonprescription drugs, or dietary supplements they use.

Pharmacokinetics

▓ Exact mechanism of action is unknown.

▓ It antagonizes dopamine D2 receptors and serotonin 5-HT2 receptors.

▓ *Metabolism:* Metabolized by multiple CYP450 enzymes, including 1A2, 2D6, and 3A4.

▓ *Half-life:* 5 to 16 hours

▓ *Excretion:* Urine (50%), feces (30%)

Precautions

▓ Hypersensitivity to drug/class

▓ Caution in case of renal impairment, hepatic impairment, dementia, Parkinson's disease, and neuroleptic malignant syndrome history

▓ There is an increased risk of fatal myocarditis, especially during, but not limited to, the first month of therapy. Promptly discontinue clozapine if myocarditis is suspected.

▓ Life-threatening agranulocytosis can occur. Baseline WBC and ANC should be done before initiation of treatment, during treatment, and for at least 4 weeks after discontinuing treatment. Every week × 6 months, then every 2 weeks for 6 more months—monthly thereafter if blood work is acceptable.

▓ Use with caution in patients with glaucoma or enlarged prostate.

▓ *Do not use in patients with*
  ▓ Myeloproliferative disorder

NOTE: For some drugs, off-label use is reported. It is the responsibility of the practitioner to evaluate the efficacy of such use.

- Uncontrolled seizure history, cardiac disease, cerebrovascular disease, hypotension, hypovolemia, dehydration, aspiration pneumonia risk; it may impair body temperature regulation, PKU (phenylalanine-containing forms), diabetes mellitus or diabetes mellitus risk, Caution is required in elderly patients, pediatric or adolescent patients, drug-induced leukopenia or neutropenia history, suicide risk.
- Granulocytopenia
- Paralytic ileus
- CNS depression
- Allergic symptoms to clozapine

Patient and Family Education
- Drug effects can linger for 7 to 8 weeks after last dose.
- Clozapine will only be provided in 1- to 4-week supplies depending on frequency of WBC monitoring. Follow-up visits and weekly blood cell counts are required to monitor therapy and to keep appointments.
- Take prescribed dose with or without food. Take with food if stomach upset occurs.
- Keep tablet in unopened blister until just before use. Remove tablet by peeling the foil from the back of the blister and then immediately place the tablet (or half tablet, if ordered) in mouth, allow the tablet to disintegrate, and then swallow with saliva.
- Do not stop taking clozapine when feeling better.
- If medication needs to be discontinued, it will be slowly withdrawn over a period of 1 to 2 weeks unless safety concerns (e.g., low WBC) require a more rapid withdrawal.
- *Immediately report to provider* if any of these conditions occur: altered mental status, change in personality or mood, chest pain, fever, flu-like symptoms, frequent urination, general body discomfort, involuntary body or facial movements, lethargy, mucous membrane sores or other signs of possible infection, muscle rigidity, pounding in the chest, rapid or difficult breathing, rapid or irregular heartbeat, seizures, sore throat, sweating, swelling of feet or ankles, unexplained fatigue, unexplained shortness of breath, unquenchable thirst, weakness, or weight gain.
- *If you have diabetes*, monitor blood glucose more frequently when drug is started or dose is changed and inform provider of significant changes in readings.
- *If you are taking antihypertensive drugs*, monitor BP at regular intervals.
- *If you have history of seizures or factors predisposing to seizures*, clozapine may cause seizures. Do not engage in any activity in which sudden loss of consciousness could cause serious risk to you or others (e.g., driving, swimming, climbing).
- *Avoid* strenuous activity during periods of high temperature or humidity.
- *Avoid* alcoholic beverages and sedatives (e.g., diazepam) while taking clozapine.
- Get up slowly from a lying or sitting position and avoid sudden position changes to prevent postural hypotension. Hot tubs and hot showers or baths may make dizziness worse.
- Take sips of water, suck on ice chips or sugarless hard candy, or chew sugarless gum if dry mouth occurs. Excess salivation can be treated, report to physician.
- Clozapine may impair your judgment, thinking, or motor skills, or it may cause drowsiness. Thus, use with caution while driving or performing other tasks requiring mental alertness until tolerance is determined.

NOTE: For some drugs, off-label use is reported. It is the responsibility of the practitioner to evaluate the efficacy of such use.

Special Populations

- *Elderly:* Caution is required due to polypharmacy and comorbid conditions. The elderly may tolerate lower doses better. Elderly with dementia-related psychosis treated with atypical antipsychotics are at higher risk of death and cerebrovascular events.
- *Renal impairment*: Use with caution.
- *Hepatic impairment*: Use with caution.
- *Cardiac impairment:* Use with caution, especially if patient is taking concomitant medication.
- *Pregnancy:* Category B. Animal studies do not show significant evidence of safety.
- *Lactation:* It is not known whether clozapine is secreted in human breast milk. Discontinuing the drug or bottle-feeding are recommended. Infants of women who choose to breastfeed while on this drug should be monitored for possible adverse effects.
- *Children:* It is not for use in children who show adverse effects. There are no controlled studies in humans. Clozapine should be used only when the potential benefits outweigh potential risks to the fetus.

NOTE: For some drugs, off-label use is reported. It is the responsibility of the practitioner to evaluate the efficacy of such use.

CYCLOBENZAPRINE (*FLEXERIL*)

Classification
Muscle relaxant

Indications
It is used to treat short-term relief of muscle spasms associated with acute painful muscle and skeletal conditions.

Available Forms
Tablet, 5 and 10 mg; capsules (extended release), 15 and 30 mg

Dosage
The daily dosage is 5 or 10 mg three times daily using immediate-release tablets or 15 or 30 mg once daily using extended-release tablets.

Administration
- The drug is to be taken by mouth with or without food.
- It should usually be administered once daily.
- Swallow the capsules whole.
- Capsules cannot be crushed or chewed. Doing so can release all of the drug at once, increasing the risk of side effects.
- The dosage is based on medical condition and response to treatment.
- Should only be used short term (for 3 weeks or less)

Side Effects
- Drowsiness, dry mouth, fatigue, headaches, and dizziness
- Nausea, vomiting, gastrointestinal upset with constipation, acid reflux, and abdominal pain
- Blurred vision, agitation/nervousness, confusion
- The patient needs to understand not to stop taking this drug especially if he or she has taken it for over 3 weeks, for it could cause withdrawal symptoms.

Drug Interactions
The following products may cause serious drug-to-drug interactions:

- Tricyclic antidepressants
- Avoid MAOIs both 2 weeks before treatment and during treatment with this medication.
- Avoid taking this drug with other products that cause drowsiness, such as alcohol, antihistamines, drugs for sleep or anti-anxiety agents, other muscle relaxants, and narcotic pain relievers.

Pharmacokinetics
- The drug is metabolized and excreted via the kidney.
- The drug is eliminated quite slowly, with an effective half-life of 18 hours (range 8–37 hours; $n = 18$).
- Plasma clearance is 0.7 L/min.

NOTE: For some drugs, off-label use is reported. It is the responsibility of the practitioner to evaluate the efficacy of such use.

Precautions
- This drug should be used in caution with patients with liver disease, hyperthyroidism, irregular heartbeat, heart block, heart failure, recent history of myocardial infarction, BPH, and glaucoma.
- It may cause dizziness or drowsiness.
- Patients are advised not to drive, use machinery, or do any activity that requires alertness until effects of the drug are known.
- The patients should not indulge in alcoholic beverages while taking this medication.

Patient and Family Education
- If patient has used an MAOI such as isocarboxazid (Marplan), tranylcypromine (Parnate), phenelzine (Nardil), or selegiline (Eldepryl, Emsam) within the past 14 days, they cannot use this drug.
- Do not use this drug if patient has a significant cardiac history with a heart rhythm disorder, congestive heart failure, heart block, or an overactive thyroid.
- This drug may impair thinking or reactions.
- Avoid driving or doing anything that requires alertness.
- Avoid drinking alcohol, which can increase side effects of cyclobenzaprine.

Special Populations
- *Pregnancy:* There are no adequate studies of use in pregnant women.
- *Nursing Mothers:* It is not known whether the drug is secreted in milk. However, since it is related to the tricyclic antidepressants, some of which are excreted in breast milk, caution is advised in using this medication in women who are breastfeeding.
- *Elderly:*
  - The plasma concentration of cyclobenzaprine is increased in the elderly.
  - The elderly may also be more at risk of CNS adverse events.
  - Cardiac events
  - Falls.
  - NOTE: For these reasons, in the elderly, cyclobenzaprine should be used only if clearly needed. In the elderly, initiate dose at 5 mg and titrate upward slowly.
- *Pediatric:* Safety and effectiveness have not been established in pediatric patients younger than 15 years of age.

NOTE: For some drugs, off-label use is reported. It is the responsibility of the practitioner to evaluate the efficacy of such use.

CYPROHEPTADINE (*PERIACTIN*)

Classification
Antihistamine

Indications
This drug is used to treat hay fever; treatment of nightmares, including nightmares related to posttraumatic stress disorder; serotonin syndrome; and in cases of hypersero-toninemia. It can also be used as a preventive measure against migraine in children and adolescents. It can relieve selective serotonin reuptake inhibitor (SSRI)–induced sexual dysfunction and drug-induced hyperhidrosis (excessive sweating). It can also be used in the treatment of cyclical vomiting syndrome and to stimulate the appetite.

Available Forms
Tablet, 4 mg; oral solution, 2 mg/5 mL

Dosage
12 mg PO followed by 2 mg q2h until symptoms improve. Do not exceed 0.5 mg/kg/day.

Administration
PO; take with food to avoid gastrointestinal (GI) distress.

Drug Interactions
There are no interactions to avoid concomitant use.

Pharmacokinetics
▦ *Absorption:* Complete; peak 6 to 9 hours
▦ *Metabolism:* Hepatic
▦ *Half-life:* 1 to 4 hours

Precautions
▦ This drug is contraindicated in narrow-angle glaucoma.
▦ Concurrent use of monoamine oxidase inhibitors
▦ Precaution must be taken in cases of bladder neck obstruction and GI obstruction.
▦ It may cause CNS depression.

Patient and Family Education
Avoid using this drug with other depressants, sleep-inducing medications unless approved by prescriber. It can cause possible dizziness and drowsiness (caution when driving or engaging in tasks requiring alertness).

Special Populations
▦ *Elderly:* It may be inappropriate for the elderly due to anticholinergic effects although for short-term use, weigh risk versus benefit.
▦ *Pregnancy:* Pregnancy category B.
▦ *Lactation:* It is not indicated.
▦ *Outcome:* Symptoms improve in 24 hours although mental confusion can last for several days.

NOTE: For some drugs, off-label use is reported. It is the responsibility of the practitioner to evaluate the efficacy of such use.

DESIPRAMINE (*NORPRAMIN*)

Classification
Tricyclic antidepressant (TCA)

Indications
Desipramine is used to treat adults with depression.

Available Forms
Tablet, 10, 25, 50, 75, 100, and 150 mg

Dosage
Adult starting dose is 50 to 75 mg daily, 25 mg for elderly. PO daily, with a maximum of 300 mg/day for hospitalized patients and 200 mg/day for outpatients. For adolescents above the age of 12 years with major depressive disorder (MDD), the dosage is 150 mg per day. This drug may be given in divided doses; it must taper slowly to discontinue.

Administration
▓ PO with a glass of water
▓ Do not abruptly stop taking the medication.
▓ Food can lessen gastrointestinal upset.
▓ Not prescribed for children
▓ Use lowest effective dose for shortest duration—shortest but adequate duration for an optimal trial. Duration is based on number of episodes of depression.

Side Effects
▓ *More common:* Drowsiness, dizziness, constipation, nausea/vomiting, urinary retention or frequency, libido changes, weight gain, general nervousness, galactorrhea, rash, and urticaria are the most common side effects of desipramine.
▓ *Less common*: Cardiac arrhythmias, extrapyramidal symptoms, clotting disturbances, worsening depression, suicidality, hyperthermia, and hypertension are the less common side effects of desipramine.

Drug Interactions
▓ Absolute contraindications include class IA antiarrhythmics, monoamine oxidase inhibitors such as phenelzine (*Nardil*), tranylcypromine (*Parnate*), isocarboxazid (*Marplan*), and selegiline (*Eldepryl*).
▓ Avoid using with cimetidine, amiodarone, clarithromycin, erythromycin, haloperidol, and St. John's wort.
▓ *Alert:* This list may not describe all possible interactions. Instruct patients to provide a list of all medicines, herbs, nonprescription drugs, or dietary supplements used, and if they smoke, drink alcohol, or use illegal drugs.

Pharmacokinetics
▓ TCAs are thought to work by inhibiting reuptake of norepinephrine and serotonin in the central nervous system, which potentiates the neurotransmitters. They also have significant anticholinergics, antihistaminic, and alpha-adrenergic activity on the cardiac system. These classes of antidepressants also possess class 1A antiarrhythmic activity, which can lead to depression of cardiac conduction, potentially resulting in heart block or ventricular arrhythmias.

NOTE: For some drugs, off-label use is reported. It is the responsibility of the practitioner to evaluate the efficacy of such use.

▧ *Metabolism:* Primarily in the liver
▧ *Excretion:* Urine
▧ *Half-life:* 7 to 60 hours with high variability due to first-pass effects of those taking the drug.

Precautions
▧ See patients as often as necessary to ensure that the drug is working on the panic attacks, determine compliance, and review side effects.
▧ Instruct patients and families to watch for worsening depression or thoughts of suicide. Also watch out for sudden or severe changes in feelings such as feeling anxious, agitated, panicky, irritated, hostile, aggressive, impulsive, severely restless, overly excited, hyperactive, or not being able to sleep. If this happens, especially at the beginning of antidepressant treatment or after a change in dose, patient should call the health care provider.
▧ Drowsiness or dizziness: Patients should not drive or use machinery or do anything that needs mental alertness until the effects of this medicine are known. Other medications that cause drowsiness can add to the drowsiness of desipramine.
▧ Caution patients not to stand or sit up quickly, especially if older. This reduces the risk of dizzy or fainting spells. Alcohol may interfere with the effect of this medicine. Avoid alcoholic drinks.
▧ Do not abruptly withdraw this drug as it may cause headache, nausea, and malaise.
▧ Advise to protect skin from ultraviolet light due to increased skin sensitivity.
▧ Caution should be exercised in the following:
  ▧ Major depressive disorder (MDD), psychosis, or bipolar affective disorder
  ▧ Contraindicated in patients with a recent myocardial infarction
  ▧ Blood dyscrasias
  ▧ Respiratory disease
  ▧ Heart disease
  ▧ Liver disease
  ▧ Seizures (convulsions)
  ▧ Psychoses or schizophrenia
  ▧ Suicidal thoughts, plans, or attempts by patients or a family member
  ▧ Monitor for hypersentivities

Patient and Family Education
▧ Store desipramine at room temperature away from moisture and heat.
▧ Stopping this medication suddenly could result in unpleasant side effects.
▧ Take the missed dose as soon as remembered. If it is almost time for the next dose, skip the missed dose and take the medicine at the next regularly scheduled time. *Do not* take extra medicine to make up the missed dose.

Special Populations
▧ *Elderly:* Older patients may be more sensitive to the effects of TCAs. The smallest effective dose should be used (beginning at 10–25 mg/day). Dose adjustment is necessary for patients with liver impairment.
▧ *Pregnancy:* Category C; unknown effects as there is limited study.
▧ *Lactation:* The drug is excreted in human breast milk, and hence should be used with caution.
▧ *Children:* It is not indicated for children; is used off label in children 6 to 12 years of age; however, alternative medications are preferred.

NOTE: For some drugs, off-label use is reported. It is the responsibility of the practitioner to evaluate the efficacy of such use.

DESVENLAFAXINE (*PRISTIQ*)

Classification
Serotonin–norepinephrine reuptake inhibitor (SNRI)

Indications
Desvenlafaxine is used to treat major depressive disorder (MDD).

Available Forms
Extended-release tablets and tablets, 50 and 100 mg, respectively.

Dosage
The starting dose is 50 mg PO, daily. Doses greater than 50 mg/day are rarely more effective; maintenance may increase adverse drug reaction risk; consider a dose of 50 mg every other day if poorly tolerated in elderly.

Administration
PO can be taken with or without food. Do not crush, cut, or chew capsule or tablet.

- Take at regular intervals.
- Caution patients not to stop taking drug except on provider's advice.
- The drug is not prescribed for children.
- Instruct patients to take missed dose as soon as possible. If it is almost time for the next dose, advise to take only that dose.

Side Effects

- *Most common:* The most common side effects are nausea, vomiting, headache, insomnia, dizziness, somnolence, decreased libido and gastrointestinal distress, sexual dysfunction, palpitations, nervousness, hypertension, hyperchidrosis, constipation, and fatigue.
- *Less common:* The less common side effects are worsening depression, suicidality, hypersensitivity reactions, urinary retention, and increased blood pressure.

Drug Interactions

- Absolute contraindications to this drug include monoamine oxidase inhibitors (MAOIs) such as phenelzine (*Nardil*), tranylcypromine (*Parnate)*, isocarboxazid (*Marplan)*, and selegiline (*Eldepryl).*
- Avoid using with other selective serotonin reuptake inhibitors (SSRIs) due to serotonin effect; SNRI drugs such as venlafaxine (*Effexor*) and all triptan agents. Exercise caution with cold medications, nonsteroidal anti-inflammatory drugs (NSAIDs), and drugs used for analgesia with opioid properties.
- *Alert:* This list may not describe all possible interactions. Instruct patients to provide a list of all medicines, herbs, nonprescription drugs, or dietary supplements used, and if they smoke, drink alcohol, or use illegal drugs.

Pharmacokinetics

- SNRI agents are potent inhibitors of neuronal serotonin and norepinephrine reuptake and weak inhibitors of dopamine reuptake.
- Relative to SSRIs, SNRI agents seem to be more effective in treating chronic pain issues that coexist with depression and may produce more stimulative effects.

NOTE: For some drugs, off-label use is reported. It is the responsibility of the practitioner to evaluate the efficacy of such use.

- Highly bound to plasma proteins and has a large volume of distribution.
- *Metabolism:* Liver inactivation via CYP 3A4
- *Excretion:* Urine 64% to 69% (45% unchanged); 11 hours (O-desmethylvenlafaxine)
- *Half-life:* 11 hours, 13 to 14 hours (moderate-to-severe hepatic impairment), 13 to 18 hours (mild to severe renal impairment), 23 hours (end-stage renal disease)
- *Peak:* 7.5 hours
- The drug is not metabolized by P450s, so has more predictable plasma levels than many other antidepressants, including venlafaxine.

Precautions
- See patients as often as necessary to ensure that the drug is working on the panic attacks, determine compliance, and review side effects.
- Make sure patients realize that they need to take prescribed doses even if they do not feel better right away. It can take several weeks before depression resolves.
- Instruct patients and families to watch for worsening depression or thoughts of suicide. Also watch for sudden or severe changes in feelings, such as feeling anxious, agitated, panicky, irritated, hostile, aggressive, impulsive, severely restless, overly excited, hyperactive, or not being able to sleep. If this happens, especially at the beginning of antidepressant treatment or after a change in dose, patient should call the health care provider.
- Drowsiness or dizziness: Patients should not drive or use machinery or do anything that needs mental alertness until the effects of this medicine are known.
- Caution patients not to stand or sit up quickly, especially if older. This reduces the risk of dizzy or fainting spells. Alcohol may interfere with the effect of this medicine. Avoid alcoholic drinks.
- Caution patients not to treat themselves for coughs, colds, or allergies without asking a health care professional for advice. Some ingredients can increase possible side effects.
- Dry mouth: Chewing sugarless gum, sucking hard candy, and drinking plenty of water may help. Contact a health care provider if the problem persists or is severe.
- Caution should be exercised in the following:
  - Bipolar disorder or a family history of bipolar disorder
  - Diabetes
  - Heart disease
  - Liver disease
  - Seizures (convulsions)
  - Suicidal thoughts, plans, or attempts by patients or a family member
  - An unusual or allergic reaction to venlafaxine, other medicines, foods, dyes, or preservatives
  - Pregnancy or trying to get pregnant
  - Breastfeeding

Patient and Family Education
- Store at room temperature. Take any unused medication after the expiration date to the local pharmacy on drug give-back day. Avoid discarding the medication into the environment.
- Try to take the medicine at the same time each day. Follow the directions on the prescription label.
- Should be taken about the same time every day, morning or evening, and can be taken with or without food.

NOTE: For some drugs, off-label use is reported. It is the responsibility of the practitioner to evaluate the efficacy of such use.

- May take up to 4 weeks to be fully effective, but patient may see symptoms of depression improving in as few as 1 to 2 weeks.
- If patient plans on becoming pregnant, discuss the benefits versus the risks of using this medicine while pregnant. This medicine is excreted in breast milk; nursing mothers should not breastfeed while taking this medicine.
- This medication should be used only when clearly needed during pregnancy. Discuss the risks and benefits with your doctor.
- If this medication is used during the last 3 months of pregnancy, newborn may have feeding or breathing difficulties, seizures, muscle stiffness, jitteriness, or constant crying.
- This medication should not be stopped unless the health care provider directs it. Report any adverse symptoms to the health care provider promptly.
- Caution should be exercised when using this drug on the elderly because they may be more sensitive to the effects of the drug.
- Similar to other SNRIs
- Do not administer with MAOIs and use caution when combining with other drugs that have activating properties.
- Use with caution in patients with a history of seizures or heart disease.

Special Populations

- *Elderly:* Older individuals tend to be more sensitive to medication side effects, such as hypotension and anticholinergic effects. Often requires adjustment of medication doses for hepatic or renal dysfunction. Elderly patients may tolerate lower doses better and there is a reduced risk of suicide. This medicine may assist in the treatment of chronic or depression-related physical pain.
- *Pregnancy:* Psychotherapy is the initial choice for most pregnant patients with mild to moderate MDD. It is a Category C drug, as there are no adequate studies during pregnancy. Particular caution with exposure (avoid if possible) during first trimester. An individual risk–benefit analysis must be done to determine appropriate treatment in pregnant women with MDD.
- *Children:* Monitor closely, as risk of suicidal ideation is greatest in adolescents. Monitor for excessive activation effects or undiagnosed bipolar disorder. Obtain consultation with a pediatric psychiatric specialist.

DEXMETHYLPHENIDATE (*FOCALIN*)

Classification
Methylphenidate (amphetamine derivative)

Indications
Dexmethyphendidate is a stimulant indicated for the treatment of attention deficit hyperactivity disorder (ADHD) in children and adults.

Available Forms
Capsule, 2.5, 5, and 10 mg; extended-release capsules, 5, 10,15, 20, 25, 30, 35, and 40 mg

Dosage
Dosage should be individualized according to the therapeutic needs and responses of the patient. All stimulant preparations should be administered at the lowest effective dosage.

■ *Children older than 6 years*: 2.5 to 10 mg PO BID; start, 2.5 mg PO BID, increase 5 to 10 mg/day every 7 days; maximum, 20 mg/day; to convert from methylphenidate, start at 50% of current methylphenidate daily dose; space doses at least 4 hours apart

■ *Adults*: 2.5 to 10 mg BID, 2.5 mg PO BID, increase 5 to 10 mg/day every 7 days; maximum, 20 mg/day; to convert from methylphenidate start at 50% of current methylphenidate daily dose; space doses at least 4 hours apart. Extended release is once daily.

Administration
Do not crush or chew the drug; it may be given with or without food.

Side Effects
Decreased appetite, dizziness, dry mouth, irritability, insomnia, upper abdominal pain, nausea and/or vomiting, weight loss, headaches, anxiety, psychiatric events, increase in manic states for bipolar patients, aggression, tics, tremors, long-term growth suppression—patients should be monitored throughout treatment, if there appears to be growth suppression, the treatment should be discontinued—rash, pyrexia, palpitations, tachycardia, elevated blood pressure (BP), sudden death, myocardial infarction, cardiomyopathy, Stevens–Johnson syndrome and toxic epidermal necrolysis, impotence, and libido changes.

Drug Interactions
There are over 242 drugs that can interact with dexmethylphenidate. Make sure to review patients' drug regimen before prescribing this drug.

Pharmacokinetics
■ Drug is absorbed by the gastrointestinal tract.
■ Amphetamines are noncatecholamine-sympathomimetic amines with central nervous system–stimulant activity.

NOTE: For some drugs, off-label use is reported. It is the responsibility of the practitioner to evaluate the efficacy of such use.

■ The mode of therapeutic action in ADHD is not known. Amphetamines are thought to block the reuptake of norepinephrine and dopamine into the presynaptic neuron and increase the release of these monoamines into the extraneural space.
■ *Metabolism:* Liver; excreted in the urine
■ *Half-life:* 2 to 4.5 hours

Precautions
■ Advanced arteriosclerosis, symptomatic cardiovascular disease, moderate to severe HTN contraindicated in glaucoma, patients with motor tics or diagnosis of Tourettes
■ Hyperthyroidism
■ Known hypersensitivity or idiosyncratic reaction to sympathomimetic amines
■ Contraindicated in patients with glaucoma agitated states.
■ Patients with a history of drug abuse: Amphetamines have a high potential for abuse. Administration of amphetamines for an extended period of time may lead to drug dependence. Particular attention should be paid to the possibility of patients obtaining this class of medication for nontherapeutic use or distribution to others, and the drugs should be prescribed or dispensed sparingly.
■ During or within 14 days following the administration of monoamine oxidase inhibitors (MAOIs), hypertensive crisis may result.
■ Use with caution in patients with preexisting psychosis.
■ Seizure history: Some studies have shown that the drug has the potential for lowering the seizure threshold.

Patient and Family Education
■ Store the drug at room temperature, protected from light.
■ Keep out of reach of children.
■ Seek medical care for any signs of heart problems (chest pain, shortness of breath), fainting, psychotic symptoms, overdose, or any other concerns.
■ Routinely assess weight and BP.
■ Treatment should be initiated at low dosages and then titrated over 2 to 4 weeks until an adequate response is achieved, or unacceptable adverse effects occur.
■ If one stimulant is not effective, another should be attempted before second-line medications are considered. Although some children benefit from daily stimulant therapy, weekend and summer "drug holidays" are suggested for children whose ADHD symptoms predominantly affect schoolwork or to limit adverse effects (e.g., appetite suppression, abdominal pain, headache, insomnia, irritability, tics).

Special Populations
■ *Elderly:* Use with caution for elderly patients with polypharmacy and comorbid conditions; the drug has not been studied for use in this population.
■ *Pregnancy:* Category C; based on animal data, drug may cause fetal harm.
■ *Lactation:* It is possibly unsafe for breatfeeding.
■ *Children:* It has not been studied in children younger than 6 years; it should not be used in children younger than 6 years.

NOTE: For some drugs, off-label use is reported. It is the responsibility of the practitioner to evaluate the efficacy of such use.

DEXTROAMPHETAMINE AND AMPHETAMINE (*ADDERALL*)

Classification
Amphetamine

Indications
The medicine is a stimulant indicated for the treatment of attention deficit hyperactivity disorder (ADHD) and narcolepsy in children and adults.

Available Forms
Extended-release capsules and tablets, 5, 7.5, 10, 12.5, 15, 20, 25, and 30 mg

Dosage
- The drug is not recommended for children younger than 3 years of age.
- In children from 3 to 5 years of age, start with 2.5 mg daily; daily dosage may be raised in increments of 2.5 mg at weekly intervals until desired response is obtained.
- In children 6 years of age and older, start with 5 mg once or twice daily; daily dosage may be raised in increments of 5 mg at weekly intervals until optimal response is obtained.
- Only in rare cases will it be necessary to exceed a total of 40 mg/day. Give first dose on awakening; additional doses (one or two) at intervals of 4 to 6 hours.
- Where possible, drug administration should be interrupted occasionally to determine whether there is a recurrence of behavioral symptoms sufficient to require continued therapy.

Narcolepsy
- Usual dose of 5 mg to 60 mg per day in divided doses, depending on the individual patient response
- The suggested initial dose for patients aged 6 to 12 years is 5 mg daily; daily dose may be raised in increments of 5 mg at weekly intervals until optimal response is obtained.
- In patients 12 years of age and older, start with 10 mg daily; daily dosage may be raised in increments of 10 mg at weekly intervals until optimal response is obtained.
- Give first dose when first awake; additional doses (one or two) at intervals of 4 to 6 hours.

  Dosage should be individualized according to the therapeutic needs and response of the patient. All stimulant preparations should be administered at the lowest effective dosage. *Adults:* 5 to 40 mg/day PO divided daily TID; start, 5 mg PO QAM or BID, increase 5 mg/day every week, give divided doses; at 4- to 6-hour intervals, maximum, 60 mg/day; doses greater than 40 mg/day rarely more effective.

Administration
Swallow capsules whole with water or other liquids. If patient cannot swallow the capsule, open it and sprinkle the medicine over a spoonful of applesauce. Swallow all of the applesauce and medicine mixture without chewing immediately. Follow with a drink of water or other liquid. Never chew or crush the capsule or the medicine inside the capsule. It can be taken with or without food.

NOTE: For some drugs, off-label use is reported. It is the responsibility of the practitioner to evaluate the efficacy of such use.

Side Effects

Decreased appetite, dizziness, dry mouth, irritability, insomnia, upper abdominal pain, nausea and/or vomiting, weight loss, headaches, anxiety, psychiatric events (increase in manic states for bipolar patients, aggression, tics, tremors), long-term growth suppression (patients should be monitored throughout treatment; if there appears to be growth suppression, the treatment should be discontinued), rash, pyrexia, palpitations, tachycardia, elevated blood pressure (BP), sudden death, myocardial infarction, cardiomyopathy, Stevens–Johnson syndrome and toxic epidermal necrolysis, impotence, and libido changes.

Drug Interactions

This drug has too many drug interactions to mention. Provider must review patients' drug regimen to determine safety.

Pharmacokinetics

▦ The drug is absorbed by the gastrointestinal tract.
▦ Amphetamines are noncatecholamine sympathomimetic amines with central nervous system–stimulant activity.
▦ The mode of therapeutic action in ADHD is not known. Amphetamines are thought to block the reuptake of norepinephrine and dopamine into the presynaptic neuron and increase the release of these monoamines into the extraneural space.
▦ *Excretion:* Urine
▦ *Half-life:* 9 *to* 14 hours
▦ *Duration:* 4 to 6 hours; onset: 30 to 60 minutes

Precautions

▦ Advanced arteriosclerosis, symptomatic cardiovascular disease, moderate-to-severe hypertension
▦ Hyperthyroidism
▦ Known hypersensitivity or idiosyncratic reaction to sympathomimetic amines
▦ Contraindicated in glaucoma
▦ Agitated states
▦ Patients with a history of drug abuse: Amphetamines have a high potential for abuse. Administration of amphetamines for an extended period of time may lead to drug dependence. Particular attention should be paid to the possibility of subjects obtaining this class of medication for nontherapeutic use or distribution to others, and the drugs should be prescribed or dispensed sparingly.
▦ During or within 14 days following the administration of monoamine oxidase inhibitors (MAOIs), hypertensive crisis may result
▦ Use with caution in patients with preexisting psychosis.
▦ Seizure history; some studies have shown that the drug has the potential for lowering the seizure threshold.

Patient and Family Education

▦ Store the drug at room temperature, protected from light.
▦ Keep out of reach of children.
▦ Seek medical care for any signs of heart problems (chest pain, shortness of breath), fainting, psychotic symptoms, overdose, or any other concerns.
▦ Routinely assess weight and BP.

NOTE: For some drugs, off-label use is reported. It is the responsibility of the practitioner to evaluate the efficacy of such use.

■ Treatment should be initiated at low dosages and then titrated over 2 to 4 weeks until an adequate response is achieved or unacceptable adverse effects occur.

■ If one stimulant is not effective, another should be attempted before second-line medications are considered. Although some children benefit from daily stimulant therapy, weekend and summer "drug holidays" are suggested for children whose ADHD symptoms predominantly affect schoolwork, or to limit adverse effects (e.g., appetite suppression, abdominal pain, headache, insomnia, irritability, tics).

Special Populations

■ *Elderly*: Use with caution for the elderly patients with polypharmacy and comorbid conditions; it has not been studied for use in this population.

■ *Pregnancy*: Category C; based on animal data, they may cause fetal harm.

■ *Lactation*: It is possibly unsafe for breastfeeding.

■ *Children*: It has not been studied in children younger than 3 years old.

DIAZEPAM (*VALIUM*)

Classification
Benzodiazepine (BZD)

Indications
Diazepam used to treat anxiety, acute alcohol withdrawal, and seizures.

Available Forms
Tablets, 2, 5, and 10 mg; oral solution, 1 mg/mL, 5 mg/mL; injection solution, 5 mg/mL; intramuscular device, 10 mg/2 mL; rectal gel, 2.5, 10, and 20 mg

Dosage
▪ Dose for anxiety or seizures is 2 to 10 mg given two to four times daily.
▪ Rectal dose is 0.2 to 0.5 mg/kg.
▪ Age of the patient determines dosage

Administration
▪ Diazepam may be taken with or without food.

Side Effects
▪ Drowsiness, fatigue, and ataxia (loss of balance)
▪ Possible paradoxical reaction with excitability, muscle spasm, lack of sleep, and rage
▪ Confusion, depression, speech problems, and double vision also are rare side effects

Drug Interactions
▪ Alcohol or medications that cause sedation may add to the sedative effects of diazepam
▪ Avoid use with other BZDs.
▪ Cimetidine (Tagamet), ketoconazole (Nizoral), itraconazole (Sporanox), omeprazole (Prilosec, Rapinex), erythromycin, clarithromycin (Biaxin), darunavir (Prezista), fluvoxamine (Luvox), and fluoxetine (Prozac) may prolong the effects of diazepam by inhibiting liver enzymes that eliminate diazepam.
▪ Dosages may need to be decreased when these drugs are used with diazepam.
▪ Carbamazepine (Tegretol), rifampin (Rifadin), and St. John's wort decrease levels of diazepam by increasing the elimination of diazepam by liver enzymes.

Pharmacokinetics
▪ Diazepam is metabolized by the liver and is excreted mainly by the kidney.
▪ Dosages of diazepam may need to be lowered in patients with abnormal kidney function.

Precautions
▪ The dosages need to be lowered in patients with abnormal kidney function.
▪ It can lead to addiction (dependency), especially when higher dosages are used over prolonged periods of time.

NOTE: For some drugs, off-label use is reported. It is the responsibility of the practitioner to evaluate the efficacy of such use.

- Abrupt discontinuation may cause symptoms of withdrawal, lightheadedness, sweating, anxiety, and fatigue.
- Seizures can occur in more severe cases of withdrawal. Therefore, after extended use, diazepam should be slowly tapered under a provider's supervision rather than abruptly stopped.
- This drug may make patient dizzy, drowsy, or cause blurred vision; use caution engaging in activities requiring alertness such as driving or using machinery.
- Limit alcoholic beverages.
- Caution is advised when using this drug in the elderly because they may be more sensitive to the effects of the drug, especially the drowsiness effect.

Patient and Family Education
Inform the patient of the following:

- Provider should be made aware of all prescription and nonprescription/herbal products used, especially of antacids, certain antidepressants drugs that cause drowsiness medicine for sleep (e.g., sedatives), muscle relaxants, and narcotic pain relievers.
- This product can affect the results of certain lab tests.
- Smoking can decrease the effectiveness of this drug.
- Not to start or abruptly stop any medicine without provider approval

Special Populations
- *Elderly*: Adjust dose according to age
- *Pregnancy*: It can cause fetal abnormalities and should not be used during pregnancy.
- *Nursing mothers*: It is excreted in breast milk and can affect nursing infants and not be used in mothers who plan to breastfeed.
- *Pediatric*: The use of this drug is not recommended.

NOTE: For some drugs, off-label use is reported. It is the responsibility of the practitioner to evaluate the efficacy of such use.

DICYCLOMINE (*BENTYL*)

Classification
Anticholinergic drug

Indications
Dicyclomine is used to treat abdominal cramping associated with opiate withdrawal.

Available Forms
Capsule, 10 and 20 mg; liquid, 10 mg/5 mL syrup; and injection, 20 mg/2 mL syrup

Dosage
Dose is 40 mg four times daily. The dosage may begin with 20 mg IM, 10 to 20 mg QID and increase after 1 week to reduce side effects.

Administration
■ PO with glass of water
■ Measure liquid medicine with a special dose-measuring spoon or cup, not a regular tablespoon.

Side Effects
Confusion, disrupted thoughts, palpitations and/or arrhythmias, decreased urination, drowsiness, dizziness, blurred vision, nausea and/or vomiting, anorexia, pruritus or rash, stuffy nose, and dry mouth are the various side effects for dicyclomine.

Drug Interactions
■ The following medications may exacerbate side effects: amantadine, antiarrhythmic agents of class 1, antihistamines, antipsychotic agents, BZDs, monoamine oxidase inhibitors, narcotic analgesics, nitrites and nitrates sympathomimetic agents, and tricyclic antidepressants.
■ The drug may antagonize the effects of antiglaucoma agents.
■ It should be avoided when intraocular pressure is present and when taking corticosteroids.
■ It may affect gastrointestinal absorption of digoxin.
■ The drug may antagonize the effects of metoclopramide.
■ Avoid the use of dicyclomine simultaneously with the use of antacids.

Pharmacokinetics
■ *Half-life:* 1.8 hour

Precautions
■ The drug may increase risk of heat stroke by decreasing sweating.

Patient and Family Education
■ Use with caution when driving or operating machinery.
■ Avoid drinking alcohol.
■ Avoid become overheated or dehydrated during exercise and hot weather.
■ Tell health care provider about all prescription and over-the-counter medications due to interaction.

NOTE: For some drugs, off-label use is reported. It is the responsibility of the practitioner to evaluate the efficacy of such use.

Special Populations

▦ *Elderly*: Use with caution among elderly patients; dosage should start at the low end.
▦ *Renal impairment*: Use with caution.
▦ *Hepatic impairment*: Use with caution.
▦ *Pregnancy*: Category B
▦ *Lactation*: Contraindicated
▦ *Children and adolescents*: Safety and efficacy have not been established.
▦ *Other*: Use with caution in patients with the following: autonomic neuropathy, hepatic/renal disease, ulcerative colitis, hyperthyroidism, hypertension, coronary heart disease, heart failure, cardiac tachyarrhythmia, hiatal hernia, and prostatic hypertrophy.

DIPHENHYDRAMINE HYDROCHLORIDE (*BENEDRYL*)

Classification
Antihistamine

Indications
This drug is used to treat rhinitis, allergy symptoms, motion sickness, Parkinson disease

Available Forms
Capsules, 25 mg, 50 mg; elixir, 12.5 mg/5 mL; injection, 50 mg/mL, strips (oral disintegrating), 12.5 and 25 mg; syrup, 12.5 mg/5 mL; tablets, 25 mg, 50 mg, tablets (orally disintegrating: 12.5 mg)

Dosage
- *Adults and children age 12 years and over:* 25 to 50 mg PO every 4 to 6 hours; maximum 300 mg daily; 10 to 50 mg IV or deep IM maximum 400 mg/daily.
- *Children aged 6 to 11 years:* 12.5 to 25 mg PO every 4 to 6 hours; maximum dose 150 mg daily. 5 mg/kg deep IM or IV divided into four doses with maximum dose 300 mg daily.
- *Children aged 2 to 5 years:* 6.25 mg PO every 4 to 6 hours with maximum dose 37.5 mg daily. 5 mg/kg deep IM or IV divided into four doses with maximum dose 300 mg daily.
- Nighttime sleep aid:
  - *Adults:* 50 mg PO at bedtime
- Nonproductive cough:
  - *Adults and children aged 12 years and over:* 25 mg of syrup PO every 4 hours not to exceed 150 mg daily.
  - *Children aged 6 to 11 years:* 12.5 mg of syrup PO every 4 hours not to exceed 75 mg daily.
  - *Children 2 to 5 years old:* 6.25 mg of syrup every 4 hours not to exceed 25 mg daily.

Administration
- PO; give with food or milk to reduce gastrointestinal (GI) distress.
- IV: do not exceed 25 mg mg/min.
- IV incompatibilities: allopurinol, amobarbital, amphotericin B, cefepime, dixamethasone, foscarnet, haloperidol lactate, phenobarbital, phenytoin, thiopental.
- IM: Give deep Injection into large muscle.
- Alternate injection sites to prevent irritation.

Side Effects
- *Central nervous system*: Seizures, drowsiness, sedation, sleepiness, dizziness, incoordination, confusion, insomnia, headache, vertigo, fatigue, restlessness, tremor, and nervousness
- *Cardiovascular*: Palpitations, hypotension, and tachycardia
- *EENT*: Diplopia, blurred vision, nasal congestion, and tinnitus

NOTE: For some drugs, off-label use is reported. It is the responsibility of the practitioner to evaluate the efficacy of such use.

▧ *GI*: Dry mouth, nausea, epigastric distress, vomiting, diarrhea, constipation, and anorexia
▧ *Genetourinary*: Dysuria, urine retention, and urinary frequency
▧ *Hematologic*: Thrombocytopenia, agranulocytosis, and hemolytic anemia
▧ *Respiratory*: Thickening of bronchial secretions
▧ *Other*: Anaphylactic shock

Drug Interactions
▧ CNS depressants may increase sedation. Use together cautiously.
▧ Monoamine oxidase inhibitors (MAOIs) may increase anticholinergic effects. Avoid using together.
▧ Other products containing diphenhydramine may increase risk of adverse reactions. Drug lifestyle: alcohol use may increase CNS depression. Discourage use together.
▧ Sun exposure may cause photosensitivity reaction. Avoid prolonged sunlight exposure.
▧ Effects of lab test results: may decrease hemoglobin level and hematocrit, may decrease granulocyte and platelet counts, may prevent reduce or mask positive result in diagnostic skin test.

Pharmacokinetics
▧ PO onset: 15 minutes, peak 1 to 4 hours, duration 5 to 8 hours
▧ IV onset immediate, peak 1 to 4 hours, duration 6 to 8 hours
▧ IM onset unknown, peak 1 to 4 hours, duration 6 to 8 hours
▧ It competes with histamine for H1 receptor sites.
▧ Prevents but does not reverse histamine-mediated responses, particularly those of bronchial tubes, GI tract, uterus, and blood vessels.
▧ It is structurally related to local anesthetics.
▧ Drug provides local anesthesia and suppresses cough reflex.

Precautions
▧ The drug is contraindicated in patients hypersensitive to the drug, newborns, premature neonates.
▧ Breastfeeding women, patients with angle-closure glaucoma, stenosing peptic ulcer, symptomatic prostatic hyperplasia, bladder neck obstruction, or pyloroduodenal obstruction, and those having an acute asthmatic attack.
▧ Avoid the use of the drug in patients taking MAOIs.
▧ Use with caution with patients with prostatic hyperplasia, asthma, chronic obstructive pulmonary disease, increased intraocular pressure, hyperthyroidism, cardiovascular (CV) disease, and hypertension.
▧ Overdose signs and symptoms are dry mouth, fixed or dilated pupils, flushing, and GI symptoms.
▧ Stop drug 4 days before diagnostic skin testing. Injection form is for IV or IM administration only.
▧ Dizziness, excessive sedation, syncope, toxicity, paradoxical stimulation, and hypotension are more likely to occur in elderly patients.

NOTE: For some drugs, off-label use is reported. It is the responsibility of the practitioner to evaluate the efficacy of such use.

Patient and Family Education

- Warn patients not to take this drug with other products containing diphenhydramine because of risk of adverse reactions.
- Take drug half hour before travel to prevent motion sickness.
- Take it with food or milk to reduce GI distress.
- Avoid alcohol and hazardous activities that require alertness until CNS effects of drug are known.
- Sugarless gum, hard candy, or ice chips may prevent dry mouth.
- Notify prescriber if tolerance develops because a different antihistamine may need to be prescribed.
- This drug can be found in many over-the-counter sleep and cold products.
- Consult prescriber before using these products.
- Warn against possible photosensitive reactions.
- Advise use of sun block when going outdoors.

Special Populations

- *Elderly*: Be mindful of disease or age-related symptoms that may contraindicate usage.
- *Pregnancy*: Category B
- *Pediatric*: Children below age 12 years should use the only as directed by prescriber.

DIVALPROEX SODIUM (*DEPACON, DEPAKENE, DEPAKOTE, DEPAKOTE ER, DEPAKOTE SPRINKLE*)

Classification
Mood-stabilizing anticonvulsant

Indications
Divalproex sodium is used for the treatment of the manic episodes of bipolar disorder, major depressive disorder (MDD), is taken long-term for prevention of both manic and depressive phases of bipolar disorder, especially the rapid-cycling variant; treatment of epilepsy, certain side effects of autism, chronic pain associated with neuropathy, and migraine headaches.

Available Forms
Tablets are supplied in three dosage strengths containing divalproex sodium equivalent to 125 mg, 250 mg, or 500 mg of valproic acid.

Dosage
Mania
- ▥ *Adults:* Initially, 750 mg daily PO in divided doses, or 25 mg/kg Depakote ER once daily. Adjust dosage based on patient's response; maximum dose for either form is 60 mg/kg daily.

To Prevent Migraine Headache
- ▥ *Adults:* Initially, 250 mg delayed-release divalproex sodium PO BID. Some patients may need up to 1,000 mg daily. Or, 500 mg Depakote ER PO daily for 1 week; then 1,000 mg PO daily.
- ▥ Adjusted dose: For elderly patients, start at lower dosage. Increase dosage more slowly and with regular monitoring of fluid and nutritional intake, and watch for dehydration, somnolence, and other adverse reactions.

Administration
- ▥ Oral: Give the drug with food or milk to reduce adverse gastrointestinal (GI) effects.
- ▥ Do not mix syrup with carbonated beverages, as the mixture may be irritating to oral mucosa.
- ▥ Capsules may be swallowed whole or opened and contents sprinkled on a teaspoonful of soft food. Patient should swallow the capsule immediately without chewing.
- ▥ Monitor drug level and adjust dosage as needed.

Side Effects
- ▥ *Central nervous system*: Asthenia, dizziness, headache, insomnia, nervousness, somnolence, tremor, abnormal thinking, amnesia, ataxia, depression, emotional upset, fever, sedation
- ▥ *Cardiovascular*: Chest pain, edema, hypertension, hypotension, tachycardia
- ▥ *EENT*: Blurred vision, diplopia, nystagmus, pharyngitis, rhinitis, tinnitus
- ▥ *Gastrointestinal*: Abdominal pain, anorexia, diarrhea, dyspepsia, nausea, vomiting, pancreatitis, constipation, increased appetite

NOTE: For some drugs, off-label use is reported. It is the responsibility of the practitioner to evaluate the efficacy of such use.

- *Hematologic*: Bone marrow suppression, hemorrhage, thrombocytopenia, bruising, petechiae
- *Hepatic*: Hepatotoxicity
- *Metabolic*: Hyperammonemia, weight gain
- *Musculoskeletal*: Back and neck pain
- *Respiratory*: Bronchitis, dyspnea
- *Skin*: Alopecia, flu syndrome, infection, erythema multiforme, hypersensitivity reactions, Stevens–Johnson syndrome, rash, photosensitivity reactions, pruritus

Drug Interactions

This drug interacts with aspirin, chlorpromazine, clonazepam, topiramate, cimetidine, felbamate, carbamazepine, lamotrigine, phenobarbital, phenytoin, rifampin, warfarin, and zidovudine. Alcohol use is discouraged.

Pharmacokinetics

- *Peak action:* Oral, between 15 minutes and 4 hour. Facilitates the effects of the inhibitory neurotransmitter gamma-aminobutyric acid
- *Half-life:* 6 to 16 hours

Precautions

- It may increase ammonia, ALT, AST, and bilirubin lab levels.
- It may increase eosinophil count and bleeding time. It may also decrease platelet, red blood cell, and white blood cell counts.
- The drug may cause false-positive results for urine ketone levels.
- It is contraindicated in patients hypersensitive to the drug and in those with hepatic disease or significant hepatic dysfunction, and in patients with a urea cycle disorder (UCD).
- Safety and efficacy of Depakote ER in children younger than age 10 years have not been established.
- Obtain liver function test results, platelet count, prothrombin time (PT) and international normalized ratio (INR) before starting therapy, and monitor these values periodically.
- Adverse reactions may not be caused by valproic acid alone because it is usually used with other anticonvulsants.
- Never withdraw a drug suddenly, because sudden withdrawal may worsen seizures. Call the prescriber at once if adverse reactions develop.
- Patients at high risk for hepatotoxicity include those with congenital metabolic disorders, mental retardation, or organic brain disease; those taking multiple anticonvulsants; and children younger than 2 years of age.
- Notify the prescriber if tremors occur; a dosage reduction may be needed.
- Weight gain is common. Monitor body mass index and assess for prediabetes and dyslipidemia.
- Sedation is common.
- Therapeutic level is 50 to 100 mcg/mL.
- When converting patients from a brand-name drug to a generic drug, use caution because breakthrough seizures may occur.
- The drug may cause thrombocytopenia or tremors.
- *Alert:* Sometimes fatal, hyperammonemic encephalopathy may occur when starting valproate therapy in patients with UCD and pancreatitis. Evaluate patients with UCD risk factors before starting valproate therapy. Patients who develop

NOTE: For some drugs, off-label use is reported. It is the responsibility of the practitioner to evaluate the efficacy of such use.

symptoms of unexplained hyperammonemic encephalopathy during valproate therapy should stop taking the drug, undergo prompt appropriate treatment, and be evaluated for underlying UCD.

▥ *Alert:* Fatal hepatotoxicity may follow nonspecific symptoms, such as malaise, fever, and lethargy. If these symptoms occur during therapy, notify the prescriber at once, because patients who might be developing hepatic dysfunction must stop taking the drug.

▥ *Alert:* Life-threatening pancreatitis has been reported following initiation of therapy as well as after prolonged use. Monitor the patient for developing symptoms and discontinue treatment if pancreatitis is suspected.

Patient and Family Education
▥ Take the drug with food or milk to reduce adverse GI effects.
▥ Do not chew capsules; irritation of mouth and throat may result.
▥ It may take several weeks or longer to optimize mood-stabilizing effects.
▥ Capsules may be swallowed whole or carefully opened and contents sprinkled on a teaspoonful of soft food. Swallow the capsule immediately without chewing.
▥ Keep drugs out of children's reach.
▥ Warn about the consequences of stopping drug therapy abruptly.
▥ Women should call their prescriber if they become pregnant or plan to become pregnant during therapy.
▥ Syrup should not be mixed with carbonated beverages; mixture may be irritating to mouth and throat.
▥ Keep drug out of children's reach.
▥ Do not stop drug therapy abruptly.
▥ Call the prescriber if malaise, weakness, lethargy, facial swelling, loss of appetite, or vomiting occurs.

Special Populations
▥ *Elderly*: Caution is advised when using this drug in the elderly due to more sensitivity to the drug. Initiate treatment at a lower dose and then escalate the dose more slowly.
▥ *Pregnancy*: Category D; this medication should only be used when clearly needed or required utmost during pregnancy.
▥ *Lactation*: The drug is secreted into breast milk. Increased risk of neural tube defects (1 in 20) and other major birth defects have been reported, especially when the fetus is exposed during first 12 weeks of pregnancy.
▥ *Children*: Caution must be exercised when using this drug in a child or adolescent.
▥ *Alert:* Antidepressants increased the risk of suicidal thinking and behavior (suicidality) in short-term studies in children and adolescents with depression and other psychiatric disorders. Caution is advised when using this drug in children because they may be more sensitive to the side effects of the drug, especially loss of appetite and weight loss. It is important to monitor weight and growth in children who are taking this drug.

NOTE: For some drugs, off-label use is reported. It is the responsibility of the practitioner to evaluate the efficacy of such use.

DONEPEZIL HYDROCHLORIDE (*ARICEPT*)

Classification
Cholinesterase inhibitor

Indications
Aricept is indicated for the treatment of dementia of the Alzheimer's type. Efficacy has been demonstrated in patients with mild, moderate, and severe Alzheimer's disease.

Available Forms
The drug is available for oral administration in film-coated tablets containing 5, 10, or 23 mg of donepezil hydrochloride. oral solution, and rapidly dissolving tablet.

Dosage
- Initially 5 mg PO once daily
- Upward titration to 10 mg/day should not occur for at least 4 to 6 weeks.
- Effective dose range is 5 to 10 mg/day.

Administration
- Orally, once daily, just prior to retiring. Swallow tablets whole; do not crush, split, or chew. It may be given with or without food.
- Rapidly dissolving tablet: Place on tongue, allow to dissolve, and then swallow.
- Oral solution: Measure dose with a calibrated oral syringe.

Side Effects
- The side effects of this drug are nausea, vomiting, diarrhea, loss of appetite, weight loss, frequent urination, muscle cramps, joint pain, swelling, or stiffness, pain, excessive tiredness, drowsiness, headache, dizziness, nervousness, depression, confusion, changes in behavior, abnormal dreams, difficulty falling asleep or staying asleep, discoloration or bruising of the skin, red, scaling, and itchy skin.
- *Serious side effects that require immediate medical attention:* Fainting, slow heartbeat, chest pain, black or tarry stools, red blood in stools, bloody vomit, vomit that looks like coffee grounds, inability to control urination, difficulty urinating or pain when urinating, lower back pain, fever, and seizures.

Drug Interactions
This medicine may interact with the following medications: other cholinesterase inhibitors, neuromuscular blockers, parasympathomimetics, amantadine, amiodarone, amoxapine, antiretroviral protease inhibitors, antimuscarinics, barbiturates, bosentan, carbamazepine, clozapine, cyclobenzaprine, digoxin, disopyramide, fluoxetine, fluvoxamine, fosphenytoin, general anesthetics, imatinib, ST I-571, ketoconazole, local anesthetics, maprotiline, nefazodone, nilotinib, nonsteroidal anti-inflammatory drugs (NSAIDs), olanzapine, orphenadrine, oxcarbazepine, paroxetine, phenothiazines, phenytoin, ranolazine, rifampin, rifapentine, sedating H1 blockers, sertraline, St. John's Wort, tricyclic antidepressants, troglitazone, cimetidine, clarithromycin, dalfopristin, delavirdine, dexamethasone, diltiazem, efavirenz, erythromycin, gefitanib, itraconazole, modafinil, nevirapine, propafenone, quinidine, verapamil, and voriconazole.

NOTE: For some drugs, off-label use is reported. It is the responsibility of the practitioner to evaluate the efficacy of such use.

Pharmacokinetics
▦ Cholinesterase inhibitor selectively inhibits acetylcholinesterase.
▦ Peak plasma levels are reached in 3 to 4 hours.
▦ Bioavailability of 100%
▦ *Half-life:* Average 70 hours

Precautions
Parasympathetic effects may occur in patients with the following conditions: asthma, coronary disease, peptic ulcer, arrhythmias, epilepsy, parkinsonism, bradycardia, and intestinal, or urinary tract obstruction could be exacerbated by the stimulation of cholinergic receptors.

Patient and Family Education
Store the drug at controlled room temperature between 15°C and 30°C (59°F–86°F).

Special Populations
▦ *Hepatic impairment:* No specific dosage adjustments are needed. Adjust dose to patient response and tolerance.
▦ *Pregnancy:* Category C; the uterus could be stimulated along with induction of labor.

DOXEPIN (*SINEQUAN, SILENOR*)

Classification
Tricyclic antidepressant (TCA)

Indications
Doxepin is used for the treatment of anxiety/depression.

Available Forms
Capsule, 10, 25, 50, 75, 100, and 150 mg; solution, 10 mg/mL

Dosage
Adults: 150 to 300 mg PO at bedtime. The initial dose is 25 to 75 mg PO at bedtime. Maximum: 300 mg/day. *Children:* Dosing is currently unavailable or not applicable.

Administration
Take this medication regularly and at the same time every day to get the most benefit. Do not stop taking this medication without consulting the health care provider. If this medicine should be taken only once a day, take at bedtime to reduce daytime sleepiness.

Side Effects
Common reactions include drowsiness, dry mouth, dizziness, constipation, blurred vision, palpitations, tachycardia, uncoordination, appetite increase, nausea/vomiting, sweating, weakness, disorientation, confusion, restlessness, insomnia, anxiety/agitation, urinary retention/frequency, rash/urticaria, pruritus, weight gain, libido changes, impotence, gynecomastia, galactorrhea, tremor, hypo/hyperglycemia, paresthesias, and photosensitivity.

Drug Interactions
- The following drugs are to be used cautiously with doxepin: antiarrhythmics class 1A, such as procainamide, quinidine gluconate, quinidine sulfate especially if coadministration is medically necessary and with risk versus benefit fully assessed by the provider, and disopyramide (*Norpace*), which may increase risk of QT prolongation.
- Cisapride (*Propulsid*) may increase risk of QT prolongation and cardiac arrhythmias; dronedarone (*Multaq*) may increase TCA levels and risk of adverse effects, increase risk of QT prolongation and cardiac arrhythmias; flumazenil (*Romazicon*) may increase risk of cardiac arrhythmias, seizures.
- Monoamine oxidase inhibitors (MAOIs) such as selegiline (*Eldepryl/Zelapar*), procarbazine (*Matulane*), phenelzine (*Nardil*), tranylcypromine (*Parnate*), isocarboxazid (*Marplan*), selegiline transdermal (*Eldepryl/Zelapar*), and rasagiline (*Azilect*), may result in central nervous system (CNS) overstimulation, hyperpyrexia, seizures, and death.
- Pimozide (*Orap*) may increase risk of CNS depression, psychomotor impairment, QT prolongation, arrhythmias, hyperpyrexia; potassium salts, such as potassium acid phosphate, potassium citrate, potassium chloride, potassium iodide,

potassium phosphate/sodium phosphate, potassium acid, phosphate/sodium acid phosphate, and potassium phosphate, are contraindicated for solid potassium dose forms. Weigh risk/benefit of thyroid protection with solid iodide salt forms; may delay solid potassium passage through gastrointestinal (GI) tract and increase risk of ulcerative/stenotic lesions.

Pharmacokinetics
■ The drug is metabolized extensively in the liver (CYP450, 2 C9/19, 2 D6) and is excreted in the urine.
■ The exact mechanism of action is unknown; it inhibits norepinephrine and serotonin reuptake.

Precautions
Determine history of allergies, especially to other TCAs or any other allergies. This medication should not be used if patient has narrow-angle glaucoma, or problems urinating (e.g., due to enlarged prostate), lung disorders (such as bronchitis, emphysema), long-term constipation, long-term heartburn, or diabetes.

Patient and Family Education
■ Take the drug with food or milk to reduce adverse GI effects.
■ Do not chew capsules; irritation of mouth and throat may result.
■ It may take several weeks or longer to optimize mood-stabilizing effects.
■ Capsules may either be swallowed whole or carefully opened and contents sprinkled on a teaspoonful of soft food.
■ Keep drugs out of children's reach.
■ Warn about the consequences of stopping drug therapy abruptly.

Special Populations
■ *Pregnancy:* Category C; use the drug with extreme caution.
■ *Lactation:* Doxepin is excreted in human milk. Due to the potential for serious adverse reactions in nursing infants from doxepin, a decision should be made whether to discontinue nursing or to discontinue the drug, taking into account the importance of the drug to the mother.
■ *Pediatric use:* Safety and effectiveness of drug in children have not been established.
■ *Elderly:* Caution is advised when using this drug in the elderly because they may be more sensitive to its side effects, especially dizziness, drowsiness, confusion, and difficulty urinating.

NOTE: For some drugs, off-label use is reported. It is the responsibility of the practitioner to evaluate the efficacy of such use.

DULOXETINE (*CYMBALTA*)

Classification
▪ Antidepressant, antianxiety
▪ Selective serotonin and norepinephrine reuptake inhibitor (SNRI)

Indications
This drug is used to treat the following:

▪ Depression, anxiety disorder
▪ Pain associated with diabetic peripheral neuropathy, or fibromyalgia

Available Forms
Delayed-release capsules, 20, 30, and 60 mg

Dosage
▪ 20 or 30 mg twice daily or 60 mg once daily
▪ Starting at 30 mg daily for 1 week before increasing to 60 mg daily may help patients adjust to the drug.
▪ There is no evidence that doses greater than 60 mg/day provide additional benefits.

Administration
▪ The drug should be swallowed whole.
▪ It should not be chewed or crushed, nor should the capsule be opened and its contents sprinkled on food or mixed with liquids.
▪ It can be given without regard to meals.

Major Depressive Disorder (MDD)
▪ A total dose of 40 mg/day (given as 20 mg twice daily) to 60 mg/day (given either once daily or as 30 mg twice daily).
▪ It may be desirable to start at 30 mg once daily for 1 week, to allow patients to adjust to the medication before increasing to 60 mg once daily.

Generalized Anxiety Disorder
▪ Starting dose for Cymbalta is 60 mg administered once daily.
▪ For some patients, start at 30 mg once daily for 1 week, to allow patients to adjust to the medication before increasing to 60 mg once daily.
▪ Although a 120-mg once-daily dose was shown to be effective, there is no evidence that doses greater than 60 mg/day confer additional benefit.

Side Effects
▪ Nausea, dry mouth, constipation, diarrhea, fatigue, difficulty sleeping, and dizziness
▪ Increased blood pressure can occur and should be monitored
▪ Seizures
▪ Sexual dysfunction (decreased sex drive and delayed orgasm and ejaculation)
▪ The dose of duloxetine should be gradually reduced when therapy is discontinued.

NOTE: For some drugs, off-label use is reported. It is the responsibility of the practitioner to evaluate the efficacy of such use.

▨ Antidepressants increased the risk of suicidal thinking and behavior (suicidality) in short-term studies in children and adolescents with depression and other psychiatric disorders.

Note: Closely observed for clinical worsening, suicidality, or unusual changes in behavior

Drug Interactions
▨ This drug is not to be used with a monoamine oxidase inhibitor or within 14 days of discontinuing the monoamine oxidase inhibitor (MAOI).
▨ Caution when using combinations of SNRIs and MAOIs for this can lead to serious, sometimes fatal, reactions, including very high body temperature, muscle rigidity, rapid fluctuations of heart rate and BP, extreme agitation progressing to delirium, and coma.
▨ Same side effects are also seen when this drug is used in combination with antipsychotics, tricyclic antidepressants, or other drugs that affect serotonin in the brain.
▨ It may increase the risk of bleeding, because duloxetine itself is associated with bleeding.
▨ Drugs that raise the pH in the gastrointestinal system (e.g., omeprazole) may cause duloxetine to be released early, whereas conditions that slow gastric emptying (e.g., diabetes) may cause premature breakdown of duloxetine.
▨ Duloxetine may reduce the breakdown of desipramine, leading to increased blood concentrations of desipramine and potential side effects.

Pharmacokinetics
▨ This drug works by preventing the reuptake of serotonin and epinephrine.
▨ This reduced uptake increases the effect of serotonin and norepinephrine in the brain.

Precautions
▨ Hepatotoxicity
▨ Discontinuation of treatment
▨ Activation of mania or hypomania

Note: Screen for risk of bipolar disorder (e.g., family history of suicide, bipolar disorder, and depression) prior to initiating treatment with Cymbalta.

▨ Seizures
▨ Effects on BP
▨ Hyponatremia
▨ Concomitant illnesses
▨ Urinary hesitancy and retention

Patient Education
▨ Check for allergies in the patient.
▨ Check whether the patient feels dizzy or drowsy after using the drug.
▨ Avoid alcoholic beverages.
▨ It may affect blood sugar levels.
▨ Before having surgery, patient must let doctor or dentist know about all the products you use (including prescription drugs, nonprescription drugs, and herbal products).

NOTE: For some drugs, off-label use is reported. It is the responsibility of the practitioner to evaluate the efficacy of such use.

Special Populations
▪ *Elderly*
- Elderly patients may be more sensitive to the effects of this medicine; monitor for hyponatremia.
- Older adults may be at greater risk for bleeding while taking this drug.

▪ *Pregnancy: Category C*
- In animal studies, duloxetine has been shown to have adverse effects on fetal development.
- There are no adequate studies in pregnant women.

▪ *Breastfeeding*
- There are no adequate studies in women for determining infant risk when using this medication during breastfeeding.
- Weigh the potential benefits against the potential risks before taking this medication while breastfeeding.
- Duloxetine is excreted in the milk of lactating women.
- As the safety of duloxetine in infants is not known, nursing while on duloxetine is not recommended

▪ *Pediatric*
- It is not recommended for pediatric use. Appropriate studies have not been performed on the relationship of age to the effects of duloxetine in the pediatric population. Safety and efficacy have not been established.

ESCITALOPRAM (*LEXAPRO*)

Classification
Antidepressant; selective serotonin reuptake inhibitor (SSRI)

Indications
For treating major depressive disorder, generalized anxiety disorder (GAD), and post-traumatic stress disorder.

Available Forms
Tablet, 5, 10, and 20 mg; oral solution: 5 mg/5 mL

Dosage
- *Adults:* Starting dose—10 to 20 mg PO, daily, may increase after 1 week to a maximum of 20 mg/day. Dose should stay at 10 mg/day.
- *Children:* Not indicated for children younger than 17 years.

Administration
- PO with a glass of water
- Take with or without food.
- Take at regular intervals, preferably in the morning.
- Caution clients not to stop taking drug except on provider's advice.
- Safety not established for children younger than 18 years in GAD.
- Instruct client to take missed dose as soon as possible. If it is almost time for the next dose, advise to take only that dose.

Side Effects
- *Most common:* Somnolence, headache, asthenia, dizziness, sweating, dry mouth, tremor, insomnia, anorexia, nervousness, anxiety, abnormal vision, change in appetite, change in sex drive or performance, diarrhea, constipation, indigestion, and nausea
- *Less common:* Suicidality, worsening depression, serotonin syndrome, seizures, hyponatremia, extrapyramidal symptoms, priapism, and acute-angle glaucoma are less common side effects of escitalopram. The other side effects are nervousness, dry mouth, constipation, asthenia, diaphoresis, anxiety, headache, drowsiness, anorexia, dyspepsia, suicide risk, fatigue, fever, palpitations, hot flashes, nasal congestion, pharyngitis, sinusitis, nausea, diarrhea, abdominal pain, vomiting, flatulence, increased appetite, sexual dysfunction, weight loss, muscle pain, upper respiratory tract, infection, cough, respiratory distress, rash, pruritus, diaphoresis and flu-like syndrome.

Drug Interactions
Most of the interactions occur with over-the-counter (OTC) cough and cold preparations.

- This medicine may also interact with the following medications:
  - Absolute contraindications include monoamine oxidase inhibitors such as phenelzine *(Nardil)*, tranylcypromine *(Parnate)*, isocarboxazid *(Marplan)*, cyproheptadine, flecainide, carbamazepine, vinblastine, insulin, lithium, tricyclic antidepressants, phenytoin, tryptophan, warfarin, and selegiline *(Eldepryl)*

NOTE: For some drugs, off-label use is reported. It is the responsibility of the practitioner to evaluate the efficacy of such use.

Avoid using with other SSRIs due to serotonin effect; serotonin-norepinephrine reuptake inhibitor highly protein-bound drugs due to increased risk of serotonin syndrome, such as desvenlafaxine *(Pristiq)* and venlafaxine *(Effexor)*; St. John's wort; haloperidol diazepam *(Valium)*; any other antidepressants; and clopidogrel *(Plavix)*. Exercise caution with cold medications, nonsteroidal anti-inflammatory (NSAIDs), and drugs used for analgesia with opioid properties.

■ Concomitant use with SSRIs, SNRIs, or tryptophan is not recommended.

■ Use caution when concomitantly consuming drugs that affect hemostasis (NSAIDs, aspirin, cimetidine, warfarin).

■ *Alert:* This list may not describe all possible interactions. Instruct clients to provide a list of all medicines, herbs, nonprescription drugs, or dietary supplements used, and whether they smoke, drink alcohol, or use illegal drugs.

Pharmacokinetics

■ *Metabolism:* Liver; CYP450: 2C19, 2D6, CYP 3A4 substrate; 2D6 (weak) inhibitor

■ *Excretion:* Only 10% excreted in urine

■ SSRIs are metabolized in the liver by cytochrome P-450 MFO microsomal enzymes.

■ Highly bound to plasma proteins and have a large volume of distribution peak plasma levels are reached in 5 hours.

■ Steady-state plasma levels are achieved in 1 week with escitalopram.

■ *Half-life:* 27 to 32 hours, but is increased by 50% in elderly clients.

Precautions

■ *Clinical worsening/suicide risk:* Monitor for clinical worsening, suicidality, and unusual change in behavior, especially during the initial few months of therapy or at times of dose changes.

■ Serotonin syndrome: Manage with immediate discontinuation and continue monitoring.

■ Discontinuation of treatment with Lexapro: A gradual reduction in dose rather than abrupt cessation is recommended whenever possible.

■ Seizures: Prescribe with care in clients with history of seizure.

■ Activation of mania/hypomania: Use cautiously in clients with a history of mania.

■ Hyponatremia: Can occur in association with syndrome of inappropriate antidiuretic hormone secretion (SIADH).

■ Abnormal bleeding: Use caution in concomitant use with NSAIDs, aspirin, warfarin, or other drugs that affect coagulation.

■ Interferes with cognitive and motor performance: Use caution when operating machinery.

■ Use in clients with concomitant illness: Use caution in clients with diseases or conditions that produce altered metabolism or hemodynamic response.

■ See client as often as necessary to ensure that the drug is working on the panic attacks, determine compliance, and review side effects.

■ Make sure clients realize that they need to take prescribed doses even if they do not feel better right away. It can take several weeks before they feel the full effect of the drug.

■ Watch out for sudden or severe changes in feelings, such as feeling anxious, agitated, panicky, irritable, hostile, aggressive, impulsive, severely restless, overly excited, and hyperactive, or not being able to sleep. If this happens, especially at the beginning of antidepressant treatment or after a change in dose, clients should call the health care provider.

NOTE: For some drugs, off-label use is reported. It is the responsibility of the practitioner to evaluate the efficacy of such use.

▩ Caution clients not to stand or sit up quickly, especially if an older client. This reduces the risk of dizziness or fainting spells. Alcohol may interfere with the effect of this medicine. Avoid alcoholic drinks.

▩ Caution clients not to treat themselves for coughs, colds, or allergies without asking health care professional for advice. Some ingredients can increase possible side effects.

▩ Dry mouth: Chewing sugarless gum or sucking hard candy and drinking plenty of water may help. Contact a health care provider if the problem does not persist, go away, or is severe.

▩ Caution should be exercised in the following:
  ▩ In clients with bipolar disorder or a family history of bipolar disorder
  ▩ Diabetes
  ▩ Heart disease
  ▩ Liver disease
  ▩ Electroconvulsive therapy
  ▩ Seizures (convulsions)
  ▩ Suicidal thoughts, plans, or attempts by client or a family member
  ▩ An unusual or allergic reaction to citalopram, sertraline, other medicines, foods, dyes, or preservatives
  ▩ Women who are pregnant or trying to get pregnant
  ▩ Breastfeeding

Patient and Family Education

▩ Store at room temperature.

▩ Try to take the medicine at the same time each day. Follow the directions on the prescription label. To get the correct dose of liquid escitalopram, measure the liquid with a marked measuring spoon or medicine cup, not with a regular tablespoon. If there is no dose-measuring device available, ask the pharmacist for one.

▩ Drug may cause dizziness or drowsiness. Warn client to avoid driving and other hazardous activities that require alertness and good psychomotor coordination until effects of drug are known.

▩ Tell client to consult prescriber before taking other prescription or OTC drugs.

▩ Advise client that full therapeutic effect may not be seen for 4 weeks or longer.

Special Populations

▩ *Elderly*: A dose of 10 mg daily is recommended for geriatric clients. The initial dose should be reduced in clients with severe renal and/or hepatic impairment. Titration upward should be slow and at intervals.

▩ *Pregnancy*: Category C; potential for persistent pulmonary hypertension if greater than 20-weeks' gestation; use in third semester may cause complications at birth.

▩ *Lactation*: The drug is excreted in human breast milk, and there are some reports of infant somnolence.

▩ *Children*: It may be given to children older than 12 years of age. Monitoring of suicidal ideations is important.

NOTE: For some drugs, off-label use is reported. It is the responsibility of the practitioner to evaluate the efficacy of such use.

ESZOPICLONE (*LUNESTA*)

Classification
Hypnotic, pyrrolopyrazine derivative; non-benzodiazepine GABA receptor agonist

Indications
Treatment of insomnia in the nondepressed patient

Available Forms
Tablet, 1, 2, and 3 mg

Dosage
Dose is 2 mg PO immediately before patient is ready for sleep. It may increase to 3 mg if clinically indicated in nonelderly patients.

Administration
▨ PO with a glass of water immediately before bedtime
▨ Drowsiness and/or dizziness will be exacerbated with concomitant alcohol consumption; alcohol should be avoided while taking this medication.
▨ Only to be used for 10 days to 2 weeks, not meant for long-term use

Side Effects
▨ Hallucinations; behavior changes; selective serotonin reuptake inhibitor (SSRI)–treated patients who take eszopiclone may experience impaired concentration, aggravated depression, and manic reaction.
▨ Side effects that usually do not require medical attention: unpleasant taste, nausea, daytime drowsiness, headache, vomiting, dizziness, infection, pain, and pharyngitis.

Drug Interactions
This medicine may interact with the following medications: antifungals, rifampin, ritonavir, SSRIs, and central nervous system depressants (including alcohol). CYP3A4 inhibitors (clarithromycin, itraconazole, ketoconazole, nefazodone, nelfinavir, troleandomycin); olanzapine may impair cognitive function.

Pharmacokinetics
This is a non-benzodiazepine hypnotic. Mechanism of action is thought to occur at the level of the GABA receptor complex. Close or connected to benzodiazepine receptors
▨ Weakly bound to plasma proteins
▨ Peak plasma levels are reached in 1 hour.
▨ Bioavailability is 80%.
▨ *Half-life:* Average is 6 hours.

Precautions
See patient as often as necessary if long-term use is indicated.

▨ Ensure that patient is aware he or she is not to exceed maximum dosage and is not taking other central nervous system depressant medications.
▨ Instruct patient to monitor for behavior changes.

NOTE: For some drugs, off-label use is reported. It is the responsibility of the practitioner to evaluate the efficacy of such use.

- ▨ If patient is drowsy or dizzy, patient should not drive, use machinery, or attempt to accomplish any task that requires mental alertness.
- ▨ Avoid alcohol, as concomitant use may exacerbate symptoms.

Patient and Family Education

Store at room temperature between 15°C and 30°C (59°F–86°F). Throw away any unused medication after the expiration date. Avoid giving with high-fat meals.

Special Populations

- ▨ *Elderly*: Recommended starting dose for elderly patients who have difficulty falling asleep is 1 mg. For elderly patients who have difficulty staying asleep, the recommended dose is 1 to 2 mg.
- ▨ *Hepatic impairment*: The starting dose should be 1 mg in patients with severe hepatic impairment. Monitor closely.
- ▨ *Pregnancy*: Category C
- ▨ *Lactation*: No human studies have been performed. Not recommended in breast-feeding mothers.
- ▨ *Children*: Safety and efficacy have not been established.

FLUOXETINE HYDROCHLORIDE (*PROZAC*)

Classification
Antidepressant

Indications
This drug is used to treat major depressive disorders (MDDs), obsessive-compulsive disorder (OCD), bulimia nervosa, Premenstrual dysphoric disorder (PMDD), post-traumatic stress disorder (PTSD), borderline personality disorder, panic disorder (short term), Raynaud phenomenon, and personality disorders.

Available Forms
Tablets, 20 mg; capsules, 10, 20, 40, 90 mg; liquid, 20 mg/5 mL

Dosage
- *Immediate release* (*Prozac Daily*): *Adults:* 20 to 80 mg PO QAM; starting dose, 10 mg PO, daily for 7 days; 20 mg PO QAM; may be increased after several weeks; maximum dose, 80 mg/day.
- *Capsule, delayed release* (*Prozac Weekly*): Pediatric dosing in 8- to 18-year-olds is 10 to 20 mg.
- *Extended release:* Not recommended for acute treatment; starting with 10 mg PO every day for 7 days. May be given to children as young as 7 years old for OCD only.

Administration
- PO with a glass of water
- Take the medicine with or without food.
- Take it at regular intervals.
- Caution patients not to stop taking drug except on provider's advice.
- Prozac Weekly may be prescribed for children as young as 7 years for selected conditions; precautions do apply.
- Prozac Weekly is not prescribed for children.
- Do not prescribe Prozac Weekly for acute treatment.
- Instruct patients to take missed dose as soon as possible. If it is almost time for the next dose, advise to take only that dose.
- Do not take fluoxetine with grapefruit juice, as it may increase blood levels of the drug.
- Avoid use of herbs that have a sedative effect.
- Fluoxetine may increase the levels of phenytoin and tricyclic antidepressants or serotonin potential such as St. John's wort. Alcohol should be avoided while using fluoxetine.
- Use of buspirone, dextromethorphan, lithium, meperidine, nefazodone, paroxetine, pentazocine, sertraline, sumatriptan, tramadol, trazodone, tryptophan, and venlafaxine can cause a serotonin syndrome.
- Fluoxetine can be taken with or without food. It should be taken in the morning to reduce nervousness and insomnia.
- Be cautious while driving, riding a bicycle, or operating machinery, as this drug causes drowsiness.

NOTE: For some drugs, off-label use is reported. It is the responsibility of the practitioner to evaluate the efficacy of such use.

Side Effects

▦ Most common: Suicidial ideation, dizziness, headache, insomnia, nervousness, anxiety, somnolence, and change in sex drive or performance are the most common side effects.

▦ Less common: The less common side effects are allergic reactions (skin rash, itching, or hives); swelling of the face, lips, or tongue; psoriasis; arthralgias; asthenia, diarrhea, anorexia; feeling faint or lightheaded, falls, nausea; dizziness, dry mouth; constipation; tremor, dyspepsia; suicidal thoughts or other mood changes; unusual bleeding or bruising; fatigue; tremor; change in appetite; increased sweating; indigestion, nausea; flu syndrome; ejaculatory dysfunction, libido decrease; rash; and abnormal vision, and vivid dreams.

Drug Interactions

Most of the interactions occur with over-the-counter cough-and-cold preparations. This medicine may also interact with the following medications:

▦ Absolute contraindications include monoamine oxidase inhibitors (MAOIs) such as phenelzine *(Nardil)*, tranylcypromine *(Parnate)*, isocarboxazid *(Marplan)*, and selegiline *(Eldepryl)*.

▦ Avoid using with other selective serotonin reuptake inhibitors (SSRIs) due to serotonin effect; serotonin-norepinephrine reuptake inhibitor (SNRI) drugs, such as desvenlafaxine *(Pristiq)* and venlafaxine *(Effexor)*; drugs with sympathomimetic properties, such as phenylpropanolamine, pseudoephedrine. Avoid using the drug with St. John's wort, haloperidol, diazepam *(Valium)*, any other antidepressants, and clopidogrel *(Plavix)*. Exercise caution with cold medications, arrhythmia medications, such as flecainide, aspirin, and other nonsteroidal anti-inflammatory drugs (NSAIDs), and drugs used for analgesia with opioid properties.

▦ *Alert:* This list may not describe all possible interactions. Instruct patients to provide a list of all medicines, herbs, nonprescription drugs, or dietary supplements used, and if they smoke, drink alcohol, or use illegal drugs. The following drugs are known to interact with fluoxetine:

　▦ Linezolid *(Zyvox)* may increase the risk of serotonin syndrome and neuroleptic syndrome, and in combination with fluvoxamine *(Luvox)* may increase rasagiline *(Azilect)* levels.

　▦ MAOIs contraindicated within 5 weeks of fluoxetine use because it may increase the risk of serotonin syndrome, neuroleptic syndrome, and in combination with fluvoxamine *(Luvox)* may increase rasagiline *(Azilect)* levels, and risk of adverse effects.

　▦ Pimozide *(Orap)* may increase the risk of bradycardia, increase pimozide levels, risk of QT prolongation, and cardiac arrhythmias.

　▦ Thioridazine *(Mellaril)* may increase thioridazine levels, risk of QT prolongation, cardiac arrhythmias, and may increase risk of syndrome of inappropriate antidiuretic hormone (SIADH), hyponatremia, serotonin syndrome, and neuroleptic and malignant syndrome.

　▦ Tramodol may increase risk of serotonin syndrome.

Pharmacokinetics

▦ *Metabolism:* Liver; CYP450 2C19, 2D6 (primary) substrate; 2C19, 3A4 (weak) inhibitor; active metabolite excreted in the urine (80%) and feces (15%)

▦ Selectively inhibits serotonin reuptake

NOTE: For some drugs, off-label use is reported. It is the responsibility of the practitioner to evaluate the efficacy of such use.

▮ *Half-life:* Fluoxetine: 2 to 3 days, norfluoxetine: 7 to 9 days
▮ See patients as often as necessary to ensure that the drug is working on the panic attacks, determine compliance, and review side effects.
▮ Make sure patients realize that they need to take prescribed doses even if they do not feel better right away. It can take several weeks before they feel the full effect of the drug.
▮ Instruct patients and families to watch for worsening depression or thoughts of suicide. Also, watch out for sudden or severe changes in feelings such as feeling anxious, agitated, panicky, irritated, hostile, aggressive, impulsive, severely restless, overly excited, hyperactive, or not being able to sleep. If this happens, especially at the beginning of antidepressant treatment or after a change in dose, patient should call the health care provider.
▮ Drowsiness or dizziness: Patients should not drive or use machinery or do anything that needs mental alertness until the effects of this medicine are known.
▮ Caution patients not to stand or sit up quickly, especially if older. This reduces the risk of dizzy or fainting spells. Alcohol may interfere with the effect of this medicine. Avoid alcoholic drinks.
▮ Caution patients not to treat themselves for coughs, colds, or allergies without asking a health care professional for advice. Some ingredients can increase possible side effects.
▮ Dry mouth: Chewing sugarless gum, sucking hard candy, and drinking plenty of water may help against a dry mouth. Contact a health care provider if the problem persists or is severe.
▮ Caution should be exercised in the following:
  ▮ Bipolar disorder or a family history of bipolar disorder
  ▮ Diabetes
  ▮ Heart disease
  ▮ Liver disease
  ▮ Electroconvulsive therapy
  ▮ Seizures (convulsions)
  ▮ Suicidal thoughts, plans, or attempts by patients or a family member
  ▮ An unusual or allergic reaction to fluoxetine, other medicines, foods, dyes, or preservatives
  ▮ Pregnancy or trying to get pregnant
  ▮ Breastfeeding mothers who are younger than 25 years
▮ *Alert:* Caution should also be exercised with the following conditions: diabetes mellitus, hyponatremia, seizures, mania/hypomania, or volume depletion.

Patient and Family Education
▮ Store at room temperature. Take any unused medication after the expiration date to the local pharmacy on drug-giveback day. Avoid discarding the medication into the environment.
▮ Discuss any worsening anxiety, aggressiveness, impulsivity, or restlessness.
▮ Report any severe, abrupt onset, or changes in symptoms to health professionals. It may be reflective of increased risk of suicidal thinking.
▮ There is an increased risk of suicidality in children, adolescents, and young adults with major depressive or other psychiatric disorder's especially during the first months of treatment.

NOTE: For some drugs, off-label use is reported. It is the responsibility of the practitioner to evaluate the efficacy of such use.

- The patient must inform health care provider of glaucoma, hypoglycemia, or abnormal bleeding tendencies.
- Therapeutic effects may take 4 weeks to fully develop, but side effects may be noticeable.
- *Alert:* Avoid the concomitant use of NSAIDs, aspirin, warfarin, and any other drugs that alter platelets within 1 week of beginning therapy.

Special Populations

- *Elderly:* No actual contraindications exist, but due to the long half-life of the drug, it has been placed on the Beers List of Potentially Inappropriate Medications for Geriatrics.
- *Renal impairment:* No adjustment is needed for those with kidney disease.
- *Hepatic impairment:* The dose may need to be decreased in patients with liver disease.
- *Pregnancy:* Category C; this is the longest-used SSRI in pregnant women. Every attempt should be made to discontinue in the third trimester secondary to development of neonatal distress on delivery.
- *Lactation:* The use of this drug is not approved for lactation and breastfeeding.
- *Children:* The drug is approved for pediatric population aged 8 years and older; only for MDD and OCD for those aged 7 years and older. Monitoring for increased suicidal ideation is critical.

NOTE: For some drugs, off-label use is reported. It is the responsibility of the practitioner to evaluate the efficacy of such use.

FLUOXETINE MALEATE (*LUVOX, LUVOX CR*)

Classification
Antidepressant, SSRI

Indications
Flioxetine maleate is used to treat obsessive-compulsive disorder, social anxiety disorder, bulimia nervosa, panic disorder, posttraumatic stress disorder, and migraine prevention.

Available Forms
Tablet, 25, 50, and 100 mg; extended-release capsule, 100 and 150 mg

Note: Some formulations not available as generic medications.

Dosage
Starting dose: 50 mg/day; maintenance: 100 mg PO nightly, dose increase by 50 mg/day weekly; maximum: 300 mg/day

Administration
- PO with a glass of water
- Take the medicine with or without food. Controlled-release tablets must remain intact and not be split or crushed prior to administration.

Side Effects
- Most common: The most common side effects are somnolence, headache, asthenia, dizziness, sweating, dry mouth, tremor, anorexia, nervousness, anxiety, abnormal vision, change in appetite, change in sex drive or performance, diarrhea, constipation, indigestion, and nausea.
- Less common: The less common side effects are suicidality, worsening depression, seizures, hyponatremia; allow 2-week washout period post-MAOI prior to initiation.
- TCAs: Plasma levels may be increased by SSRIs, so add extrapyramidal symptoms, priapism, and acute-angle glaucoma.

Drug Interactions
Note black box warnings!

Most of the interactions occur with over-the-counter cough-and-cold preparations. This medicine may also interact with the following medications:

- Absolute contraindications include MAOIs such as phenelzine *(Nardil)*, tranylcypromine *(Parnate)*, isocarboxazid *(Marplan)*, and selegiline *(Eldepryl)*.
- Use with caution and in low doses.
- ASA and nonsteroidal anti-inflammatory drugs (NSAIDs): There is an increased risk of bleeding.
- Central nervous system depressants: It may increase depressant effects.
- Other SSRIs or Serotonin antagonist and reuptake inhibitors (SARIs): It may cause serotonin syndrome in combination with other medications, such as tramadol, high-dose triptans, or the antibiotic linezolid.

NOTE: For some drugs, off-label use is reported. It is the responsibility of the practitioner to evaluate the efficacy of such use.

▦ Use with caution in patients taking blood thinners *(Coumadin)*, other antidepressants, antihistamines, lithium, TCAs, and certain antibiotics, such as erythromycin, clarithromycin, azithromycin; serotonin-norepinephrine reuptake inhibitor drugs, such as desvenlafaxine *(Pristiq)* and venlafaxine *(Effexor)*; drugs with sympathomimetic properties, such as phenylpropanolamine, pseudoephedrine, St. John's wort, haloperidol; diazepam *(Valium)*, and any other antidepressants; clopidogrel *(Plavix)* and lansoprazole *(Prevacid)*; for these medications pharmacokinetics and dynamics may change.

▦ Exercise caution with cold medications, NSAIDs, and drugs used for analgesia with opioid properties.

▦ *Alert:* This list may not describe all possible interactions. Instruct patients to provide a list of all medicines, herbs, nonprescription drugs, or dietary supplements used, and if they smoke, drink alcohol, or use illegal drugs.

▦ MAOIs: When this drug interacts with MAOIs there is an extreme risk for serotonin syndrome.

▦ Take at regular intervals.

▦ Caution patients not to stop taking drug except on provider's advice.

▦ This drug is not prescribed for children.

▦ Instruct patients to take missed dose as soon as possible. If it is almost time for the next dose, advise to take only that dose.

Pharmacokinetics

▦ This drug is highly bound to plasma proteins and has a large volume of distribution.

▦ It is readily absorbed in the gastrointestinal tract, metabolized in the liver, and excreted in the urine. Dosages may be decreased in patients with liver or kidney disease.

▦ Caution is advised for elderly clients.

▦ *Metabolism:* The liver metabolizes the drug extensively; CYP1A2, CYP2Cp, CYP3A4, CYP4501A2, 2D6 inhibitor.

▦ *Peak plasma levels:* Reached in 3 to 8 hours.

▦ *Excretion:* 85% (urine primarily); 2% unchanged

▦ *Half-life:* 15.6 hours, 17.4 to 25.9 hours (elderly)

Precautions

▦ Adverse effects and side effects are commonly observed before therapeutic effects.

▦ Many side effects are dose dependent and may improve over time.

▦ Taper discontinuation to avoid withdrawal symptoms.

▦ See patients as often as necessary to ensure that the drug is working on the panic attacks, determine compliance, and review side effects.

▦ Make sure patients realize that they need to take prescribed doses even if they do not feel better right away. It can take several weeks before they feel the full effect of the drug.

▦ Instruct patients and families to watch for worsening depression or thoughts of suicide. Also, watch out for sudden or severe changes in feelings, such as feeling anxious, agitated, panicky, irritated, hostile, aggressive, impulsive, severely restless, overly excited, hyperactive, or not being able to sleep. If this happens, especially at the beginning of antidepressant treatment or after a change in dose, patient should call the health care provider.

NOTE: For some drugs, off-label use is reported. It is the responsibility of the practitioner to evaluate the efficacy of such use.

▣ Drowsiness or dizziness: Patients should not drive or use machinery or do anything that needs mental alertness until the effects of this medicine are known.

▣ Caution patients not to stand or sit up quickly, especially if older. This reduces the risk of dizziness or fainting spells. Alcohol may interfere with the effect of this medicine. Avoid alcoholic drinks.

▣ Caution patients not to treat themselves for coughs, colds, or allergies without asking a health care professional for advice. Some ingredients can increase possible side effects.

▣ Dry mouth: Chewing sugarless gum, sucking hard candy, and drinking plenty of water may help against a dry mouth. Contact health care provider if the problem persists or is severe.

▣ Caution should be exercised in the following:
  ▪ Bipolar disorder or a family history of bipolar disorder
  ▪ Diabetes
  ▪ Heart disease
  ▪ Liver disease
  ▪ Electroconvulsive therapy
  ▪ Seizures (convulsions)
  ▪ Suicidal thoughts, plans, or attempts by patients or a family member
  ▪ An unusual or allergic reaction to fluvoxamine, other medicines, foods, dyes, or preservatives
  ▪ Pregnancy or trying to get pregnant
  ▪ Breastfeeding

Patient and Family Education

▣ The medicine should be taken about the same time every day, morning or evening, and can be taken with or without food (with food if there is any stomach upset).

▣ It may start with half of lowest effective dose for 3 to 7 days, then increase to lowest effective dose to diminish side effects.

▣ Administration time may be adjusted based on observed sedating or activating drug effects.

▣ The drug may take up to 4 to 8 weeks to show its maximum effect at this dose, but some may see symptoms of dysthymia improving in as little as 2 weeks.

▣ If patient plans on becoming pregnant or is pregnant, discuss the benefits versus the risks of using this medicine while pregnant.

▣ As this medicine is excreted in the breast milk, nursing mothers should not breastfeed while taking this medicine without prior consultation with a psychiatric nurse practitioner or psychiatrist. Newborns may develop symptoms, including feeding or breathing difficulties, seizures, muscle stiffness, jitteriness, or constant crying.

▣ Do not stop taking this medication unless the health care provider directs. Report side effects or worsening symptoms to the health care provider promptly.

▣ The medication should be tapered gradually when changing or discontinuing therapy.

▣ Dosage should be adjusted to reach remission of symptoms and treatment should continue for at least 6 to 12 months following last reported dysthymic experience, duration based on number of episodes.

▣ Caution is advised when using this drug in the elderly because they may be more sensitive to the effects of the drug. Elderly patients should receive a lower starting dose.

NOTE: For some drugs, off-label use is reported. It is the responsibility of the practitioner to evaluate the efficacy of such use.

▦ Keep these medications out of the reach of children and pets.
▦ Store at room temperature. After the expiration date, take any unused medication to the local pharmacy on drug-giveback day. Avoid discarding the medication into the environment. Watch carefully for signs of suicidal ideation.

Special Populations

▦ *Elderly*: Older individuals tend to be more sensitive to medication side effects, such as hypotension and anticholinergic effects. They often require adjustment of medication doses for hepatic or renal dysfunction. SSRIs with shorter half-lives (e.g., paroxetine) may be more desirable for geriatric populations than SSRIs with longer half-lives (e.g., fluoxetine). SSRIs have been associated with increased risk of falls in nursing home residents and neurologic effects in patients with Parkinson's disease. Elderly patients are more prone to SSRI-induced hyponatremia.
▦ *Renal and hepatic impairment*: Initial dose should be reduced in patients with severe renal and/or hepatic impairment. Titration upward should be slow and at intervals.
▦ *Pregnancy*: Psychotherapy is the initial choice for most pregnant patients with major depressive disorder. Most SSRIs are Category C drugs, due to adverse effects; first trimester teratogenicity has been observed in animal studies. If continued during pregnancy, dosage may need to be increased to maintain euthymia due to physiologic changes associated with pregnancy. Neonatal withdrawal and serotonin syndrome may occur in third trimester, persistent pulmonary hypertension occurs if more than 20-week gestation.
▦ *Lactation*: It is generally considered safe; substantial human data show no or minimal risk to breast-milk production or to the infant.
▦ *Children*: Initial SSRI dosing is not indicated for children. Increasing doses may require more gradual increments, and discontinuation may require a more gradual taper.

FLUPHENAZINE, FLUPHENAZINE HYDROCHLORIDE (*MODECATE, MODECATE CONCENTRATE*), FLUPHENAZINE DECANOATE (*PROLIXIN*)

Classification
Antipsychotic drug, typical, first-generation, phenothiazine

Indications
Psychosis

Available Forms
Tablet, 1, 2.5 (scored), 5 (scored), and 10 mg (scored); decanoate for long-acting IM or SC administration, 25 mg/mL; short-acting IM injection, 2.5 mg/mL; elixir, 2.5 mg/5 mL; oral concentrate, 5 mg/mL

Dosage
- *Oral*: Initial, 0.5 to 10 mg/day in divided doses; maximum, 40 mg/day
- *IM (short-acting)*: Initial: 1.25 mg; 2.5 to 10 mg/day can be given in divided doses every 6 to 8 hours; maximum dose, generally 10 mg/day
- *Fluphenazine decanoate (long-acting)*: Initial: 12.5 to 25 mg (0.5–1 mL); subsequent doses and intervals determined in accordance with the patient's response; generally no more than 50 mg/2 mL given at no shorter interval than 3 weeks.

Administration
- Oral solution should not be mixed with drinks containing caffeine, tannic acid (tea), or pectinates (apple juice).
- Prolixin Elixir (fluphenazine hydrochloride elixir USP) 0.5 mg/mL (2.5 mg per 5 mL teaspoonful)
- IM decanoate: use dry, 21-gauge needle. May be given subcutaneously.
- Onset of action is at 24 to 72 hours after administration with significant antipsychotic actions evident within 48 to 96 hours.

Side Effects
Motor side effects from blockage of D2 in striatum; seizures, neuromalignant syndrome, leukopenia, agranulocytosis, aplastic anemia, thrombocytopenia, elevations in prolactin from blockage of D2 in the pituitary; worsening of negative and cognitive symptoms due to blockage of D2 receptors in the mesocortical and mesolimbic dopamine pathways; sedation, blurred vision, constipation, dry mouth; weight gain; dizziness, hypotension; possible increased incidence of diabetes or dyslipidemia with conventional antipsychotics is unknown; neuroleptic-induced deficit syndrome; akathisia; extrapyramidal symptoms, parkinsonism, tardive dyskinesia (TD); galactorrhea, amenorrhea; sexual dysfunction; priapism; decreased sweating, depression; hypotension, tachycardia, syncope.

Drug Interactions
- It may decrease the effects of levodopa and dopamine agonists.
- It may increase effects of antihypertensive drugs except for guanethidine, whose actions may be antagonized by fluphenazine.
- Concurrent use with central nervous system depressants may produce additive effects.

NOTE: For some drugs, off-label use is reported. It is the responsibility of the practitioner to evaluate the efficacy of such use.

■ Antacids may inhibit absorption. Administer the dosage at least 2 hours apart.

■ Additive anticholinergic effects may occur if used with atropine or related compounds.

■ Alcohol and diuretics increase the risk of hypotension.

■ Some patients on neuroleptics and lithium developed an encephalopathic syndrome similar to Neuroleptic malignant syndrome (NMS).

■ Interaction with St. John's wort increases risk of photosensitivity

■ Use with epinephrine may lower blood pressure.

Pharmacokinetics

■ *Half-life:* Oral formulation—approx. 15 hours; IM formulation—approximately 6.8 to 9.6 days.

■ *Peak*: PO—30 minutes; IM decanoate—unknown; IM—90 to 120 minutes; subcutaneous—unknown

Precautions

■ Some neuroleptics and lithium have caused an encephalopathic syndrome similar to NMS in some patients.

■ Fluphenazine and epinephrine may lower BP.

■ Additive anticholinergic effects may occur if used with atropine or related compounds.

■ Alcohol and diuretics may increase the risk of hypotension.

■ Do not use if the patient is in a comatose state.

■ Do not use if there is proven allergy or sensitivity to fluphenazine.

■ It may lower seizure threshold; fluphenazine has severe reactions to insulin, glaucoma, prostatic hyperplasia.

Patient and Family Education

■ Inform your provider of all drug allergies.

■ Take the dose exactly as prescribed by the provider. Do not take in larger or smaller amounts or for longer than recommended.

■ Fluphenazine can be taken with or without food.

■ Avoid becoming overheated or dehydrated during exercise and in hot weather. You may be more prone to heat stroke.

■ Avoid getting up too fast from a sitting or lying position. Get up slowly and steady yourself to prevent a fall.

■ Avoid drinking alcohol.

■ Stop using this medication and call provider immediately if you have very stiff (rigid) muscles, high fever, sweating, confusion, fast or uneven heartbeats, tremors; feel like you might pass out; have jerky muscle movements you cannot control, trouble swallowing, problems with speech; have blurred vision, eye pain, or see halos around lights; have increased thirst and urination, excessive hunger, fruity breath odor, weakness, nausea, and vomiting; have fever, chills, body aches, flu symptoms; or have white patches or sores inside your mouth or on your lips.

■ Do not stop taking the drug suddenly without first talking to your provider, even if you feel fine. You may have serious side effects if you stop taking the drug suddenly.

■ Call provider if symptoms do not improve or get worse.

■ Store at room temperature away from moisture and heat.

NOTE: For some drugs, off-label use is reported. It is the responsibility of the practitioner to evaluate the efficacy of such use.

Special Populations

- ◾ *Elderly*: Lower initial dose (1–2.5 mg/day) and slower titration in elderly patients. Elderly are more susceptible to adverse effects. It is not approved for treatment of elderly patients with dementia-related psychosis, and such patients are at increased risk of cardiovascular events and death.
- ◾ *Renal impairment*: Use with caution and with slower titration.
- ◾ *Hepatic impairment*: Use with caution and with slower titration.
- ◾ *Cardiac impairment*: Cardiovascular toxicity can occur, especially orthostatic hypotension.
- ◾ *Pregnancy*: Category C; some animal studies have demonstrated adverse effects; there are no controlled studies in humans. Infants whose mothers took a phenothiazine during pregnancy have exhibited EPS, jaundice, hyperreflexia, and hyporeflexia. Psychotic symptoms may worsen during pregnancy, necessitating some form of treatment. Atypical antipsychotics may be preferable.
- ◾ *Lactation*: Drug crosses to the infant through breast milk; dystonia, TD, and sedation have been observed in the infant. Recommend discontinuing drug or bottle-feed.
- ◾ *Children and adolescents*: Safety and efficacy of fluphenazine are not established for children and adolescents. Decanoate and enanthate injectable formulations are contraindicated in children younger than 12 years. It is generally considered second-line treatment after trial with atypical antipsychotics.

NOTE: For some drugs, off-label use is reported. It is the responsibility of the practitioner to evaluate the efficacy of such use.

FLURAZEPAM (*DALMANE, DALMADORM*)

Classification
Benzodiazepine (BZD)

Indications
Flurazepam is used for the treatment of insomnia.

Available Forms
Capsule, 15 and 30 mg

Dosage
15 to 30 mg PO immediately before patient is ready for sleep.

Administration
▪ PO with a glass of water at bedtime
▪ Drowsiness and/or dizziness will be exacerbated with concomitant alcohol consumption; alcohol should be avoided while taking this medication.
▪ Caution clients not to stop taking drug abruptly if used long term.

Side Effects
▪ Hallucinations; behavior changes.
▪ Side effects that usually do not require medical attention: nausea, daytime drowsiness, headache, vomiting, dizziness, diarrhea, dry mouth, and nervousness.

Drug Interactions
This medicine may interact with the following medications: antifungals; central nervous system depressants (including alcohol); digoxin; macrolides; phenytoin.

Pharmacokinetics
▪ BZD, hypnotic
▪ Mechanism of action is thought to occur at the level of the gamma-aminobutyric acid receptor complex.
▪ Highly bound to plasma proteins.
▪ Peak plasma levels are reached in 0.50 to 2 hours.
▪ The drug is metabolized by CYP450 3A4 and excreted through the urine.
▪ Average half-life of patent drug is 2 to 3 hours, half-life of metabolite is 40 to 114 hours.

Precautions
▪ See patient as often as necessary if long-term use is indicated.
▪ Ensure that patient is aware he or she is not to exceed maximum dosage.
▪ Instruct patient to monitor for behavior changes.
▪ If patient is drowsy or dizzy, patient should not drive, use machinery, or attempt to accomplish any task that requires mental alertness.
▪ Avoid alcohol, as concomitant use may exacerbate symptoms.

NOTE: For some drugs, off-label use is reported. It is the responsibility of the practitioner to evaluate the efficacy of such use.

Patient and Family Education

■ Store at room temperature between 20°C and 25°C (59°F–77°F).
■ Discard unused medication after the expiration date.

Special Populations

■ *Elderly*: The elderly are more sensitive to hypnotics. Use lowest effective dose, maximum 15 mg. Due to sedation and increased risk of falls, all BZDs are placed on Beers List of Potentially Inappropriate Medications for Geriatrics.
■ Modify dosage accordingly in patients with hepatic function impairment, typical 15 mg maximum dose.
■ *Pregnancy*: Category X; absolute contraindication
■ *Lactation*: No human studies have been performed. Not recommended in breast-feeding mothers. Drug is excreted in breast milk.
■ *Children*: This drug is not for use in children younger than 15 years of age.

NOTE: For some drugs, off-label use is reported. It is the responsibility of the practitioner to evaluate the efficacy of such use.

GALANTAMINE HYDROBROMIDE (*RAZADYNE, RAZADYNE ER*)

Classification
Anti-Alzheimer; cholinesterase inhibitor

Indications
This medicine is used to treat mild to moderate Alzheimer's disease.

Available Forms
Capsules (extended release), 8, 16, and 24 mg; oral solution, 4 mg/mL, tablets, 4, 8, and 12 mg; immediate-release tablet, and oral solution

Dosage
■ *IR tablets:* Initially, 4 mg PO BID. After 4 weeks, it may be increased to 8 mg PO BID.
■ *ER capsules:* 8 mg PO daily in the morning; after 4 weeks it may be increased to 16 mg PO daily in morning. Dosage range from 16 to 24 mg in divided doses.
■ *Oral solution:* Equivalent to the immediate-release tablets.

Administration
■ It can be administered orally.
■ Take it with food to limit drug intolerance.

Side Effects
■ Nausea, vomiting, diarrhea, loss of appetite, stomach pain, heartburn, weight loss, extreme tiredness, dizziness, pale skin, headache, uncontrollable shaking of a part of body, depression, difficulty falling asleep or staying asleep, runny nose.
■ *Serious side effects that require medical attention:* Difficulty urinating, blood in the urine, pain or burning while urinating, seizures.
■ Bradycardia, AV block, fainting; shortness of breath; black and tarry stools; red blood in the stools; bloody vomit; vomit that looks like coffee grounds.

Drug Interactions
This medicine may interact with the following medications: cholinesterase inhibitors; conivaptan; fluoxetine; neuromuscular blockers; parasympathomimetics; paroxetine; amantadine; amiodarone; amoxapine; antiretroviral protease inhibitors; antimuscarinics; aprepitant, fosaprepitant; barbiturates; cimetidine; clarithromycin; clozapine; cyclobenzaprine; delavirdine; digoxin; disopyramide; efavirenz; erythromycin; fluconazole; fluvoxamine; general anesthetics; imatinib, STI-571; itraconazole; ketoconazole; local anesthetics; maprotiline; nefazodone; nilotinib; olanzapine; orphenadrine; phenothiazines; sedating H-1 blockers; St. John's wort; tricyclic antidepressants; troglitazone; troleandomycin; voriconazole; beta-blockers; bosentan; carbamazepine; phenytoin; quinidine; rifabutin; diltiazem; fosphenytoin; nevirapine; nicardipine; nonsteroidal anti-inflammatory drugs; oxcarbazepine; rifampin; rifapentine; terbinafine; verapamil; and zafirlukast.

Pharmacokinetics
■ Cholinesterase inhibitor, reversible inhibitor of acetylcholinesterase
■ Peak plasma levels are reached in approximately 1 hour

NOTE: For some drugs, off-label use is reported. It is the responsibility of the practitioner to evaluate the efficacy of such use.

- Bioavailability is 90%
- *Half-life:* Average 7 hours

Precautions
- If treatment is stopped for several days with the intent to restart, then patient should be started back with the initial dose and then slowly retitrated to the highest tolerated dose.
- Use this drug with caution in patients with moderate hepatic impairment.
- Patients should be cautioned about engaging in tasks that require mental alertness, such as operating heavy machinery or driving, until reasonably certain that the drug does not affect them adversely.
- Use this drug with caution with pulmonary disease.
- Use this drug with caution in patients with cardiac disease.
- It may exacerbate symptoms of Parkinson's disease.

Patient and Family Education
Store galantamine at room temperature and away from excess heat and moisture. Throw away any medication that is outdated or no longer needed.

Special Populations
Hepatic impairment: Not recommended in patients with hepatic dysfunction.
Renal impairment: Not recommended in patients with renal impairment.

GUANFACINE HYDROCHLORIDE (*INTUNIV, TENEX*)

Classification
Antihypertensive; selective alpha-2A-adrenergic receptor agonist; centrally acting antihypertensive with alpha-2-adrenoceptor agonist properties in tablet form for oral administration

Indications
Selective alpha-2a-adrenergic receptor agonist indicated for the treatment of attention deficit hyperactivity disorder in children and adolescents aged 6 to 17 years. It can also be used for Tourette syndrome.

Available Forms
Capsule, 1, 2, and 3 mg

Dosage
▪ *Children: 6 to 17 years:* 1 to 4 mg PO daily; start, 1 mg PO daily, increase by 1 mg/day every week; alternate, 0.05 to 0.12 mg/kg PO daily
▪ *Adults:* It is used in adults for hypertension.

Administration
Do not give with high-fat meals; do not cut/crush/chew; taper dose by 1 mg/day every 3 to 7 days to discontinue.

Side Effects
Somnolence; headache; fatigue; upper abdominal pain; nausea; irritability; dizziness; hypotension; decreased appetite; dry mouth; constipation; syncope; AV block, bradycardia, sinus arrhythmia; dyspepsia; chest pain; asthma; emotional lability, anxiety, depression, insomnia, nightmares, and sleep changes.

Drug Interactions
▪ Avoid use with other central nervous system depressant drugs due to increased potential for sedation.
▪ The administration of guanfacine concomitantly with a known microsomal enzyme inducer (phenobarbital or phenytoin) to patients with renal impairment reportedly resulted in significant reductions in elimination half-life and plasma concentration.
▪ In such cases, therefore, more frequent dosing may be required to achieve or maintain the desired hypotensive response.

Pharmacokinetics
▪ Guanfacine is a selective alpha-2A-adrenergic receptor agonist that has a 15 to 20 times higher affinity for this receptor subtype than for the alpha-2B or alpha-2C subtypes.
▪ It is a known antihypertensive agent. By stimulating alpha-2A-adrenergic receptors, guanfacine reduces sympathetic nerve impulses from the vasomotor center to the heart and blood vessels, resulting in decreased peripheral vascular resistance and a reduction in heart rate.
▪ Time to peak plasma concentration is 5 hours.
▪ *Metabolism:* Liver, excreted in urine
▪ *Half-life:* 18 hours

NOTE: For some drugs, off-label use is reported. It is the responsibility of the practitioner to evaluate the efficacy of such use.

Precautions

- Hypersensitivity to guanfacine or concomitant use with other products containing guanfacine *(Tenex)*.
- This drug is not for use in children younger than 6 years; safety beyond 2 years of treatment has not been established.
- Geriatric populations—not labeled for use

Patient and Family Education

- Swallow whole with water, milk, or other liquid.
- Store at room temperature.
- Do not take with a high-fat meal—plasma concentrations will increase.
- Use with caution when operating heavy equipment or machinery until response to treatment is known.
- Avoid use with alcohol.
- Avoid dehydration and becoming overheated.
- Have blood pressure and heart rate assessed before administering drug.
- Taper dose by 1 mg/day every 3 to 7 days to discontinuing (abrupt cessation may cause increased plasma catecholamines, rebound hypertension, nervousness/ anxiety).

Special Populations

- *Elderly*: There is no adult dosing for this medication.
- *Pregnancy*: Category B
- *Lactation*: Safety unknown
- *Children*: For use in ages 6 to 17 years; use with caution.

NOTE: For some drugs, off-label use is reported. It is the responsibility of the practitioner to evaluate the efficacy of such use.

HALOPERIDOL DECANOATE, HALOPERIDOL LACTATE (*HALDOL*)

Classification
Phenylbutylpiperadine derivative, first-generation (typical) antipsychotic

Indications
Haloperidol is used to treat psychotic disorders and control motor tics and verbal tics in adults and children who have Tourette's disorder (condition characterized by hiccups, motor or verbal tics). It is also used to treat severe behavioral problems, such as explosive, aggressive behavior or hyperactivity in children who cannot be treated with psychotherapy or with other medications.

Available Forms
Tablet (scored), 0.5, 1, 2, 5, 10, and 20 mg; concentrate, 2 mg/mL; solution, 1 mg/mL; injection, 5 mg/mL (immediate release); decanoate injection, 50-mg haloperidol as 50 mg/mL, haloperidol decanoate, 100-mg haloperidol as 141.04 mg/mL.

Dosage
- *Oral*: 1 to 20 mg/day; max, 60 mg/day
- *Immediate-release injection*: 2 to 5 mg each dose, sometimes given every 2 to 4 weeks
- Decanoate injection: 10 to 20 times the effective daily dose of oral formulation, administered every 4 weeks

Drug Interactions
Dopamine agonists may diminish therapeutic effect. Carbamazepine increases metabolism of haloperidol. Caution must be exercised with other agents that prolong QT interval. Anticholinergics may increase glaucoma, buspirone may increase haloperidol level. Never give with lithium (acute renal insufficiency), methyldopa: may cause dementia, rifampin: decreases haloperidol level.

Administration
- *Oral:* Once daily or in divided doses at the beginning of treatment during rapid escalation; increase as needed based on patient's body weight, symptoms and provider assessment.
- *Immediate-release injection:* Initial dose 2 to 5 mg; subsequent doses may be given as often as every hour; patient should be switched to oral administration as soon as possible.
- *Decanoate injection:* Initial dose 10 to 15 times the effective oral dose for patients maintained on low antipsychotic doses (up to equivalent of 10 mg/day oral haloperidol). Initial dose may be as high as 20 times previous oral dose for patients maintained on higher antipsychotic doses: maximum, 100 mg. If higher dose is required, the remainder can be administered 3 to 7 days later. Administer total dose every 2 to 4 weeks.
- Patient must stay hydrated.
- Haloperidol is frequently dosed too high. High CYP2D6 inhibitor. Doses may actually worsen negative symptoms of schizophrenia and increase extrapyramidal symptoms (EPS) side effects.

NOTE: For some drugs, off-label use is reported. It is the responsibility of the practitioner to evaluate the efficacy of such use.

Side Effects

Neuroleptic-induced deficit syndrome; akathisia; EPS, parkinsonism, tardive dyskinesia, tardive dystonia; galactorrhea, amenorrhea; dizziness, sedation; dry mouth, constipation, urinary retention, blurred vision; decreased sweating; hypotension, tachycardia, hyperlipidemia; weight gain; rare neuroleptic malignant syndrome (NMS); rare seizures; rare jaundice, agranulocytosis, leukopenia; haloperidol with anticholinergics may increase intraocular pressure; reduces effects of anticoagulants; plasma levels of haloperidol lowered by rifampin; may enhance effects of antihypertensive agents; and haloperidol with lithium may contribute to development of encephalopathic syndrome.

Drug Interactions

- It may decrease the effects of levodopa, dopamine agonists.
- It may increase the effects of antihypertensive drugs, except for guanethidine.
- Addictive effects with central nervous system (CNS) depressants, dose of other should be reduced.
- It may interact with some pressor agents (epinephrine) to lower blood pressure.

Pharmacokinetics

- *Absorption:* Injection—100%; oral—60% to 70%
- *Onset:* IM and IV, 30 to 60 minutes
- *Duration:* 2 to 6 hours; decanoate—2 to 4 weeks
- *Metabolism:* Hepatic 50% to 60% glucuronidation
- *Half-life:* Approximately 12 to 36 hours; decanoate—3 weeks. PO—24 hours, IM—21 hours.
- *Excretion:* Urine 30%, feces 15%; PO—3 to 6 hours, IV—unknown, IM decanoate—3 to 9 days, IM lactate—10 to 20 minutes

Precautions

- Keep patient recumbent for at least 30 minutes following injection to minimize hypotensive effects.
- Discontinue the use of haloperidol if patient develops symptoms of NMS.
- Use with caution in patients with respiratory depression.
- It may alter cardiac conduction and prolong QT interval.
- There is a risk of EPS and tardive dyskinesia and hyperprolactinemia.
- Seizures
- Excessive sedation problems
- Avoid extreme heat exposure.
- The patient may experience rapid shift to depression if used to treat mania.
- Patients with thyrotoxicosis may experience neurotoxicity.
- Do not use this drug with Lewy body dementia or Parkinson's disease.
- Use with caution in patients with QTc prolongation, hypothyroidism, familial long-QT syndrome.
- Do not use if there is a proven allergy to haloperidol.

Patient and Family Education

- Maintain adequate hydration.
- Avoid contact (liquid) with skin; may cause contact dermatitis.
- Do not take within 2 hours of antacid.

NOTE: For some drugs, off-label use is reported. It is the responsibility of the practitioner to evaluate the efficacy of such use.

■ Take exactly as prescribed.

■ Avoid getting up too fast from sitting or lying position. Get up slowly and steady yourself to prevent a fall.

■ Avoid drinking alcohol.

■ Stop using this medication and call provider immediately if you have very stiff (rigid) muscles, high fever, sweating, confusion, fast or uneven heartbeats, tremors; feel like you might pass out; have jerky muscle movements you cannot control, trouble swallowing, problems with speech; have blurred vision, eye pain, or seeing halos around lights; have increased thirst and urination, excessive hunger, fruity breath odor, weakness, nausea and vomiting; have fever, chills, body aches, flu symptoms, or have white patches or sores inside mouth or on lips.

■ Do not stop taking drug suddenly without first talking to provider, even if you feel fine. May have serious side effects if you stop taking the drug suddenly.

■ Call provider if symptoms do not improve, or get worse.

■ Store at room temperature away from moisture and heat.

Special Populations

■ *Elderly*: Elderly patients are at an increased risk of death; use with extreme caution.

■ Lower doses should be used and patient monitored closely. Do not use in elderly patients with dementia.

■ *Lactation*: Breastfeeding is not recommended.

■ *Other renal impairment*: Use with caution in patients with myasthenia gravis, Parkinson's disease, and seizures.

■ *Hepatic impairment*: Use with caution.

■ *Cardiac impairment*: Because of risk of orthostatic hypertension, use with caution.

■ *Pregnancy*: Category C; some animal studies show adverse effects, no controlled studies in humans. Neonates exposed during third trimester may present with extrapyramidal symptoms, and withdrawal symptoms, breathing and feeding difficulties

■ *Lactation*: Category C

■ *Children and adolescents*: Safety and efficacy not established. Not intended for use with children under age 3 years. Generally consider as second line, not first line.

NOTE: For some drugs, off-label use is reported. It is the responsibility of the practitioner to evaluate the efficacy of such use.

HYDROXYZINE HYDROCHLORIDE (*ATARAX, VISTARIL*), HYDROXYZINE PAMOATE (*VISTARIL*)

Classification
Anxiolytic

Indications
Hydroxyzine is used to treat anxiety.

Available Forms

Hydroxyzine hydrochloride
- ▓ Capsules, 10, 25, and 50 mg
- ▓ Injection, 25 mg/mL, 50 mg/mL
- ▓ Syrup, 2 mg/mL, 10 mg/5 mL
- ▓ Tablets, 10, 25, and 50 mg

Hydroxyzine pamoate
- ▓ Capsules, 25 and 50 mg
- ▓ Oral suspension, 25 mg/5 mL

Dosages
- ▓ *Adults*: 50 to 100 mg PO QID or 50 to 100 mg IM QID
- ▓ *Children age 6 years and older*: 50 to 100 mg PO daily in divided doses;
- ▓ *Children younger than 6 years*: 50 mg PO daily in divided doses

Preoperative and Postoperative Adjunctive Therapy for Sedation
- ▓ *Adults*: 50 to 100 mg PO or IM
- ▓ *Children*: 0.6 mg/kg PO or IM

Pruritus
- ▓ *Adults*: 25 mg PO or IM TID or QID
- ▓ *Children age 6 years and older*: 50 to 100 mg PO daily in divided doses
- ▓ *Children younger than age 6 years*: 50 mg PO daily in divided doses

Administration
- ▓ PO: Give without regard for meals.
- ▓ Shake suspension well before giving.
- ▓ IM: Parenteral form (hydroxyzine hydrochloride) is for IM use only, use Z-track injection.
- ▓ Never give IV or subcutaneously.
- ▓ Aspirate IM injection carefully to prevent inadvertent IV injection. Inject deeply into a large muscle.

Side Effects
- ▓ *Central nervous system*: Drowsiness, involuntary motor activity
- ▓ *Gastrointestinal*: Dry mouth, constipation
- ▓ *Skin*: Pain at IM injection site
- ▓ *Other*: Hypersensitivity reactions

NOTE: For some drugs, off-label use is reported. It is the responsibility of the practitioner to evaluate the efficacy of such use.

Drug Interactions
▓ *Anticholinergics*: May cause additive effects. Use together cautiously.
▓ *CNS depressants*: May increase CNS depression. Use together cautiously, may need dosage adjustments.
▓ *Epinephrine*: May inhibit and reverse vasopressor effect of epinephrine. Avoid using together.
▓ *Drug-lifestyle*: Alcohol use: May increase CNS depression. Discourage use together.
▓ *Effects on lab test results*: May cause false increase in urinary 17-hydroxycorticosteroid level. May cause false-negative skin allergen tests by reducing or inhibiting the cutaneous response to histamine.

Pharmacokinetics
▓ It suppresses activity in certain essential regions of the subcortical area of the CNS. PO onset 15 to 30 minutes, peak 2 hours, duration 4 to 8 hours.
▓ IM onset is unknown, peak unknown, duration 4 to 6 hours. Half-life is 3 hours.

Precautions
▓ Contraindicated in patients hypersensitive to the drug, patients in early pregnancy, and breasteeding women.
▓ Overdose signs and symptoms: Hypersedation.

Patient and Family Education
▓ If patient is taking other CNS drugs, watch for oversedation.
▓ Look alike/sound alike: Hydroxyurea, hydrogesic, or hydralazine./ Vistaril with Restoril
▓ Warn patients to avoid hazardous activities that require alertness and good coordination until effects of drug are known.
▓ Avoid use of alcohol while taking the drug. Sugarless gum, hard candy, or ice chips may prevent dry mouth.

Special Populations
▓ *Pregnancy*: Not recommended; warn women of childbearing age to avoid use during pregnancy and breastfeeding.
▓ *Pediatrics:* Unknown
▓ *Elderly*: Elderly patients may be more sensitive to adverse anticholinergic effects; monitor these patients for dizziness, excessive sedation, confusion, hypotension, and syncope.

NOTE: For some drugs, off-label use is reported. It is the responsibility of the practitioner to evaluate the efficacy of such use.

IBUPROFEN (*MOTRIN*)

Classification
Nonsteroidal anti-inflammatory drug (NSAID)

Indications
Ibuprofen is used to treat generalized pain associated with opiate withdrawal.

Available Forms
Tablet, 100, 200, 400, 600, and 800 mg; chewable tablets, 50 and 100 mg; oral suspension, 100 mg/5 mL, 40 mg/5 mL

Dosage
Dose is 1,200 to 3,200 mg daily divided as follows: 300 mg QID or 400, 600, or 800 mg TID or QID; maximum, not to exceed 3,200 mg/day.

Administration
▥ PO with meals or milk to reduce gastrointestinal (GI) upset.
▥ *Missed dose:* Take as soon as remembered. Skip the missed dose if it is almost time for the next scheduled dose. Do not take extra medicine.

Side Effects
The side effects of ibuprofen are heartburn, nausea, vomiting, constipation, bloating, GI ulceration, and occult blood loss.

Drug Interactions
▥ Heparin may prolong bleeding time.
▥ It may increase lithium toxicity.
▥ Garlic, ginger, and ginkgo may increase bleeding time.

Pharmacokinetics
▥ *Metabolism:* Liver
▥ *Excretion:* Eliminated in urine (50%–60%; <10% unchanged)
▥ *Bioavailability:* 80% to 100%
▥ *Onset:* 30 to 60 minutes
▥ *Peak:* 120 minutes (tablets); 62 minutes (chewable); 47 minutes (suspension)
▥ *Half-life*: 2 to 4 hours

Precautions
▥ Watch for toxic hepatitis, peptic ulcer disease, and anaphylaxis.

Patient and Family Education
▥ Notify health care provider immediately of passage of dark tarry stools, coffee ground emesis, or other GI distress.
▥ Do not take with aspirin.
▥ Avoid alcohol and NSAIDs.

NOTE: For some drugs, off-label use is reported. It is the responsibility of the practitioner to evaluate the efficacy of such use.

Special Populations

- ▨ *Elderly*: There are no contraindications for the use of this drug in the elderly population.
- ▨ *Renal impairment*: Use with caution.
- ▨ *Hepatic impairment*: Use with caution; it may require smaller dosage.
- ▨ *Pregnancy*: Category B
- ▨ *Lactation*: There are no contraindications for the use of this drug in breastfeeding mothers.
- ▨ *Children and adolescents*: Whether the drug is safe to use under age 6 years has not been established.

ILOPERIDONE (*FANAPT*)

Classifications
Antipsychotic; dopamine and serotonin antagonist

Indication
Iloperidone is used to treat schizophrenia.

Available Forms
Tablets, 1, 2, 4, 6, 8, 10, and 12 mg

Dosage
- *Adults*: Initially, 1 mg PO BID
- Increase as needed as per dosing schedule: 2 mg PO BID on day 2; 4 mg PO BID on day 3; 6 mg PO BID on day 4; 8 mg PO BID on day 5; 10 mg PO BID on day 6; 12 mg PO BID on day 7.
- Maximum dosage is 12 mg PO BID.
- For patients taking CYP2D6 inhibitors and CYP3A4 inhibitors, reduce dosage by half.

Administration
Give drug with or without food.

Side Effects
- *Central nervous system*: Somnolence, akathisia, parkinsonism, agitation, dystonia, dizziness, insomnia, anxiety, restlessness, seizures, and fatigue
- *Cardiovascular*: Tachycardia,
- *EENT*: Blurred vision
- *Gastrointestinal*: Nausea, vomiting, dyspepsia, abdominal pain, diarrhea, dysphasia, and decreased appetite
- *Metabolic*: Dyslipidemia, hyperglycemia, weight gain
- *Musculoskeletal*: back pain, skin, rash, and pruritus

Drug Interactions
This medicine may interact with the following medications:

- Alpha blockers may enhance antihypertensive effects.
- Centrally acting drugs may increase CNS effects.
- Dextromethorphan may increase dextromethorphan level. Avoid use together.
- Avoid use with alcohol.
- Effects on lab test results: It may decrease hematocrit.

Pharmacokinetics
- It may antagonize dopamine type 2 and serotonin type 2.
- Onset unknown, peak 2 to 4 hours, duration unknown; half-life: 18 to 37 hours

---

NOTE: For some drugs, off-label use is reported. It is the responsibility of the practitioner to evaluate the efficacy of such use.

Precautions
- Avoid use with drugs known to prolong QT interval and in elderly patients with dementia-related symptoms.
- Overdose signs and symptoms are prolonged QT interval, drowsiness, sedation, tachycardia, and hypotension.
- Obtain baseline blood pressure, monitor regularly. Life-threatening hyperglycemia may occur in patients taking atypical antipsychotics.
- Monitor complete blood count (CBC) frequently during first few months of therapy and discontinue if white blood cell (WBC) drops with no underlying cause.
- Monitor potassium and magnesium levels at baseline and periodically in patients at risk for electrolyte imbalance.
- Drug may lower seizure threshold in patients with history of seizures.

Patient and Family Education
- Take drug on regular basis and do not skip doses.
- Periodic blood tests will be needed to monitor tolerance to the drug.
- Monitor weight and diet.
- Tell patients to avoid alcohol, warn against driving until effects of drug are know, and immediately report sudden change in body temperature, blood pressure, or irregular heartbeat.
- Monitor patients for tardive dyskinesia.
- Monitor for orthostatic hypotension.
- Monitor for signs of neuromalignant syndrome.
- Check CBC, renal function, and prolactin level periodically.
- Discontinue if severe neutropenia develops.
- Monitor for metabolic changes.
- Assess patients for risk of suicide ideation.

Special Populations
- *Elderly*: Patients with dementia-related psychosis are at increased risk for death.
- Antipsychotics are not approved for treatment of dementia-related psychosis. Use cautiously in patients with hyperlipidemia diabetes or risk for diabetes, or seizures.
- Use cautiously in patients with known CV disease and preexisting low WBC counts.
- *Pregnancy:* Category C
- *Pediatric*: Iloperidone is not indicated for use in children.

NOTE: For some drugs, off-label use is reported. It is the responsibility of the practitioner to evaluate the efficacy of such use.

IMIPRAMINE (*TOFRANIL*)

Classification
Tricyclic antidepressant

Indications
Imipramine is used to treat adults with depression/anxiety.

Available Forms
■ *Tofranil:* Tablet, 25 and 50 mg
■ *Tofranil PM:* Capsule, 75, 100, 125, and 150 mg; tablet, 10, 25, and 50 mg

Dosage
■ *Adults:* Starting dose, 25 to 75 mg PO nightly and increase by 25 to 50 mg/day every 3 to 4 days; maintenance dose, typically in divided doses, 75 to 300 mg/day.
■ *Elderly:* 100 mg/day; it can be given in divided doses. Must taper dose gradually to discontinue.
■ *Children:* For depression: Start, 1.5 mg/kg/day PO divided TID, increase by 1 to 1.5 mg/kg/day every 3 to 4 days; maximum, 5 mg/kg/day. *More than 12 years*: Start, 30 to 40 mg/day PO divided TID–QID and increase by 10 to 25 mg/day every 3 to 4 days; maximum, 100 mg/day if used for antidepressant effect.

Administration
Oral formulations require TID–QID.

■ PO with a glass of water
■ Do not crush, cut, or chew extended-release tablets.
■ Do not abruptly stop taking the medication.
■ It is not prescribed for children except when used for nocturnal enuresis and depression in children as young as 6 years.
■ Use lowest effective dose for shortest duration dosing.

Side Effects
The side effects of this drug are similar to that of amitriptyline.

■ *More common:* Drowsiness, dizziness, constipation; nausea/vomiting, urinary retention or frequency, libido changes, weight gain, general nervousness, and galactorrhea are the most common side effects.
■ *Less common:* Cardiac arrhythmias, extrapyramidal symptoms, clotting disturbances, worsening depression, suicidality, hyperthermia, and hypertension are the less common side effects.
■ Fatigue, sedation, and weight gain
■ Sexual dysfunction

Drug Interactions
This medicine may interact with the following medications:

■ Absolute contraindications include class 1A antiarrhythmics, monoamine oxidase inhibitors (MAOIs) such as phenelzine (Nardil), tranylcypromine (Parnate), isocarboxazid (Marplan), and selegiline (Eldepryl).
■ Avoid using with cimetadine, amiodarone, clarithromycin, haldoperidol, and St. John's wort.

NOTE: For some drugs, off-label use is reported. It is the responsibility of the practitioner to evaluate the efficacy of such use.

▨ *Alert:* This list may not describe all possible interactions. Instruct patients to provide a list of all medicines, herbs, nonprescription drugs, or dietary supplements used, and whether they smoke, drink alcohol, or use illegal drugs.

▨ MAOIs: Risk for extreme hypertension

▨ Central nervous system depressants (e.g., alcohol): TCAs increase effects.

▨ Direct-acting adrenergic agonists (e.g., epinephrine): TCAs increase effects.

▨ Anticholinergic drugs (e.g., antihistamines): TCAs increase effects. Do not use in combination.

▨ Selective serotonin reuptake inhibitors (SSRIs) and other medications: serotonin syndrome

Pharmacokinetics

▨ TCAs are thought to work by inhibiting reuptake of norepinephrine and serotonin in the CNS, which potentiates the neurotransmitters. They also have significant anticholinergics, antihistaminic, and alpha-adrenergic activity on the cardiac system. These classes of antidepressants also possess class 1A antiarrhythmic activity, which can lead to depression of cardiac conduction potentially resulting in heart block or ventricular arrhythmias.

▨ *Metabolism:* This drug is metabolized extensively by the liver to the active metabolite desipramine form by CYP450 2D6. Also metabolized by CYP450 1A2.

▨ *Excretion:* Primarily in urine, up to less than 5% unchanged, also excreted in the bile/feces.

▨ *Peak:* 1 to 2 hours

▨ *Onset:* After 2 weeks

▨ *Half-life:* 6 to 18 hours

Precautions

▨ See patients as often as necessary to ensure that the drug is working on the panic attacks, determine compliance, and review side effects.

▨ Instruct patients and families to watch for worsening depression or thoughts of suicide. Also, watch out for sudden or severe changes in feelings, such as feeling anxious, agitated, panicky, irritated, hostile, aggressive, impulsive, severely restless, overly excited, hyperactive, or not being able to sleep. If this happens, especially at the beginning of antidepressant treatment or after a change in dose, patient should call the health care provider.

▨ Drowsiness or dizziness: Patients should not drive or use machinery or do anything that needs mental alertness until the effects of this medicine are known. Other medications that cause drowsiness can add to the drowsiness of imipramine.

▨ Caution patients not to stand or sit up quickly, especially if older. This reduces the risk of dizzy or fainting spells. Alcohol may interfere with the effect of this medicine. Avoid alcoholic drinks.

▨ Do not abruptly withdraw this drug as it may cause headache, nausea, and malaise.

▨ Advise to protect skin from ultraviolet light due to increased skin sensitivity.

▨ Grapefruit and grapefruit juice may interact with imipramine.

▨ Caution should be exercised in the following:
  ▨ Major depressive disorder (MDD), psychosis, or bipolar affective disorder
  ▨ Contraindicated in patients with a recent myocardial infarction
  ▨ Blood dyscrasias
  ▨ Respiratory disease
  ▨ Heart disease

NOTE: For some drugs, off-label use is reported. It is the responsibility of the practitioner to evaluate the efficacy of such use.

- Liver disease
- Seizures (convulsions)
- Suicidal thoughts, plans, or attempts by patients or a family member
- An unusual or allergic reaction to imipramine, other medicines, foods, dyes, or preservatives
- Overdose may result in lethal cardiotoxicity or seizure.
- Use with caution in patients having a history of seizure or heart disease.
- Avoid in patients with a history of cardiac arrhythmia. Monitor with EKG.

Patient and Family Education
- Store imipramine at room temperature away from moisture and heat.
- Stopping this medication suddenly could result in unpleasant side effects.
- Take the missed dose as soon as remembered. If it is almost time for the next dose, skip the missed dose and take the medicine at the next regularly scheduled time. Do not take extra medicine to make up the missed dose.
- It should be taken about the same time every day, with or without food. It may cause prolonged sedation. Do not drive until the effect of this medication is known.
- Administration time may be adjusted based on observed sedating or activating drug effects.
- It may take up to 4 to 8 weeks to show its maximum effect, but patient may see symptoms of dysthymia improving in as little as 2 weeks.
- If patient plans on becoming pregnant, discuss the benefits versus the risks of using this medicine while pregnant.
- As this medicine is excreted in breast milk, nursing mothers should not breastfeed while taking this medicine without prior consultation with a psychiatric nurse practitioner or psychiatrist. Newborns may develop symptoms, including feeding or breathing difficulties, seizures, muscle stiffness, jitteriness, or constant crying.
- Do not stop taking this medication unless the health care provider directs. Report symptoms to the health care provider promptly.
- Drug should be tapered gradually.
- Treatment should continue for at least 6 to 12 months following last reported dysthymic experience.
- Keep these medications out of the reach of children and pets.

Special Populations
- *Elderly:* Older patients tend to be more sensitive to the medication side effects, such as hypotension and anticholinergic effects. They often require adjustment of medication doses for hepatic or renal dysfunction TCAs. Dose adjustment is necessary for geriatric patients, and in patients with liver impairment
- *Pregnancy:* Category D; some clinical reports of congenital malformations, but no direct causal link. Not recommended in pregnancy, as there are no adequate studies showing potential for side effects during pregnancy.
- *Lactation:* This drug is excreted in human breast milk; alternative medications are recommended.
- *Children:* Tofranil is indicated. The drug is not recommended for children younger than 6 years old with nocturnal enuresis or with depression. Monitor for suicidal ideation with depression. Tofranil PM is not approved for use in children under the age of 12 years.

NOTE: For some drugs, off-label use is reported. It is the responsibility of the practitioner to evaluate the efficacy of such use.

ISOCARBOXAZID (*MARPLAN*)

Classification
Monoamine oxidase inhibitor (MAOI)

Indications
This drug is used as an antidepressant and anxiolytic.

Available Forms
Tablet, 10 mg

Dosage
Starting dose: 20 mg/day; maintenance dose: 20 to 60 mg/day, in divided doses.

Administration
PO, TID–QID dosing. After 1 week, may increase by up to 20 mg/week to maximum 60 mg/day.

Side Effects
▪ Hypertensive crisis, secondary to excessive consumption of dietary tyramine (e.g., soft cheeses, aged fish, aged meat, and avocados).
▪ Central nervous system stimulation
▪ Orthostatic hypotension
▪ Sexual dysfunction

Drug Interactions
▪ Selective serotonin reuptake inhibitors (SSRIs), serotonin-norepinephrine reuptake inhibitors (SNRIs), and tricyclic antidepressants (TCAs): There is a risk for extreme hypertension.
▪ Indirect-acting adrenergic agonists (e.g., ephedrine): It increases MAOI effects.
▪ Antihypertensive drugs may dangerously lower blood pressure.

Pharmacokinetics
Duration of action: May last 2 to 3 weeks following discontinuation due to irreversible monoamine oxidase inhibition.

Precautions
▪ Adverse effects and side effects are commonly observed before therapeutic effects.
▪ Dietary restrictions require substantial patient adherence.

Patient and Family Education
▪ This drug should be taken about the same time every day, with or without food.
▪ Substantial education required on dietary changes and importance of dietary adherence.
▪ Patient should advise all health care providers that he or she is on an MAOI prior to initiating new medications.

NOTE: For some drugs, off-label use is reported. It is the responsibility of the practitioner to evaluate the efficacy of such use.

- Administration time may be adjusted based on observed sedating or activating drug effects.
- It may take up to 4 to 8 weeks to show its maximum effect, but some may see symptoms of dysthymia depression improving in as little as 2 weeks.
- Do not take the drug in case of pregnancy or trying to get pregnant.
- As this medicine is excreted in the breast milk, nursing mothers should not breast-feed while taking this medicine. Newborns may develop symptoms, including feeding or breathing difficulties, seizures, muscle stiffness, jitteriness, or constant crying.
- Report potential side effects to the health care provider promptly.
- Keep these medications out of the reach of children and pets.

Special Populations

- *Elderly*: There is a requirement for lower drug dose in adult patients over 65 years. Due to common need for polypharmacy, drug is not recommended.
- *Pregnancy*: Psychotherapy is the initial choice for most pregnant patients with major depressive disorder (MDD). This drug is generally not recommended during pregnancy.
- *Children*: It is not recommended for children less than 16 years of age.

LAMOTRIGINE (*LAMICTAL, LAMICTAL CD, LAMICTAL ODT, LAMICTAL XR*)

Classification
Anticonvulsant, mood-stabilizing anticonvulsant

Indications
Indication only for maintenance, not acute phase.

Available Forms
Tablet, 25, 100, 150, and 200 mg; chewable tablet, 2, 5, and 25 mg; tablet (oral disintegrating), 25, 50, 100, and 200 mg; tablet (extended release), 25, 50, 100, 200, and 300 mg

Dosage
Starting dose for adults is 25 mg by mouth every day for 2 weeks; then 50 mg every day for 2 weeks; then 100 mg every day for 1 week; maximum, 200 mg/day.

Administration
- Discontinue medicine at first sign of a rash.
- This medicine should be taken as directed and is well tolerated in the recommended doses.
- Individuals taking this medicine should carry an identification card to alert medical personnel who might be caring for them.
- The potential carcinogenic, mutagenic, and fertility effects are unknown.
- This is a category C drug and should be used in pregnancy if the potential benefit outweighs the risk. It is not known whether the drug is excreted in breast milk so caution should be exercised when it is administered to nursing women.
- Pediatric use under the age of 18 years has not been established. Individuals taking opioid-containing medicines, such as cough-and-cold preparations, antidiarrheal preparations, and opioid analgesics with lamotrigine may not benefit from these medicines.
- Concomitant use is unknown.
- This drug does not interfere with drug testing using urine samples.

Side Effects
Dizziness, headache, diplopia, ataxia, asthenia, nausea, blurred vision, somnolence, rhinitis, rash, pharyngitis, vomiting, cough, flu syndrome, dysmenorrhea, uncoordination, insomnia, diarrhea, fever, abdominal pain, depression, tremor, anxiety, vaginitis, speech disturbance, seizures, weight loss, photosensitivity, nystagmus, constipation, and dry mouth.

Drug Interactions
Avoid using the following drugs with this medicine:
- Oral progesterone contraceptives (may decrease hormonal contraceptive levels).
- Etonogestrel subdermal implant (may decrease hormonal contraceptive levels).
- Ginkgo biloba, Eun-haeng, fossil tree, ginkyo, icho, ityo, Japanese silver apricot, kew tree, maidenhair tree, salisburia, silver apricot, ginkgo (may decrease anticonvulsant efficacy).
- Medroxyprogesterone acetate (may decrease hormonal contraceptive levels).

NOTE: For some drugs, off-label use is reported. It is the responsibility of the practitioner to evaluate the efficacy of such use.

- Acetaminophen (may decrease effects of lamotrigine).
- Valproate may decrease clearance of lamotrogine (increases lamotrogine level and decreases valproate level).
- Oxcarbazepine, phenobarbital, phenytoin, and primodone (may decrease lamotrigine level).
- St. John's wort (may decrease lamotrigine levels as clearance is increased).
- Folate inhibitors (methotrexate, sulfamethoxazole, and trimethoprim) may have an additive effect.

Pharmacokinetics

The drug is metabolized by the liver (CYP450). It is excreted in the urine (94%) and feces (2%).

- *Peak plasma:* 1 to 5 hours
- *Bioavailability:* 98%
- *Half-life:* 14.5 to 70.25 hours

Precautions

Discontinue medicine at first sign of a rash. Incidence is 0.8% in children 2 to 6 years of age and 0.3% in adults. Most life-threatening rashes occur and may occur at any time during treatment.

- Caution should be exercised when administering this medicine to patients with suicide risk, pregnancy, hepatic impairment, renal impairment, and hypersensitivity to antiepileptic drugs.
- Individuals taking opioid-containing medicines, such as cough-and-cold preparations, antidiarrheal preparations, and opioid analgesics may not benefit from these medicines.
- This drug may cause aseptic meningitis.

Patient and Family Education

- Do not stop taking this drug suddenly; it must be tapered by your health care provider.
- Notify your health care provider immediately if your depression symptoms increase.
- High risk of nonadherence due the need to take the medication twice daily.

Special Populations

- *Elderly:* Caution should be exercised when administering this drug to the elderly.
- *Renal impairment:* For moderate to severe impairment, decrease dose by 25%. If there is severe impairment, decrease dose by 50%.
- *Pregnancy:* Category C drug. Animal studies show adverse fetal effect(s) but no controlled human studies.
- *Lactation:* It is considered unsafe for breastfeeding mothers. Medication administration requires cessation of breastfeeding.
- *Children:* It is not recommended for children due to severe limitations.

NOTE: For some drugs, off-label use is reported. It is the responsibility of the practitioner to evaluate the efficacy of such use.

LEVOMILNACIPRAN (*FETZIMA*)

Classification
Antidepressant (serotonin–norepinephrine reuptake inhibitor [SNRI])

Indications
Levomilnacirpan is for major depressive disorder (MDD) in adults.

Available Forms
Extended-release capsules, 20, 40, 80, and 120 mg

Dosage
▪ 20 mg PO daily for 2 days initially; then increase to 40 mg PO daily.
▪ Dose effect: Increase dose in increments of 40 mg/day at intervals of 2 or more days; not to exceed 120 mg/day.
▪ Initiated at 20 mg once daily for 2 days and then increased to 40 mg once daily.

Administration
▪ Swallow the extended-release capsule in whole.
▪ The medication can be taken with or without food.
▪ Avoid abrupt withdrawal of this drug. Slowly titrate off drug.

Side Effects
▪ Nausea, constipation, vomiting, hyperhidrosis, increased heart rate, erectile dysfunction, tachycardia, palpitations; hypertension, urinary hesitation.
▪ Hypersensitivity
▪ Suicidal thoughts and behaviors in adolescents and young adults
▪ Serotonin syndrome
▪ Elevated blood pressure (BP)
▪ Elevated heart rate
▪ Abnormal bleeding
▪ Narrow-angle glaucoma
▪ Urinary hesitation or retention
▪ Activation of mania/hypomania
▪ Seizure
▪ Hyponatremia

Drug Interactions
▪ Use levomilnacirpan with caution in patients who are on monoamine oxidase inhibitors (MAOIs). Allow at least 14 days after MAOI discontinuation before starting levomilnacipran.
▪ There is an increased risk of serotonin syndrome with other serotonergic drugs or with drugs that impair serotonin metabolism.
▪ There is an increased risk of bleeding with concomitant nonsteroidal anti-inflammatory drugs (NSAIDs), aspirin, and anticoagulants; there is a need to monitor the same.
▪ Concomitant strong CYP3A4 inhibitors adjust dose.
▪ Avoid alcohol.
▪ Use with caution with other central nervous system (CNS)-active drugs, or drugs that can increase BP or heart rate.

NOTE: For some drugs, off-label use is reported. It is the responsibility of the practitioner to evaluate the efficacy of such use.

Pharmacokinetics

▪ The exact mechanism of action of levomilnacipran is unknown.
▪ It is thought to be related to the potentiation of serotonin and norepinephrine in the CNS, through inhibition of reuptake at serotonin and norepinephrine transporters.

Precautions

▪ There is an increased risk of suicidal thinking and behavior in children, adolescents, and young adults.
▪ Monitor for serotonin syndrome especially if patient is on other serotonergic agents; thoroughly review patient medications for other serotonergic MAOIs, tricyclic antidepressants, selective serotonin reuptake inhibitors (SSRIs).
▪ Use caution with patients who have history of bipolar disorder, mania, or hypomania, hypertension, cardiovascular disease, seizures, tachyarrhythmias, obstructive urinary disorders, seizure disorder.
▪ Monitor BP and heart rate; reduce dose or discontinue if elevation persists.
▪ Use of this drug can increase risk of bleeding caution with use of NSAIDs, aspirin, or anticoagulants.
▪ If patients are taking diuretics, monitor the patients' volume/electrolytes. There is an increased risk of hyponatremia.

Patient and Family Education

▪ Patients should be monitored closely for changes in behavior, clinical worsening, and suicidal tendencies; this should be done during initial 1 to 2 months of therapy and dosage adjustments.
▪ The patient's family should communicate any abrupt changes in behavior to the health care provider.
▪ Be aware of all drug interactions and notify provider if medications change.
▪ Make sure patient and family are aware of all side effects.
▪ Monitor creatinine clearance (CrCl) in patients with existing renal impairment: moderate (CrCl 30–59 mL/min): maximum 80 mg once daily; severe (CrCl 15–29 mL/min): maximum 40 mg once daily.

Special Populations

▪ *Elderly*
  ▪ SSRIs and SNRIs, including Fetzima, have been associated with cases of clinically significant hyponatremia in elderly patients, who may be at greater risk for this adverse event.
  ▪ Monitor patients' renal and liver function regularly.
▪ *Pregnancy*
  ▪ Category C: There are no adequate and well-controlled studies of Fetzima in pregnant women.
  ▪ Neonates exposed to dual reuptake inhibitors of serotonin and norepinephrine (such as Fetzima), or SSRIs late in the third trimester have developed complications that can arise immediately upon delivery.
▪ *Children and Young Adults*
  ▪ Clinical studies on the use of Fetzima in pediatric patients have not been conducted; therefore, the safety and effectiveness of Fetzima in the pediatric population have not been established. Fetzima is not approved for use in pediatric patients.

NOTE: For some drugs, off-label use is reported. It is the responsibility of the practitioner to evaluate the efficacy of such use.

LISDEXAMFETAMINE DIMESYLATE (*VYVANSE*)

Classification
Central nervous system (CNS) stimulant

Indications
Stimulant indicated for the treatment of attention deficit hyperactivity disorder (ADHD) in children and adults.

Available Forms
Capsule, 20, 30, 40, 50, 60, 70 mg

Dosage
Dosage should be individualized according to the therapeutic needs and response of the patient. All stimulant preparations should be administered at the lowest effective dosage.

■ *Children: 6 to 12 years old:* 30 mg PO QAM; maximum, 70 mg/day; may increase dose 10 to 20 mg/day every week; use lowest effective dose.
■ *Adults:* 30 mg QAM; maximum, 70 mg/day; may increase dose 10 to 20 mg/day every week; use lowest effective dose.

Administration
Swallow capsules whole with water or other liquids. If patient cannot swallow the capsule, open it and mix with water. Follow with a drink of water or other liquid. It can be taken with or without food. Avoid afternoon doses; the drug has the potential for insomnia.

Side Effects
■ Decreased appetite, dizziness, dry mouth, irritability, insomnia, upper abdominal pain, nausea and/or vomiting, weight loss, headaches, and anxiety
■ Psychiatric events: increase in manic states for bipolar patients, aggression, tics, and tremors.
■ Long-term growth suppression: patients should be monitored throughout treatment, if there appears to be growth suppression, the treatment should be discontinued.
■ Rash, pyrexia, palpitations, tachycardia, elevated blood pressure, sudden death, myocardial infarction, cardiomyopathy, Stevens–Johnson syndrome and toxic epidermal necrolysis, impotence, and libido changes

Drug Interactions
The medication may interact with urinary acidifying agents, monoamine oxidase inhibitors (MAOIs), adrenergic blockers, antihistamines, antihypertensives, veratrum alkaloids, ethosuximide, tricyclic antidepressants, meperidine, phenobarbital, phenytoin, chlorpromazine, Haldol, lithium, norepinephrine, and propoxyphene.

Pharmacokinetics
■ This drug is absorbed by the gastrointestinal tract.

NOTE: For some drugs, off-label use is reported. It is the responsibility of the practitioner to evaluate the efficacy of such use.

■ The mode of therapeutic action in ADHD is not known. Amphetamines are thought to block the reuptake of norepinephrine and dopamine into the presynaptic neuron and increase the release of these monoamines into the extraneural space.

■ Prodrug converted to dextroamphetamine.

■ *Metabolism:* Liver; mainly excreted in the urine (96%).

■ *Time to peak:* 1 hour

■ *Half-life:* Less than 0.5 hours

Precautions

■ Advanced arteriosclerosis, symptomatic cardiovascular disease, and moderate-to-severe hypertension

■ Hyperthyroidism

■ Known hypersensitivity or idiosyncratic reaction to sympathomimetic amines

■ Glaucoma

■ Agitated states

■ Patients with a history of drug abuse: Amphetamines have a high potential for abuse. Administration of amphetamines for an extended period of time may lead to drug dependence. Particular attention should be paid to the possibility of patients obtaining this class of medication for nontherapeutic use or distribution to others, and the drugs should be prescribed or dispensed sparingly.

■ During or within 14 days following the administration of MAOIs, hypertensive crisis may result.

■ Use with caution in patients with preexisting psychosis.

■ Seizure history: Some studies have shown the potential for lowering the seizure threshold.

Patient and Family Education

■ Store the drug at room temperature, protected from light.

■ Keep it out of reach of children.

■ Seek medical care for any signs of heart problems (chest pain, shortness of breath), fainting, psychotic symptoms, overdose, or any other concerns.

■ Routinely assess weight and BP.

■ Treatment should be initiated at low doses and then titrated over 2 to 4 weeks until an adequate response is achieved or unacceptable adverse effects occur.

■ If one stimulant is not effective, another should be attempted before second-line medications are considered. Although some children benefit from daily stimulant therapy, weekend and summer "drug holidays" are suggested for children whose ADHD symptoms predominantly affect schoolwork or to limit adverse effects (e.g., appetite suppression, abdominal pain, headache, insomnia, irritability, tics).

Special Populations

■ *Elderly:* Use caution with polypharmacy and comorbid conditions; has not been studied for use in this population.

■ *Pregnancy:* Category C; based on animal data, they may cause fetal harm.

■ *Lactation:* Possibly unsafe.

■ *Children:* not recommended due to strict limitations

NOTE: For some drugs, off-label use is reported. It is the responsibility of the practitioner to evaluate the efficacy of such use.

LITHIUM CARBONATE, LITHIUM CITRATE (*CIBALITH-S*, *ESKALITH*, *LITHOBID*)

Classification
First-line nonanticonvulsant mood stabilizer

Indications
This drug is used to treat mania in bipolar disorder. Initially, lithium is often used in conjunction with antipsychotic drugs as it can take up to a month for it to have an effect. Lithium is also used as prophylaxis for depression and mania in bipolar disorder. It is sometimes used for other psychiatric disorders, such as cycloid psychosis, borderline personality disorder, and major depressive disorder.

Available Forms
Capsule, 150, 300, and 600 mg; slow-release tablet, 300 mg; controlled-release tablet, 300 and 450 mg; syrup, 300 mg (8 mEq lithium/5 mL)

Dosage
Adults: 300 to 600 mg/day PO up to QID, or 900-mg controlled-release tablet PO every 12 hours. Increase dosage based on blood levels. Recommended therapeutic lithium levels are 1 to 1.5 mEq/L for acute mania and 0.6 to 1.2 mEq/L for maintenance therapy.

Administration
- Oral
- Give the drug after meals with plenty of water to minimize gastrointestinal upset.
- Do not crush controlled-release tablets.

Side Effects
- *Central nervous system*: Fatigue, lethargy, coma, epileptiform seizures, tremors, drowsiness, headache, confusion, restlessness, dizziness, psychomotor retardation, blackouts, electroencephalogram changes, impaired worsened mental syndrome, impaired speech, ataxia, and incoordination
- *Cardiovascular*: Arrhythmias, bradycardia, reversible EKG changes, and hypotension
- *EENT*: Tinnitus and blurred vision
- *Gastrointestinal*: Vomiting, anorexia, diarrhea, thirst, nausea, metallic taste, dry mouth, abdominal pain, flatulence, and indigestion
- *Genitourinary*: Polyuria, renal toxicity with long-term use, glycosuria, decreased creatinine clearance (CrCl), and albuminuria.
- *Hematologic*: Leukocytosis with leukocyte count of 14,000 to 18,000/mm.
- *Metabolic*: Transient hyperglycemia, goiter, hypothyroidism, and hyponatremia
- *Musculoskeletal*: Muscle weakness
- *Skin*: Pruritus, rash, diminished or absent sensation, drying and thinning of hair, psoriasis, acne, and alopecia
- *Other*: Ankle and wrist edema

Drug Interactions
- Angiotensin-converting enzyme inhibitors, aminophylline, sodium bicarbonate, urine alkalizers, calcium channel blockers (verapamil), carbamazepine, fluoxetine,

---

NOTE: For some drugs, off-label use is reported. It is the responsibility of the practitioner to evaluate the efficacy of such use.

methyldopa, nonsteroidal anti-inflammatory drugs, probenecid, neuromuscular blockers, thiazide diuretics, and diuretics

▦ Diuretics, especially loop diuretics, may inhibit lithium elimination, and increase lithium toxicity.

▦ Caffeine may decrease lithium levels and drug effects. Advise patients who ingest large amounts of caffeine.

Pharmacokinetics

▦ Probably alters chemical transmitters in the CNS, possibly by interfering with ionic pump mechanisms in brain cells, and may compete with or replace sodium ions. The peak action is between 30 minutes and 1 hour; extended release, 4 to 12 hours.

▦ *Bioavialability*: 95% to 100% (immediate release/syrup); 60% to 905% (extended release)

▦ *Excretion*: Urine (95%–99%)

▦ *Half-life:* 18 hours (adolescents); 36 hours (elderly)

Precautions

▦ Lithium may increase glucose and creatinine levels.

▦ It may decrease sodium, T3, T4, and protein-bound iodine levels.

▦ It may increase white blood cell and neutrophil counts.

▦ It is contraindicated if therapy cannot be closely monitored.

▦ Avoid using the drug in pregnant patients unless benefits outweigh risks.

▦ Use with caution in patients receiving neuromuscular blockers and diuretics; in elderly or debilitated patients; and in patients with thyroid disease, seizure disorder, infection, renal or CV disease, severe debilitation or dehydration, or sodium depletion.

▦ *Alert:* Drug has a narrow therapeutic margin of safety. Determining drug level is crucial to the safe use of the drug. Do not use the drug in patients who cannot have regular tests done. Monitor levels 8 to 12 hours after the first dose, the morning before the second dose is given, two or three times weekly for the first month, and then weekly to monthly during maintenance therapy.

▦ When the drug level is less than 1.5 mEq/L, adverse reactions are usually mild.

▦ Monitor baseline EKG, thyroid studies, renal studies, and electrolyte levels.

▦ Check fluid intake and output, especially when surgery is scheduled.

▦ Weigh patient daily; check for edema or sudden weight gain.

▦ Adjust fluid and salt ingestion to compensate if excessive loss occurs from protracted diaphoresis or diarrhea. Under normal conditions, patient's fluid intake should be 2.5 to 3 L daily; patient should follow a balanced diet with adequate salt intake.

▦ Check urine-specific gravity and report levels below 1.005, which may indicate diabetes insipidus.

▦ Drug alters glucose tolerance in diabetics. Monitor glucose level closely.

▦ Perform outpatient follow-up of thyroid and renal functions every 6 to 12 months. Palpate thyroid to check for enlargement.

Patient and Family Education

▦ Tell the patient to take the drug with plenty of water and after meals to minimize GI upset.

▦ Explain the importance of having regular blood tests to determine drug levels; even slightly high values can be dangerous.

NOTE: For some drugs, off-label use is reported. It is the responsibility of the practitioner to evaluate the efficacy of such use.

- Warn patients and caregivers to expect transient nausea, large amounts of urine, thirst, and discomfort during the first few days of therapy and to watch for evidence of toxicity (diarrhea, vomiting, tremor, drowsiness, muscle weakness, incoordination).
- Instruct patients to withhold one dose and call the prescriber if signs and symptoms of toxicity appear, but do not stop drug abruptly.
- Warn patients to avoid hazardous activities that require alertness and good psychomotor coordination until the CNS effects of drug are known.
- Tell patients not to switch brands or take other prescription or over-the-counter drugs without the prescriber's guidance.
- Tell patients to wear or carry medical identification at all times.

Special Populations

- *Elderly*: Initial dose reduction and possibly lower maintenance doses due to age-related changes and sensitivity to side effects.
- *Pregnancy*: Category D; positive evidence of fetal harm has been demonstrated.
- *Children*: It is not approved in children younger than 12 years of age; use with caution and monitor closely for side effects and suicidality. Children may experience more frequent and severe side effects.

LOPERAMIDE (*IMODIUM*)

Classification
Antidiarrheal drug

Indications
Loperamide treats diarrhea associated with opiate withdrawal.

Available Forms
Capsule, 1 and 2 mg; oral solution, 1 mg/5 mL, 1 mg/7.5 mL

Dosage
The dosage is 4 mg (two capsules) followed by 2 mg (one capsule) after each unformed stool. Daily dose should not exceed 16 mg (eight capsules). Clinical improvement is usually observed within 48 hours.

Administration
- PO with a full glass of water
- The drug may be taken with or without food.
- *Missed dose:* Take as soon as remembered. Skip the missed dose if it is almost time for the next scheduled dose. Do not take extra medicine.

Side Effects
Anaphylactic reactions (rare); stomach pain/bloating; diarrhea that is bloody, watery, or worsening; flu-like symptoms with skin reaction/rash; dizziness; fatigue; constipation; mild stomach pain; mild skin pruritus and rash.

Drug Interactions
When given concurrently with saquinavir, the therapeutic efficacy of saquinavir should be closely monitored.

Pharmacokinetics
- *Bioavailability:* 0.3%
- *Onset:* 1 to 3 hours
- *Half-life:* 11 hours
- *Excretion:* Feces (30%–40%); urine (1%)

Precautions
- Discontinue the use of this drug if the patient has constipation, abdominal distention, or ileus develop.

Patient and Family Education
- Do not take if stools are bloody, black, or tarry.
- Do not use this medication to treat diarrhea caused by antibiotic use.
- Drink extra water to prevent dehydration.
- It may take up to 48 hour for symptoms to improve.
- Call health care provider if symptoms do not improve after treatment for 10 days.
- Exercise caution when driving or operating machinery.

NOTE: For some drugs, off-label use is reported. It is the responsibility of the practitioner to evaluate the efficacy of such use.

Special Populations

■ *Elderly:* No dose adjustments required

■ *Renal impairment:* No dose adjustments required

■ *Hepatic impairment*: Use with caution; monitor for signs of central nervous system toxicity.

■ *Pregnancy:* Category C

■ *Lactation:* Contraindicated

■ *Children and adolescents*: Use with caution; monitor fluid and electrolyte balance.

NOTE: For some drugs, off-label use is reported. It is the responsibility of the practitioner to evaluate the efficacy of such use.

LORAZEPAM (*ATIVAN*)

Classification
Benzodiazepine (BZD)

Indications
Lorazepam is used for anxiety and sedation during hypnosis.

Available Forms
Tablet, to be taken orally, contains 0.5, 1, or 2 mg of lorazepam; oral concentrate, 2 mg/mL; injectable solution, 2 mg/mL, 4 mg/mL.

Dosage
▪ The dosage of 2 to 6 mg/day is given in divided doses, the largest dose should be taken before bedtime
▪ Daily dosage may vary from 1 to 10 mg/day.
▪ For anxiety, most patients require an initial dose of 2 to 3 mg/day given BID or TID.
▪ For insomnia due to anxiety or transient situational stress, a single daily dose of 2 to 4 mg may be given, usually at bedtime.
▪ For elderly or debilitated patients, an initial dosage of 1 to 2 mg/day in divided doses is recommended, to be adjusted as needed and tolerated.
▪ The dosage of Ativan (lorazepam) should be increased gradually when needed to help avoid adverse effects. When higher dosage is indicated, the evening dose should be increased before the daytime doses.

Administration
▪ Lorazepam can be given PO, IM, and IV. Missed doses need to be given as soon as possible; however, if it is time for the next dose, do not administer a double dose.
▪ If a dose is missed, it should be taken as soon as possible. If it is time for the next dose, skip the missed dose and resume usual dosing schedule.

Side Effects
Dizziness, weakness, and unsteadiness; a few other side effects include nausea, constipation, fatigue, and sedation.

Drug Interactions
▪ Increased central nervous system (CNS)-depressant effects when administered with other CNS depressants, such as alcohol, barbiturates, antipsychotics, sedative/hypnotics, anxiolytics, antidepressants, narcotic analgesics, sedative antihistamines, anticonvulsants, and anesthetics.
▪ Use caution when combining clozapine and lorazepam for they may produce marked sedation, excessive salivation, hypotension, ataxia, delirium, and respiratory arrest.
▪ Administration of lorazepam with valproate results in increased plasma concentrations and reduced clearance of lorazepam.
▪ Administration of lorazepam with probenecid may result in a more rapid onset or prolonged effect of lorazepam due to increased half-life and decreased total clearance.

NOTE: For some drugs, off-label use is reported. It is the responsibility of the practitioner to evaluate the efficacy of such use.

▥ Administration of theophylline or aminophylline may reduce the sedative effects of BZDs, including lorazepam.

Pharmacokinetics

▥ The drug enhances gamma-aminobutyric acid (GABA).
▥ The drug is metabolized by the liver, enhances GABA effects, which inhibits the transmission of nerve signals and thus reduces nervous excitation.
▥ *Bioavailability:* 90%
▥ *Peak plasma:* 2 hours
▥ *Half-life:* 14 hours

Contraindications

The drug is contraindicated in patients with

▥ hypersensitivity to BZDs or to any components of the formulation
▥ acute narrow-angle glaucoma

Precautions

Avoid abrupt withdrawal for long-term use, use of alcohol in depressed patients, intra-arterial administration, and use in drug-abuse patients.

Patient and Family Education

▥ Notify health care provider if there are problems with the liver or kidneys, alcohol or drug consumption, glaucoma, lung problems, or if treated for psychiatric disorders.
▥ Herbs with sedative effects should be avoided.
▥ Alcoholic beverages should be avoided. Lithium with lorazepam can cause children's body temperature to drop.
▥ Use of CNS depressants can cause respiratory depression.
▥ Lorazepam should never be shared with another person, especially someone who has a history of drug abuse or addiction. Keep the medication in a secure place where others cannot get to it.
▥ It is dangerous to try to purchase lorazepam on the Internet or from vendors outside of the United States.
▥ Medications distributed from Internet sales may contain dangerous ingredients, or may not be distributed by a licensed pharmacy.
▥ Samples of lorazepam purchased on the Internet have been found to contain haloperidol (Haldol), a potent antipsychotic drug with dangerous side effects.
▥ For more information, contact the U.S. Food and Drug Administration or visit www.fda.gov/buyonlineguide.
▥ Store in a tightly closed container and keep at room temperature away from excess heat and moisture.

NOTE: For some drugs, off-label use is reported. It is the responsibility of the practitioner to evaluate the efficacy of such use.

Special Populations

- *Elderly*: Caution is advised. Due to its sedative property effect and increased risk of falls, all BZDs are included on Beers List of Potentially Inappropriate Medications for Geriatrics.
- *Renal impairment:* No adjustment is needed if using the oral form; however, dose may need to be adjusted if using the IV form.
- *Hepatic impairment:* May require decreasing the dose, and if patient has hepatic failure or impaired liver function, use should be avoided.
- *Pregnancy*: Category D. This drug should not be used in women who are pregnant. Lorazepam is associated with an increased risk of birth defects.
- *Lactation:* Should not be used in women who are breastfeeding.
- *Children*: Safety has not been established in children under 12 years; long-term effects are unknown in children younger than 12 years old.

LURASIDONE HYDROCHLORIDE (*LATUDA*)

Classification
Antipsychotic; dopamine and serotonin receptor antagonist

Indications
Lurasidone hydrochloride is used to treat schizophrenia.

Available Forms
Tablet, 40 and 80 mg

Dosage
▨ *Adults*: Initially, 40 mg once daily
▨ The dosage may increase to maximum of 80 mg daily.
▨ For patients with moderate to severe renal disease or hepatic impairment, or if taken concomitantly with CYP3A4 inhibitor, maximum dose is 40 mg daily.

Administration
This drug should be administered with food (at least 350 calories).

Pharmacokinetics
▨ Efficacy mediated through antagonism at the dopamine type 2 and serotnin type 2 receptors.
▨ Onset unknown, peaks in 1 to 3 hours, duration unknown.
▨ *Half-life:* 18 hours
▨ Effects on lab test results: It may increase prolactin, total cholesterol, triglyceride, glucose, serum creatinine, aspartate aminotransferase, alanine aminotransferase, and creatine kinase levels. It may decrease white blood cells, neutrophil, and granulocyte counts.

Side Effects
▨ *Central nervous system*: Somnolence, akathisia, parkinsonism, agitation, dystonia, dizziness, insomnia, anxiety, restlessness, seizures, and fatigue.
▨ *Cardiovascular*: Tachycardia
▨ *EENT*: Blurred vision
▨ *Gastrointestinal*: Nausea, vomiting, dyspepsia, abdominal pain, diarrhea, dysphasia, and decreased appetite
▨ *Metabolic*: Dyslipidemia, hyperglycemia, and weight gain
▨ *Musculoskeletal*: Back pain, rash, and pruritus

Drug Interactions
▨ Antihypertensives may increase risk of hypotension, centrally acting drugs: may increase risk of adverse effects.
▨ Moderate inhibitors of CYP3A4 may significantly reduce lurasidone level.
▨ Strong inducers of CYP3A4 may significantly increase lurasidone level.
▨ Drug/lifestyle: Alcohol use may increase risk of adverse effects (cognitive impairment).

NOTE: For some drugs, off-label use is reported. It is the responsibility of the practitioner to evaluate the efficacy of such use.

Patient and Family Education

- Take drug on regular basis and do not skip doses.
- Periodic blood tests will be needed to monitor tolerance to the drug.
- Monitor weight and diet.
- Tell patient to avoid alcohol, warn against driving until effects of drug are known, and immediately report sudden change in body temperature, blood pressure, or irregular heartbeat.
- Monitor patients for tardive dyskinesia.
- Monitor for orthostatic hypotension.
- Monitor for signs of neuromalignant syndrome.
- Check complete blood count, renal function, and prolactin level periodically.
- Discontinue if severe neutropenia develops.
- Monitor for metabolic changes.
- Assess patients for risk of suicide ideation.

Special Populations

- *Pregnancy:* Category B; use cautiously in pregnant or breastfeeding women.
- *Elderly*
  - Patients with dementia-related psychosis are at increased risk for death.
  - Antipsychotics are not approved for treatment of dementia-related psychosis. Use the drug cautiously in patients with hyperlipidemia, diabetes, or risk for diabetes or seizures.
  - Use cautiously in patients with known CV disease, prexisting low WBC counts.
- *Pediatrics:* Latuda is not indicated for use in children.

MEMANTINE HYDROCHLORIDE (*NAMENDA, NAMENDA XR*)

Classification
N-methyl-D-aspartate (NMDA) receptor antagonist

Indications
This drug is used to treat moderate to severe Alzheimer's disease.

Available Forms
Immediate-release tablet, 5 and 10 mg; oral solution, 2 mg/mL; extended-release capsule, 7, 14, 21, and 28 mg

Dosage
▩ *Oral dosage: Immediate-release tablets or oral solution:* 5 mg PO once daily, titrate slowly to increase the dose by 5 mg/week over a 3-week period to achieve target dose of 10 mg PO BID at week 4.
▩ *Extended-release capsules:* 7 mg PO once daily; increase dose in increments at minimum intervals of 1 week up to the target dose of 28 mg once daily, making sure previous dose is well tolerated before advancing.

Administration
▩ The drug can be administered orally.
▩ Take the drug with or without food.
▩ Do not cut/divide/chew.
▩ The contents of the extended-release capsules can be sprinkled on applesauce.

Side Effects
Extreme tiredness, dizziness, confusion, headache, sleepiness, constipation, vomiting, pain anywhere in the body, especially the back, and coughing. *Serious side effects that may require medical attention:* Shortness of breath, hallucination, Stevens–Johnson syndrome, seizures, cataracts, conjunctivitis, cerebrovascular accident (CVA), heart failure, and suicidal ideation.

Drug Interactions
This medication may interact with dofetilide, procainamide, quinidine, acetazolamide, adefovir, alkalinizing agents, amantadine, antimuscarinics, bromocriptine, cimetidine, dextromethorphan, digoxin, entecavir, ketamine, lamivudine, levodopa, metformin, methazolamide, midodrine, morphine, pergolide, pramipexole, quinine, ropinirole, trimethoprim, trospium, vancomycin, amiloride, hydrochlorothiazide, nicotine, ranitidine, and triamterene.

Pharmacokinetics
▩ *Peak concentration:* Immediate-release—3 to 7 hours; extended-release—9 to 12 hours
▩ *Bioavailability:* 100%
▩ It can be detected in the cerebrospinal fluid 30 minutes after IV infusion.
▩ *Half-life:* Average 60 to 80 hours
▩ *Excretion:* Urine (74%)

NOTE: For some drugs, off-label use is reported. It is the responsibility of the practitioner to evaluate the efficacy of such use.

Precautions

▓ This drug should be used with caution in patients with severe hepatic disease and renal failure.

▓ Memantine has not been evaluated in patients with known seizure disorders. Patients who are taking memantine and have seizures or a history of seizure disorder should be monitored closely.

Patient and Family Education

▓ Do not divide, cut, or chew the capsules.

▓ Contents of the capsule may be sprinkled on applesauce.

▓ Store memantine at room temperature and away from excess heat and moisture.

▓ Throw away any medication that is outdated or no longer needed.

▓ Take the missed dose as soon as remembered. However, if it is almost time for the next dose, skip the missed dose and continue regular dosing schedule. Do not take a double dose to make up for a missed one.

Special Populations

▓ *Hepatic impairment:* In patients with mild to moderate hepatic impairment, no dose adjustments are needed; however, caution is advised when using this drug in patients with severe hepatic dysfunction.

▓ *Renal impairment:* In patients with CrCl 30 mL/min or greater, no adjustment is needed; if CrCl is 5–29 mL/min based on Cockcroft–Gault equation, a target dose of 5 mg PO twice daily of immediate release is recommended or a target dose of 14 mg/day of the extended-release capsule is recommended. Not recommended for patients with CrCl less than 5 mL/min.

METHADONE HCl (*METHADOSE ORAL CONCENTRATE*)

Classification
Partial opioid agonist

Indications
Detoxification treatment of opioid and maintenance treatment for opiate dependence.

Available Forms
Oral concentrate, 10 mg/1 mL dispersable tablets for oral suspension too.

Dosage
▦ *Short-term detoxification*: Titrated to a daily dose of 40 mg in divided doses.
▦ *Maintenance treatment*: 80 to 120 mg/day; single initial doses are 20 to 30 mg with 5 to 10 mg if needed not to exceed 40 mg on day 1.

Administration
▦ PO with a full glass of water.
▦ Dissolvable tablet must be dissolved in liquid prior to consumption.
▦ May be taken with or without food.
▦ *Missed dose*: Take as soon as remembered. Skip the missed dose if it is almost time for the next scheduled dose. Do not take extra medicine.

Side Effects
Dizziness, sedation; nausea, vomiting, sweating; bradycardia, palpitations; dysphoria, euphoria; respiratory depression, and pulmonary edema

Drug Interactions
Avoid CNS depressants, other agents that can cause constipation, and medications that can confound the QTc risk.

▦ May experience withdrawal symptoms when given opioid antagonists, mixed agonist/antagonists, and partial agonists.
▦ Antiretroviral agents result in increased clearance and decreased plasma levels.
▦ Rifampin may cause decrease in serum levels and possible withdrawal symptoms.
▦ Phenytoin may cause up to 50% decrease in serum levels, leading to withdrawal symptoms.
▦ St. John's wort, phenobarbital, and carbamazepine may result in withdrawal symptoms.

Pharmacokinetics
▦ *Half-life*: 8 to 59 hours

Precautions
▦ Death has been reported when methadone is abused in conjunction with BZDs.
▦ Caution should be used when giving drugs capable of inducing electrolyte disturbance that may prolong the QT interval.
▦ Should not be abruptly discontinued

NOTE: For some drugs, off-label use is reported. It is the responsibility of the practitioner to evaluate the efficacy of such use.

- Use with caution in hypothyroidism, Addison's disease, prostatic hypertrophy, and respiratory insufficiency.
- May result in hypotension in patients who have inability to maintain stable blood pressure.
- Use with extreme caution with head injuries.

Patient and Family Education

- Take exactly as prescribed. Do not take in larger or smaller amounts or for longer than recommended.
- Can be taken with or without food.
- Exercise caution when driving or operating machinery due to sedative effects of medication.
- Do not drink alcohol while taking methadone.
- Do not stop taking the drug abruptly.

Special Populations

- *Elderly*: Use with caution due to sedative effects.
- *Renal impairment*: Use with caution.
- *Hepatic impairment*: Use with caution.
- *Pregnancy:* Category C. There are no controlled studies of methadone use in pregnant women that can be used to establish safety.
- *Lactation:* Some drug is found in mother's breast milk: discontinue drug or bottle feed.
- *Children and adolescents*: Safety and efficacy have not been established.

METHADONE HCl (*METHADOSE ORAL CONCENTRATE, DOLOPHINE, METHADOSE*)

Classification
Partial opioid agonist

Indications
Methadone HCl can be used for detoxification treatment of opioid abuse and maintenance treatment for opiate dependence. Oral methadone can only be dispensed by certified treatment programs or during inpatient care for conditions other than concurrent opioid addiction.

Available Forms
Oral concentrate, 10 mg/1 mL; dispersible, tablets, 40 mg (maintenance); injection, 10 mg/mL; oral solution, 5 mg/mL, 10 mg/mL, 10 mg/mL (concentrate); tablet, 5 and 10 mg

Dosage
▪ *Short-term detoxification:* Titrated to a daily dose of 40 mg in divided doses.
▪ *Maintenance treatment:* 80 to 120 mg/day; initial dose should not exceed 30 mg. Maintenance dose 20 to 120 mg daily.

Administration
▪ PO with a full glass of water; oral form of the drug is half as potent as injected dose.
▪ *Parenteral:* IM injection is preferred. Use rotating sites. Subcutaneous injection may also be used.
▪ Oral form is legally required in maintenance programs. Completely dissolve the medication in 0.5 cup orange juice or powdered citrus drink.
▪ It may be taken with or without food.
▪ *Missed dose:* Take as soon as remembered. Skip the missed dose if it is almost time for the next scheduled dose. Do not take extra medicine.

Side Effects
Dizziness, sedation; nausea, vomiting, sweating; bradycardia, palpitations; dysphoria, euphoria; respiratory depression, pulmonary edema, seizures, arrhythmias, prolonged QT interval, cardiac arrest, heart failure hypomagnesemia, and respiratory arrest.

Drug Interactions
▪ Patients may experience withdrawal symptoms when given opioid antagonists, mixed agonist/antagonists, and partial agonists.
▪ Antiretroviral agents result in increased clearance and decreased plasma levels.
▪ Rifampin may cause a decrease in serum levels and possible withdrawal symptoms.
▪ Phenytoin may cause up to 50% decrease in serum levels, leading to withdrawal symptoms.
▪ St. John's wort, phenobarbital, and carbamazepine may result in withdrawal symptoms.

NOTE: For some drugs, off-label use is reported. It is the responsibility of the practitioner to evaluate the efficacy of such use.

Pharmacokinetics

■ *Half-life*: 8 to 59 hours
■ *Time to peak*: 1 to 7.5 hours. PO—90 to 120 minutes; parenteral—1 to 2 hours
■ *Excretion*: Urine

Precautions

■ Death has been reported when methadone is abused in conjunction with benzodiazepines.
■ Caution should be used when giving drugs capable of inducing electrolyte disturbance that may prolong the QT interval.
■ Methadone should not be abruptly discontinued.
■ Use with caution in hypothyroidism, Addison's disease, prostatic hypertrophy, and respiratory insufficiency.
■ It may result in hypotension in patients who have inability to maintain stable blood pressure.
■ Use the drug with extreme caution with head injuries.

Patient and Family Education

■ Take the drug exactly as prescribed. Do not take in larger or smaller amounts or for longer than recommended.
■ Methadone can be taken with or without food.
■ Exercise caution when driving or operating machinery due to sedative effects of medication.
■ Do not drink alcohol.
■ Do not stop taking the drug abruptly.

Special Populations

■ *Elderly:* Use with caution due to sedative effects.
■ *Renal impairment:* Use with caution.
■ *Hepatic impairment:* Use with caution.
■ *Pregnancy:* Category C; there are no controlled studies of methadone use in pregnant women that can be used to establish safety.
■ *Lactation:* Some drug is found in mother's breast milk; discontinue drug or opt for bottle feed.
■ *Children and adolescents:* Safety and efficacy have not been established.

NOTE: For some drugs, off-label use is reported. It is the responsibility of the practitioner to evaluate the efficacy of such use.

METHOCARBAMOL (*ROBAXIN*)

Classification
Central nervous system depressant with sedative and musculoskeletal relaxant properties

Indications
■ This drug is used to treat muscle spasms/pain.
■ It is used along with rest, physical therapy, and other treatment.

Available Forms
■ 500 and 750 mg tablets
■ Injection solution

Dosage
Oral
■ 500 mg: *Adults*: Initial dosage: three tablets QID
■ Maintenance dosage: Two tablets QID
■ 750 mg: *Adults*: Initial dosage: two tablets QID
■ Maintenance dosage: One tablet q4h or two tablets TID

IV/IM
Rate of injection should not exceed 3 mL/min, that is, one 10 mL vial in approximately 3 minutes.

Administration
Oral
■ The recommended dose is 6 g a day for the first 48 to 72 hours of treatment.
■ For severe conditions, 8 g a day may be administered.
■ Dosage can usually be reduced to approximately 4 g a day.

IM/IV
■ The injectable form is hypertonic, watch to prevent vascular extravasation.
■ If blood is aspirated into the syringe discard it, for it does not mix with the hypertonic solution.
■ The total dosage should not exceed 30 mL (three vials) a day for more than 3 consecutive days except in the treatment of tetanus.
■ Use caution in patients with seizure disorders.

Side Effects
■ Anaphylactic reaction, angioneurotic edema, fever, and headache
■ Bradycardia, flushing, hypotension, syncope, and thrombophlebitis
■ Dyspepsia, jaundice (including cholestatic jaundice), nausea, and vomiting
■ Leukopenia
■ Hypersensitivity reactions
■ Amnesia, confusion, diplopia, dizziness or lightheadedness, drowsiness, insomnia, mild muscular incoordination, nystagmus, sedation, seizures (including grand mal), and vertigo
■ Blurred vision, conjunctivitis, nasal congestion, metallic taste, pruritus, rash, and urticaria

NOTE: For some drugs, off-label use is reported. It is the responsibility of the practitioner to evaluate the efficacy of such use.

Serious Side Effects
These side effects need to be reported immediately:

- Fever, chills, flu symptoms
- Slow heart rate
- Feeling like you might pass out
- Seizure (convulsions) or
- Jaundice (yellowing of your skin or eyes)

Less Serious Side Effects
- Dizziness, spinning sensation, drowsiness
- Headache, confusion, memory problems, loss of balance, or coordination;
- Nausea, vomiting, upset stomach
- Flushing (warmth, redness, or tingly feeling)
- Blurred vision, double vision, eye redness
- Sleep problems (insomnia)
- Stuffy nose or
- Mild itching or rash

Drug Interactions
- Use this drug with caution in patients with myasthenia gravis receiving anticholinesterase agents.
- Using methocarbamol together with ethanol can increase nervous system side effects, such as dizziness, drowsiness, and difficulty concentrating.

Pharmacokinetics
- The plasma clearance of methocarbamol ranges between 0.20 and 0.80 L/h/kg, the mean plasma elimination half-life ranges between 1 and 2 hours, and the plasma protein binding ranges between 46% and 50%.
- Methocarbamol is metabolized via dealkylation and hydroxylation.
- Conjugation of methocarbamol also is likely.
- Essentially all methocarbamol metabolites are eliminated in the urine.
- Small amounts of unchanged methocarbamol also are excreted in the urine.

Precautions
- Long-term studies to evaluate the carcinogenic potential of methocarbamol have not been performed.
- No studies have been conducted to assess the effect of methocarbamol on mutagenesis or its potential to impair fertility.

Patient and Family Education
- Some people may also experience impairment in thinking and judgment.
- Avoid or limit the use of alcohol while on methocarbamol.
- Avoid activities requiring mental alertness, such as driving or operating hazardous machinery, until you know how the medication affects you.
- Inform provider about all other medications, including vitamins and herbs.
- Patient needs to be reminded not to stop using this medication without first talking to provider.

NOTE: For some drugs, off-label use is reported. It is the responsibility of the practitioner to evaluate the efficacy of such use.

Special Populations

■ *Elderly*
  ■ Elimination half-life of methocarbamol is prolonged.
  ■ Fraction of bound methocarbamol is decreased in the elderly.
  ■ Renal clearance of methocarbamol is reduced in those with impaired renal function

■ *Pregnancy Category C*
  ■ It is also not known whether the drug can cause fetal harm when administered to a pregnant woman or effect reproduction capacity.

■ *Nursing Mothers:* It is not known whether the drug is excreted in human milk, and hence it should be used with caution.

■ *Pediatric Use:* Safety and effectiveness in pediatric patients below the age of 16 years have not been established.

NOTE: For some drugs, off-label use is reported. It is the responsibility of the practitioner to evaluate the efficacy of such use.

METHYLPHENIDATE (*METHYLIN*, COMBINE WITH INFORMATION ABOUT PATCH FOR READIBILITY)

Classification
Methylphenidate (amphetamine derivative)

Indications
This drug is used primarily to treat narcolepsy and attention deficit hyperactivity disorder (ADHD).

Available Forms
Tablets, 2.5, 5, 10, and 20 mg; capsule, 10, 20, 30, 40, 50, and 60 mg; chewable, 2.5, 5, and 10 mg; oral solution, 5 mg/5 mL, 10 mg/10 mL; extended release, Metadate CD—10, 20, 30, 40, 50, and 60 mg; Ritalin LA—10, 20, 30, and 40 mg; Concerta: 18, 27, 36, and 54 mg; sustained release, Ritalin SR tablets—20 mg

Dosage
- ▥ 5 to 15 mg PO BID. Start with 10 mg; increase to the therapeutic needs and response of the patient. All stimulant preparations should be administered at the lowest effective dose.
- ▥ *Children older than 6 years:* 20 to 60 mg PO QAM; start, 20 mg PO QAM; increase 10 to 20 mg/day every week. Give divided doses at 4- to 6-hour intervals.

Administration
- ▥ PO chewable tablet only.
- ▥ Metadate CD or Ritalin LA may be swallowed whole or contents sprinkled onto small amount of cool applesauce and taken immediately.
- ▥ Give drug *after* meals to reduce appetite suppressant effects. Give last dose at least 6 hours before bedtime.

Side Effects
- ▥ Decreased appetite, dizziness
- ▥ Palpitations, stroke, myocardial infarction, sudden death in patients with structural cardiac defects, hypertension, arrhythmia, overstimulation, restlessness, seizures, infection, abnormal thinking, weight loss, somnolence, changes in libido, urticaria, dry mouth, irritability, insomnia, upper abdominal pain, nausea and/or vomiting, headaches, and anxiety
- ▥ Psychiatric events: increase in manic states for bipolar patients, aggression, tics, tremors
- ▥ Long-term growth suppression: patients should be monitored throughout treatment, if there appears to be growth suppression, the treatment should be discontinued.
- ▥ Rash, pyrexia, palpitations, tachycardia, elevated blood pressure (BP), sudden death, myocardial infarction, cardiomyopathy
- ▥ Stevens–Johnson syndrome, toxic epidermal necrolysis, impotence, and libido changes
- ▥ Thrombocytopenia, purpura, and leucopenia
- ▥ *Side effects that usually do not require medical attention*: Anxiety, insomnia, diarrhea, constipation, dizziness, nausea, nervousness, rhinitis, and dry mouth

NOTE: For some drugs, off-label use is reported. It is the responsibility of the practitioner to evaluate the efficacy of such use.

Contraindications

Advanced arteriosclerosis, symptomatic cardiovascular disease, moderate to severe hypertension, hyperthyroidism, glaucoma, history of drug abuse, agitated states, or within 14 days of monoamine oxidase inhibitors (MAOIs).

Drug Interactions

This drug may interact with urinary acidifying agents; the following medications: central nervous system (CNS) depressants (including alcohol); MAOIs; selective serotonin reputake inhibitors; adrenergic blockers; antihistamines; antihypertensives; CNS stimulants; veratrum alkaloids; ethosuximide; tricyclic antidepressants; meperidine; phenobarbital; phenytoin; warfarin chlorpromazine; Haldol; lithium; norepinephrine; propoxyphene, caffeine.

Pharmacokinetics

- Stimulant; blocks reuptake of NE and dopamine; stimulates CNS similar to amphetamines.
- The drug is absorbed by the gastrointestinal tract.
- The mode of therapeutic action in ADHD is not known. Amphetamines are thought to block the reuptake of norepinephrine and dopamine into the presynaptic neuron and increases the release of these monoamines into the extraneuronal space.
- Food prolongs time to maximum concentration by 2.5 hours.
- Peak plasma levels are reached in 6 to 8 hours.
- *Half-life:* Average is 12 hours (mean half-life average shortened by 1–2 hours in children).
- *Metabolism:* Liver, mainly excreted in the urine
- *Half-life:* 3 to 4 hours

Precautions

- See client as often as necessary to ensure drug is promoting positive cognitive and behavioral results.
- Advise the patient to report any new rashes immediately.
- Discontinue the drug immediately if any rash is reported.
- Advise patient of risk for transient psychotic-like symptoms (ideas of reference, paranoid delusions, and auditory hallucinations) and aggressive behaviors.
- Client may develop drug tolerance or dependence. Drug has high street value.
- Advanced arteriosclerosis, symptomatic cardiovascular disease, moderate to severe hypertension.
- Hyperthyroidism
- Known hypersensitivity or idiosyncratic reaction to sympathomimetic amines
- Glaucoma
- Agitated states
- Patients with a history of drug abuse: amphetamines have a high potential for abuse.
- Patients may experience transient palpitations and EKG changes.
- Avoid using in clients with left ventricular hypertrophy or mitral valve prolapse.
- During or within 14 days following the administration of MAOIs, hypertensive crisis may result.
- Use with caution in patients with preexisting psychosis.

NOTE: For some drugs, off-label use is reported. It is the responsibility of the practitioner to evaluate the efficacy of such use.

▦ Seizure history: Some studies have shown the potential for lowering the seizure threshold.

▦ There is potential for growth inhibition in pediatric clients.

▦ Advise patient not to suddenly discontinue medication, taper off.

Patient and Family Education

▦ Do not operate heavy machinery or equipment until reasonably certain that drug will not affect ability to engage in such activities.

▦ Discontinue medication immediately if rash is noted and follow up with provider.

▦ Store the drug at room temperature between 15°C and 30°C (59°F–86°F). Throw away any unused medication after the expiration date.

▦ The patient may experience palpitations.

▦ Have patient monitor BP at home and notify provider of persistent BP elevations.

▦ Discontinue or hold medication in presence of chest pain and do not restart until reassessed by provider.

▦ The patient may experience transient blurred vision.

▦ Keep it out of reach of children.

▦ Seek medical care for any signs of heart problems (chest pain, shortness of breath), fainting, psychotic symptoms, overdose, or any other concerns.

▦ Routinely assess weight and BP.

▦ Treatment should be initiated at low doses and then titrated over 2 to 4 weeks until an adequate response is achieved or unacceptable adverse effects occur.

▦ If one stimulant is not effective, another should be attempted before second-line medications are considered. Although some children benefit from daily stimulant therapy, weekend and summer "drug holidays" are suggested for children whose ADHD symptoms predominantly affect schoolwork, or to limit adverse effects (e.g., appetite suppression, abdominal pain, headache, insomnia, irritability, tics).

Special Populations

▦ *Elderly*: The elderly more sensitive to stimulants. Use lowest effective dose. Caution with polypharmacy and comorbid conditions.

▦ *Hepatic impairment:* Modify dose by one half accordingly.

▦ *Pregnancy:* Category C; based on animal data, they may cause fetal harm.

▦ *Lactation:* Excreted in breast milk; no human, possibly unsafe, studies have been performed. It is not recommended in breastfeeding mothers.

▦ *Children*: For use in children 12 years of age or older. The drug has not been studied in children younger than 6 years; should not be used in children younger than 3 years.

METHYLPHENIDATE TRANSDERMAL (METHYLPHENIDATE HYDROCHLORIDE, *CONCERTA, METADATE CD, METADATE ER, METHYLIN ER, RITALIN, RITALIN LA, RITALIN SR, DAYTRANA PATCH)*

Classification
Methylphenidate (amphetamine derivative), central nervous system (CNS) stimulant, piperidine derivative

Indications
The drug is indicated for the treatment of attention deficit hyperactivity disorder (ADHD) in children and adults.

Available Forms
Transdermal patch, 10, 15, 20, and 30 mg/9-hr patch.

Dosage
- Dosage should be individualized according to the therapeutic needs and response of the patient. All stimulant preparations should be administered at the lowest effective dosage.
- *Children Older Than 6 years:* One patch daily × 9 hours, off × 15 hours; start, 10 mg/9-hr patch daily, may increase to next-size patch every 7 days; maximum, 30 mg/9-hr patch daily.
- *Adults 18 to 65 years old:* One patch daily × 9 hours, off × 15 hours; start, 10 mg/9-hr patch daily, may increase to next-size patch every 7 days; maximum, 30 mg/9-hr patch daily.

Administration
Apply same titration when converting from oral; apply to hip 2 hours before desired effect; drug effects may persist 5 hours after patch removal; rotate sites; do not alter/cut patch. Hold patch in place for 30 seconds using palm of hand after which area is waterproof. If patch comes off another one may be applied but not to exceed total time of 9 hr/day.

Side Effects
- Decreased appetite, dizziness, dry mouth, irritability, insomnia, upper abdominal pain, nausea and/or vomiting, weight loss, headaches, and anxiety
- Psychiatric events: increase in manic states for bipolar patients, aggression, tics, and tremors
- Long-term growth suppression: patients should be monitored throughout treatment, if there appears to be growth suppression, the treatment should be discontinued
- Rash and pyrexia
- Palpitations, tachycardia, elevated blood pressure (BP), sudden death, myocardial infarction, and cardiomyopathy
- Stevens–Johnson syndrome and toxic epidermal necrolysis, impotence, libido changes, and skin irritation

NOTE: For some drugs, off-label use is reported. It is the responsibility of the practitioner to evaluate the efficacy of such use.

Drug Interactions

The drug may interact with urinary acidifying agents, monoamine oxidase inhibitors (MAOIs), adrenergic blockers, antihistamines, antihypertensives, veratrum alkaloids, ethosuximide, tricyclic antidepressants, meperidine, phenobarbital, phenytoin, chlorpromazine, Haldol, lithium, norepinephrine, and caffeine propoxyphene.

Pharmacokinetics

- The drug is absorbed by the gastrointestinal tract.
- Noncatecholamine sympathomimetic amines with CNS-stimulant activity
- The mode of therapeutic action in ADHD is not known. Thought to block the reuptake of norepinephrine and dopamine into the presynaptic neuron and increase the release of these monoamines into the extraneural space.
- *Metabolism:* Liver, mainly excreted in the urine
- *Peak plasma:* 7.5 to 10.5 hours
- *Onset:* 2 hours
- *Half-life:* 3.5 hours

Precautions

- Advanced arteriosclerosis, symptomatic cardiovascular disease, moderate to severe hypertension, arrhythmias, thrombocytopenia, leukopenia, respiratory cough
- Hyperthyroidism
- Known hypersensitivity or idiosyncratic reaction to sympathomimetic amines
- Glaucoma
- Agitated states
- Patients with a history of drug abuse have a high potential for abuse with this drug. Particular attention should be paid to the possibility of patients obtaining this class of medication for nontherapeutic use or distribution to others, and the drugs should be prescribed or dispensed sparingly.
- During or within 14 days following the administration of MAOIs, hypertensive crisis may result.
- Use with caution in patients with preexisting psychosis.
- Seizure history: Some studies have shown the potential for lowering the seizure threshold.

Patient and Family Education

- Store the drug at room temperature, protected from light.
- Keep it out of reach of children.
- Seek medical care for any signs of heart problems (chest pain, shortness of breath), fainting, psychotic symptoms, overdose, or any other concerns.
- Routinely assess weight and BP.
- Treatment should be initiated at low doses and then titrated over 2 to 4 weeks until an adequate response is achieved or unacceptable adverse effects occur.
- Dispose of properly, away from children or animals (remnant medication may persist on patch).
- If one stimulant is not effective, another stimulant should be attempted before second-line medications are considered. Although some children benefit from daily stimulant therapy, weekend and summer "drug holidays" are suggested for children whose ADHD symptoms predominantly affect schoolwork or to limit adverse effects (e.g., appetite suppression, abdominal pain, headache, insomnia, irritability, tics).

NOTE: For some drugs, off-label use is reported. It is the responsibility of the practitioner to evaluate the efficacy of such use.

Special Populations

■ *Elderly:* Caution with polypharmacy and comorbid conditions; has not been studied for use in this population.
■ *Pregnancy:* Category C; based on animal data, they may cause fetal harm.
■ *Lactation:* Possibly unsafe
■ *Children:* It has not been studied in children younger than 6 years; should not be used in children younger than 3 years.

MIDAZOLAM HYDROCHLORIDE *(VERSED)*

Classification
Benzodiazepine (BZD), anxiolytic

Indications
This drug is used for relaxation during hypnotic sessions, preoperative procedures, to reduce anxiety, and induce amnesia and somnolence.

Available Forms
Syrup (liquid), 2 mg/mL; injectable form, 1 and 5 mg/mL; preservative-free solution

Dosage
IM, IV, PO; schedule IV drug; requires a prescription with a maximum of five refills/6 months.

Procedural IV Dosing
- *Adults under 60 years:* 1 mg IV every 2 to 3 minutes with a maximum of 2.5 mg/ dose; cumulative doses over 5 mg are rarely needed.
- *Over 60 years:* Maximum dose is 1.5 mg total. Cumulative doses over 3.5 mg are rarely needed.
- *Children 6 months to 5 years:* 0.05 to 0.1 mg/kg × 1; repeat every 2 to 3 minutes as needed. Maximum 0.6 mg/kg total. Cumulative dose rarely over 6 mg.
- *Children 6 to 12 years:* 0.025 to 0.05 mg/kg × 1; repeat every 2 to 3 minutes before procedure; maximum dose 0.4 mg; cumulative dose rarely above 10 mg.
- *Children over 12 years:* 0.5 to 2 mg IV × 1; repeat every 2 to 3 minutes when needed. Cumulative dose above 10 mg is rarely needed. May be mixed in same syringe with morphine sulfate, meperidine, atropine or scopaolamine. When mixing infusion, use 5mg/ml vial and dilute to 0.5 mg/mL with D5W or normal saline.

Oral
- *Children above 6 years:* 0.25 to 0.5 mg/kg PO × 1 with a maximum of 20 mg. Give 20 to 30 minutes before procedure. *Children below 6 years:* may need up to 1 mg/kg/ dose.

IM
Note: Deep IM into large muscle
- *Children above 6 years:* 0.1 to 0.15 mg/kg IM × 1 with maximum of 0.5 mg/kg total; cumulative dosing over 10 mg is rarely needed. Give 15 to 30 minutes before procedure.
- Given by slow IV administration (more than 2 minutes) with careful attention to proper venous placement to avoid extravasation.

Side Effects
Nausea, vomiting, reduced heart rate, cough, and pain at injection site. Serious side effects include difficulty breathing, irregular heart rate, allergic reactions, respiratory depression and/or cardiac arrest, airway obstruction, oxygen desaturation, apnea, and sometimes death.

NOTE: For some drugs, off-label use is reported. It is the responsibility of the practitioner to evaluate the efficacy of such use.

Drug Interactions

■ Substrate of CYP3A4 (major). Avoid concomitant use with efavirenz, protease inhibitors, fluconazole, isoniazid, macrolide antibiotics, propofol, and certain statins. Avoid grapefruit juice with oral syrup.

■ The sedative effect of IV midazolam is accentuated by any other drugs that may depress the central nervous system (CNS), particularly narcotics such as morphine.

■ Caution is also advised when midazolam is administered concomitantly with drugs that are known to inhibit the P450 34A enzyme system, such as cimetidine (*Tagamet*), erythromycin, diltiazem (*Cardizem*), verapamil (*Calan/Isoptin/Verelan*), ketoconazole, and itraconazole (*Sporanox*).

■ Both cimetidine and ranitidine increased the mean steady-state concentration of blood level for midazolam.

■ Erythromycin doubled the half-life of midazolam.

■ No significant adverse interactions have been noted with commonly used premedications or drugs used during anesthesia, including atropine, scopolamine, diazepam, hydroxyzine, succinylcholine, or topical local anesthetics. Grapefruit juice may increase bioavailability of oral drug, St. John's wort may decrease drug level.

Pharmacokinetics

■ *Absorption:* Oral—rapid
■ *Peak:* PO—45 to 60 minutes, IM—15 to 60 minutes, IV—rapid
■ *Onset:* IM—15 minutes; IV—1 to 5 minutes; PO—30 to 60 minutes
■ *Duration:* Mean—2 hours; up to 6 hours
■ *Metabolism:* Hepatic via CYP3A4; 95% protein binding
■ Metabolized by the liver (CYP450: 3A4 substrate) and excreted in the urine (90%) and feces (2%)
■ Drug binds to BZD receptors and enhances gamma-aminobutyric acid effects.
■ *Half-life:* 2 to 6 hours; prolonged in cirrhosis, congestive heart failure, obesity, elderly

Precautions

■ There is a possibility for loss of consciousness.

■ It may cause severe respiratory depression or apnea; appropriate resuscitative equipment must be available.

■ Titrate dose cautiously.

■ Decrease dose by 30% if narcotics or other CNS depressants are given. Caution must be exercised in patients with compromised respiratory function or renal or hepatic impairment.

■ Use the drug only in hospital/ambulatory care setting with continuous respiratory and cardiac monitoring, appropriate ventilation/intubation equipment, and personnel trained/skilled in airway management.

■ One dedicated person other than practitioner performing the procedure should continuously monitor deeply sedated pediatric patients.

■ Reactions such as agitation, involuntary movements, hyperactivity, and combativeness have been reported in adult and pediatric patients.

■ Should such reactions occur, caution should be exercised before continuing administration.

NOTE: For some drugs, off-label use is reported. It is the responsibility of the practitioner to evaluate the efficacy of such use.

Patient and Family Education

■ Avoid use of alcohol or prescription or over-the-counter sedatives; driving; or tasks that require alertness for a minimum of 24 hours after administration.

■ There may be some loss of memory following administration.

■ Tell practitioner if the patient is pregnant or a nursing mother.

■ Midazolam is associated with a high incidence of partial or complete impairment of recall for the next several hours.

■ Do not mix alcohol or any other depressant drug and midazolam without the health care provider's knowledge.

■ Do not operate hazardous machinery or a motor vehicle until the effects of the drug have subsided or until 1 full day after anesthesia.

Special Populations

■ *Elderly*: Glaucoma, angle closure, chronic obstructive pulmonary disease, and congestive heart failure are contraindications to the sedative effects decreased for elderly or debilitated patients. Due to its sedative property and increased risk of falls, all BZDs are included on Beers List of Potentially Inappropriate Medications for Geriatrics.

■ *Pregnancy*: Pregnancy category D; has shown positive evidence of human fetal risk.

■ *Lactation*: No breastfeeding for 24 hours after administration. Safety unknown as there is inadequate literature to assess risk.

■ *Renal impairment*: The drug should be used with caution and renal function should be checked prior to beginning treatment with dose adjustment as necessary.

■ *Hepatic impairment*: The drug should be used with caution and liver function should be checked prior to beginning treatment with dose adjustment as necessary.

■ *Children*: Use caution in neonates, as rapid IV injection can cause severe hypotension and seizures.

NOTE: For some drugs, off-label use is reported. It is the responsibility of the practitioner to evaluate the efficacy of such use.

MIRTAZAPINE (*REMERON,* ALSO *REMERON SOLTAB*)

Classification
Noradrenergic and specific serotonergic antidepressant (NaSSA), antidepressant, tetra-cyclic antidepressant

Indications
Mirtazapine is used to treat depression.

Available Forms
Tablet, 7.5, 15, 30, and 45 mg; oral disintegrating tablets: 15, 30, 45 mg tablets

Dosage
- *Starting dose*: 5 to 15 mg nightly; titrate up to 15 to 45 mg/day
- *Adults:* 15 to 45 mg PO at bedtime; initial dose is usually 15 mg PO at bedtime.
- *Children:* Not indicated for children.

Administration
PO, with or without food, at bedtime

Side Effects
- *Serious:* Agranulocytosis
- Anticholinergic effects; blood dyscrasias: neutropenia and agranulocytosis; ortho-static hypotension or hypertension; somnolence and sedation, dizziness, tremor, confusion; increased risk for hyperlipidemia; dry mouth; significant appetite increase and weight gain (greater than 7% body mass); asthenia; decreased appe-tite, hypercholesteremia, constipation, hyperglyceridemia; influenza-like symp-toms; abnormal dreams, abnormal thinking; tremor; confusion; peripheral edema; myalgia; back pain; and urinary frequency.

Drug Interactions
- Serotonin agents (i.e., Linezolid)
- *Sedatives:* Effects may be exacerbated by use of other sedatives. Diazepam=avoid use altogether.
- *Monoamine oxidase inhibitors (MAOIs):* Risk for drug toxicity
- *Central nervous system stimulants* (e.g., amphetamines)
- Given PO; regular tablet is given with water.
- To take the disintegrating tablets (*RemeronolTab*), keep the tablet in its blister pack until ready to use. Open the package and peel the foil from the tablet blister. Do not push a tablet through the foil or it may break the tablet. Using dry hands, remove the tablet, place in mouth, and let it dissolve. Do not swallow the tablet whole. Do not chew it. Swallow several times and flush it away with water.

Pharmacokinetics
- The drug is metabolized extensively in the liver (CYP450 1A2, 2C9, 2D6, and 3A4) and excreted in the urine (85%) and feces (15%). Prolonged half-life of 20 to 40 hours, which is increased further in patients with hepatic or renal impairment.
- *Peak plasma*: 2 hours
- *Bioavailability*: 50%

NOTE: For some drugs, off-label use is reported. It is the responsibility of the practitioner to evaluate the efficacy of such use.

Precautions

■ Caution should be exercised if the patient has the following conditions: bipolar disorder, hypotension, cerebrovascular diagnosis, hypovolemia, seizure threshold disorder, dehydration.

■ *Anticholinergic drugs* (e.g., antihistamines): Increase effects

■ Use with caution in patients with hepatic impairment or renal impairment.

■ *Patients at risk for seizure disorders:* This drug may lower seizure threshold.

■ Monitor with complete blood count and history for signs of agranulocytosis or severe neutropenia.

■ Low incidence of sexual dysfunction.

■ Usually dosed at bedtime due to associated drowsiness (may be helpful in patients with insomnia or anxiety).

■ It may alter liver function.

■ Adverse effects and side effects are commonly observed before therapeutic effects.

Patient and Family Education

■ Take 60 to 90 minutes prior to bedtime, due to associated drowsiness. Do not drive until the effect of this medication is known.

■ It may cause stomach upset or blood pressure changes (particularly with getting up suddenly).

■ This medication may increase appetite or craving for carbohydrates. Monitoring diet and exercise is important.

■ It may take up to 4 to 8 weeks to show its maximum effect at this dose, but some may see symptoms of depression improving in as little as 2 weeks.

■ If the patient is planning on becoming pregnant or is pregnant, discuss the benefits versus the risks of using this medicine while pregnant.

■ As this medicine is excreted in the breast milk, nursing mothers should not breast-feed while taking this medicine without prior consultation with a psychiatric nurse practitioner or psychiatrist. Newborns may develop symptoms, including feeding or breathing difficulties, seizures, muscle stiffness, jitteriness, or constant crying.

■ Do not stop taking this medication unless the health care provider directs. Report side effects or worsening symptoms to the health care provider promptly.

■ Dosage should be adjusted to reach remission of symptoms and treatment should continue for at least 4 to 9 months following remission of symptoms.

■ Avoid discontinuing the drug without tapering the dosage.

■ Talk to the health care provider about any other medications in use. Mirtazapine is not Food and Drug Administration approved for use in the elderly because they may be more sensitive to the effects of the drug. Elderly patients should receive a lower starting dose.

■ Keep these medications out of the reach of children and pets.

Special Populations

■ *Elderly:* Older individuals tend to be more sensitive to medication side effects, such as hypotension and anticholinergic effects. They often require adjustment of medication doses for hepatic or renal dysfunction. Recommended to begin at lower dosage.

■ *Pregnancy:* Contraindicated in pregnancy

■ *Children:* Not recommended. Black box warning: Not approved for use in children

NOTE: For some drugs, off-label use is reported. It is the responsibility of the practitioner to evaluate the efficacy of such use.

- There is an increased risk of suicidality in children, adolescents, and young adults, especially during the first months of treatment. Mirtazapine is not approved by the FDA for use in children. Use only after consultation with psychiatric specialist.
- *Renal impairment:* Dosage has not been defined.
- *Hepatic impairment:* Dosage has not been defined.

MODAFINIL (*PROVIGIL*)

Classification
Stimulant, nonamphetamine

Indications
Used primarily to treat sleep disorders that result in excessive sleepiness such as narcolepsy, obstructive sleep apnea despite use of continuous positive airway pressure (CPAP), hypopnea syndrome, and shift work sleep disorder.

Available Forms
Tablet, 100 and 200 mg

Dosage
200 mg PO when prepared for long periods of wakefulness. Maximum dose is 400 to 800 mg; rarely more effective with dosing greater than 200 mg.

Administration
■ PO with a glass of water.
■ Take with or without food in the morning.

Side Effects
■ Hypertension; arrhythmia; cataplexy; dysmenorrhea; dyspnea; infection; abnormal thinking; weight loss

Important: Watch for Stevens Johnson syndrome rash—not approved for pediatrics for any reason because of this. Discontinue at first sign of rash.

■ *Side effects that usually do not require medical attention*: anxiety; back pain; diarrhea; dizziness; dyspepsia; headache; insomnia; nausea; nervousness; or rhinitis.

Drug Interactions
Modafinil may interact with the following medications: central nervous system (CNS) depressants (including alcohol); monoamine oxidase inhibitors (MAOIs); macrolides; phenytoin; estrogen, antifungals that use cytochrome P450 3A4 (CYP 3A4). Modafinil is an inducer of 3A4 itself, so interactions are harder to predict.

Pharmacokinetics
■ Stimulant, exact mechanism of action unknown. Believed to have similar wake-promoting actions as sympathomimetic agents.
■ Rapid absorption in absence of food
■ Peak plasma levels are reached in 2 to 4 hours
■ Steady state reached within 2 to 4 days of dosing
■ *Half-life*: Average is 15 hours once steady state is reached

Precautions
■ See client as often as necessary to ensure drug is promoting wakefulness, determine compliance and review side effects.

NOTE: For some drugs, off-label use is reported. It is the responsibility of the practitioner to evaluate the efficacy of such use.

- Advise patient to report any new rashes immediately.
- Discontinue drug immediately if any rash is reported.
- Advise patient of risk for transient psychosis-like symptoms (ideas of reference, paranoid delusions, and auditory hallucinations).
- May experience transient palpitations and electrocardiogram (EKG) changes.
- Avoid using in clients with left ventricular hypertrophy or mitral valve prolapse.

Patient and Family Education
- Avoid alcohol
- Do not operate heavy machinery or equipment until reasonably certain that drug will not affect ability to engage in such activities.
- Discontinue medication immediately if rash is noted and follow-up with provider.
- May experience palpitations
- Have patient monitor blood pressure (BP) at home and notify provider of persistent BP elevations.
- Store at room temperature between 20°C and 25°C (68°F–77°F).

Special Populations
- *Older adults*: more sensitive to stimulants. Use lowest effective dose.
- *Hepatic impairment*: modify dose by one-half accordingly.
- *Pregnancy*: Category C
- *Lactation*: no human studies have been performed. Not recommended in breast-feeding mothers.
- *Children*: not for use in pediatric patients.

Recurrence Rate
- Rate of relapse for those who have been in treatment is approximately 90%.
- Majority of relapses take place within 3 months following treatment.

Patient Education
- Educate on importance of joining a support group. Information available online for worldwide support groups, including NA, AA, and CA.
- Teach about relapse prevention. Encourage CBT to increase coping skills and individual therapy to enhance personal insight.
- Patients taking disulfiram (Antabuse) must be advised to avoid alcohol and any substances that contain alcohol. This includes mouthwash, colognes, and cough syrups; should also be sure in case of emergency to tell care providers that they are on this medication. Some medications may contain alcohol.

Medical/Legal Pitfalls
- Rates of suicide are three to four times more prevalent in people who abuse alcohol or drugs as compared to the general population.
- Individuals withdrawing from substances are at great risk for depression. When not properly treated, depression can lead to suicide.
- Individuals being treated for abuse may have a history of seeing multiple health care professionals and obtain medications ("doctor shopping"). Such practice may lead to accidental and/or intentional overdose.

NOTE: For some drugs, off-label use is reported. It is the responsibility of the practitioner to evaluate the efficacy of such use.

MODAFINIL (*PROVIGIL, ALERT-C*)

Classification
Stimulant, nonamphetamine, analeptic

Indications
Modafinil is used primarily to treat sleep disorders that result in excessive sleepiness such as narcolepsy, obstructive sleep apnea, hypopnea syndrome, multiple sclerosis (MS) related fatigue, and shift work sleep disorder.

Available Forms
Tablet, 100 and 200 mg

Dosage
200 mg PO when prepared for long periods of wakefulness. Maximum dose is 400 mg. Rarely more effective with dosing greater than 200 mg.

Administration
▦ PO with a glass of water
▦ Take the drug with or without food.

Side Effects
▦ Suicidal ideation, asthma, hypertension, arrhythmia, cataplexy, dysmenorrhea, dyspnea, infection, abnormal thinking, weight loss, urinary tract infection, hematuria, and pyuria
▦ *Side effects that usually do not require medical attention*: Anxiety, back pain, diarrhea, dizziness, dyspepsia, headache, insomnia, nausea, nervousness, rhinitis, and syncope.

Drug Interactions
Drug may interact with the following medications: antifungals, central nervous system (CNS) depressants (including alcohol), monoamine oxidase inhibitors, macrolides, phenytoin, estrogen, cyclosporine, selective serotonin reputake inhibitors, tricyclic antidepressants, CNS stimulants, theophylline, carbamazepine, diazepam, hormonal contraceptives, phenytoin, and warfarin.

Pharmacokinetics
▦ It is a stimulant, and the exact mechanism of action is unknown. It is believed to have similar wake-promoting actions as sympathomimetic agents.
▦ Rapid absorption in absence of food.
▦ Peak plasma levels are reached in 2 to 4 hours.
▦ Steady state reached within 2 to 4 days of dosing.
▦ *Excretion*: Urine (80%)
▦ *Half-life*: Average is 15 hours once steady state is reached.

Precautions
▦ See client as often as necessary to ensure drug is promoting wakefulness, determine compliance, and review side effects.
▦ Advise patient to report any new rashes immediately.

NOTE: For some drugs, off-label use is reported. It is the responsibility of the practitioner to evaluate the efficacy of such use.

▪ Discontinue drug immediately if any rash is reported.
▪ Advise patient of risk for transient psychotic symptoms (ideas of reference, paranoid delusions, and auditory hallucinations).
▪ The patient may experience transient palpitations and EKG changes.
▪ Avoid using in clients with left ventricular hypertrophy or mitral valve prolapse.

Patient and Family Education

▪ Do not operate heavy machinery or equipment until reasonably certain that drug will not affect ability to engage in such activities.
▪ Discontinue medication immediately if rash is noted and follow up with provider.
▪ The patient may experience palpitations.
▪ Have the patient monitor blood pressure (BP) at home and notify provider of persistent BP elevations.
▪ Store the drug at room tssemperature between 20°C and 25°C (68°F–77°F).

Special Populations

▪ *Elderly*: The elderly are more sensitive to stimulants. Use lowest effective dose.
▪ *Hepatic impairment*: Modify dose by one half accordingly.
▪ *Pregnancy*: Category C
▪ *Lactation*: No human studies have been performed. It is not recommended in breast-feeding mothers.
▪ *Children*: Not for use in pediatric patients under the age of 16 years for any reason.

NALOXONE HYDROCHLORIDE (*NARCAN*)

Classification
Opioid antagonist and antidote

Indications
Naloxone hydrochloride is used to counter the effects of opiate overdose, for example, heroin or morphine overdose. Naloxone is specifically used to counteract life-threatening depression of the central nervous system and respiratory system.

Available Forms
Injection, 0.4 mg, 1 mg/mL

Dosage
Adults:
It may be administered intravenously, intramuscularly, or subcutaneously.

- The most rapid onset of action is achieved by IV administration, which is recommended in emergency situations.
- IV infusion: Narcan (naloxone) may be diluted for IV infusion in normal saline or 5% dextrose solutions.
- An initial dose of 0.4 mg to 2 mg of Narcan (naloxone) may be administered intravenously.
- If the desired degree of counteraction and improvement in respiratory functions are not obtained, it may be repeated at 2- to 3-minute intervals.
- Intramuscular or subcutaneous administration may be necessary if the IV route is not available.
- For the partial reversal of opioid depression following the use of opioids during surgery, smaller doses of Narcan (naloxone) are usually sufficient.
- The dose of Narcan (naloxone) should be titrated according to the patient's response.
- For the initial reversal of respiratory depression, Narcan (naloxone) should be injected in increments of 0.1 to 0.2 mg intravenously at 2- to 3-minute intervals to the desired degree of reversal, that is, adequate ventilation and alertness without significant pain or discomfort. Larger than necessary dosing of Narcan (naloxone) may result in significant reversal of analgesia and increase in blood pressure.
- Similarly, too rapid reversal may induce nausea, vomiting, sweating, or circulatory stress.

Children:
Opioid Overdose—Known or Suspected
- The usual initial dose in children is 0.01 mg/kg body weight given IV If this dose does not result in the desired degree of clinical improvement, a subsequent dose of 0.1 mg/kg body weight may be administered. If an IV route of administration is not available, Narcan (naloxone) may be administered IM or SC in divided doses. If necessary, Narcan (naloxone) can be diluted with sterile water for injection.

Postoperative Opioid Depression
Follow the recommendations and cautions under Adult Postoperative Depression. For the initial reversal of respiratory depression, Narcan (naloxone) should be injected

in increments of 0.005 mg to 0.01 mg intravenously at 2- to 3-minute intervals to the desired degree of reversal.

Administration
SC, IM, or IV. *Adults:* 0.4 to 2 mg IV, IM, or SC. Repeat every 2 to 3 minutes as needed. If patient does not respond after 10 mg has been administered, question diagnosis of opoid-induced toxicity. *Neonates:* 0.01 mg/kg IV, IM or SC every 2 to 3 minutes as needed.

Side Effects
Common reactions include tachycardia, hypertension, hypotension, nausea, vomiting, tremor, withdrawal symptoms, diaphoresis, pulmonary edema, and irritability. Common side effects in children are seizures, ventricular fibrillation, ventricular tachycardia, and pulmonary edema (pediatric).

Drug Interactions
This medicine may also interact with:

■ Topiramate (may increase risk of CNS depression and psychomotor impairment).
■ Tramadol and tramadol/acetaminophen (may not reverse all symptoms of overdose, increase risk of seizures).
■ This drug blocks effects of all opioids, including opioid-containing cough suppressants and opioid analgesics.

Pharmacokinetics
■ The drug is metabolized in the liver and is excreted in the urine.
■ The drug antagonizes the various opioid receptors.
■ *Half-life:* 64 minutes (adults), 3 hours (neonates)
■ *Peak:* Parenteral—5 to 15 minutes

Precautions
Caution is advised in patients with cardiovascular disease, opioid addiction, hepatic impairment, or renal impairment, and in patients on cardiotoxic drugs.

Patient and Family Education
Stop using naloxone and call the doctor if chest pain, lightheadedness, seizure, or difficulty breathing develops.

Special Populations
■ *Renal impairment:* No adjustment is needed.
■ *Hepatic impairment:* Caution is advised in children with hepatic impairment; dosing not defined.
■ *Pregnancy:* Category B drug
■ *Lactation:* Safety in lactation is unknown. Caution is advised.
■ *Children:* Dose adjustment may be required in children with renal impairment. Caution is advised in children with hepatic impairment.

NOTE: For some drugs, off-label use is reported. It is the responsibility of the practitioner to evaluate the efficacy of such use.

NALTREXONE (*REVIA, VIVITROL*)

Classification
Opioid antagonist, opoid-cessation agent

Indications
Naltrxone is used primarily in the management of narcotic drug and alcohol dependence and opioid addictions.

Available Forms
Tablet, 50 mg; injection, 380 mg

Dosage
- If there is any question of occult opioid dependence, perform analoxone challenge test and do not initiate Revia (naltrexone) therapy until the naloxone challenge is negative.
- Treatment of alcoholism
- A dose of 50 mg once daily is recommended for most patients (see Special Populations).
- The placebo-controlled studies that demonstrated the efficacy of Revia (naltrexone) as an adjunctive treatment of alcoholism used a dose regimen of Revia (naltrexone) 50 mg once daily for up to 12 weeks.
- Other dose regimens or durations of therapy were not evaluated in these trials.

Treatment of Opioid Dependence
Initiate treatment with Revia (naltrexone) using the following guidelines:

- Treatment should not be attempted unless the patient has remained opioid free for at least 7 to 10 days.
- Self-reporting of abstinence from opioids in opioid addicts should be verified by analysis of the patient's urine for absence of opioids.
- The patient should not be manifesting withdrawal signs or reporting withdrawal symptoms.
- If there is any question of occult opioid dependence, perform a naloxone challenge test. If signs of opioid withdrawal are still observed following naloxone challenge, treatment with Revia (naltrexone) should not be attempted.
- The naloxone challenge can be repeated in 24 hours.
- Treatment should be initiated carefully, with an initial dose of 25 mg of Revia (naltrexone). If no withdrawal signs occur, the patient may be started on 50 mg a day thereafter.
- Subcutaneous and intramuscular injections can be given.

  Note: Individual patients, especially those with opioid dependence, may respond to lower doses of naloxone. In some cases, 0.1 mg IV naloxone has produced a diagnostic response.

Alternative Dosing Schedules
- Once the patient has been started on Revia (naltrexone), 50 mg every 24 hours will produce adequate clinical blockade of the actions of parenterally administered

---

NOTE: For some drugs, off-label use is reported. It is the responsibility of the practitioner to evaluate the efficacy of such use.

opioids (i.e., this dose will block the effects of a 25-mg IV heroin challenge). A flexible approach to a dosing regimen may need to be employed in cases of supervised administration.

■ Thus, patients may receive 50 mg of Revia (naltrexone) every weekday with a 100-mg dose on Saturday, 100 mg every other day, or 150 mg every third day.
■ The degree of blockade produced by (naltrexone) may be reduced by these extended dosing intervals.
■ There may be a higher risk of hepatocellular injury with single doses above 50 mg, and use of higher doses and extended dosing intervals should balance the possible risks against the probable benefits (see Special Populations).

Administration
■ Take with a full glass of water.
■ This drug may be taken with or without food unless stomach upset occurs.
■ Do not stop taking drug without provider's advice.
■ Do not take opioids while on this medicine.
■ *Missed dose:* Take the medication as soon as remembered. If it is almost time for the next dose, skip the missed dose and wait until next regularly scheduled dose. Do not take extra medicine to make up the missed dose.

Side Effects
Depression, nervousness, irritability, sedation/somnolence, suicidal attempt/ideation, skin rash, pharyngitis, hepatocellular injury, aches, pains, change in sex drive or performance, feeling anxious, dizzy, restlessness, fearful, headache, loss of appetite, nausea, runny nose, sinus problems, sneezing, stomach cramps, and trouble sleeping.

Drug Interactions
This medicine may also interact with the following medications:

■ Central nervous system depressants
■ Tramadol (*Rybix/Ryzolt/Ultram*) and tramadol/acetaminophen may not reverse all symptoms of overdose, increase risk of seizures, block effects of all opioids, including opioid-containing cough suppressants.
■ Carry an identity card or medical identity bracelet stating that you are taking medication.
■ Thioridazine may cause lethargy and somnolence with concurrent use.
■ Patients may not experience significant benefit from concurrent use of opioid-containing medicines, such as cold-and-cough preparations, antidiarrheal preparations, and opioid analgesics.

Pharmacokinetics
■ Opioid antagonists, such as naltrexone, are metabolized in the liver.
■ They are completely absorbed from the GI tract.
■ Elimination is primarily by glomerular filtration.
■ Naltrexone and its metabolites may undergo enterohepatic recirculation.
■ Elimination from the system takes 5 to 10 days. Initial peak is within 2 hours, followed by a second peak 2 to 3 days later.
■ Measurable levels can occur for more than 1 month after initial dosing.

NOTE: For some drugs, off-label use is reported. It is the responsibility of the practitioner to evaluate the efficacy of such use.

■ Exposure is three- to fourfold higher with IM administration compared to oral administration.

■ Pure opioid receptor antagonist

■ Subject to significant first-pass metabolism

■ *Half-life:* 4 hours; IM: 2 to 3 days

Precautions

■ Do not drive, operate machinery, or do anything that requires mental alertness until it is known how this drug exerts its effects.

■ Caution individuals not to stand or sit up quickly, as dizziness is a side effect of this medicine.

■ Check liver enzyme levels.

■ Do not initiate treatment until confirmed abstinence from opioids for 7 to 10 days.

■ Urine drug screen is often not sufficient proof that patient is opioid free; therefore, health care provider may choose to give naloxone challenge before beginning treatment and periodically thereafter.

■ Tell individual not to take any medicine that contains opioids during treatment, as this could cause serious injury, coma, or death.

■ Avoid pregnancy and nursing while taking this medicine.

■ Attempts by patient to overcome blocking effects by using large amounts of opiates may result in life-endangering opioid intoxication.

Patient and Family Education

■ *Missed dose:* Take the medication as soon as remembered. If it is almost time for the next dose, skip the missed dose and wait until next regularly scheduled dose. Do not take extra medicine to make up the missed dose.

■ Use caution when driving or operating machinery.

■ If stomach upset occurs, take with food.

■ Wear medical identification indicating naltrexone use.

■ This drug may increase sensitivity to lower doses of opioids; large doses of heroin or any other opiate may cause coma and death.

■ Do not take this medicine within 7 to 10 days of taking an opioid drug.

■ Exercise caution when driving or performing other tasks requiring mental alertness and coordination.

■ Stop taking the medicine if any of the following develops: allergic reaction, stomach pain lasting more than a few days, white bowel movements, dark urine, or yellowing of eyes.

■ Combine with psychotherapy or other counseling methods for full treatment effect.

■ Notify health care provider if there is shortness of breath, coughing, or wheezing, as naltrexone *(Vivitrol)* injections may cause allergic pneumonia.

■ Nausea may result after a naltrexone *(Vivitrol)* injection.

Special Populations

■ *Elderly:* Trials of subjects over 65 years of age did not include sufficient numbers to determine the safety and efficacy in the geriatric population.

■ *Hepatic impairment*: Use the drug with caution due to hepatotoxic effects. Caution is advised in children with hepatic impairment. It is contraindicated in acute hepatitis and hepatic failure.

NOTE: For some drugs, off-label use is reported. It is the responsibility of the practitioner to evaluate the efficacy of such use.

- ▦ *Renal impairment:* Caution advised.
- ▦ *Pregnancy:* Category C; the safety and efficacy of this medicine has not been established.
- ▦ *Lactation*: Nursing mothers should not take this medicine, as it has a potential for serious adverse effects in infants. The safety and efficacy of this medicine has not been established.
- ▦ *Children*: Safety and effectiveness has not been established in the pediatric population.

NICOTINE (*NICOTROL NS, NICOTROL INHALER, COMMIT, HABITROL, NICODERM, NICOTROL PROSTEP, NICORETTE GUM, NICORETTE DS*), VARENICLINE (*CHANTIX*)

Classification
Nicotinic receptor agonist

Indications
Nicotine is commonly used to treat tobacco nicotine dependence.

Available Forms
Gum, 2 and 4 mg; lozenges, 2 and 4 mg; spray, 0.5 mg; inhaler, 4 mg; transdermal patch, 7, 14, and 21; 5, 10, and 15; and 11 and 22 mg/day.

Dosage
▪ *Oral:* Chew and park one piece of gum when you feel the urge to smoke. Repeat as needed to up to 30 pieces/day.
▪ *Topical:* Apply one transdermal patch every 24 hours as follows:
  ▫ *Habitrol and Nicoderm:* 21 mg/day for 6 weeks, then 14 mg/day for 2 weeks, then 7 mg/day for 2 weeks. For patients with cardiovascular (CV) disease, who weigh less than 45 kg, or who smoke less than half a pack per day: 14 mg/day for 6 weeks, then 7 mg/day for 4 weeks.
  ▫ *Prostep:* 22 mg/day for 4 to 8 weeks, then 11 mg/day for 2 to 4 weeks. For patients with CV disease, who weigh less than 45 kg, or who smoke less than ½ pack per day: 11 mg/day for 4 to 8 weeks.
  ▫ *Nicotrol:* Wear patch for 16 hr/day; 15 mg/day for 4 to 12 weeks, then 10 mg/day for 2 to 4 weeks, then 5 mg/day for 2 to 4 weeks.

Administration
▪ Chew gum as directed.
▪ Remove old patch before applying new one.
▪ Apply patch to nonhairy skin surface.
▪ Patches are heat sensitive; store at or below 30°C.

Side Effects
Headaches, dizziness, lightheadedness; insomnia, irritability; tachycardia, palpitations; sore mouth, throat, tingling of tongue; skin rash, pruritus; runny nose, nasal irritation, and watery eyes.

Drug Interactions
Nicotine can cause increased serum concentrations of caffeine, clozapine, olanzapine., theophylline, insulin, propranolol, and acetaminophen. Coffee and cola may decrease absorption of gum.

Pharmacokinetics
▪ *Half-life:* 30 to 120 minutes (3 to 4 hours for transdermal)
▪ *Peak plasma:* Spray—4 to 15 minutes, gum—25 to 30 minutes, patch—2 to 10 hours.
▪ *Excretion:* Urine (30%)

NOTE: For some drugs, off-label use is reported. It is the responsibility of the practitioner to evaluate the efficacy of such use.

Precautions

Contraindicated immediately post myocardial infarction, severe angina pectoris, or in case of life-threatening arrhythmias.

Patient and Family Education

■ Chew gum and park for 30 minutes at a time to get full effect.
■ Chew only one piece of gum at a time.
■ Discontinue use of patch if local skin reaction occurs.
■ Smoking while using the patch increases adverse reactions.

Special Populations

■ *Elderly:* Use with caution; can cause unsavory reactions.
■ *Renal impairment:* No contraindications
■ *Hepatic impairment*: No contraindications known
■ *Pregnancy:* Category D (nasal spray, transdermal patch); category C (gum)
■ *Lactation:* Use only if benefits outweigh the risk associated.
■ *Children and adolescents*: Safety and efficacy not established; long-term effects in children/adolescents are unknown.

NORTRIPTYLINE HYDROCHLORIDE (*PAMELOR, AVENTYL*)

Classification
Tricyclic antidepressant (TCA)

Indications
The drug is used to treat adults with depression/anxiety and postherpetic neuralgia.

Available Forms
Capsule, 10, 25, 50, and 75 mg; oral solution, 10 mg/5 mL (480 mL)

Dosage
- *Adults:* Starting dose, 25 to 50 mg/day; maintenance PO dose, typically 50 to 200 mg/day if used for antidepressive effects. PO in three to four divided doses nightly and increase by 25 to 50 mg/day every 2 to 3 days.
- *Elderly:* Dose is 10 to 25 mg PO nightly and increase by 10 to 25 mg/day every 2 to 3 days; maximum, 150 mg/day. Once tolerated, may be given once per day in divided doses at bedtime. Must taper the dose gradually to discontinue.
- *Children:* Not indicated, black box warning for use under age 16 years.

Administration
- PO with a glass of water
- Do not abruptly stop taking the medication.
- Approved in children with enuresis and depression as young as 6 years.
- Use lowest effective dose for shortest duration.

Side Effects
- Similar to amitriptyline; cardiac arrhythmias, fatigue, sedation, and weight gain; sexual dysfunction.
- *More common:* Drowsiness, dizziness, constipation; nausea/vomiting, urinary retention or frequency, libido changes, weight gain, general nervousness, galactorrhea, gynecomastia, rash, seizures, and urticaria.
- *Less common:* Cardiac arrhythmias, cerebrovascular accident (CVA), heart block, myocardial infarction, agranulocytosis, thrombocytopenia, and hypoglycemia.
- Extrapyramidal symptoms, clotting disturbances, worsening depression, suicidiality, hyperthermia, and hypertension.

Drug Interactions
This medicine may interact with the following:
- *Monoamine oxidase inhibitors (MAOIs):* Risk for extreme hypertension
- Selective serotonin reuptake inhibitor: Risk with use of Clonidine.
- *Central nervous system (CNS) depressants* (e.g., alcohol): TCAs increase effects.
- *Direct-acting adrenergic agonists* (e.g., epinephrine): TCAs increase effects.
- *Anticholinergic drugs* (e.g., antihistamines): TCAs increase effects with the following medications.
- Absolute contraindications include class IA antiarrhythmics; MAOIs, such as phenelzine (*Nardil*), tranylcypromine (*Parnate*), isocarboxazid (*Marplan*), and selegiline (*Eldepryl*).

NOTE: For some drugs, off-label use is reported. It is the responsibility of the practitioner to evaluate the efficacy of such use.

▪ Avoid using with cimetadine, amiodarone, clarithromycin, erythromycin, haldo-peridol, St. John's wort, evening primrose oil, Sam-E.
▪ *Alert:* This list may not describe all possible interactions. Instruct patients to provide a list of all medicines, herbs, nonprescription drugs, or dietary supplements used, and whether they smoke, drink alcohol, or use illegal drugs.

Pharmacokinetics

▪ *Metabolism:* The drug is metabolized to an inactive form by CYP450; TCAs are thought to work by inhibiting reuptake of norepinephrine and serotonin in the CNS, which potentiates the neurotransmitters. They also have significant anticholinergic, antihistaminic, and alpha-adrenergic activity on the cardiac system. These classes of anstidepressants also possess class 1A antiarrhythmic activity, which can lead to depression of cardiac conduction potentially resulting in heart block or ventricular arrhythmias. Extensively metabolized by liver CYP 2D6 substrate.
▪ *Excretion:* Urine primarily, feces
▪ Peak plasma: 7 to 8 hours
▪ *Half-life:* Approximately 18 to 24 hours

Precautions

▪ See patients as often as necessary to ensure that the drug is working on the panic attacks, determine compliance, and review side effects, which are commonly observed before therapeutic effects.
▪ Many side effects are dose dependent and may improve over time.
▪ Overdose may result in lethal cardiotoxicity
▪ Monitor with routine EKG.
▪ Instruct patients and families to watch for worsening depression or thoughts of suicide. Also watch out for sudden or severe changes in feelings, such as feeling anxious, agitated, panicky, irritated, hostile, aggressive, impulsive, severely restless, overly excited, hyperactive, or not being able to sleep. If this happens, especially at the beginning of antidepressant treatment or after a change in dose, patient should call the health care provider.
▪ Drowsiness or dizziness: Patients should not drive or use machinery or do anything that needs mental alertness until the effects of this medicine are known.
▪ Caution patients not to stand or sit up quickly, especially if older. This reduces the risk of dizziness or fainting spells. Alcohol may interfere with the effect of this medicine. Avoid alcoholic drinks.
▪ Do not abruptly withdraw this drug as it may cause headache, nausea, and malaise.
▪ Advise to protect skin from ultraviolet light due to increased skin sensitivity.

Caution should be exercised in the following:

▪ Major depressive disorder (MDD), psychosis, or bipolar affective disorder
▪ Contraindicated in patients with a recent myocardial infarction
▪ Blood dyscrasias
▪ Respiratory disease
▪ Heart disease
▪ Liver disease
▪ Seizures (convulsions)
▪ Suicidal thoughts, plans, or attempts by patients or a family member
▪ An unusual or allergic reaction to imipramine, other medicines, foods, dyes, or preservatives

NOTE: For some drugs, off-label use is reported. It is the responsibility of the practitioner to evaluate the efficacy of such use.

Patient and Family Education

- Should be taken about the same time every day, with or without food. It may cause prolonged sedation. Do not drive until the effect of this medication is known.
- Administration time may be adjusted based on observed sedating or activating drug effects.
- It may take up to 4 to 8 weeks to show its effects, but patient may see symptoms of depression improving in as little as 2 weeks.
- If patient plans on becoming pregnant, discuss the benefits versus the risks of using this medicine while pregnant.
- As this medicine is excreted in the breast milk, nursing mothers should not breast-feed while taking this medicine without prior consultation with a psychiatric nurse practitioner or psychiatrist. Newborns may develop symptoms, including feeding or breathing difficulties, seizures, muscle stiffness, jitteriness, or constant crying.
- Do not stop taking this medication unless the health care provider directs. Report symptoms to the health care provider promptly.
- Drug should be tapered gradually when discontinued.
- Dosage should be adjusted to reach remission of symptoms and treatment should continue for at least 4 to 9 months following remission of symptoms.
- Keep these medications out of the reach of children and pets.
- Store nortriptyline at room temperature away from moisture and heat.
- Stopping this medication suddenly could result in unpleasant side effects.
- Take the missed dose as soon as remembered. If it is almost time for the next dose, skip the missed dose and take the medicine at the next regularly scheduled time. *Do not* take extra medicine to make up the missed dose.

Special Populations

- *Elderly:* Older individuals may be more sensitive to medication side effects, such as hypotension and anticholinergic effects. Often require adjustment of medication doses for hepatic or renal dysfunction. The smallest effective dose is necessary for patients with melancholia, liver impairment, and unipolar depression. However, cardiac side effects and fall risk are of great concern in this population. Side effects may be more pronounced and require decreased dosage.
- *Pregnancy:* Category D; not recommended in pregnancy. Some clinical reports of congenital malformations, but no direct causal link. Alternative medications are recommended.
- *Lactation:* Excreted in human breast milk, bottle feed if possible or use with caution.
- *Children:* Not recommended

NOTE: For some drugs, off-label use is reported. It is the responsibility of the practitioner to evaluate the efficacy of such use.

OLANZAPINE (*ZYPREXA*, *ZYPREXA ZYDIS*), OLANZAPINE PAMOATE (*ZYPREXA RELPREVV*)

Classification
Second-generation (atypical) antipsychotic; dibenzapine derivative

Indications
Olanzapine is used to treat schizophrenia, monotherapy, or combination therapy for acute mixed or manic episodes associated with bipolar I disorder, maintenance mono-therapy of bipolar I disorder, and agitation associated with schizophrenia or bipolar I disorder.

Available Forms
Tablet: 2.5, 5, 7.5, 10, 15, and 20 mg; orally disintegrating tablet (ODT): 5, 10, 15, and 20 mg. *Symbyax* (olanzapine/floxetine combinationolanzapine–fluoxetine combina-tion: capsule, 6 mg/25 mg, 6 mg/50 mg, 12 mg/25 mg, 12 mg/50 mg; injection: 10 mg, extended-release injection: 210 mg base vial, 300 mg base vial, 405 mg base vial, *Zyprexa*: Injection, 10 mg one vial; tablets, 10, 15, 20 mg tablets; *Zyprexa zydis*: 5, 10, 15, 20 mg tablets

Dosage
■ 5 to 10 mg/day, up to maximum 20 mg/day (PO oral or IM)
■ 6 to 12 mg/olanzapine/25 to 50 mg fluoxetine (olanzapine–fluoxetine combination)
■ Extended release injection: 150 to 300 mg; IM every 2 weeks or 405 mg IM every 4 weeks
■ *Children aged 13 years and older*: 2.2 to 5 mg PO once daily to maintenance dose of 10 mg/day

Administration
■ Injectable formulation may be more easily administered to patient with acute agi-tated, aggressive psychosis, and delusional disorder.
■ Tablets and combination capsules may be given with or without food.
■ Advise patient to take the missed dose as soon as he or she remembers. Skip the missed dose if it is almost time for the next scheduled dose. Do not take extra medi-cine to make up the missed dose.
■ Store at room temperature away from moisture, heat, and light.

Side Effects
The drug can increase risk for diabetes and dyslipidemia; dizziness, sedation; weight gain; dry mouth, constipation, dyspepsia; suicide attempt, leucopenia peripheral edema; joint pain, back pain, metabolic syndrome, chest pain, extremity pain, abnor-mal gait, ecchymosis; tachycardia; orthostatic hypotension (usually during initial dose titration); hyperglycemia; increased risk of death and cerebrovascular events in elderly with dementia-related psychosis; tardive dyskinesia (rare); rash on exposure to sunlight; neuroleptic malignant syndrome (rare); seizures.

Drug Interactions
■ It may increase effects of antihypertensive medications and drugs that affect the QTc.
■ It may antagonize levodopa and dopamine agonists.

NOTE: For some drugs, off-label use is reported. It is the responsibility of the practitioner to evaluate the efficacy of such use.

- Antihypertensives, carbamezapine, ciprofloxin, diazepam, and fluoxetine (even though combination formula Symbyax)
- Metoclopramide
- There may need to be a reduced dose if given with CYP450 1A2 inhibitors (e.g., fluvoxamine).
- There may also need to increase dose if given with CYP450 1A2 inducers (e.g., cigarette smoke, carbamazepine).
- *Alert:* This list may not describe all possible interactions. Instruct clients to provide a list of all the medicines, herbs, nonprescription drugs, or dietary supplements they use.

Pharmacokinetics
- *Metabolism:* Metabolites are inactive.
- *Metabolism:* Through direct glucoxidation and CYP450 oxidation
- *Peak:* 6 hours (PO), 15 to 45 minutes (IM)
- *Excretion:* Urine (57%), feces (30%)
- *Half-life:* 21 to 54 hours; 30 days for extended-release injection

Precautions
- Use with caution in patients with conditions that predispose to hypotension (dehydration, overheating). Watch closely for hypotension if given IM formulation.
- Use with caution in patients with prostatic hypertrophy, narrow angle-closure glaucoma, and paralytic ileus.
- Use with caution in patients who are at risk for aspiration pneumonia.
- IM formulation is not recommended to be given with parenteral benzodiazepines. If patients need a parenteral BZD, it should be given at least 1 hour after IM formulation olanzapine (*Zyprexa*).
- Ativan often administered concomitantly in acute psychotic episodes in crisis ERs or psychiatric hospitalization
- *Do not use if there is a proven allergy.*
- *Do not give IM formulation:*
    - If patient has unstable medical condition (e.g., acute myocardial infarction, unstable angina pectoris, severe hypotension, and/or bradycardia, sick sinus syndrome, recent heart surgery).
    - If patient has known risks of narrow angle-closure glaucoma.

Patient and Family Education
- Take exactly as prescribed by the provider. Do not take in larger or smaller amounts or for longer than recommended.
- It can be taken with or without food.
- For olanzapine orally disintegrating tablets, ODTs, keep the tablet in its blister pack until patient is ready to take it. Open the package and peel back the foil from the tablet blister. Do not push a tablet through the foil. Using dry hands, remove the tablet and place directly on the tongue; it will begin to dissolve right away. Do not swallow the tablet whole. Allow it to dissolve in the mouth without chewing. If desired, drink liquid to help swallow the dissolved tablet.
- *If you have diabetes*: Check blood sugar levels on a regular basis while taking olanzapine.

NOTE: For some drugs, off-label use is reported. It is the responsibility of the practitioner to evaluate the efficacy of such use.

▪ You can gain weight or have high cholesterol and triglycerides while taking this drug, especially if a teenager. Your blood will need to be tested often.

▪ Do not stop taking the drug suddenly without first talking to provider, even if you feel fine. You may have serious side effects if you stop taking the drug suddenly.

▪ Call provider if symptoms do not improve or get worse.

▪ Store at room temperature away from moisture, heat, and light.

Special Populations

▪ *Elderly:* Black box warning: in elderly, risk of cardiovascular or infection-related death. Not indicated for dementia-related psychosis.

  ▪ The elderly may tolerate lower doses better. Elderly with dementia-related psychosis treated with atypical antipsychotics are at higher risk of death and cerebrovascular events. It can increase incidence of stroke.

  ▪ If IM formulation is given, the recommended starting dose is 2.5 to 5 mg. A second injection of 2.5 to 5 mg may be given 2 hours after the first injection. No more than three injections should be administered within 24 hours.

▪ *Renal impairment:* No dose adjustment is required for oral formulation. Consider lower starting dose (5 mg) for IM formulation. It is not removed by hemodialysis.

▪ *Hepatic impairment:* Starting oral dose, 5 mg for patients with moderate to severe hepatic function impairment; increase dose with caution. Consider lower starting dose (5 mg) for IM formulation. Check patient liver function tests a few times a year.

▪ *Cardiac impairment:* Use with caution because of risk of orthostatic hypotension.

▪ *Pregnancy:* Category C; some animal studies show adverse effects. There are no controlled studies in humans. It should be used only when the potential benefits outweigh potential risks to the fetus. Olanzapine may be preferable to anticonvulsant mood stabilizers if treatment is required during pregnancy. Neonates exposed in third trimester at risk for extrapyramidal symptoms and withdrawal, severe feeding and breathing difficulty. Use only if benefits outweigh the risks.

▪ *Lactation:* It is not known if olanzapine is secreted in human breast milk. It is recommended to either discontinue drug or bottle feed.

▪ *Children and adolescents:*

  ▪ Probably safe and effective for behavioral disturbances in this population.

  ▪ Higher risk of suicide in young adults aged 18 to 24 during first 2 months of treatment

  ▪ Not for use under age 13 years

  ▪ IM formulation has not been studied in patients younger than 18 years, and is not recommended for use in this population.

  ▪ Should be monitored more frequently than adults

NOTE: For some drugs, off-label use is reported. It is the responsibility of the practitioner to evaluate the efficacy of such use.

OXAZEPAM (*SERAX*)

Classification
Benzodiazepine (BZD)

Indications
Oxazepam is used for the treatment of alcohol withdrawal, sedation during hypnosis, and to treat anxiety.

Available Forms
Capsule, 10, 15, and 30 mg

Dosage
- ▦ 30 to 60 mg/day in three to four divided doses
- ▦ *Adults:* Anxiety: 10 to 30 mg PO TID or QID
- ▦ *Elderly:* 10 to 15 mg PO TID or QID

Administration
- ▦ PO with a full glass of water
- ▦ Oxazepam may be taken with or without food.
- ▦ Write prescription for the shortest duration possible in order to prevent potential dependence.
- ▦ *Missed dose:* Take as soon as remembered. Skip the missed dose if it is almost time for the next scheduled dose. Do not take extra medicine.
- ▦ If discontinuing the drug, health care provider will gradually taper.
- ▦ Dose may need to be gradually decreased to avoid side effects such as seizures.
- ▦ When used for an extended period, this medication may not work as well and may require different dosing.
- ▦ Stop smoking while taking this drug as it may decrease the effectiveness of oxazepam.

Side Effects
The side effects are clumsiness or unsteadiness, confusion, unusual risk behaviors; hyperactivity; hallucinations; jaundice; lightheadedness, dizziness, drowsiness, and slurred speech; weakness; confusion; nervousness, hyperexcitability; hypersalivation, dry mouth; and hallucinations (rare).

Drug Interactions
- ▦ Increased central nervous system (CNS) depressive effects when taken with other CNS depressants.
- ▦ Precautions: Black box warning: Not used much due to high risk of hepatic failure.
- ▦ Use with caution in patients with pulmonary impairment/disease.
- ▦ History of substance abuse increases risk of dependency; use with caution in patients with history of substance abuse.
- ▦ Some patients present with disinhibiting behaviors after administration.
- ▦ Do not use with patients with narrow-angle glaucoma.
- ▦ Some depressed patients may experience worsening of suicidal thoughts.
- ▦ Oxazepam should not be used with sodium oxybate as it may increase the risk of CNS and respiratory depression.

NOTE: For some drugs, off-label use is reported. It is the responsibility of the practitioner to evaluate the efficacy of such use.

■ Probenecid may be used with great caution; may increase the risk of CNS depression (aripiprazole, dexmedetomidine, and propofol). It may increase oxazepam levels and risk of toxicity. The health care provider needs to be notified prior to taking drugs that cause drowsiness, such as antihistamines (diphenhydramine), anti seizure drugs (carbamazepine), medicine for sleep (sedatives), muscle relaxants, narcotic pain relievers (codeine), psychiatric medicines (phenothiazines such as chlorpromazine, or tricyclics such as amitriptyline), and/or tranquilizers.

Pharmacokinetics

The drug is metabolized in the liver (CYP450). Enhances the gamma-aminobutyric acid effects.

■ *Half-life:* 2.8 to 5.7 hours
■ *Excreton:* Urine
■ *Peak plasma:* 3 hours
■ *Precautions:* Monitor complete blood count and liver profiles. Serious reactions include leukopenia, hepatic impairment, and abuse.

Patient and Family Education

■ Take exactly as prescribed.
■ Tell the provider if treated for another psychiatric illness, such as depression.
■ Refrain from driving or operating dangerous machinery until the effect of this drug is known.
■ The drug can be taken with or without food.
■ Exercise caution when driving or operating machinery due to sedative effects of medication.
■ Do not drink alcohol for it can cause serious problems.
■ There is a potential for dependence on the drug, so extra care is given if increasing the dose or abruptly discontinuing it.
■ If pregnant during therapy or intend to become pregnant, communicate this information to the health care provider.
■ Avoid alcohol.
■ Do not abruptly stop taking this medication.

Special Populations

■ *Elderly:* Caution should be exercised and the initial dose should be the lowest possible due to the drowsiness effect. Initial dose of 30 mg in three divided doses: It can increase up to 60 mg/day in three to four doses if needed. Because of its sedative property and increased risk of falls, all BZDs are included on Beers List of Potentially Inappropriate Medications for Geriatrics.
■ *Renal impairment:* Use with caution. May increase drug levels.
■ *Hepatic impairment:* Use with caution. Due to its short half-life, it is a preferred BZD for those with liver disease.
■ *Pregnancy:* Category D; do not use unless benefits outweigh risks.
■ *Lactation:* Some caution advised with breastfeeding.
■ *Children:* Drug is found in mother's breast milk; discontinue drug or bottle-feed.
■ *Children and adolescents: Under 6 years:* Safety and efficacy has not been established. Long-term effects for children and adolescents unknown. Absolute dosage for pediatric patients 6 to 12 years of age has not been established.

NOTE: For some drugs, off-label use is reported. It is the responsibility of the practitioner to evaluate the efficacy of such use.

OXCARBAZEPINE (*CARBATROL*)

Classification
Anticonvulsant

Indications
- Partial seizures with complex symptomatology
- Generalized tonic-clonic seizures (grand mal)
- Mixed seizure patterns that include the above, or other partial or generalized seizures.
- Absence seizures (petit mal) do not appear to be controlled by carbamazepine.

Available Forms
- Extended-release capsule, 100, 200, 300 mg

Dosage
Adults and Children Above 12 Years of Age
Initial
- The dosage is 200 mg twice daily.
- Increase at weekly intervals by adding up to 200 mg/day until the optimal response is obtained.
- It should not exceed 1,000 mg per day in children 12 to 15 years of age, and 1,200 mg daily in patients above 15 years of age.
- Doses up to 1,600 mg daily have been used in adults.

Maintenance
Adjust dosage to the minimum effective level, usually 800 to 1,200 mg daily.

Children Below 12 Years of Age
- Children taking total daily dosages of immediate-release carbamazepine of 400 mg or greater may be converted to the same total daily dosage of carbamazepine extended-release, using a twice daily regimen.
- Optimal clinical response is achieved at daily doses below 35 mg/kg.
- If positive response has not been achieved, plasma levels should be measured to determine the therapeutic range.

Administration
- A low initial daily dosage with gradual increase is advised.
- As soon as adequate control is achieved, the dosage may be reduced very gradually to the minimum effective level.
- Capsules may be opened and the beads sprinkled over food.
- The drug should not be crushed or chewed.
- Carbatrol (carbamazepine extended-release) can be taken with or without meals.

Side Effects
Hemopoietic System
- Aplastic anemia, agranulocytosis, pancytopenia, bone marrow depression, thrombocytopenia, leukopenia, leukocytosis, eosinophilia, acute intermittent porphyria

NOTE: For some drugs, off-label use is reported. It is the responsibility of the practitioner to evaluate the efficacy of such use.

Skin
- Toxic epidermal necrolysis
- Stevens–Johnson syndrome
- Pruritic and erythematous rashes, urticaria, photosensitivity reactions, alterations in skin pigmentation, exfoliative dermatitis, erythema multiforme and nodosum, purpura, aggravation of disseminated lupus erythematosus, alopecia, and diaphoresis
- Hirsutism (rare)

Cardiovascular System
- Congestive heart failure, edema, aggravation of hypertension, hypotension, syncope and collapse, aggravation of coronary artery disease
- Arrhythmias and AV block
- Thrombophlebitis, thromboembolism
- Adenopathy or lymphadenopathy

Gastrointestinal System
- Abnormal liver function tests
- Cholestatic and hepatocellular jaundice, hepatitis

Respiratory System
- Dyspnea
- Pneumonitis
- Pneumonia

Genitourinary System
- Urinary frequency, acute urinary retention, oliguria with elevated blood pressure, azotemia, renal failure, and impotence
- Albuminuria, glycosuria, elevated blood urea nitrogen, and microscopic deposits in the urine have also been reported.

Nervous System
- Dizziness, drowsiness, disturbances of coordination, confusion, headache, fatigue, blurred vision, hallucinations, diplopia, nystagmus, speech disturbances, abnormal involuntary movements, peripheral neuritis and parenthesis, depression with agitation, talkativeness, tinnitus, and hyperacusis.

Digestive System
- Nausea, vomiting, gastric distress and abdominal pain, diarrhea, constipation, anorexia, and dryness of the mouth and pharynx, including glossitis and stomatitis

Eyes
- Lens opacities
- Conjunctivitis

Musculoskeletal System
- Aching joints and muscles
- Leg cramps

NOTE: For some drugs, off-label use is reported. It is the responsibility of the practitioner to evaluate the efficacy of such use.

Metabolism
- Fever and chills
- Inappropriate antidiuretic hormone secretion syndrome
- hyponatremia and confusion
- Decreased levels of plasma calcium have been reported

Other
- Elevated levels of cholesterol, high-density lipoprotein (HDL) cholesterol, and triglycerides

Drug Interactions
- This drug has many drug to drug interactions. Patients need to be educated on this fact and to always check with provider *before* taking any over-the-counter meds, including vitamins and herbal supplements.
- The following drugs have been shown to increase plasma levels of this drug: Acetazolamide, azole antifungals, cimetidine, clarithromycin(1), dalfopristin, danazol, delavirdine, diltiazem, erythromycin, fluoxetine, fluvoxamine, grapefruit juice, isoniazid, itraconazole, ketoconazole, loratadine, nefazodone, niacinamide, nicotinamide, protease inhibitors, propoxyphene, quinine, quinupristin, troleandomycin, valproate(1), verapamil, and zileuton
- The following drugs have been shown to decrease plasma levels of this drug: Cisplatin, doxorubicin HCl, felbamate, rifampin, phenobarbital, phenytoin, primidone, methsuximide, and theophylline

Pharmacokinetics
- Carbamazepine is metabolized in the liver.
- Half-life is also variable.
- Average half-life range is from 35 to 40 hours and 12 to 17 hours on repeated dosing.
- Oral clearance following a single dose was 25 ± 5 mL/min and following multiple dosing was 80 ± 30 mL/min.

Precautions
- Aplastic anemia and agranulocytosis
- Suicidal behavior and ideation

Patient and Family Education
- Signs and symptoms of hematologic problem, such as fever, sore throat, rash, ulcers in the mouth, easy bruising, petechial or purpuric hemorrhage.
- The patients are advised to report to provider immediately if any such signs or symptoms appear.
- The drug may increase the risk of suicidal thoughts and behavior
- Be alert for the emergence or worsening of symptoms of depression, any unusual changes in mood or behavior, or the emergence of suicidal thoughts, behavior, or thoughts about self-harm.
- Behaviors of concern should be reported immediately to providers.
- Dizziness and drowsiness may occur, caution about the hazards of operating machinery or automobiles.

NOTE: For some drugs, off-label use is reported. It is the responsibility of the practitioner to evaluate the efficacy of such use.

- It may interact with some drugs.
- Report the use of any other prescription or nonprescription medication or herbal products.

Special Populations

- *Elderly:* Unknown
- *Pregnancy:* Category D
- *Breastfeeding*
  - Transferred to breast milk and during lactation
  - Discontinue nursing or discontinue the drug
- *Pediatric*
  - It is effective in the management of children with epilepsy.
  - Therapeutic range (4 to 12 mcg/mL) is the same in children and adults for a 6-month treatment period.
  - No research on long-term use

PERPHENAZINE (*TRILAFON*)

Classification
Antipsychotic, phenothiazine class

Indications
Perphenazine is used to treat schizophrenia.

Available Forms
Tablets, 2, 4, 8, and 16 mg

Dosage
- In nonhospitalized patients: Adults and children older than 12 years—initially 4 to 8 mg PO TID, reduce the dosage as soon as possible to minimum effective dose.
- Schizophrenia in hospitalized patients: Adults and children older than age 12 years—initially, 8 to 16 mg PO BID, TID, or QID.
- Increase the dosage to 64 mg daily as needed.
- Severe nausea and vomiting: Adults—8 to 16 mg PO daily in divided doses up to 24 mg

Administration
- Store tablets in tight, light-resistant container.
- Obtain baseline blood pressures before starting therapy and monitor regularly. Watch for orthostatic hypotension.

Side Effects
- *Central nervous system*: seizures, neuromalignant syndrome, extrapyramidal symptoms, tardive dyskinesia, sedation, drowsiness
- *Cardiovascular*: orthostatic hypotension, tachycardia, EKG changes
- *EENT*: blurred vision, ocular changes, nasal congestion
- *Gastrointestinal*: dry mouth, constipation, nausea, vomiting, diarrhea
- *Genitourinary*: urinary retention, dark-colored urine, menstrual irregularities, inhibited ejaculation; hematologic: leukopenia, agranulocytosis, thrombocytopenia
- *Hepatic*: cholestatic jaundice
- *Metabolic*: weight gain
- *Skin*: mild photosensitivity reactions
- *Other*: gynecomastia

Drug Interactions
- Antacids may inhibit absorption or oral phenothiazines
- Separate doses by at least 2 hours.
- Atropine, phosphorus insecticides: it may increase anticholinergic effects.
- Barbiturates: It may decrease phenothiazine effect.
- CNS depressants may increase CNS depression.
- Fluoxetine, paroxetine, sertraline, and tricyclic antidepressants may increase phenothiazine level.
- Lithium: This drug may increase neurologic adverse effects.
- Drug–herb: St. John's wort: The drug my cause photosensitivity reactions. Drug–lifestyle: Alcohol use may increase CNS depression. Sun exposure may increase risk of photosensitivity reactions.

NOTE: For some drugs, off-label use is reported. It is the responsibility of the practitioner to evaluate the efficacy of such use.

Pharmacokinetics

■ Perphenazine may exert antipsychotic effects by blocking postsynaptic dopamine receptors in the brain.

■ Onset, peak, and duration unknown

Precautions

■ The drug is contraindicated in those with CNS depression, blood dyscrasia, bone marrow depression, and liver damage.

■ Use the drug cautiously in patients with alcohol withdrawal, psychotic depression, suicidal ideation, severe adverse reactions to other phenothiazines, renal impairment, CV disease, and respiratory disorders.

■ Neonates exposed to antipsychotics in the third semester of pregnancy are at risk of developing extrapyramidal symptoms and withdrawal signs and symptoms following delivery. Use the drug during pregnancy only if the benefit to the mother justifies the risk to the fetus.

■ Overdose signs and symptoms: The signs and symptoms of perphenazine overdose are stupor, coma seizures in children, tachycardia, prolonged QRS or QT interval, AV block, torsades de pointes, ventricular arrhythmia, hypotension, and cardiac arrest.

Patient and Family Education

■ Warn patients about activities that require alertness or coordination until effect of drug is known.

■ Advise patients to avoid alcohol while taking this medication.

■ Have patients report signs of urinary retention or constipation.

■ Tell patients to wear sun block and stay hydrated if exposed to sunlight.

■ Patients can relieve dry mouth with sugarless gum or hard candy. They should carry bottled water with them at all times and drink when thirsty.

Special Populations

■ *Elderly*: Elderly patients with dementia-related psychosis treated with conventional or atypical antipsychotics are at increased risk for death. Antipsychotics are not approved for treatment of dementia-related psychosis.

■ *Pregnancy*: Category C

■ *Pediatric*: Not for use in children under age 12 years.

NOTE: For some drugs, off-label use is reported. It is the responsibility of the practitioner to evaluate the efficacy of such use.

PHENOBARBITAL

Classification
Nonselective central nervous system (CNS) depressant

Indications
It is primarily used as a sedative hypnotic.

Available Forms
Oral Tablets
15, 30, and 100 mg

Oral Elixir
- It contains 20 mg of phenobarbital per teaspoon (5 mL).
- Preserve and dispense in tight, light-resistant containers.
- Store at controlled room temperature 15°C to 30°C (59°F–86°F).

Dosage
- Adult oral dosage:
  - Daytime sedative: 30 to 120 mg daily in two to three divided doses
  - Bedtime hypnotic: 100 to 320 mg
  - Anticonvulsant: 50 to 100 mg two to three times daily
- Pediatric oral dosage: 1 to 3 mg/kg

Administration
- Dosages of phenobarbital must be individualized with full knowledge of their particular characteristics and recommended rate of administration.
- Factors of consideration are the patient's age, weight, and condition.
- IV routes should be used only when oral administration is impossible or impractical.

Side Effects
- Restless muscle movements in your eyes, tongue, jaw, or neck
- Slow heartbeat, shallow breathing
- Feeling light-headed, fainting
- A fever or a sore throat
- Sores in your mouth
- Easy bruising or bleeding
- Broken blood vessels under your skin
- Drowsiness or dizziness
- Problems with memory or concentration
- Excitement, irritability, aggression, or confusion (especially in children

Drug Interactions
Note: Many reports exist of significant drug interactions. *Always use with caution.*

- *Anticoagulants:* It causes a decrease in anticoagulant activity as measured by the prothrombin time.
- *Corticosteroids:* Phenobarbital appears to enhance the metabolism of exogenous corticosteroids. Therapy may require dosage adjustments if phenobarbital is added to or withdrawn from their dosage regimen.

NOTE: For some drugs, off-label use is reported. It is the responsibility of the practitioner to evaluate the efficacy of such use.

▒ *Griseofulvin:* This drug interferes with the absorption of orally administered griseofulvin; here by, decreasing its blood level.

▒ *Doxycycline:* It shortens the half-life of doxycycline for as long as 2 weeks after barbiturate therapy is discontinued.

▒ *Phenytoin, sodium valproate, valproic acid:* Its effect is not predictable; phenytoin and phenobarbital blood levels should be monitored frequently if these drugs are given concurrently.

▒ *CNS depressants:* The concomitant use of other CNS depressants, including other sedatives or hypnotics, antihistamines, tranquilizers, or alcohol, may produce additive depressant effects.

▒ *Monoamine oxidase inhibitors (MAOIs):* MAOIs prolong the effects of phenobarbital probably because the metabolism of the phenobarbital is inhibited.

▒ *Estradiol, estrone, progesterone, and other steroidal hormones:* It may decrease the effect of estradiol by increasing its metabolism.

Pharmacokinetics

▒ Phenobarbital is absorbed orally, rectally, or through parenteral administration.

▒ The rate of absorption is increased if the sodium salt is ingested as a dilute solution or taken on an empty stomach.

▒ Duration of action, related to the rate at which phenobarbital is redistributed throughout the body, varies among persons and in the same person from time to time.

▒ Long-acting phenobarbital has onset of action of 1 hour or longer and duration of actions of 10 to 12 hours.

▒ Rapidly distributed to all tissues and fluids with high concentrations in the brain, liver, and kidneys.

▒ Lowest lipid solubility, lowest plasma binding, lowest brain protein binding, the longest delay in onset of activity, and the longest duration of action in the barbiturate class

▒ Half-life of 53 to 118 hours (mean: 79 hours); for children and newborns the plasma half-life is 60 to 180 hours (mean: 110 hours).

▒ Phenobarbital is metabolized primarily by the liver and excreted in the urine.

Precautions

▒ This drug may be habit forming.

▒ Tolerance and psychological and physical dependence may occur with continuing use.

▒ Use with caution, if at all, in patients who are mentally depressed, have suicidal tendencies, or a history of drug abuse.

▒ Elderly or debilitated patients may react to phenobarbital with marked excitement, depression, and confusion. In some persons, phenobarbital repeatedly produces excitement rather than depression.

▒ Use with caution in patients with hepatic damage.

▒ Phenobarbital should not be administered to patients showing the premonitory signs of hepatic coma.

Note: Periodic laboratory evaluation of complete blood count, Metabolic panels including liver and renal monitoring is essential.

Patient and Family Education
- Phenobarbital can make birth control pills less effective.
- Never stop using phenobarbital suddenly.
- Provider should be notified if patient wants to discontinue the medication.
- Increased seizures can occur if drug is suddenly stopped; the provider can decrease dose slowly to wean off drug.
- Be aware that memory has been affected. In some instances, short-term memory loss occurs.
- Phenobarbital may be habit forming.
- Medication should be kept in a secure place where others cannot get to it.

Special Populations
- *Elderly:* Use with caution in the elderly, as they may be more sensitive to its effects.
- *Pregnancy: Category D*
  - Reports of infants suffering from long-term phenobarbital exposure in utero included the acute withdrawal syndrome of seizures and hyperirritability from birth to a delayed onset of up to 14 days.
  - An association exists between exposure to barbiturates prenatally and an increased incidence of brain tumors.
- *Breastfeeding:* Small amounts of phenobarbital are excreted in the milk.
- *Pediatrics*
  - Phenobarbital should not be used in children younger than 12 years.
  - Safety and effectiveness in these children have not been confirmed.

NOTE: For some drugs, off-label use is reported. It is the responsibility of the practitioner to evaluate the efficacy of such use.

QUETIAPINE FUMARATE (*SEROQUEL, SEROQUEL XR*)

Classification
Atypical antipsychotic (second generation); dibenzothiazepine

Indications
Quetiapine fumarate is used to treat schizophrenia, depressive episodes associated with bipolar disorder, monotherapy or combination therapy for acute manic episodes associated with bipolar I disorder, major depressive disorder, adjunctive therapy, obsessive-compulsive disorder, and acute and maintenance treatment of schizophrenia.

Available Forms
▦ Tablet, 25, 50, 100, 200, 300, 400 mg; extended-release tablet, 50, 150, 200, 300, 400 mg
▦ Film coated; oral: quetiapine fumarate 25, 50, 100, 150, 200, 300, and 400 mg tablets
▦ Oral: quetiapine fumarate 25, 50, 100, 150, 200, 300, and 400 mg tablets

Dosage
▦ Dose is 400 to 800 mg/day in one (*Seroquel XR*) or two (*Seroquel*) doses for schizophrenia and bipolar mania.
▦ Dose is 300 mg once per day for bipolar depression.
▦ Dose for the initial 5 days of therapy is 50 mg (day 1), 100 mg (day 2), 200 mg (day 3), 300 mg (day 4), and 400 mg (day 5). After day 5, the dose should be adjusted within the recommended dose range of 400 to 600 mg/day based on response and tolerability.
▦ *Adults:* Initial dose is 25 mg twice daily, with increases in total daily dose of 25 to 50 mg divided into two or three doses on the second and third days, as tolerated, to a total dose range of 300 to 400 mg daily by the fourth day. It can be given at a maximum dose of 800 mg/day.
▦ *Elderly:* Initial dose is 25 mg/day. The dose should be increased daily in increments of 25 to 50 mg to an effective dose, depending on the clinical response and tolerability of the patient.

Administration
▦ Tablets may be given with or without food.
▦ Take this medicine with a full glass of water.
▦ Advise patient not to crush, chew, or break an extended-release tablet. Swallow the pill whole. Breaking the pill may cause too much of the drug to be released at one time.
   ▦ Advise patient to take the missed dose as soon as remembered. Skip the missed dose if it is almost time for the next scheduled dose. Do not take extra medicine to make up the missed dose.

NOTE: For some drugs, off-label use is reported. It is the responsibility of the practitioner to evaluate the efficacy of such use.

Side Effects

The drug can increase risk for diabetes and dyslipidemia; dizziness, sedation, palpitations; blurred vision; dry mouth, constipation, dyspepsia, abdominal pain, weight gain; tachycardia; hyperglycemia; increased risk of death and cerebrovascular events in elderly with dementia-related psychosis; palpitations; fatigue; asthenia; somnolence; dizziness; cough; orthostatic hypotension (usually during initial dose titration); neuroleptic malignant syndrome (rare); and seizures (rare leukopenia).

Drug Interactions

This medicine may interact with the following:

- Alcohol and other central nervous system depressants may increase CNS depression.
- It my increase hypotensive effects of antihypertensives.
- The drug may increase the clearance of hepatic enzyme inducers, such as phenytoin.
- It may also decrease total free thyroxine (T4); serum levels of quetiapine may be increased.
- However, no dose adjustment is required.
- *Alert:* This list may not describe all possible interactions. Instruct clients to provide a list of all the medicines, herbs, nonprescription drugs, or dietary supplements they use.
- It may increase serum cholesterol, triglycerides, aspartate aminotransferase, alanine transaminase, white blood cell count, and gamma-glutamyl transpeptidase (GGT) levels
- It may produce false-positive results.

Pharmacokinetics

- *Metabolism:* Metabolites are inactive. Blocks dopamine and serotonin 5-HT2 receptors.
- *Onset:* Unknown
- *Peak:* 1.5 hour; PO—1.5 hours, extended release—6 hours
- *Bioavailability:* 100%
- *Metabolism:* The drug is metabolized by the liver into the metabolite, *N* -desalkyl-quetiapine. The CYP enzymes responsible for the metabolism of quetiapine are CYP2D6 and CYP3A4.
- *Excretion:* It is primarily excreted in the urine (73%) and the remaining amount of the drug is excreted in the feces (27%).
- *Half-life:* 6 to 7 hours; 6 hours for PO, 7 to 12 hours for extended release

Precautions

- Use the drug with caution in patients who are at risk for aspiration pneumonia.
- It is not approved for children under age 10 years.
- It may increase suicidal ideation in children through those age 24 years of age.
- The manufacturer recommends examining for cataracts before and every 6 months after starting quetiapine.
- Use the drug with caution in patients with Alzheimer's dementia, history of breast cancer, cardiovascular disease, cerebrovascular disease, dehydration, hepatic impairment, seizures, and hypothyroidism.

NOTE: For some drugs, off-label use is reported. It is the responsibility of the practitioner to evaluate the efficacy of such use.

- *Do not use the drug if there is a proven allergy.*
- *Contraindications:* None known

Patient and Family Education
- Take as much drug exactly as prescribed by the provider. Do not take it in larger or smaller amounts or for longer than recommended.
- It can be taken with or without food.
- Quetiapine can cause side effects that may impair thinking or reactions. Be careful if you drive or do anything that requires you to be awake and alert.
- Quetiapine may cause high blood sugar (hyperglycemia). Talk to provider if any signs of hyperglycemia, such as increased thirst or urination, excessive hunger, or weakness. If diabetic, check blood sugar levels on a regular basis.
- Drink fluids often, especially during physical activity.
- Avoid becoming overheated or dehydrated during exercise and in hot weather. You may be more prone to heat stroke.
- Avoid getting up too fast from a sitting or lying position. Get up slowly and steady yourself to prevent a fall.
- *Avoid alcohol intake.*
- *Stop using this medication and call provider immediately* if you have very stiff (rigid) muscles, high fever, sweating, confusion, fast or uneven heartbeats, tremors; feel like you might pass out; have jerky muscle movements you cannot control, trouble swallowing, problems with speech; have blurred vision, eye pain, or see halos around lights; have increased thirst and urination, excessive hunger, fruity breath odor, weakness, nausea and vomiting; have fever, chills, body aches, flu symptoms; or have white patches or sores inside your mouth or on your lips.
- Do as ordered; do not stop taking the drug suddenly without first talking to the health care provider, even if you feel fine. You may have serious side effects if you stop taking the drug suddenly.
- Call provider if symptoms do not improve or get worse.
- Store at room temperature away from moisture and heat.
- Avoid tasks that require alertness and motor skills until response to drug is established.

Special Populations
Black box warning for elderly patients with dementia due to increased risk of death.

- *Elderly:* Generally lower dose is used (e.g., 25–100 mg twice a day) in the elderly. Higher dose can be used if it can tolerated. Elderly with dementia-related psychosis treated with atypical antipsychotics are at higher risk of death and cerebrovascular events.
- *Renal impairment:* No dose adjustment is required.
- *Hepatic impairment:* Dose may need to be reduced.
- *Cardiac impairment:* Use with caution because of risk of orthostatic hypotension.
- *Pregnancy:* Category C; some animal studies show adverse effects. There are no controlled studies in humans. It should be used only when the potential benefits outweigh potential risks to the fetus. Quetiapine may be preferable to anticonvulsant mood stabilizers if treatment is required during pregnancy.
- *Lactation: Not recommended.* It is not unknown whether the drug is secreted in human breast milk. It is recommended to either discontinue drug or bottle-feed.

NOTE: For some drugs, off-label use is reported. It is the responsibility of the practitioner to evaluate the efficacy of such use.

Infants of women who choose to breastfeed while on this drug should be monitored for possible adverse effects.

▦ *Children and adolescents:* Not for use in children younger than 13 years of age.

▦ Should be monitored more frequently than adults. May tolerate lower doses better.

▦ Watch for activation of suicidal ideation. Inform parents or guardian of this risk so they can help monitor the risk. There is an increased risk of suicidal thinking and behavior in children and adolescents with major depressive disorder and other psychiatric disorders.

NOTE: For some drugs, off-label use is reported. It is the responsibility of the practitioner to evaluate the efficacy of such use.

RISPERIDONE (*RISPERDAL, RISPERDAL M-TAB, RISPERDAL CONSTA*)

Classification
Atypical antipsychotic (second generation); benzisoxazole derivative

Indications
This drug is used for the treatment of schizophrenia (age 13 and older), monotherapy, or combination therapy for acute, mixed, or manic episodes associated with bipolar I disorder (age 10 and older), Tourette syndrome, obsessive compulsive disorder (OCD), and treatment of irritability associated with autistic disorder in children and adolescents aged 5 to 16 years.

Available Forms
Tablet, 0.25, 0.5, 1, 2, 3, 4 mg; orally disintegrating tablet, 0.25, 0.5, 1, 2, 3, 4 mg; liquid, 1 mg/mL (30-mL bottle); long-acting depot microspheres formulation for deep intramuscular (IM) formulation, 12.5, 25 mg vial/kit, 37.5 mg vial/kit, 50 mg vial/kit.

Dosage
Schizophrenia
- *Adults:* Drug may be given once or twice daily. Initial dosing is generally 2 mg/day. Increase dosage at intervals not less than 24 hours, in increments of 1 to 2 mg/day, as tolerated, to a recommended dose of 4 to 8 mg/day PO for adults with acute psychosis. Periodically and bipolar disorder. Maximum daily dose = 16 mg.
- Dose is 0.5 to 2.0 mg/day PO for children and elderly.
- Dose is 25 to 50 mg IM; reassess every 2 weeks to determine the need for maintenance treatment.
- *Adolescents aged 13 to 17:* Start treatment with 0.5 mg once daily, given as a single daily dose in either morning or evening. Adjust dose, if indicated, at intervals not less than 24 hours, in increments of 0.5 or 1 mg/day, as tolerated, to a recommended dose of 3 mg/day. There are no data to support use beyond 8 weeks.

Irritability, Including Aggression, Self-Injury, and Temper Tantrums Associated With an Autistic Disorder
- *Adolescents and children aged 5 and older who weigh 20 kg (44 lb) or more:* Initially, 0.5 mg PO once daily or divided BID; after 4 days, increase dose to 1 mg. Increase dosage further in 0.5-mg increments at intervals of at least 2 weeks.
- *Children aged 5 and older who weigh less than 20 kg:* Initially, 0.25 mg PO once daily or divided BID. After 4 days, increase dose to 0.5 mg. Increase dosage further in 0.25-mg increments at intervals of at least 2 weeks. Increase the dosage cautiously in children who weigh less than 15 kg (33 lb).

Administration
- Give drug PO with food. Place M-Tab directly on tongue.
- Advise patient to take the missed dose as soon as remembered. Skip the missed dose if almost time for the next scheduled dose.
- Open package by peeling off foil backing with dry hands.
- Measure the liquid form of risperidone with a special dose-measuring spoon or cup, not a regular tablespoon.
- Do not mix the liquid form with cola or tea.

NOTE: For some drugs, off-label use is reported. It is the responsibility of the practitioner to evaluate the efficacy of such use.

▒ Phenylalanine contents of orally disintegrating tablets are as follows: 0.5-mg tablet contains 0.14 mg phenylalanine; 1-mg tablet contains 0.28 mg phenylalanine; 2-mg tablet contains 0.56 mg phenylalanine; 3-mg tablet contains 0.63 mg phenylalanine; 4-mg tablet contains 0.84 mg phenylalanine.

Intramuscular
▒ Continue oral therapy for the first 3 weeks of IM injection therapy until injections take effect, then stop oral therapy.
▒ To reconstitute IM injection, inject premeasured diluent into vial and shake vigorously for at least 10 seconds. Suspension appears uniform, thick, and milky; particles are visible, but no dry particles remain. Use drug immediately or refrigerate for up to 6 hours after reconstitution. If more than 2-minutes pass before injection, shake vigorously again. See manufacturer's package insert for more detailed instructions.
▒ Refrigerate IM injection kit and protect it from light. Drug can be stored at temperature less than 77°F (25°C) for no more than 7 days before administration.

Side Effects
This drug can increase risk for diabetes and dyslipidemia, extrapyramidal symptoms (dose dependent), hyperprolactinemia (dose dependent), dizziness. These side effects can occur at low doses with pseudolactation occurring.

▒ Akathisia, somnolence, dystonia, headache, insomnia, headache, agitation, anxiety; nausea, sedation, weight gain, constipation, abdominal pain; tachycardia; sedation; sexual, parkinsonism dysfunction; hyperglycemia; increased risk of death and cerebrovascular events in elderly with dementia-related psychosis; tardive dyskinesia; suicide attempt, dizziness, fever, hallucination, mania, impaired concentration, abnormal thinking and dreaming, tremor, hypoesthesia, fatigue, depression, nervousness, neuromalignant syndrome, and suicide attempt.
▒ Tachycardia, chest pain, orthostatic hypotension (rare, usually during initial dose, titration); neuroleptic malignant syndrome seizures (rare); peripheral edema, syncope, and hypertension
▒ Rhinitis, sinusitis, pharyngitis, and ear disorder
▒ Constipation, nausea, vomiting, dyspepsia, abdominal pain, anorexia, dry mouth, increased saliva, and diarrhea
▒ Urinary incontinence, increased urination, abnormal orgasm, vaginal dryness, weight gain, hyperglycemia, and weight loss
▒ Arthralgia, back pain, leg pain, and myalgia
▒ Coughing, dyspnea, and upper respiratory infection
▒ Rash, dry skin, photosensitivity reactions, acne, and injection site pain
▒ Injury and decreased libido

Drug Interactions
▒ It may increase effects of antihypertensive medications.
▒ It may antagonize levodopa and dopamine agonists.
▒ Plasma levels of risperidone may be reduced if given in conjunction with antihypertensives and carbamazepine.
▒ Plasma levels of risperidone may be increased if given in conjunction with central nervous system (CNS) depressants, dopamine agonists, levodopa, fluoxetine, or paroxetine.

NOTE: For some drugs, off-label use is reported. It is the responsibility of the practitioner to evaluate the efficacy of such use.

- ▓ Plasma levels of risperidone may be increased if given in conjunction with clozapine, but no dose adjustment is required. Avoid using together as may increase toxicity of these drugs.
- ▓ Methadone: This drug may decrease methadone levels.
- ▓ Theophylline: This drug may decrease theophylline levels.
- ▓ Trazodone: This drug may increase trazodone level.
- ▓ Rifampin, rifabentine may decrease ritonavir levels.
- ▓ St. John's wort may substantially reduce drug levels. Using the two together is contraindicated.
- ▓ Oral contraceptives: It may reduce effectiveness of contraceptive.
- ▓ *Alert:* This list may not describe all possible interactions. Instruct clients to provide a list of all the medicines, herbs, nonprescription drugs, or dietary supplements they use.

Pharmacokinetics

- ▓ *Elimination*: 7 to 8 weeks after last injection (long-acting formulation)
- ▓ *Metabolism:* Metabolites are active; the drug is metabolized by CYP450 2D6. Blocks dopamine and 5-HT two receptors in the brain.
- ▓ *Half-life*: 3–24 hours (oral formulation); 3 to 6 days (long-acting formulation)
- ▓ *Peak action*: 2 hours
- ▓ *Excretion:* Urine (70%), feces (14%)
- ▓ *Duration of effect:* Unknown.

Precautions

- ▓ Use with caution in patients with conditions that predispose to hypotension (dehydration, overheating).
- ▓ It may increase prolactin level.
- ▓ It may decrease hemoglobin level and hematocrit.
- ▓ Sun exposure may increase risk of photosensitivity reactions.
- ▓ It is contraindicated in patients hypersensitive to drug and in breastfeeding women.
- ▓ Use cautiously in patients with prolonged QT interval, cerebrovascular disease, dehydration, hypovolemia, history of seizures, or conditions that could affect metabolism or hemodynamic responses.
- ▓ Use cautiously in patients exposed to extreme heat.
- ▓ Use cautiously in patients at risk for aspiration pneumonia.
- ▓ Priapism has been reported.
- ▓ *Do not use if there is a proven allergy.*
- ▓ Use IM injection cautiously in those with hepatic or renal impairment.
- ▓ *Alert*: Obtain baseline blood pressure (BP) measurements before starting therapy, and monitor pressure regularly. Watch for orthostatic hypotension, especially during first-dose adjustment.
- ▓ *Alert:* Fatal cerebrovascular adverse events (stroke, transient ischemic attacks) may occur in elderly patients with dementia. Drug is not safe or effective in these patients.
- ▓ Monitor patient for tardive dyskinesia, which may occur after prolonged use. It may not appear until months or years later and may disappear spontaneously or persist for life, despite stopping drug.

NOTE: For some drugs, off-label use is reported. It is the responsibility of the practitioner to evaluate the efficacy of such use.

▧ Life-threatening hyperglycemia may occur in patients taking atypical antipsychotics. Monitor patients with diabetes regularly.

▧ Monitor patient for weight gain.

▧ Periodically reevaluate drug's risks and benefits, especially during prolonged use.

▧ *Alert:* Watch for evidence of neuroleptic malignant syndrome (NMS) (extrapyramidal effects, hyperthermia, autonomic disturbance), which is rare but can be fatal.

▧ *Alert:* Monitor patient for symptoms of metabolic syndrome (significant weight gain and increased body mass index, hypertension, hyperglycemia, hypercholesterolemia, and hypertriglyceridemia).

Patient and Family Education

▧ Take exactly as prescribed by the provider. Do not take in larger or smaller amounts or for longer than recommended.

▧ It can be taken with food.

▧ You may be more sensitive to temperature extremes (very hot or cold conditions) when taking this medication. Avoid getting too cold, or becoming overheated or dehydrated.

▧ Drink plenty of fluids, especially in hot weather and during exercise.

▧ Risperidone can cause side effects that may impair thinking or reactions. Be careful if you drive or do anything that requires you to be awake and alert.

▧ Risperidone may cause high blood sugar (hyperglycemia). Talk to your provider if any signs of hyperglycemia, such as increased thirst or urination, excessive hunger, or weakness occur. If diabetic, check blood sugar levels on a regular basis.

▧ The risperidone orally disintegrating tablet may contain phenylalanine. Talk to your provider before using this form of risperidone if you have PKU.

▧ *Avoid drinking alcohol.* It can increase some of the side effects.

▧ Do *not* mix the liquid form with cola or tea.

▧ *Stop using this medication and call provider immediately* if you have fever, stiff muscles, confusion, sweating, fast or uneven heartbeats, restless muscle movements in face or neck, tremor (uncontrolled shaking), trouble swallowing, feeling light-headed, or fainting.

▧ Do not stop taking the drug suddenly without first talking to provider, even if you feel fine. You may have serious side effects if you stop taking the drug suddenly.

▧ Call provider if symptoms do not improve or get worse.

▧ Store the drug at room temperature away from moisture, light, and heat. Do not freeze the liquid form of risperidone.

▧ Warn patient to avoid activities that require alertness until effects of drug are known.

▧ Warn patient to rise slowly, avoid hot showers, and use other precautions to avoid fainting when starting therapy.

▧ Advise patient to use caution in hot weather to prevent heatstroke.

▧ Tell patient to take drug with food.

▧ Instruct patient to keep the ODT in the blister pack until just before taking it. Use dry hands to peel a part of the foil to expose the tablet; do not attempt to push it through the foil. After opening the pack, dissolve the tablet on tongue without cutting or chewing.

Special Populations

▧ *Elderly:*

▧ Initially, 0.5 mg orally once a day; then increase to 0.5 mg twice a day. Titrate once a week for doses above 1.5 mg twice a day.

NOTE: For some drugs, off-label use is reported. It is the responsibility of the practitioner to evaluate the efficacy of such use.

- Long-acting risperidone: 25 mg every 2 weeks. Oral administration should be continued for 3 weeks after the first injection.
- Elderly with dementia-related psychosis treated with atypical antipsychotics are at higher risk of death and cerebrovascular events. Black box warning for elderly patients with dementia.

■ *Renal impairment:*
- Initially, 0.5 mg orally twice a day for the first week. Increase to 1 mg twice a day during the second week.
- Long-acting risperidone should not be given to patients with renal function impairment unless they can tolerate at least 2 mg/day orally.
- Long-acting risperidone should be given 25 mg every 2 weeks. Oral administration should be continued for 3 weeks after the first injection.

■ *Hepatic impairment:*
- Initially, 0.5 mg orally twice a day for the first week. Increase to 1 mg twice a day during the second week.
- Long-acting risperidone should not be given to patients with hepatic function impairment unless he or she can tolerate at least 2 mg/day orally.
- Long-acting risperidone should be given 25 mg every 2 weeks. Oral administration should be continued for 3 weeks after the first injection.

■ *Cardiac impairment:* Use with caution because of risk of orthostatic hypotension. There is a greater risk of stroke if given to elderly patients with atrial fibrillation.

■ *Pregnancy:* Category C; some animal studies show adverse effects. There are no controlled studies in humans. It should be used only when the potential benefits outweigh potential risks to the fetus. Risperidone may be preferable to anticonvulsant mood stabilizers if treatment is required during pregnancy. Effects of hyperprolactinemia on the fetus are unknown.

■ *Lactation:* Drug is secreted in human breast milk. It is recommended to either discontinue the drug or bottle-feed.

■ *Children and adolescents:* This drug is not for use in children under age 5.

NOTE: For some drugs, off-label use is reported. It is the responsibility of the practitioner to evaluate the efficacy of such use.

RIVASTIGMINE TARTRATE (*EXELON, EXELON PATCH*)

Classification
Cholinesterase inhibitor; anti-Alzheimer's

Indications
The drug is used for treatment of the following:

▪ Mild to moderate dementia of the Alzheimer's type
▪ Mild to moderate dementia associated with Parkinson's disease

Available Forms
Capsule, 1.5, 3, 4.5, 6 mg; oral solution, 2 mg/mL; patch, 4.6, 9.5, 13 mg/24 hr

Dosage
Oral: Starting dose, 1.5 mg PO BID; after 2 weeks, if the dose is well tolerated, may be increased to 3 mg BID. Dose may be increased to 6 mg BID. The maximum dose is 6 mg BID (12 mg/day).

Transdermal: Starting dose, one 4.6 mg/24-hour patch transdermally daily. After 4 weeks, may increase to the 9.5 mg/24-hr patch.

Administration
▪ *Oral:* This drug should be taken with meals in divided doses in the morning and evening. It may be swallowed directly from the syringe provided, or may be mixed with a small amount of water, cold fruit juice, or soda. Oral solution and capsules may be interchanged at equal doses.
▪ *Patch:* Remove previous transdermal patch before placing a new one.

Side Effects
▪ Nausea, vomiting, loss of appetite, heartburn or indigestion, stomach pain, weight loss, diarrhea, constipation, gas, weakness, dizziness, headache, extreme tiredness, lack of energy, tremor or worsening of tremor, increased sweating, difficulty falling asleep or staying asleep, bradycardia, and confusion.
▪ *Serious side effects that may require medical attention:* Fainting, black and tarry stools, red blood in stools, bloody vomit, vomit that looks like coffee grounds, difficult or painful urination, seizures, depression, anxiety, aggressive behavior, hearing voices or seeing things that do not exist, uncontrollable movements and muscle contractions, and Stevens–Johnson syndrome.

Drug Interactions
This medicine may interact with the following medications: amantadine, other cholinesterase inhibitors, neuromuscular blockers, orphenadrine, cyclobenzaprine, parasympathomimetics, disopyramide, sedating H-1 blockers, amoxapine, antimuscarinics, clozapine, digoxin, general anesthetics, local anesthetics, maprotiline, nicotine, nonsteroidal anti-inflammatory drugs (NSAIDs), olanzapine, phenothiazines, nicotine(smoking)-may increase drug clearance, and tricyclic antidepressants.

Pharmacokinetics
Selective inhibitor of brain acetylcholinesterase and butylcholinesterase

NOTE: For some drugs, off-label use is reported. It is the responsibility of the practitioner to evaluate the efficacy of such use.

Oral

■ Peak plasma concentrations reached in approximately 1 hour.
■ Bioavailability after a 3-mg dose is 36%, indicating a significant first pass effect.
■ It should be taken with food to enhance bioavailability.
■ *Half-life*: 1.5 hours
■ *Duration*: 10 hours

Topical

■ Peak plasma concentrations are typically reached in 8 hours (range from 8–16 hours).
■ Steady state of medication is affected by body weight.
■ Approximately 50% of the drug load is released from the transdermal system over 24 hours.
■ *Half-life*: 3 hours
■ *Duration*: 24 hours
■ *Excretion*: Urine (97%)

Precautions

Patients with a carbamate hypersensitivity should be cautious; rivastigmine is a carbamate derivative.

Patient and Family Education

Oral

■ Store at 25°C (77°F); excursions permitted to 15°C to 30°C (59°F–86°F).
■ Store the drug in a tight container. Store the solution in an upright position.
■ Do not place rivastigmine solution in the freezer or allow to freeze.
■ When oral solution is combined with cold fruit juice or soda, the mixture is stable at room temperature for up to 4 hours.
■ Throw away any medication that is outdated or no longer needed.

Patches

■ Apply once daily to clean, dry, hairless, intact skin.
■ It may applied to the back, chest, or upper arm.
■ Rotate application sites daily. Do not apply to the same site more than once every 14 days.
■ Apply patch at approximately the same time every day. Remove the old patch before replacing with a new one.
■ Patch may be worn while swimming, bathing, showering, or in hot weather.
■ Avoid excessive sunlight or saunas.

Special Populations

■ *Elderly*: Use with caution; check liver and kidney functions.
■ *Hepatic impairment:* Use with caution
■ *Cardiac impairment:* Use with caution
■ *Pregnancy:* Category C; some effects of on the fetus are unknown.
■ *Lactation*: unknown effects
■ *Children and adolescents*: This drug is not for use in children.

NOTE: For some drugs, off-label use is reported. It is the responsibility of the practitioner to evaluate the efficacy of such use.

SERTRALINE HYDROCHLORIDE (*ZOLOFT*)

Classification
Antidepressant, selective serotonin reuptake inhibitor (SSRI)

Indications
Sertraline is used primarily to treat depression but may also be used for obsessive-compulsive disorder (OCD), personality disorders (PD), posttrauma stress, premenstrual dysphoric disorder (PMDD), or social anxiety, panic disorder.

Available Forms
Capsule, 25, 50, 100 mg; tablet, 25, 50, and 100 mg; concentrate solution, 20 mg/mL (60 mL)

Dosage
Starting dose is 25 mg daily, after 1 week increase to 50 mg.; maintenance dose, 50 to 75 mg incrementally; maximum, 200 mg daily

Administration
- PO with a glass of water.
- Take the drug with or without food.
- Take it at regular intervals.
- It may be prescribed for children as young as 6 years of age for selected conditions (25 mg/day); *precautions do apply.*
- Instruct patients to take missed dose as soon as possible. If it is almost time for the next dose, advise to take only that dose.

Side Effects
Displays some inhibition of dopamine reuptake, which may be beneficial to some patients (e.g., those experiencing hypersomnia, low energy, or mood reactivity), but problematic to others (e.g., causing overactivation in patients with panic disorder). Sertraline hydrochloride may cause more gastrointestinal side effects than other drugs in its class.

- Nervousness, headache, and nausea, insomnia; serotonin syndrome; dry mouth, easy bruising, or excess perspiration; diarrhea
- Withdrawal syndrome (including neonatal withdrawal syndrome): Symptoms may include dizziness, muscle aches, headache, nausea, vomiting, gait instability, agitation, and/or "electric shock" sensations, and suicidal behavior.
  - Sexual dysfunction (more than 50% of men and women)
  - Hyponatremia (e.g., in geriatric patients taking diuretics)
  - Side effects are most common during the first or second week of therapy. Starting with a lower dosage and gradually increasing it, and taking the medication with food will limit some of these side effects.
  - *Most common*: Dizziness, headache, insomnia, somnolence, and change in sex drive or performance
  - *Less common*: Allergic reactions (skin rash, itching, or hives); swelling of the face, lips, or tongue; feeling faint or lightheaded; falls; hallucination; loss of contact with reality; seizures; suicidal thoughts or other mood changes; unusual

NOTE: For some drugs, off-label use is reported. It is the responsibility of the practitioner to evaluate the efficacy of such use.

bleeding or bruising; unusually weak or tired; vomiting; change in appetite; diarrhea; increased sweating; indigestion; nausea; myalgia, and tremors

Drug Interactions

- *Monoamine oxidase inhibitors (MAOIs)*: Extreme risk for serotonin syndrome. Allow 2-week washout period post-MAOI prior to initiation.
- *Tricyclic Antidepressants (TCAs)*: Plasma levels may be increased by SSRIs, so add with caution in low doses.
- *Aspirin and nonsteroidal anti-inflammatory drug (NSAIDs)*: Increased risk of bleeding
- *Central nervous system depressants*: It may increase depressant effects.
- *SSRIs or serotonin antagonist and reuptake inhibitors (SARIs)*: It may cause serotonin syndrome in combination with the following medications: tramadol, high-dose triptans, or the antibiotic linezolid. Cimetidine may decrease clearance of sertraline.
- Use with caution in patients taking blood thinners (*Coumadin*); other antidepressants; antihistamines; lithium' TCAs; and certain antibiotics, such as erythromycin, clarithromycin, or azithromycin.
- Absolute contraindications include MAOIs, such as phenelzine (*Nardil*), tranylcypromine (*Parnate*), isocarboxazid (*Marplan*), and selegiline (*Eldepryl*).
- Avoid using with serotonin–norepinephrine reuptake inhibitor agents, triptans, and other SSRI agents.
- Caution with aspirin, NSAIDs (e.g., ibuprofen or naproxen), COX inhibitors, other anti-inflammatory drugs.
- *Alert*: This list may not describe all possible interactions. Instruct patients to provide a list of all medicines, herbs, nonprescription drugs, or dietary supplements used, and if they smoke, drink alcohol, or use illegal drugs.

Pharmacokinetics

- This drug is highly bound to plasma proteins and has a large volume of distribution.
- It is readily absorbed in the GI tract; SSRIs are metabolized in the liver, and excreted in the urine. Dosages may be decreased in patients with liver or kidney disease.
- Caution advised in elderly clients.
- *Metabolism*: It is metabolized in the liver by cytochrome P450 microsomal enzymes.
- *Peak plasma levels*: 2 to 10 hours
- *Half-life*: Variable, but most SSRIs have half-lives of 20 to 26 hours. They are highly bound to plasma proteins and have a large volume of distribution.
- Addition of serotonergic medications to a patient's regimen must not occur until 2 to 3 weeks after discontinuation of an SSRI (some recommend a 5-week "washout" period for fluoxetine prior to initiation of an MAOI).
- *Metabolism*: Liver: CYP 2C19, 2D6, 3A4 substrate; 2D6 (weak), 3A4 (weak) inhibitor.
- *Excretion*: Urine 40% to 45% (none unchanged); feces 40% to 45% (12%–14% unchanged)

Precautions

- This drug may cause sedation and mental clouding.
- Use this drug with caution in patients with liver, kidney, or cardiovascular disease.
- Adverse effects and side effects are commonly observed before therapeutic effects.
- Many side effects are dose dependent and may improve over time.
- Taper discontinuation to avoid withdrawal symptoms.

NOTE: For some drugs, off-label use is reported. It is the responsibility of the practitioner to evaluate the efficacy of such use.

▪ *Elderly*: The elderly may require decreased dosage.

▪ See patients as often as necessary to ensure that the drug is working on the panic attacks, determine compliance, and review side effects.

▪ Make sure patients realize that they need to take prescribed doses even if they do not feel better right away. It can take several weeks before they feel the full effect of the drug.

▪ Instruct patients and families to watch for worsening depression or thoughts of suicide. Also, watch out for sudden or severe changes in feelings, such as feeling anxious, agitated, panicky, irritated, hostile, aggressive, impulsive, severely restless, overly excited, hyperactive, or not being able to sleep. If this happens, especially at the beginning of antidepressant treatment or after a change in dose, patient should call the health care provider.

▪ Drowsiness or dizziness: Patients should not drive or use machinery or do anything that needs mental alertness until the effects of this medicine are known.

▪ Caution patients not to stand or sit up quickly, especially if older. This reduces the risk of dizziness or fainting spells. Alcohol may interfere with the effect of this medicine. Avoid alcoholic drinks.

▪ Caution patients not to treat themselves for coughs, colds, or allergies without asking a health care professional for advice. Some ingredients can increase possible side effects.

▪ For dry mouth, chewing sugarless gum or sucking hard candy and drinking plenty of water may help. Contact your health care provider if the problem persists or is severe.

▪ Caution should be exercised in the following:
  ▫ Bipolar disorder or a family history of bipolar disorder
  ▫ Diabetes
  ▫ Heart disease
  ▫ Liver disease
  ▫ Electroconvulsive therapy
  ▫ Seizures (convulsions)
  ▫ Suicidal thoughts, plans, or attempts by patients or a family member
  ▫ An unusual or allergic reaction to sertraline, other medicines, foods, dyes, or preservatives
  ▫ Pregnancy or trying to get pregnant
  ▫ Breastfeeding

Patient and Family Education

▪ It should be taken about the same time every day, morning or evening, and can be taken with or without food (with food if there is any stomach upset).

▪ It may start with half of lowest effective dose for 3 to 7 days, then increase to lowest effective dose to diminish side effects.

▪ Administration time may be adjusted based on observed sedating or activating drug effects.

▪ It may take up to 4 to 8 weeks to show its maximum effect at this dose, but some may see symptoms of dysthymia improving in as little as 2 weeks.

▪ If patient plans on becoming pregnant or is pregnant, discuss the benefits versus the risks of using this medicine while pregnant.

▪ As this medicine is excreted in the breast milk, nursing mothers should not breast-feed while taking this medicine without prior consultation with a psychiatric nurse

NOTE: For some drugs, off-label use is reported. It is the responsibility of the practitioner to evaluate the efficacy of such use.

practitioner or psychiatrist. Newborns may develop symptoms, including feeding
or breathing difficulties, seizures, muscle stiffness, jitteriness, or constant crying.

▪ Do not stop taking this medication unless the health care provider directs. Report
side effects or worsening symptoms to the health care provider promptly.

▪ The medication should be tapered gradually when changing or discontinuing
therapy.

▪ Dosage should be adjusted to reach remission of symptoms and treatment should
continue for at least 6 to 12 months following last reported dysthymic experience.

▪ Caution is advised when using this drug in the elderly because they may be more
sensitive to the effects of the drug. Elderly patients should receive a lower starting
dose.

▪ Keep these medications out of the reach of children and pets.

▪ Store the drug at room temperature. Take any unused medication after the expiration date to the local pharmacy on drug-giveback day. Avoid throwing the medication into the environment.

▪ Discuss any worsening anxiety, aggressiveness, impulsivity, or restlessness.

▪ Patients or families should report any severe, abrupt onset or changes in symptoms
to health professionals. This may be reflective of increased risk of suicidal thinking.

▪ Caution for the concomitant use of NSAIDs, aspirin, and any other drugs that alter
platelets.

Special Populations

▪ *Elderly:* Older individuals tend to be more sensitive to medication side effects,
such as hypotension and anticholinergic effects. They often require adjustment of
medication doses for hepatic or renal dysfunction. SSRIs with shorter half-lives or
less P-450 inhibition may be more desirable (e.g., citalopram) for geriatric populations than SSRIs with longer half-lives (e.g., *fluoxetine*). SSRIs have been associated
with increased risk of falls in nursing home residents and neurologic effects in
patients with Parkinson's disease. Elderly patients are more prone to SSRI-induced
hyponatremia.

▪ *Hepatic impairment:* Dose adjustment is necessary.

▪ *Pregnancy:* Psychotherapy is the initial choice for most pregnant patients with
major depressive disorder (MDD). Most SSRIs are Category C drugs, due to
adverse effects; risks are observed in animal studies. Sertraline has been found to
have lower cord blood levels than other SSRIs, although the clinical significance
is unknown. Thus, an individual risk-benefit analysis must be done to determine
appropriate treatment in pregnant women with depressive disorder (DD). If continued during pregnancy, SSRI dosage may need to be increased to maintain euthymia
due to physiologic changes associated with pregnancy.

▪ *Lactation:* Adverse reactions have not been reported; however, long-term effects
have not been studied, and the manufacturer recommends caution.

▪ *Children:* Initial SSRI dosing approved for use in children is 50% of the adult dose.
Increasing doses may require more gradual increments, and discontinuation may
require a more gradual taper. Psychiatric consultation is recommended due to
black box warning of children 12 years or older; however, monitoring for increased
suicidal ideation using SSRI therapy in children is critical.

Black box warning: Only for use in children 6 years or older for OCD.

TACRINE HYDROCHLORIDE (*COGNEX*)

Classification
Cholinesterase inhibitor

Indications
For the treatment of mild to moderate dementia of the Alzheimer type.

Available Forms
Capsule, 10, 20, 30, 40 mg

Dosage
- 40 mg daily (10 mg QID).
- Maintain this dose for at least 4 weeks with every-other-week monitoring of transaminase levels beginning at week 4 of therapy. Increase dose to 80 mg (20 mg QID) if patient is tolerating treatment.

Administration
Oral capsules; store at room temperature. Take prescribed doses at regular intervals between meals but take with food if GI disturbance occurs. Consistency in administration times is necessary to avoid decrease in effectiveness and increase in side effects.

Side Effects
- *Central nervous system*: Dizziness and headache
- *Cardiovascular*: Hypo- or hypertension
- *Dermatologic*: Rash
- *EENT*: Rhinitis
- *Gastrointestinal*: Nausea/vomiting, diarrhea, dyspepsia, and anorexia
- *Genitourinary*: Urinary incontinence or frequency
- *Metabolic*: Weight decrease
- *Musculoskeletal*: Myalgia
- *Respiratory*: Coughing

Drug Interactions
This drug may interact with cimetidine, fluvoxamine, levodopa, and theophylline.

Pharmacokinetics
- Inhibits reversible cholinesterase in CNS, leading to increased concentrations of acetylcholine.
- Absorbed after oral administration. Food decreases bioavailability about 30% to 40%.
- The drug is metabolized by cytochrome P450 system. Elimination time is 2 to 4 hours.
- Hepatic impairment may reduce effectiveness.
- Plasma concentrations are about 50% higher in women than in men.
- Smokers get one third less effectiveness of the drug; contraindications: jaundice, rash, fever.

For some drugs, off-label use is reported. It is the responsibility of the practitioner to evaluate the efficacy of such use.

Precautions

Precaution must be undertaken for the following scenarios:

▓ Patients with history of abnormal liver function
▓ Patient may be carcinogenic
▓ Overdosage: cholinergic crisis

Patient Education

▓ Effectiveness may lessen over time.
▓ Medication needs to be taken as directed.
▓ Advise patient of the usual side effects.

Special Populations

▓ *Pregnancy*: Category C
▓ *Elderly*: For use in elderly with mild to moderate dementia of the Alzheimer's type.
▓ *Children*: Safety and efficacy not established in any dementing illness.

TEMAZEPAM (*RESTORIL*)

Classification
Benzodiazepine (BZD) hypnotic

Indications
Temazepam is used for the treatment of insomnia, especially, short term: 7 to 10 days.

Available Forms
Capsule, 7.5, 15, 22.5, and 30 mg

Dosage
The dosage is 15 to 30 mg/day PO immediately before patient is ready for sleep.

Administration
■ PO with a glass of water; take 15 to 20 minutes before bedtime.
■ Drowsiness and/or dizziness will be exacerbated with concomitant alcohol consumption; alcohol should be avoided while taking this medication.
■ Caution clients not to stop taking drug abruptly if used long term.

Side Effects
■ Hallucinations, behavior changes
■ *Side effects that usually do not require medical attention*: Nausea, daytime drowsiness, headache, vomiting, dizziness, diarrhea, dry mouth, nervousness, confusion, euphoria, hangover, vertigo, anaphylaxis, angioedema, and drug dependence.

Drug Interactions
This medicine may interact with the following medications:

■ Antacids may decrease sedative effects.
■ Digoxin: This drug may increase digoxin level.
■ Diphenhydramine: It may increase effects of both drugs.
■ Probenicid: Probenicid causes rapid or prolonged temazepam effects.
■ Theophylline: Decreases sedative effects, antifungals; central nervous system (CNS) depressants (including alcohol)
■ Herbs: Calendula, kava, lemon balm, and valerian may enhance sedative effect.

Pharmacokinetics
■ BZD, hypnotic
■ Mechanism of action is thought to occur at the level of the gamma-aminobutyric acid (GABA) receptor complex; acts on limbic system, thalamus and hypothalamus.
■ Highly bound to plasma proteins
■ Peak plasma levels are reached in 1.2 to 1.6 hours.
■ *Half-life*: Average is 8 to 12 hours.
■ *Excretion*: Urine

Precautions
■ See patient as often as necessary if long-term use is indicated.

For some drugs, off-label use is reported. It is the responsibility of the practitioner to evaluate the efficacy of such use.

▦ Ensure that the patient is aware of the fact that he or she is not to exceed maximum dosage.
▦ Instruct patient to monitor for behavior changes.
▦ If patient is drowsy or dizzy, patient should not drive, use machinery, or attempt to accomplish any task that requires mental alertness.
▦ Avoid alcohol, as concomitant use may intensify side effects of CNS depression.

Patient and Family Education
▦ Store the drug at room temperature between 20°C and 25°C (59°F–77°F).
▦ Discard unused medication after the expiration date.

Special Populations
▦ *Elderly*: The elderly are more sensitive to hypnotics. Use lowest effective dose, recommended 7.5 mg/day. Due to sedation and increased risk of falls, all BZDs are placed on Beers List of Potentially Inappropriate Medications for Geriatrics.
▦ *Hepatic impairment*: Modify dosage accordingly.
▦ *Pregnancy*: Category X
▦ *Lactation*: No human studies have been performed. It is not recommended in breast-feeding mothers. Drug is excreted in breast milk.
▦ *Children*: It is not for use in children less than 18 years of age.

For some drugs, off-label use is reported. It is the responsibility of the practitioner to evaluate the efficacy of such use.

THIORIDAZINE HYDROCHLORIDE (*MELLARIL*)

Black box warning: Not prescribed due to severe black box warnings of prolonged QTc interval and sudden death. Not in formularies.

Classification
Antipsychotic drug, typical (first generation)

Indications
This drug is used to treat schizophrenia.

Available Forms
Tablet, 10, 25, 50, 100 mg

Dosage
The dosage is 200 to 800 mg in divided doses.

Administration
■ The dose of 50 to 100 mg three times a day; increase gradually; maximum 800 mg/day in divided doses.
■ Start low and go slow as QTc prolongation is dose dependent.

Side Effects
Motor side effects due to blocking of D2 in the striatum; elevations in prolactin due to blocking of D2 in the pituitary; worsening of negative and cognitive symptoms; sedation, blurred vision, constipation, dry mouth; weight gain; dizziness, hypotension; increased incidence of diabetes or dyslipidemia; potentially dangerous QTc prolongation; neuroleptic malignant syndrome (rare); jaundice (rare); agranulocytosis; seizure (rare); ventricular arrhythmias and sudden death; increased risk of death and cerebrovascular events in elderly patients with dementia-related psychosis.

Drug Interactions
■ The drug may decrease effects of levodopa and dopamine agonists.
■ It may increase effects of antihypertensive drugs.
■ The drug may enhance QTc prolongation interval of other drugs that do the same.
■ Paroxetine, fluoxetine, duloxetine, bupropion, sertraline, citalopram, and other CYP450 2D6 agents can raise thioridazine to dangerous levels.
■ Fluvoxamine, propranolol, and pindolol can inhibit metabolism and raise to dangerous levels.
■ When used with a barbiturate, it may cause respiratory depression/arrest.
■ Additive effects between thioridazine and central nervous system depressants.
■ There is an increased risk of hypotension with alcohol and diuretics.
■ It can cause compensatory tachycardia and MI.
■ Encephalopathic syndrome similar to neuroleptic malignant syndrome may develop when used with lithium.

For some drugs, off-label use is reported. It is the responsibility of the practitioner to evaluate the efficacy of such use.

Pharmacokinetics

■ CYP450 2D6 metabolizes thioridazine.
■ Duration: 4 to 5 days
■ *Half-life*: Approximately 10 hours

Precautions

■ With signs of neuroleptic malignant syndrome, treatment must be discontinued immediately.
■ *Do not augment* with other psychotropic agents.
■ QTc prolongation may lead to Torsades de Pointes–type arrhythmia or sudden death.
■ Use with caution in patients with respiratory disorders, glaucoma, or urinary problems.
■ Antiemetic effect can mask overdose.
■ Use the drug with caution in alcohol withdrawal or convulsive disorders because it may lower seizure threshold.
■ Use it with caution with Parkinsonism or Lewy body dementia.
■ Monitor for pigmentary retinopathy especially at higher doses.
■ Use the drug with caution in patients with bradycardia or those who are taking drugs that can induce bradycardia (beta-blockers, clonidine, digitalis).
■ Use it with caution in patients with hypokalemia and/or magnesemia (diuretic, stimulant laxatives, IV amphotericin B, glucocorticoids, and tetracosactide).
■ *Do not use* if patient suffers from the following conditions: coma, extremes of hypotension or hypertension, QTc interval greater than 450 msec or taking an agent that also prolongs QTc, cardiac arrhythmia, recent acute myocardial infarction (AMI), uncompensated heart failure, or taking drugs that inhibit thioridazine metabolism (CYP450 inhibitors).

Patient and Family Education

■ Take exactly as prescribed by the provider. Do not take in larger or smaller amounts or for longer than recommended.
■ It can be taken with or without food.
■ *Avoid becoming overheated or dehydrated during exercise and in hot weather*. You may be more prone to heat stroke.
■ *Avoid getting up too fast from a sitting or lying position*. Get up slowly and steady yourself to prevent a fall.
■ *Avoid drinking alcohol*.
■ *Stop using this medication and call provider immediately* if you have very stiff (rigid) muscles, high fever, sweating, confusion, fast or uneven heartbeats, tremors; feel like you might pass out; have jerky muscle movements you cannot control, trouble swallowing, problems with speech; have blurred vision, eye pain, or see halos around lights; have increased thirst and urination, excessive hunger, fruity breath odor, weakness, nausea and vomiting; have fever, chills, body aches, flu symptoms; or have white patches or sores inside your mouth or on your lips.
■ Do not stop taking drug suddenly without first talking to provider, even if you feel fine. You may have serious side effects if you stop taking the drug suddenly.
■ Call provider if symptoms do not improve or get worse.
■ Store the drug at room temperature away from moisture and heat.
■ Caution is needed in taking this medication if you have any of the following conditions: narrow-angle glaucoma, prostatic hypertrophy, or cardiovascular disease.
■ Annual eye examinations are recommended.

For some drugs, off-label use is reported. It is the responsibility of the practitioner to evaluate the efficacy of such use.

Special Populations

■ *Elderly*: The elderly may tolerate lower doses better, and are more sensitive to adverse effects. It is not approved for treatment of elderly patients with dementia-related psychosis, and such patients are at increased risk of cardiovascular events and death.

■ *Renal impairment*: Use with caution.

■ *Hepatic impairment*: Use with caution.

■ *Cardiac impairment:* Avoid in patients with QTc prolongation, recent AMI, and uncompensated heart failure. *Risk/benefit ratio may not justify use* in cardiac impairment.

■ *Pregnancy:* Category C; some animal studies have demonstrated adverse effects; there are no controlled studies in humans. Psychotic symptoms may worsen during pregnancy, necessitating some form of treatment. Atypical antipsychotics may be preferable.

■ *Lactation:* It is not known whether it is secreted in human breast milk, but assumed so. Recommended to discontinue thioridazine or bottle-feed.

■ *Children and adolescents*: Safety and efficacy not established in children and adolescents but risk/benefit ratio may justify use. Start at initial dose of 0.5 mg/kg/day and increase gradually. Maximum dose is 3 mg/kg/day.

THIOTHIXENE (*NAVANE*)

Classification
Antipsychotic, thioxanthene

Available Forms
Capsule, 1, 2, 5, 10 mg

Indications
Thiothixene is used to treat mild to moderate to severe psychosis.

Dosages
- Mild to moderate psychosis: adults and children age 12 and older: initially 2 mg PO TID.
- Increase gradually to 15 mg daily as needed.
- Severe psychosis: Adults and children age 12 and older: Initially, 5 mg PO BID.
- Increase gradually to 20 to 30 mg daily as needed. Maximum dose is 60 mg daily.

Administration
- Give drug without regard to food as per dosing schedule.
- Monitor for tardive dyskinesia, which may occur at any time but especially after prolonged use. It may persist even though the drug was stopped.
- Watch for evidence of neuromalignant syndrome.
- Watch for orthostatic hypotension.
- Withhold dose and notify prescriber if jaundice, blood dyscrasia, or persistent extrapyramidal symptoms develop, especially in pregnant women.

Pharmacokinetics
Unknown. Probably blocks dopamine receptors in brain. Onset, peak, and duration: unknown.

Side Effects
- *Central nervous system:* Neuroleptic malignant syndrome, seizures, extrapyramidal reactions, sedation, tardive dyskinesia, pseudoparkinsonism, dizziness, and drowsiness.
- *Cardiovascular:* Orthostatic hypotension, tachycardia, dystonia, and EKG changes.
- *EENT:* Blurred vision, nasal congestion, and ocular changes
- *Gastrointestinal:* Dry mouth and constipation
- *Genitourinary:* Urine retention, menstrual irregularities, breast enlargement, and inhibited ejaculation
- *Hematologic:* Agranulocytosis, transient leukopenia, and leukocytosis
- *Hepatic:* Jaundice
- *Metabolic:* Weight gain and hyperprolactinemia
- *Skin:* Mild photosensitivity reactions, allergic reactions, and exfoliative dermatitis
- *Other:* Gynecomastia

Drug Interactions
- Central nervous system (CNS) depressants: It may increase CNS depression. Use together cautiously.

For some drugs, off-label use is reported. It is the responsibility of the practitioner to evaluate the efficacy of such use.

■ Alcohol use may increase CNS depression.

■ The drug may increase liver enzyme levels.

■ It may increase or decrease white blood cell (WBC) counts.

■ It may decrease granulocyte counts.

■ The drug may cause false-positive results for urinary porphyria, urobilinogen, amylase, and 5-hydroxyindoleacetic acid tests that use human chorionic gonadotropin (HCG).

Precautions

■ Contraindicated in patients hypersensitive to drug and in those with CNS depression, circulatory collapse, coma, or blood dyscrasias.

■ Use with caution in patients with history of seizure disorder and in those undergoing alcohol withdrawal.

■ Use cautiously in elderly or debilitated patients and in those with CV disease (may cause sudden drop in blood pressure), hepatic disease, heat exposure, glaucoma, or prostatic hyperplasia.

■ Neonates exposed in third trimester are at risk for developing extrapyramidal symptoms and withdrawal symptoms following delivery.

■ Use in pregnancy only if potential benefit to mother justifies risk to the fetus.

Patient Education

■ Discourage use of alcohol.

■ Warn patients to avoid activities that require alertness or good coordination until effects of drug are known.

■ Drowsiness and dizziness usually subside after first few weeks.

■ Have patient report signs of urinary retention or constipation.

■ Sun exposure may increase photosensitivity reactions.

■ Relieve dry mouth with sugarless gum or hard candy.

Special Populations

■ *Pregnancy*: Category C.

■ *Elderly*: Black box warning: Not approved for use in elderly dementia-related psychosis.

■ *Pediatric*: Not recommended for use in children below age 12 years.

TRAZODONE HYDROCHLORIDE (*DESYREL, OLEPTRO*)

Classification
Serotonin-2 antagonist/reuptake inhibitor; antidepressant, triazolopyridine derivative

Indications
Trazodone is used to treat major depressive disorder, depression, insomnia, and to prevent migraine. It is the most prescribed medication for sleep in the United States.

Available Forms
Tablet, 50, 100, 150 (*Desyrel*), 300 mg; extended-release tablet (scored), 150, 300 mg

Dosage
For insomnia, start at 50 mg at night; starting dose of 150 mg/day in divided doses. Dose may be increased by 50 mg every 3 to 4 days; maintenance dose 75 to 400 mg TID with increases of 50 mg/day every 3 to 4 days. Maximum dose 400 mg/day (outpatient) to 600 mg/day (inpatient).

Children: Black box warning: not approved for use in children.

Administration
Orally, taking with food decreases some side effects and increases absorption. Scored extended-relief tablets may be broken in half, but should not be crushed or chewed.

Side Effects
The side effects are sedation, hypotension, nausea; may aid patients experiencing selective serotonin reuptake inhibitor (SSRI)/serotonin–norepinephrine reuptake inhibitor (SNRI)-induced insomnia. Rare occurrences of priapism have been reported. This should be discussed with male clients. The most common reactions to this drug include somnolence, xerostomia, headache, sedation, dizziness, nausea/vomiting, blurred vision, fatigue, diarrhea, constipation, edema, abdominal discomfort, myalgia/arthralgia, nasal congestion, weight changes, confusion, ataxia, sexual dysfunction, syncope, tremor, ocular irritation, malaise, and hypertension.

Drug Interactions
SSRIs may increase plasma concentrations. It may intensify the hypotensive effects of antihypertensive agents—"decreased dosage of HTN agent may be required." Patients taking monoamine oxidase inhibitors (MAOIs) should not take this drug.

Pharmacokinetics
The drug is metabolized by CYP450 3A4 to an active metabolite in the liver and 75% is excreted in the urine (less than 1% unchanged) and 20% in the feces. It inhibits CNS uptake of serotonin, not a tricyclic derivative.

- *Peak:* One hour (without food); 2.5 hours (with food)
- *Onset:* Six weeks (for antidepression); 1 to 3 hours (for sleep aid)
- *Half-life:* Parent drug, 7 to 8 hours; active metabolite

For some drugs, off-label use is reported. It is the responsibility of the practitioner to evaluate the efficacy of such use.

Precautions

- ▦ Do not use with MAOIs.
- ▦ Use with caution in patients with history of seizures.
- ▦ Use with caution in patients at risk for undiagnosed hyponatremia, bipolar disorder, priapism bleeding risk, volume depletion, alcohol use, cardiac disease, and QT prolongation.

Patient and Family Education

Notify the health care provider if the patient feels more depressed after initiation of therapy. Do not use alcohol while taking this drug. Do not stop taking this drug without talking to the health care provider.

Special Populations

- ▦ *Elderly*: Older individuals tend to be more sensitive to medication side effects, such as hypotension and anticholinergic effects. They often require adjustment of medication doses for hepatic or renal dysfunction. The elderly may be more sensitive to side effects and require a lower dosing regimen. Use the drug with caution due to sedative effects.
- ▦ *Pregnancy*: Psychotherapy is the initial choice for most pregnant patients with mild to moderate MDD. Category C; not advised during pregnancy as there are no adequate studies (similar to nefazodone). Animal studies show adverse fetal effect(s), but no controlled human studies have been conducted.
- ▦ *Lactation*: There is limited information in animals and/or humans that demonstrates no risk/minimal risk of adverse effects to infant/breast milk production.
- ▦ *Children*: Not indicated for children.
- ▦ *Renal impairment*: Renal dosing is not defined.
- ▦ *Hepatic impairment*: Caution is advised in hepatic impairment.

TRIAZOLAM (*HALCION*)

Note: Rarely prescribed due to high risk of abuse. Not in most formularies.

Classification
Benzodiazepine (BZD) hypnotic

Indications
Triazolam is used for the treatment of insomnia.

Available Forms
Tablet, 0.125 and 0.25 mg

Dosage
The dosage is 0.125 to 0.5 mg PO immediately before patient is ready for sleep. Maximum dose: 0.5 mg PO QHS.

Administration
▪ PO with a glass of water
▪ Drowsiness and/or dizziness will be exacerbated with concomitant alcohol consumption; alcohol should be avoided while taking this medication.
▪ Caution clients not to stop taking drug abruptly if used long term.

Side Effects
▪ Hallucinations, behavior changes
▪ *Side effects that usually do not require medical attention*: Nausea, daytime drowsiness, headache, vomiting, dizziness, diarrhea, dry mouth, nervousness, lightheadedness, and ataxia.

Drug Interactions
This medicine may interact with the following medications: antifungals; central nervous system depressants (including alcohol), digoxin, macrolides, and phenytoin.

Pharmacokinetics
▪ BZD, hypnotic
▪ Mechanism of action is thought to occur at the level of the GABA receptor complex.
▪ Highly bound to plasma proteins
▪ Peak plasma levels are reached in 1 to 2 hours.
▪ Metabolized by CYP450 3A4, glucuronic acid conjugation
▪ Onset: 15 to 30 minute
▪ Duration: 6 to 7 hours
▪ Excretion: Urine
▪ *Half-life:* Average is 1.5 to 5.5 hours

Precautions
▪ See patient as often as necessary if long-term use is indicated.
▪ Ensure that patient is aware that he or she is not to exceed maximum dosage.
▪ Instruct patient to monitor for behavior changes.

For some drugs, off-label use is reported. It is the responsibility of the practitioner to evaluate the efficacy of such use.

- If patient is drowsy or dizzy, patient should not drive, use machinery, or attempt to accomplish any task that requires mental alertness.
- Avoid alcohol, as concomitant use may exacerbate symptoms.

Patient and Family Education
- Store at room temperature between 20°C and 25°C (59°F–77°F).
- Throw away any unused medication after the expiration date.

Special Populations
- *Elderly*: The eldery are more sensitive to hypnotics. Use lowest effective dose, typically 0.125 mg. Due to sedation and increased risk of falls, all BZDs are placed on Beers List of Potentially Inappropriate Medications for Geriatrics.
- *Hepatic impairment:* Modify dosage accordingly.
- *Pregnancy*: Category X; absolute contraindication
- *Lactation*: No human studies have been performed. Not recommended in breast-feeding mothers. Drug is excreted in breast milk.
- *Children*: Not for use in children younger than 18 years of age.

ZALEPLON (*SONATA*)

Classification
Non-benzodiazepine (BZD) gamma-aminobutyric acid (GABA) receptor agonist

Indications
Zaleplon is used for the short-term (7–10 days) treatment for insomnia in the nondepressed patient.

Available Form
Capsule, 5 and 10 mg

Dosage
Five to 10 mg PO (range 5–20 mg/day) immediately before patient is ready for sleep.

Administration
■ PO with a glass of water
■ Avoid taking the drug within 2 hours of a fatty meal.
■ Drowsiness and/or dizziness will be exacerbated with concomitant alcohol consumption; alcohol should be avoided while taking this medication.

Side Effects
Complex Sleep Behavior
■ Hallucinations; behavior changes; selective serotonin reuptake inhibitors-treated patients taking zaleplon may experience impaired concentration, aggravated depression, and manic reaction; may cause amnesia. In most cases, memory problems can be avoided if zaleplon is taken only when the patient is able to get more than 4 hours of sleep before being active.
■ *Side effects that usually do not require medical attention*: Nausea, daytime drowsiness, headache, vomiting, dizziness, and diarrhea.

Drug Interactions
This medicine may interact with the following medications: antifungals, chlorpromazine, flumazenil, clarithromycin, rifamycin, ritonavir, SSRIs, central nervous system depressants (including alcohol), amiodarone, and verapamil.

Pharmacokinetics
Non-BZDs are hypnotics of the pyrazolopyrimidines class. Mechanism of action is thought to occur at the level of the GABA-BZ receptor complex.
■ Peak plasma levels are reached in 1 hour.
■ Bioavailability is 30%.
■ *Peak*: 1 hour
■ *Duration*: Shorter than zolpidem
■ *Excretion*: Urine (70%), feces (175)
■ *Half-life*: Average is 1 hour.

NOTE: For some drugs, off-label use is reported. It is the responsibility of the practitioner to evaluate the efficacy of such use.

Precautions
- Ensure that patient is aware that he or she is not to exceed maximum dosage.
- Patient should not take this medication unless prepared to sleep for at least 4 hours.
- Instruct patient to monitor for behavior changes.
- If patient is drowsy or dizzy, patient should not drive, use machinery, or attempt to accomplish any task that requires mental alertness.
- Avoid alcohol, as concomitant use may exacerbate symptoms.

Patient and Family Education
Store the drug at room temperature. Throw away any unused medication after the expiration date. An FDA–approved patient medication guide, which is available with the product information, must be dispensed with this medication.

Special Populations
- *Elderly*: The elderly are more sensitive to hypnotics. Use no more than 5 mg.
- *Hepatic impairment*: Modify dosage accordingly in patients with hepatic function impairment.
- *Pregnancy*: Category C
- *Lactation*: No human studies have been performed. It is not recommended in breast-feeding mothers.
- *Children*: Safety and efficacy have not been established.

ZIPRASIDONE (*GEODON*)

Classification
Second-generation (atypical) antipsychotic

Indications
This drug is used for the treatment of schizophrenia, delaying relapse in schizophrenia, acute agitation in schizophrenia (intramuscular), acute mania/mixed mania, other psychotic disorders, bipolar maintenance, and bipolar depression.

Available Forms
Capsule, 20, 40, 60, and 80 mg; injection, 20 mg/mL

Dosage
- Dose is 160 mg (80 BID) for all indications mg/day in divided doses, PO for schizophrenia.
- The dosage is 80 to 160 mg/day in divided doses, PO for bipolar.
- *Acute agitation*: 10 to 20 mg IM (doses of 10 mg may be administered every 2 hours, doses of 20 mg may be administered every 4 hours; with major depressive disorder max: 40 mg). Not to be administered for more than 3 consecutive days.

Administration
- Take this medication with a meal.
- Dosing at 20 to 40 mg twice a day is too low and activating, perhaps due to potent 5HT2C antagonist properties. Reduce activation by increasing the dose to 60 to 80 mg twice a day.
- Best efficacy in schizophrenia and bipolar disorder is at doses greater than 120 mg/day.
- Measure body mass index monthly for 3 months, then quarterly.
- Monitor fasting triglycerides monthly for several months in patients at high risk for metabolic complications.
- Blood pressure, fasting plasma glucose, fasting lipids within 3 months and then annually, but earlier and more frequently for patients with diabetes or who have gained more than 5% of initial weight.

Side Effects
- Nausea, constipation, dyspepsia, cough, anorexia, myalgia
- Dizziness, sedation, and hypotension, especially at high doses
- Motor side effects (rare)
- Possible increased incidence of diabetes or dyslipidemia is unknown.

Drug Interactions
- It may enhance the effects of antihypertensive drugs.
- It may antagonize levodopa with dronedarone, artemether, lumefantrine, meto clopramide, nilotinib, primozide, quinine, thioridazine, tetrabenazine, and dopamine agonists.
- It may also enhance QTc prolongation of other drugs capable of prolonging QTc interval agents.

NOTE: For some drugs, off-label use is reported. It is the responsibility of the practitioner to evaluate the efficacy of such use.

Pharmacokinetics

■ *Protein binding*: Greater than 99%
■ *Metabolism*: The drug is metabolized by CYP450 3A4. Hepatic via aldehyde oxidase, less than one third is via cytochrome P450 system.
■ *Absorption*: Must be given orally with food to obtain 60% bioavailability; 100% (IM).
■ *Onset:* PO, 6 to 8 hours; 30 minuts to 2 hours
■ *Duration:* 2 hours
    ■ Peak: 6 to 8 hours (PO), less than 60 minutes (IM)
    ■ Excretion: Urine (20%), feces (66%)
■ *Half-life:* 6.6 hours

Precautions

■ The drug prolongs QTc interval more than some other antipsychotics.
■ Use with caution in patients with conditions that predispose to hypotension (dehydration, overheating).
■ Priapism has been reported.
■ Dysphagia has been associated with antipsychotic use and should be used cautiously in patients at risk for aspiration pneumonia.
■ Do not use the drug if patient is taking agents capable of prolonging QTc interval (pimozide, thioridazine, selected antiarrhythmics, moxifloxacin, sparfoxacin).
■ Do not use it if there is a history of QTc prolongation, cardiac arrhythmia, recent acute myocardial infarction, prolonged QT congenital.
■ Long QT syndrome, recent myocardial infarction, uncompensated heart failure, or other QTc-prolonging arrhythmias.
■ Do not use it if there is a proven allergy to ziprasidone.
■ EPS, neuroleptic malignant syndrome (NMS), temperature regulation, dementia, electrolyte imbalance
■ Use IM formulation with caution in patients with renal impairment due to accumulation of cyclodextrin.
■ Seizures, excessive sedation

Patient and Family Education

■ Take oral formulation with a meal of a few hundred calories (e.g., turkey sandwich and a piece of fruit) to enhance the absorption.
■ *Avoid becoming overheated or dehydrated during exercise and in hot weather.* You may be more prone to heat stroke.
■ *Avoid getting up too fast from a sitting or lying position.* Get up slowly and steady yourself to prevent a fall.
■ *Avoid drinking alcohol.*
■ *Stop using this medication and call provider immediately* if you have very stiff (rigid) muscles, high fever, sweating, confusion, fast or uneven heartbeats, tremors; feel like you might pass out; have jerky muscle movements you cannot control, trouble swallowing, problems with speech; have blurred vision, eye pain, or see halos around lights; have increased thirst and urination, excessive hunger, fruity breath odor, weakness, nausea and vomiting; have fever, chills, body aches, flu symptoms; or have white patches or sores inside your mouth or on your lips.
■ *Do not stop taking* the drug suddenly without first talking to provider, even if you feel fine. You may have serious side effects if you stop taking the drug suddenly.
■ Call provider if symptoms do not improve or get worse.
■ Store the drug at room temperature away from moisture and heat.

NOTE: For some drugs, off-label use is reported. It is the responsibility of the practitioner to evaluate the efficacy of such use.

Special Populations

▨ *Elderly*: Some patients may tolerate lower doses better. Elderly patients with dementia-related psychosis treated with atypical antipsychotics are at an increased risk of death compared to placebo.

▨ *Renal impairment*: No dose adjustment is necessary.

▨ *Hepatic impairment*: No dose adjustment is necessary.

▨ *Cardiac impairment*: Contraindicated in patients with a known history of QTc prolongation, recent AMI, and uncompensated heart failure.

▨ *Pregnancy:* Category C; some animal studies show adverse effects. There are no controlled studies in humans.

▨ *Lactation:* It is not known whether it is secreted in breast milk. Either discontinue the use of the drug or bottle-feed.

▨ *Children and adolescents*: Early data suggest that it may be safe and effective for behavioral disturbances in children and adolescents.

NOTE: For some drugs, off-label use is reported. It is the responsibility of the practitioner to evaluate the efficacy of such use.

ZOLPIDEM (*AMBIEN*)

Classification
Non-benzodiazepine GABA receptor agonist

Indications
This drug is used for the treatment of insomnia.

Available Forms
Tablet, 5, 10 mg; tablet (ER), 6.25, 12.5 mg; tablet (SL), 1.75, 3.5, 5, 10 mg; oral spray, 5 mg/spray

Dosage
The dose of 5 to 10 mg PO immediately before patient is ready for sleep. Maximum 10 mg/day. One may use 12.5 mg *Ambien ER* in patients who have difficulty staying asleep.

Administration
- PO with a glass of water
- Take at least 2 hours after a meal.
- Drowsiness and/or dizziness will be exacerbated with concomitant alcohol consumption; alcohol should be avoided while taking this medication.
- Caution clients not to stop taking drug abruptly if used long term.

Side Effects
- Hallucinations, sedation; behavior changes; selective serotonin reuptake inhibitors–treated patients taking zolpidem may experience impaired concentration, aggravated depression, and manic reaction.
- *Side effects that usually do not require medical attention:* Nausea, daytime drowsiness, headache, vomiting, dizziness, and diarrhea.

Drug Interactions
This medicine may interact with the following medications: antifungals, chlorpromazine, flumazenil, imipramine, rifamycin, ritonavir, SSRIs, and CNS depressants (including alcohol).

Pharmacokinetics
- Non-BZDs hypnotic of the imidazopyridine class. Mechanism of action is thought to occur at the level of the GABA receptor complex.
- Highly bound to plasma proteins.
- Peak plasma levels are reached in 1.6 hours.
- *Half-life*: Average is 2.6 hours (PO).
- *Excretion*: Urine (48%–67%), feces (29%–42%)

Precautions
- See patient as often as necessary if long-term use is indicated.
- Ensure that patient is aware that he or she is not to exceed maximum dosage.
- Instruct patient to monitor for behavior changes.

NOTE: For some drugs, off-label use is reported. It is the responsibility of the practitioner to evaluate the efficacy of such use.

- ▦ If patient is drowsy or dizzy, patient should not drive, use machinery, or attempt to accomplish any task that requires mental alertness.
- ▦ Avoid alcohol, as concomitant use may exacerbate symptoms.

Patient and Family Education
- ▦ Store at room temperature between 20 °C and 25 °C (59 °F–77 °F).
- ▦ Discard unused medication after the expiration date.
- ▦ An FDA-approved patient medication guide, which is available with the product information, must be dispensed with this medication.

Special Populations
- ▦ *Elderly*: The elderly are more sensitive to hypnotics. Use no more than 5 mg.
- ▦ *Hepatic impairment*: Modify dosage accordingly.
- ▦ *Pregnancy*: Category C
- ▦ *Lactation*: No human studies have been performed. Not recommended in breast-feeding mothers.
- ▦ *Children*: Safety and efficacy have not been established.

NOTE: For some drugs, off-label use is reported. It is the responsibility of the practitioner to evaluate the efficacy of such use.

ZONISAMIDE (*ZONEGRAN*)

Classification
Mood-stabilizing anticonvulsant

Available Forms
Capsule, 25, 50, and 100 mg

Dosage
Children 2 to 16 years: It is not recommended for children younger than 16 years of age.
Adults: Initially, 100 mg once daily; then increase to 200 mg once daily after 2 weeks. Further increases to 300 mg once daily and 400 mg once daily can be made with a minimum of 2 weeks between adjustments. Maximum dose: 600 mg once daily.
Elderly: Initially, 100 mg once daily; then increase to 200 mg once daily after 2 weeks. Further increases to 300 mg once daily and 400 mg once daily can be made with a minimum of 2 weeks between adjustments

Administration
■ The drug may be given with or without food.
■ Do not crush or break capsules. Swallow capsules whole.
■ Do not give to patients who are allergic to sulfonamides.

Side Effects
The side effects are drowsiness, dizziness, fatigue, confusion, irritability, impaired memory/concentration, diplopia, insomnia, speech difficulties, dyspepsia, diarrhea, anorexia, headache, and abdominal pain.

Drug Interactions
■ Alcohol and CNS depressants may increase sedative effect.
■ Carbamazepine, phenobarbital, phenytoin, and valproic acid may increase metabolism and decrease effect of drug.

Pharmacokinetics
■ *Onset:* 4 days
■ *Peak:* 2 to 6 hours
■ *Metabolism:* It is metabolized in the liver into metabolites, N-acetyl zonisamide, and 2-sulfamoylacetyl phenol. The CYP enzyme responsible for the metabolism of zonisamide is CYP3A4.
■ *Excretion:* Primarily excreted in the urine.
■ *Half-life:* 63 hours
■ *Precautions:* Contraindications: Allergy to sulfonamides
■ *Cautions:* Renal and hepatic impairment

Patient and Family Education
■ Avoid tasks that require alertness and motor skills until response to drug is established.
■ Avoid alcohol.
■ Instruct patient to report if rash, back/abdominal pain, blood in urine, fever, sore throat, ulcers in mouth, or if easy bruising occur.

NOTE: For some drugs, off-label use is reported. It is the responsibility of the practitioner to evaluate the efficacy of such use.

Special Populations

▨ *Elderly*: No age-related precautions for the elderly, but lower doses recommended.

▨ *Pregnancy:* Category C

▨ *Lactation*: Not known whether the drug is distributed in breast milk. It is not recommended for breastfeeding patients.

▨ *Children*: Safety and efficacy of this drug not established in children younger than 16 years of age.

Index

CPSIA information can be obtained
at www.ICGtesting.com
Printed in the USA
LVHW021915080119
603173LV00011B/210/P